3rd edition

W. B. SAUNDERS COMPANY

PHILADELPHIA · LONDON · TORONTO

MODERN PRACTICE
IN CROWN AND BRIDGE
PROSTHODONTICS

JOHN F. JOHNSTON, D.D.S., M.S.D., F.A.C.D.

University Professor Emeritus of Dentistry

RALPH W. PHILLIPS, A.B., M.S., D.Sc., F.A.C.D.

Assistant Dean of Research
Research Professor and Chairman
Department of Dental Materials

ROLAND W. DYKEMA, D.D.S., M.S.D., F.A.C.D.

Professor and Chairman
Department of Fixed and Removable Partial Prosthodontics

INDIANA UNIVERSITY SCHOOL OF DENTISTRY

W. B. Saunders Company: West Washington Square
Philadelphia, PA 19105

1 St. Anne's Road
Eastbourne, East Sussex BN21 3UN, England

1 Goldthorne Avenue
Toronto, Ontario M8Z 5T9, Canada

Listed here is the latest translated edition of this book together
with the language of the translation and the publisher.

Spanish — Editorial Mundi S.A.I.C. yF. Buenos Aires, Argentina

Modern Practice in Crown and Bridge Prosthodontics   ISBN 0-7216-5172-0

Print No.:   18   17   16   15   14   13   12   11   10

This Book Is Dedicated to Our Wives

LAVONNE JOHNSTON
DOROTHY PHILLIPS
DOROTHY DYKEMA

Without their constant help and understanding, their militant defense of our shortcomings and subtle bolstering of our egos, completion of this project would have been impossible.

PREFACE TO
THE THIRD EDITION

The Third Edition of *Modern Practice in Crown and Bridge Prosthodontics* has been revised and reorganized to include the discussion of new materials and techniques and to emphasize the progress in established methods of procedure.

The authors have maintained a conservative (although expanded and further diversified) philosophy and approach toward clinical operations that will meet the needs of both student and practicing dentist. The technician who follows the prescribed techniques, or achieves the designated end results by other means, can have a happy relationship with the profession.

Since publication of the Second Edition the authors have had the good fortune to attend courses given by Dr. David Shooshan, Dr. Kenneth Morrison, Dr. Bruce Smith, Mr. John McLean, and Dr. George Mumford, and to participate in courses given in many parts of the country. This has given us new ideas and clarified and focused our thinking.

We acknowledge with thanks the extensive help given us by Dr. Ray Maesaka (Chairman for undergraduate clinical Fixed Partial Prosthodontics at IUPUI, consultant in that area), Dr. Donald Cunningham, Dr. Sumiya Hobo, Dr. Paul Lew, Dr. George Simpson, Mrs. Isabelle Ezzell, Mr. Calvin Linton, Mrs. Patrick Barrett, and Mr. Richard Scott and his staff. Chancellor M. K. Hine, formerly dean, and Dean Ralph McDonald have been co-operative and indulgent. We are grateful to all these people, and to the manufacturers, listed in the appendix, who have provided illustrations.

Lavonne Johnston has continued to read, search, rewrite, edit, and type the manuscript. Once again her efforts have made the completion of this book possible and we are deeply appreciative of her labors.

THE AUTHORS

PREFACE TO
THE SECOND EDITION

In this second edition, *Modern Practice in Crown and Bridge Prosthodontics* has been expanded and portions have been reorganized.

Additional space and increased emphasis have been given to more advanced and diversified techniques that will appeal to the practicing dentist. In the material on ceramics there is much that will be of assistance to the technician.

Despite the introduction of new and advanced information, however, we have retained a conservative approach to clinical operations and have kept firmly in mind the needs of the student. We have also, in this revision, attempted to conform closely to the nomenclature approved by *Current Clinical Dental Terminology*.

During the past five years, it has been the privilege of the authors to attend or to participate in teaching courses in all sections of the country. This provided many opportunities to visit crown and bridge departments and to discuss concepts and techniques, always to our benefit. Especially noteworthy were the contacts with Dr. Donald Smith, Professor Emeritus of Crown and Bridge Dentistry of the University of Southern California, Dr. Ernest Granger, at the University of Pennsylvania, and Dr. Charles Stuart, at the University of Kentucky.

Material was generously made available for our use by the following men: Dr. Miles R. Markley, Dr. R. E. Going, Dr. Frank A. Eich, Dr. R. E. Baker, Dr. P. N. Kondon, Dr. Harry Lundeen, Dr. Bailey Davis, Dr. Fredrick A. Hohlt, Dr. William Gilmore, Dr. Robert E. Willey, and Mr. Russell J. Jones.

We acknowledge with thanks the permission given by Drs. Donald Spees, Lloyd Phillips, John Borkowski, Dwain Love, and Stefan Wittner for use of their preparation outlines; our appreciation goes, too, to others who responded later to our questionnaire.

Willing co-operation was forthcoming from Mr. Richard Scott and his staff in making the illustrations. Drs. Thomas Connell, James Grimes, and Sumiya Hobo gladly provided many new drawings.

Drs. George Mumford and Ray Maesaka have been extremely helpful in the selection and development of material to be used in the area of ceramics and in the chapter on Dentistry for the Young-age Group.

Dean Maynard K. Hine graciously acquiesced in an occasional change of schedules made necessary by pressures connected with this text.

Many manufacturers, listed in the Appendix, have contributed illustrations.

We are deeply grateful to all these prople.

The authors appreciate the courtesy of the Virginia State Dental Association, The C. V. Mosby Company, the Tennessee State Dental Association, and the Year Book Medical Publishers, Inc., in giving their consent for the reuse of material previously published in the *Virginia Dental Journal, The Journal of Prosthetic Dentistry*, the *Journal of the Tennessee State Dental Association*, and *Practical Dental Monographs.*

Typing, reading copy, rewriting, research, and editing once again have been done by Lavonne Johnston. Without her keen interest, dedication, and the untold hours devoted to this project, our endeavors would have fallen short of our goal. To her we extend well deserved recognition.

THE AUTHORS

CONTENTS

CONTENTS xiii

INTRODUCTION

Dentistry is one of the health sciences encompassing the study and application of measures designed to prevent deterioration of the oral apparatus, and the use of pertinent clinical procedures that will serve for the betterment of those treated. Among its many ramifications are the relief of pain, the treatment of oral diseases, the maintenance of masticatory efficiency, and the maintenance or restoration of the esthetic qualities of the mouth and face. One of the functions of dental practice, and one that is frequently overlooked, is to combine and co-ordinate research and educational, preventive, and clinical efforts so that an ever-increasing number of people can avoid wearing complete dentures.

Clinical preventive dentistry may be divided into several phases or specialties. The order in which these can be administered most effectively to achieve retention or stabilization of the dentition is as follows: (1) education of the patient and treatment for the control of caries, (2) operative dentistry, and (3) periodontics (these first three are closely interrelated); (4) the planning and construction of bridges; (5) the designing and insertion of removable partial dentures after the mouth has been adequately prepared; (6) endodontics; (7) surgery; and (8) orthodontics. (Numbers 6, 7, and 8 will be employed often as adjuncts to expedite 2, 3, 4, and 5.)

If the patient reports to the dentist early in life and is convinced of the dividends to be earned from a policy of preventive therapy, correct mouth hygiene, and prompt repair of the tooth when a carious lesion has penetrated the enamel, there should be little need later for major restorative operations. If a tooth must be lost, it is the duty of the dentist to inform the patient that the space should be filled as soon after surgery as healing and shaping of the ridge tissue occur. Too often such a suggestion is not made, or, if made at all, it is done in a halfhearted manner. The significance of keeping the arches intact is not stressed, nor are the sequelae from lack of replacement discussed and presented emphatically.[1] Since the loss of one tooth can effect changes in positions and contact relationships of all teeth remaining in the mouth, the desirability of replacing the missing tooth, and of *recommending such services at the same time* that the removal of the tooth is advised, becomes obvious. "Replacing a tooth can be more important than saving the tooth."[2]

1

The following quotations succinctly summarize the popularity and momentous potentialities of the fixed partial denture prosthesis:

". . . In my own experience the fixed bridge, where indicated and properly installed, has been found the most successful, not only from the standpoint of health and natural function, but from the standpoint of appearance and lasting qualities. The fixed bridge is the easiest to care for, comes nearer to satisfying the patient's pride and peace of mind, and seems more nearly a part of his natural masticatory mechanism than any removable appliance."[3]

"Patients do appreciate the effort to provide the same service to all, regardless of cost. They respond by offering to do their part. There is no doubt that improvement in the dentist's aptitude and skill and in his ability to construct restorations of the highest specifications will result in a better type of practice. People in a community learn quickly who is a good dentist and who is a poor one."[3]

REFERENCES

1. Brown, L. W., Jr.: Dentistry's zone of silence. J.A.D.A., 55:843, Dec. 1957.
2. Adams, J. W.: Personal communication.
3. Grubb, H. D.: Partial dentures with precision attachments. J.A.D.A., 42:154, Feb. 1951.

chapter 1

PREOPERATIVE STUDY

In order that subsequent discussions may be understood and methods and meanings may be grasped readily, terminology must be clarified.[1]

DEFINITIONS OF TERMS

Crown and bridge prosthodontics is the science and art of the complete restoration of a single tooth, or the replacement of one or more teeth by a nonremovable partial denture.

A **crown** is a restoration that reproduces the entire surface anatomy of the clinical crown of a tooth (Fig. 1–1). It may be a metal casting, a metal casting with a veneer of tooth-colored porcelain or resin, or a so-called jacket crown constructed of porcelain or resin. The prepared tooth stump may be sound, or it may be partially rebuilt by a cast metal core or a cast core and post, cemented to the remaining tooth structure, or by amalgam. Occasionally small areas of the tooth stump may be restored with resin or zinc phosphate cement.

A **bridge** is a nonremovable prosthesis, or fixed partial denture, rigidly attached to one or more abutment teeth, replacing one or more lost or missing teeth (Fig. 1–2).

A **removable bridge** is a prosthesis, or removable partial denture, entirely supported under occlusal force by natural teeth and maintained in position by clasps or other attachments. It replaces one or more, usually more, missing teeth and should be bilateral in its retention (Fig. 1–3).

A **partial denture** is a removable prosthesis replacing one or more missing teeth, which receives its major support under occlusal force from the structures underlying its base.[2] It is kept in position by clasps and rests or intracoronal attachments (Fig. 1–4).

A bridge may be divided into four component parts:

The **abutment** is the natural tooth (usually two or more) or a root that supports the prosthesis and to which it is attached.

The **retainer** is the restoration, rebuilding the prepared abutment tooth, by which the bridge is attached to the abutment and to which the pontic is connected.

(Text continues on page 9)

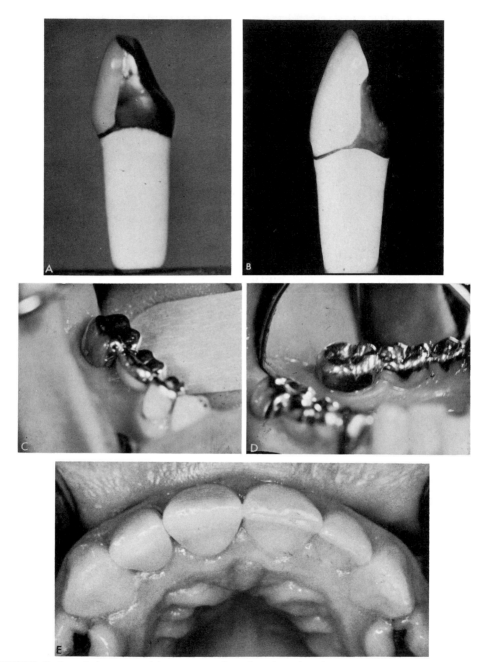

FIGURE 1–1. *A*, A crown with a veneer of tooth-colored resin.

 B, A crown with a bonded porcelain veneer.

 C and *D*, Full veneer gold crown retainers on second molar abutments (buccal and lingual views).

 E, Porcelain jacket crowns on right central and lateral incisors.

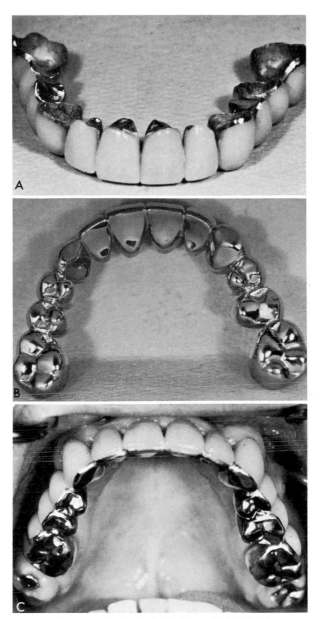

FIGURE 1–2. *Eight views of eight bridges.*

A, A twelve-unit maxillary bridge with veneered gold crown retainers on the right first molar, right cuspid, left cuspid, left second bicuspid, and left first molar. All units are veneered with resin except the incisors, on which Steele's facings were used.

B, The twelve-unit bridge, or fixed partial denture, from the occlusal. Notice the size and position of the solder joints, the form of the embrasures, and the spillways crossing the marginal ridges.

C, The twelve-unit bridge cemented to the abutments.

(*Continued*)

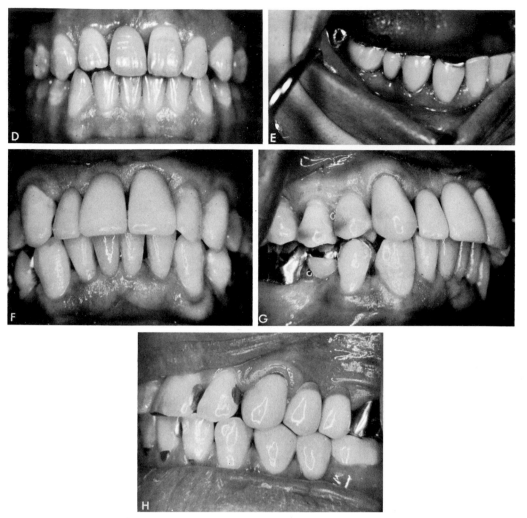

D, A three-unit bridge replacing the maxillary right central incisor. It is retained by pin-ledges on the left central and right lateral incisor abutments.

E, A three-unit bridge replacing a mandibular right second bicuspid. The retainers are veneered gold crowns on the first bicuspid and first molar. There is a separate veneered gold crown on the cuspid and a single-unit full veneer gold crown on the second molar.

F, A maxillary four-unit bridge with bonded porcelain veneer crown retainers on the right cuspid and left central. The right lateral and central incisor pontics are bonded porcelain veneers. The occluding three-unit mandibular bridge has pinledge retainers on the right lateral and left central incisors. The pontic has a Steele's facing with porcelain incisal. The abutments were realigned orthodontically.

G, Diagonal view of bridges in *F*. Mandibular posterior three-unit bridge with full veneer gold crown on molar and three-quarter crown on first bicuspid. Pontic has gold occlusal surface and glazed Steele's Sanitarypontic porcelain facing in contact with ridge tissue.

H, Maxillary posterior four-unit bridge retained by a full veneer gold crown on molar and a porcelain veneered gold crown on cuspid. Cervical collar of gold was covered by gingival tissue within three weeks after cementation. Bicuspid pontics are veneered with porcelain. Cervicals of veneers are stained pink to shorten exposed buccal surfaces. Mandibular three-unit posterior bridge with porcelain veneered retainers on molar and bicuspid abutments. Pontic has porcelain veneer.

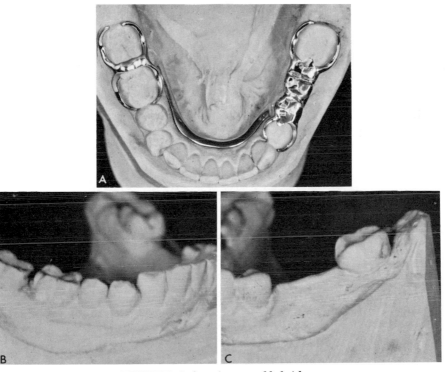

FIGURE 1–3. *A removable bridge.*

A, Occlusal view, bridge in place.

B, Groove cut above contact areas of approximating inlays to make room for clasp to cross occlusion.

C, Guiding planes on molar and bicuspid. Rest seat in molar.

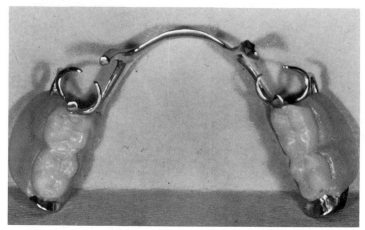

FIGURE 1–4. A partial denture. This is a bilateral distal extension (Class I) removable partial denture with two Roach-Akers clasps and two secondary retainers.

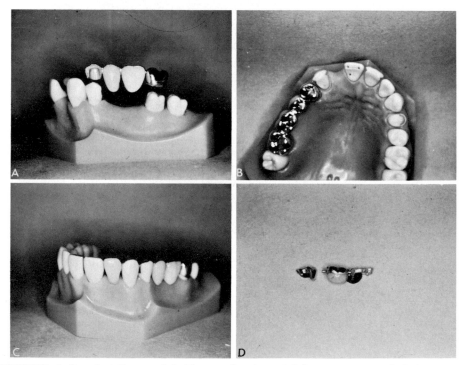

FIGURE 1–5. *A*, A four-unit bridge, or fixed partial denture, suspended above a model and displaying its component parts. The retainers are a partial veneer crown above the first bicuspid abutment and a full veneer gold crown above the second molar abutment. The pontics replace the second bicuspid and first molar. The joints, or connectors, are solder.

B, An occlusal view of the four-unit bridge, showing the reduction from normal tooth form in the dimensions of the pontics. Two other abutments can be seen. The upper right cuspid is prepared for a partial veneer, or three-quarter, crown; the right central will receive a pinledge. The left central incisor preparation is for a partial veneer crown; the left first bicuspid will be restored with a veneered gold crown.

C, The bridge (*A*) seated, with the pontics in contact with the ridge tissue, but without pressure against it. A labial view of the upper right anterior bridge replacing the lateral incisor. Retainers and abutments are discussed under *B*.

D, The subocclusal rest, one type of nonrigid connector.

The **pontic** is the substitute for the lost tooth, esthetically and functionally; usually, although not necessarily, it occupies the space formerly filled by the natural tooth (Fig. 1-5).

The **joint,** or **connector,** is the part of a dental bridge that unites the retainer with the pontic or that joins the individual units of the bridge. It may be rigid, e.g., the solder joint, or nonrigid, as are the subocclusal and dovetail occlusal rests.

REQUIREMENTS OF BRIDGE CONSTRUCTION

There are two kinds of requirements in bridge construction. The first is a concept of certain intangibles that may be defined as an appreciation of (1) forces developed by the oral mechanism, and of the capability of the tooth and its supporting structures to resist them, (2) modifications of normal tooth form that are designed to reduce forces or increase resistance to them, and (3) establishing and maintaining normal tissue tone.

The second requirement exacts a superior level of technical proficiency and concern in (1) the removal of caries from the abutment or from any associated tooth, the loss of which might affect the design or life of the bridge; (2) the sterilization or cleansing of the tooth surface; (3) the protection of the pulp during preparation of the tooth and construction of the bridge; (4) the restoration of the tooth surface in such a way that it will function normally and comfortably and not abuse the supporting structures; (5) the restoration of multiple areas of occlusion; and (6) a comprehensive and applicable knowledge of tooth form and esthetic tooth alignment.[3]

The construction of crowns and bridges, especially bridges, where and when they are needed, must be considered an accessory to preventive dentistry. Discernment and dexterity are more of a requisite here than in any other segment of this profession. Anatomy, ceramics, the chemistry of resins, colorimetry, dental materials, metallurgy, periodontics, phonetics, physics, radiology, and tooth form—all these must be aptly applied for successful diagnosis and practice in the field of crown and bridge prosthodontics. Adams[4] has stated that the preparation of an upper cuspid for a partial veneer crown is the most significant test of a dentist's clinical skill. While this opinion may not be accepted universally, undeniably the construction of a complicated bridge is a challenge.

The beginning student may feel that he is confronted with, and confounded by, a bewildering jumble of facts, many with exceptions attached, and with a multitude of technical procedures, each of which is subdivided into numbered steps for its execution. Although much of this must be memorized to provide a doctrinal background so that initial laboratory and clinical operations may lead to some understanding and be done with dispatch, perception and application soon become automatic. Many of the items discussed later in the text under examination can be observed and accomplished simultaneously with the steps in procedure. Each has a special purpose; the order in which these are noted is not indicative of their relative influence.

BENEFITS DERIVED FROM INSTALLATION OF A BRIDGE

If a bridge is built soon after the loss of a tooth, the patient should benefit in many ways. The bridge should contribute to mastication; it should augment the ability of the patient to enunciate; it should restore and preserve contacts between the abutments and the approximating teeth, and also all others in the arch; and it should maintain the positions of the opposing teeth and the normal tone of the supporting structure.

When a space is unfilled for a long time, there will be some shifting of positions of the teeth approximating the edentulous area and possibly extrusion of the opposing teeth (Figs. 1–6 and 1–7).[5] Even here a bridge should substantially aid mastication, help reinstate contacts of appropriate strength, size, and location, and improve the health of the alveolus and periodontium and prevent further injury to them. Any bridge at all times should create the illusion of natural teeth.

INDICATIONS FOR BRIDGES

A bridge is indicated whenever there are properly distributed and healthy teeth to serve as the abutments, provided that these teeth have suitable crown-root ratios and that after radiographic, diagnostic cast, and oral exami-

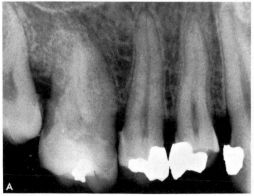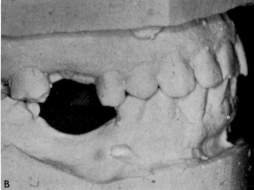

FIGURE 1-6. *A*, Radiograph of maxillary right posterior showing first molar extruded so that alveolar process contained only conical apical half of root. Extension of crown beyond occlusal plane was so great that correction was not advisable. Second molar tipped mesially into distal surface cervical concavity of first molar. Extraction advised.

B, Diagnostic casts showing relation of maxillary and mandibular edentulous spaces.

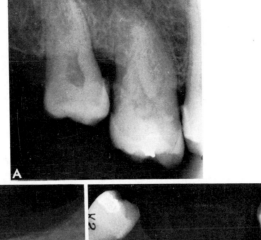

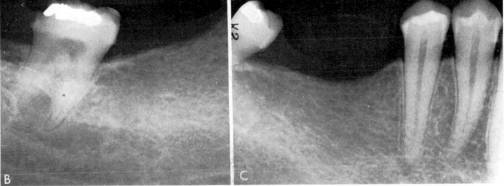

FIGURE 1-7. *A*, Radiograph showing maxillary second molar. Crown-root ratio, root form, and space length all point to fixed partial dentures. (See *B* in Figure 1-6).

B, Mandibular molar (see *B* in Figure 1-6) has poor root form, although crown-root ratio is 1:1½. Crown form and length and space length contraindicate fixed prosthesis.

C, Bicuspids have 1:2½ crown-root ratio, and splinted would give good support for a bridge. Since the left quadrant is intact, situation calls for occluding fixed prostheses.

nations seem capable of sustaining the additional load. These criteria may be defined as follows:

Proper distribution ordinarily means the presence of an abutment tooth (or teeth) at each end of the edentulous space, and an intermediate abutment (pier) when in the posterior the over-all length of the prosthesis will include the area of more than five teeth.

A tooth is considered *healthy* if the supporting bony structure is not being dissipated by alveolar atrophy (Fig. 1-8); if the soft tissue and periodontal membrane are in normal condition; and if the pulp is vital and responds typically to accepted stimuli, or, when the tooth is pulpless, if the root canals are adequately filled and the apical alveolus is not resorbed. A tooth may be carious and be restored to health by treatment. Gingivitis and other irregular conditions must be eliminated or controlled.

Crown-root ratio or periodontal support may be determined and evaluated by the application of a rule hereinafter designated as "Ante's law,"[6] which states that "in fixed bridgework the combined pericemental area of the abutment teeth should be equal to or greater in pericemental area than

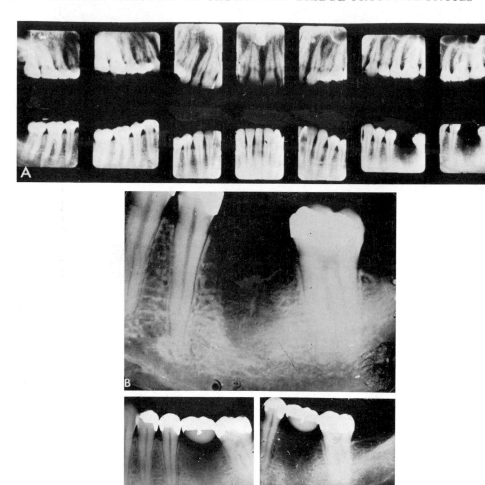

FIGURE 1–8. *Radiographs.*

A, A full mouth radiograph showing healthy alveolar structure.

B, A detail of the radiograph shown in *A*, illustrating acceptable alveolar bone, good crown-root ratio, and normal periodontal membrane.

C, The same area shown in *B* two years after placement of the three-unit fixed partial denture, or bridge. The abutment teeth are healthy. Ante's law and crown-root ratio are demonstrated satisfactorily. The pontic has a cast gold occlusal and a Sanitarypontic facing; the connectors are a distal solder joint and an anterior subocclusal rest.

the tooth or teeth to be replaced." While there may be some deviation from this rule, the pericemental area of the abutments often being as much as 15 or 20 per cent less than an equal amount, it should be computed when planning a bridge. The accepted and desired crown-root ratio is 1:1½ in linear measurement.[7] (See Figure 1–8*B*.) Here, also a less favorable proportion frequently can be acceptable when there is an absence of mobility and the patient has a healthy mouth and supporting tissue and an occlusion that at that time is nondestructive.

Radiographic examination will disclose the crown-root ratio, the presence of periodontal pockets, the quality and thickness of the periodontal membrane, rarefied apical areas, root contour, depth of caries, and height of the alveolus.

Examination of diagnostic casts (Fig. 1-9) will help ascertain the long-axis relationship of the proposed abutment teeth, mesial and distal space width, relationship of the opposing teeth to the abutments and to the spaces, tipping, adverse forces, the amount of tooth reduction necessary to arrive at retentive preparations and compatible paths of insertion, and sometimes the association of the gingival line to the cementoenamel junction.

Oral examination will reveal tissue tone, evidences of premature contact, extent of caries, depth of the gingival crevice, minute details of tooth form, and in lateral and protrusive excursions it will show relationships in occlusion that may not be discernible from articulated casts.

The designated abutment teeth may be deemed capable of sustaining the anticipated load if the considered opinion of the operator would suggest success after reviewing distribution, health, crown-root ratio, radiographic and oral examinations, and his previous experience. However, there may be intangible or external factors, such as eating or smoking habits, that could motivate against construction.

Long bridges and splints are being advocated for the stabilization of

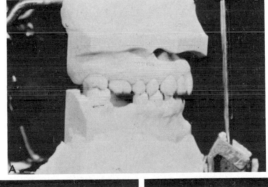

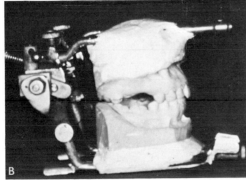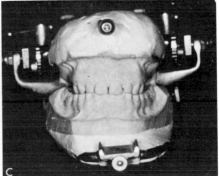

FIGURE 1-9. *Diagnostic casts.*

A, Lower first molar missing; second bicuspid rotated; upper molar extruded but can be reduced; plus vertical overlap. Bridge indicated.

B and *C*, Note position of upper right third molar and length of space. Bridge contraindicated.

teeth in the patient with advanced periodontal disease. Undoubtedly too many dentists avoid such treatment, but conversely an enthusiastic few overestimate the efficacy of these procedures. As a result too many patients are misled. Sound restorative judgment should be exercised.

CONTRAINDICATIONS TO BRIDGES

A bridge is contraindicated (1) when the space to be filled is of such length that the additional load generated from the occlusion of the pontics will impair the health of the tissues around the teeth that may be designated as abutments; (2) when the space length will require, for rigidity, a beam of such dimensions that embrasures will be greatly reduced in area and the underlying tissue overprotected; (3) when a previous prosthesis has shown that the associated mucous membrane reacts unfavorably to such an environment; (4) when, in the anterior, there has been such a loss of alveolar process that the pontics in the fixed prosthesis would be excessively long and unsightly or when a contoured partial denture base would be needed to restore face form; (5) when the fixed prosthesis would occlude with natural teeth or with a fixed prosthesis only on one end for half or less of its length; and (6) when there may be some question as to the ability of the remaining supporting structure around the abutment teeth to accept any additional load without bilateral bracing.

A bridge must be built so that it will restore arch form and occlusion. If the form of the prosthesis is an arc of a circle, a lever arm will be projected unless the span is segmented by a pier. The point of greatest leverage on the bridge must be supported by an abutment, or the areas of retention must be extended in each direction away from the space far enough to counteract the lever arm and establish counterbalancing retention (Figs. 1-10 and 1-11).[8]

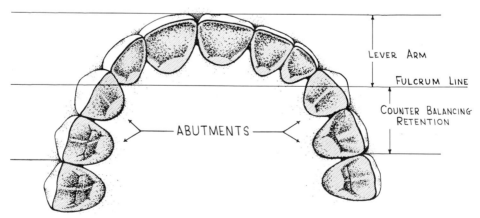

FIGURE 1-10. Lever arm and extended retention. A drawing of a clinical nine-unit anterior bridge illustrating the fulcrum line running through the tips of the cuspid abutments; the length of the lever 'arm from the fulcrum line to the most anterior point on any pontic; and the distal extension of retention onto the first bicuspids, included as abutments. If one of the central incisors had remained to serve as a pier, counterbalancing retention, derived from the first bicuspids, would have been unnecessary.

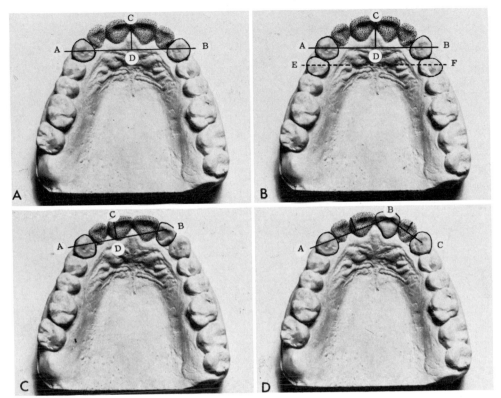

FIGURE 1-11. *A,* Line AB represents the fulcrum line around which the bridge tends to rotate or tip when force is applied to the incisal edges of the pontics of a bridge replacing all four maxillary incisors. Line CD is the lever arm. The longer the lever arm, the greater is the resultant force that tends to tip the bridge. This force often causes gradual anterior drifting and tipping of the cuspid abutments, together with periodontal breakdown, and tends to offset the retentive qualities of the abutment preparations.

B, The use of the first bicuspids as abutments in addition to the cuspids will offset the effect of the lever arm by providing retention and support, which is located to the distal of the line of rotation.

C, Allowing a lateral incisor to remain when constructing an extensive anterior bridge effectively shortens the lever arm. However, in most cases the adjacent cuspid still will be needed for adequate support and retention and to compensate for the lever arm.

D, The use of an intermediate abutment in the form of a central incisor creates two fulcrum lines, AB and BC, and considerably shorter lever arms. When one lever arm is subjected to force, the opposite terminal abutment tends to compensate for the leverage produced. Seldom will both lever arms be in function at the same time.

The shape and length of the root of the abutment must meet certain specifications. A long root, with flattened, parallel sides, is vital for a good abutment. When the root is round or conical, the stability of the tooth will be lessened, and when this is coupled with a lack of length, the terminus of a fixed prosthesis should not be attached to a single tooth.

When the proposed abutments have exposed root areas that are sensitive and that cannot be covered by the retainers, the construction of a bridge often is contraindicated, because the added stress may aggravate the sensitivity. If improvement can be effected, usually it is obtained by a removable bridge with bilateral bracing.

If the height or quantity of the alveolar process and periodontal membrane around the tooth to be used as an abutment is being reduced by some adverse force, the bridge should not be made unless such activity can be restrained both before and after construction.

Mouth hygiene cannot be sustained unless a bridge receives painstaking attention. If a mouth shows habitual lack of care and the patient does not respond to counsel for improvement, then the effort, time, and expense attending the construction and cementation of a bridge may be wasted. If it is impossible for a person to observe strict oral hygiene because of a physical handicap, a fixed prosthesis is contraindicated.

When the supporting bone has receded or the occlusion may be destructive, a removable bridge, designed to have bilateral retention and bracing, should take precedence over a unilateral fixed bridge.

Adolescent Mouths

Bridges may be contraindicated in the mouths of adolescents when the teeth are not yet in occlusion or when the pulps are excessively large, prohibiting retentive preparations. When a bridge is constructed under the latter circumstance, it may possibly be considered as temporary, to be remade when the patient is more mature and the pulps have decreased in size. The teeth then must be reprepared for a new bridge. At times it is wiser to build a space maintainer designed to hold the abutments and opposing teeth in position. This should be mandatory if the teeth have not made contact with the opposing arch.

Aged Mouths

Bridges are contraindicated in the mouths of elderly patients when there is a noticeable lack of resiliency in the periodontal membrane and when, through abrasion, the increased size of the occluding surfaces has intensified the forces to be absorbed by the thin or dense periodontal membrane and rigid alveolar process. The several exceptions here will be prompted by the length and location of the space; the general mouth condition; the radiographic evidence concerning the periodontal membrane and the alveolar process; and the general physical condition of the patient, his desire for a more complete chewing apparatus, and his reaction to other types of prostheses.

Abnormal Occlusion

A bridge is contraindicated where the occlusion is abnormal and closure produces forces that will react adversely on the supporting structures (Fig.

FIGURE 1-12. Maxillary bicuspids missing, space closed. Mandibular first bicuspid in center of opposing space. Cuspid abutment has end-to-end relationship with occluding cuspid. Molar abutment occludes only on mesial half. Lower first bicuspid must be recontoured to permit correct shaping of upper pontic. Incisal edge of cuspid abutment must have additional thickness of metal in incisal of retainer. Molar retainer must have circumferential retention to support molar.

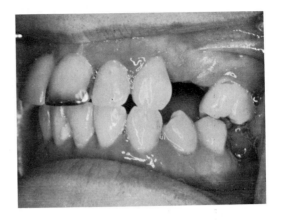

1-12).[9] Such a relationship may preclude construction of pontics that have acceptable form or it may rotate one or more of the abutments to such an extent that the stability of the retainers will be uncertain. If these faults cannot be adjusted or eliminated by inlays, crowns, or equilibration,[10] there should be few deviations from this rule.

The use of a rotated tooth in bridge construction may be debatable. Quite likely it will be awkward to prepare. Retentive form, occlusion, and esthetics must be cleverly contrived. However, when the operator puts forth the effort to overcome the objectionable features, many such teeth will serve well as abutments.

*   *   *   *   *   *

The demands placed upon all the materials and fabricated restorations and prostheses used and placed in the oral cavity are heroic. Occlusal forces are in the magnitude of thousands of pounds per square inch. Temperature changes induced by foods and liquids are instantaneous and may be as much as 65° C. The pH alters swiftly from alkalinity to acidity. The oral environment is warm and moist and conducive to corrosion. The soft tissues and the dental pulp are easily traumatized and irritated, calling for constant vigilance.

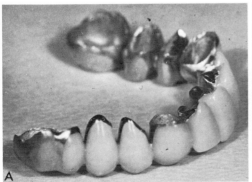 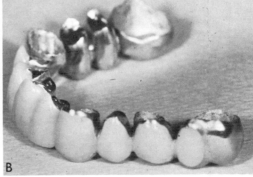

FIGURE 1-13. Correct design. Lateral views of the twelve-unit bridge shown in Figure 1-2. Note the minimal ridge covering areas on the pontics, the embrasure form, and size and location of the joints.

Because of these and many other exacting conditions that must be met by materials and techniques, the oral environment and the problems it causes continue to intrigue the scientist, and research is proceeding at an accelerated rate. It is conceivable that very soon the criteria favorable to all oral operations will become more inclusive.

When it is designed correctly and constructed competently (Fig. 1-13), a fixed partial prosthesis begets a happy patient. There is a growing acceptance of bridge construction by the public and the profession. Advances in armamentarium, resulting in indirect techniques and more freedom for the patient, have contributed to this acceptance. Participation in this movement is a rewarding experience for all concerned.

REFERENCES

1. Boucher, C. O., ed.: Current Clinical Dental Terminology. St. Louis, The C. V. Mosby Company, 1963.
2. Applegate, O. C.: Essentials of Removable Partial Denture Prosthesis. 3rd ed. Philadelphia, W. B. Saunders Company, 1965, p. 5.
3. Grubb, H. D.: Fixed bridgework. J. Pros. Den., *3*:121, Jan. 1953.
4. Adams, J. W.: Lecture, Postgraduate course, Indiana University School of Dentistry, April 1954.
5. Brown, L. W., Jr.: Dentistry's zone of silence. J.A.D.A., *55*:843, Dec. 1957.
6. Ante, I. H.: The fundamental principles of abutments. Michigan State D. Soc. Bul., *8*:14, July 1926.
7. Smith, G. P.: Objectives of a fixed partial denture. J. Pros. Den., *11*:463, May–June 1961.
8. Dykema, R. W.: Fixed partial prosthodontics. J. Tennessee D. A., *42*:309, Oct. 1962.
9. Simpson, R. L.: Failures in crown and bridge prosthodontics. J.A.D.A., *47*:154, Aug. 1953.
10. Nuttall, E. B.: Diagnosis and correction of occlusal disharmonies in preparation for fixed restorations. J.A.D.A., *44*:399, April 1952.

Gilmore, H. W.: Textbook of Operative Dentistry. St. Louis, The C. V. Mosby Company, 1967.
Klaffenbach, A. O.: Biochemical restoration and maintenance of the permanent first molar space. J.A.D.A., *45*:633, Dec. 1952.
Shooshan, E. D.: Adequate operative dentistry and its significance in maintaining oral health. J. Pros. Den., *6*:710, Sept. 1956.
Tylman, S. D.: To what degree can the partially edentulous patient be rehabilitated biologically and mechanically by means of crowns and fixed bridges? J. Ontario D. A., *30*:255, 314, Aug. and Oct. 1953.
Yurkstas, A. A.: The effect of missing teeth on masticatory performance and efficiency. J. Pros. Den., *4*:120, Jan. 1954.
Yurkstas, A. A., Fridley, H. H., and Manly, R. S.: A functional evaluation of fixed and removable bridgework. J. Pros. Den., *1*:570, Sept. 1951.

chapter 2

DIFFERENTIAL DIAGNOSIS AND DETERMINATION AND PLANNING OF TREATMENT

Diagnosis consists of the recognition of an abnormality and a thorough investigation of the severity of a condition and the reason why it has occurred. Treatment, or correction, must be based on a case study that ignores no phase of the over-all situation and follows the most promising course to its culmination.

There are five steps in diagnosis and selection of treatment:

(1) a comprehensive study of existing conditions;

(2) an evaluation of the potential of the remaining teeth and their supporting structures, as related to (a) the load to which the abutments will be subjected and their abilities to sustain this load, and (b) the relative retentive and esthetic qualities of retainer preparations on the abutments;

(3) a discriminating assessment of the relationship of one arch to the other, with the optimal load-bearing ability of the bridge structure;

(4) an eventual selection of a method of restoration that gives consideration to the esthetic requirements imposed by the patient as well as his caries index, oral hygiene, and anticipated co-operation,[1, 2, 3, 4, 5] and

(5) a plan of treatment that will accomplish this satisfactorily.

The existing vertical dimension and maxillo-mandibular relationship are accepted and maintained in the majority of cases, and in the construction of either a fixed or a removable prosthesis the most conservative approach is always attempted. The authors define "conservative" to mean *conservation of tooth structure and the surface enamel* unless the caries index, the need for maximal retention, the presumable susceptibility to caries, or the most effective position of a clasp requires that a tooth be crowned.

19

THE IMPORTANCE AND METHODS OF
TREATMENT PLANNING

Rules must be established as a starting point for the selection and planning of treatment, but it must be remembered that the ideal case is seldom found. While this chapter and others will refer to many instances of minor divergence from suggested procedures, there can be no change in the basic principles of selection, planning, construction, and maintenance.

Step-by-step treatment planning is imperative in order that teeth may be preserved, time saved, costs kept to a minimum, and the most satisfactory (or most practical) type of restoration inserted. A "most satisfactory or practical" restoration means one that will produce the maximum in chewing efficiency for the longest period of time, with the least tendency toward a destructive

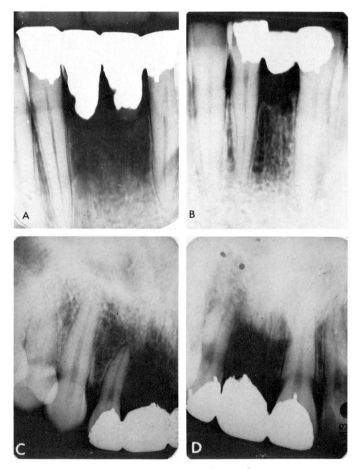

FIGURE 2-1. *Radiographs.*

A, Mandibular lateral incisors with high alveolar process and good crown-root ratio.

B, Support is reduced on central incisor abutment, but because of short span is still acceptable without splinting.

C and *D*, Maxillary lateral incisor with almost 1:1 ratio, but because of spacing, short span, and crown-root ratio of central, it was considered safe. Bridge has been worn for 18 years with no apparent change.

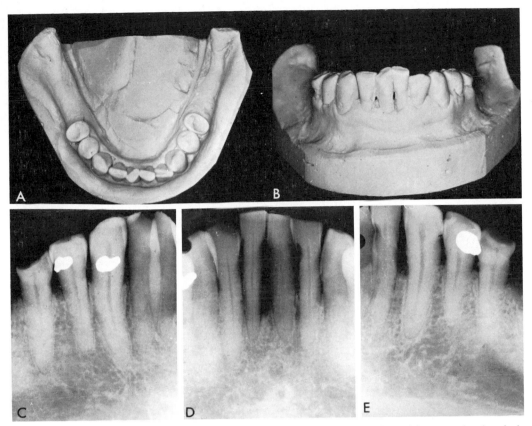

FIGURE 2-2. *A,* Occlusal view of mandibular cast. Second bicuspids severely abraded.

B, Labial view. Central incisors extruded. Cuspids and bicuspids abraded by occluding porcelain denture teeth.

C, Left bicuspids and cuspid have good supporting alveolus and good crown-root ratio

D, Central incisors mobile; right lateral poor; left lateral two-thirds denuded on mesial.

E, Right bicuspids and cuspid have acceptable bony support. It was recommended that all incisors be extracted, and that a treatment bite rim with anterior teeth be worn to increase posterior vertical dimension and to permit mandible to reposition.

Two treatment plans might be considered: (1) A ten-unit bridge would splint all remaining teeth and could be contoured for retention and support of a Class I removable partial denture. (2) If the lower anterior ridge receded grossly, the bicuspids and cuspid on each side could be splinted and contoured to retain and support a Class I, Mod. I, partial denture.

With either plan of treatment, vertical dimension of the second bicuspids must be increased. The second plan could be successful because of occlusion with maxillary complete denture.

influence on the abutments, the opposing teeth, and their supporting structures.

Dr. Howard Raper[6] expresses his concept of a dental restoration in this way: "It is a mechanical repair, a treatment for a local disease, and a prophylactic against a systemic disease."

In order that a restoration or prosthesis can be made to coincide with Dr. Raper's definition, all phases of the construction must be considered in advance. He has implied that there must be properly placed contact areas with adequate strength; correct contour of proximal, buccal, and lingual

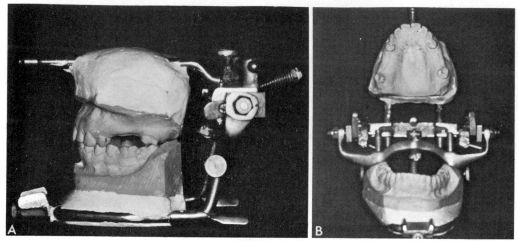

FIGURE 2-3. *Diagnostic casts.*

A, Long maxillary posterior space; distal abutment tipped mesially.

B, Distal abutments are third molars; one is tipped buccally; spaces are long. Removable bridge indicated and constructed.

surfaces; harmonious occlusal carving; marginal fit with no overextension or other discrepancies; and protection of the cusps to prevent fracture of the buccal or lingual walls.

These things cannot be accomplished without diagnosis and formulation of a plan of treatment that will fix in the mind of the operator all the existing limitations and all the modifications that may be inaugurated to overcome them.[7, 8, 9] These steps entail examination of radiographs (Figs. 2–1 and 2–2), diagnostic casts (Fig. 2–3), and the mouth (Fig. 2–4); consultation with the patient; exploration of the carious or otherwise dubious abutment and associated teeth; an understanding of the periodontal factors; consideration of the feasibility of orthodontic positioning of abutment or opposing teeth; and arrangement of appointments so that prepared teeth will be left unrestored for minimal periods only.[10] Likewise, the time surrendered by the patient must fit into the schedule of the dentist, yet disrupt the patient's normal routine as little as possible.

Radiographic Examination

Radiographs should reveal the status quo in all sections of the mandible or maxilla and many times in the temporomandibular joint. Edentulous spaces should be examined for residual roots and rarefied areas. The radiographs should be scrutinized to appraise the amount and quality of the supporting structure. The root areas within the alveolar process should be measured and compared in length to the portion of the tooth extending beyond the crest of the alveolus. The thickness of the periodontal membrane should be observed for evidence signifying abnormal pressure not in line with the long axis of the tooth. Apical rarefaction should be noted. The

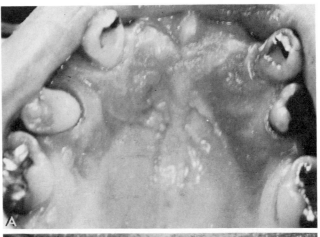

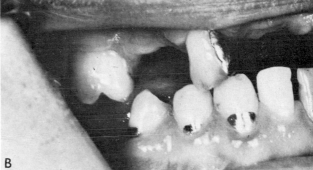

FIGURE 2-4. *Examination of the mouth.*

A, B, and *C.* Six teeth that must be explored and evaluated before making decision regarding treatment plan. Position of cuspid and caries index suggested orthodontic repositioning of cuspid abutment and veneered gold crowns as retainers.

D, Labial view showing upper left cuspid locked to lingual of mandibular teeth.

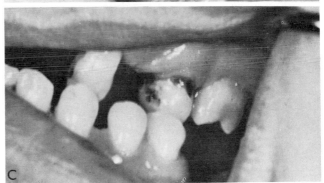

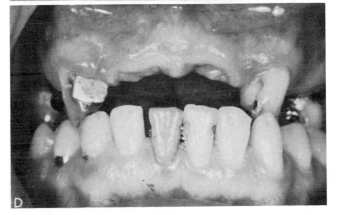

continuity of the cortical layer should be inspected for alveolar atrophy. In addition, the long-axis relationship of the proposed abutment teeth should be calculated.

An acceptable situation radiographically would be one in which (1) the root length within the alveolar process is greater than the combined lengths of crown and root outside it (Fig. 2–5); (2) the alveolar process in the edentulous area is well filled (although there can be exceptions to this following recent extraction); (3) the periodontal membrane appears to be of uniform thickness and not undergoing undue lateral stress; and (4) the long-axis relationship of the abutment teeth is within 25 to 30 degrees of being parallel. Construction of the bridge still may be termed acceptable, even if the alveolus has receded beyond the prescribed ratio, provided examination shows that splinting can be done (Figs. 2–6, 2–7, and 2–8).

A situation would be termed nonacceptable (1) if the radiographs disclose manifestations contrary to the above; (2) when there is apical resorp-

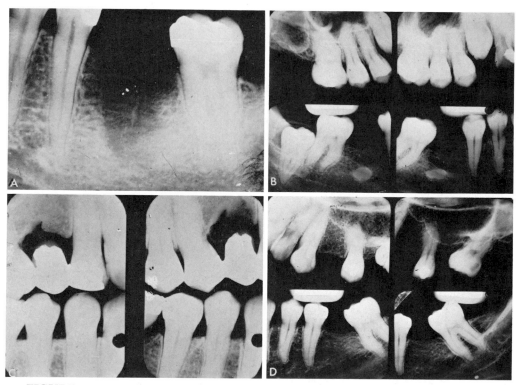

FIGURE 2–5.   *A*, Root length, crown-root ratio, edentulous area, and periodontal membrane of uniform thickness show bicuspid and molar to be good risks for abutments.

B and *C*, Radiograph shows retained maxillary cuspid and mandibular third molar and root fragment (?) in alveolus of mandibular space. Cuspid and molar were removed; sockets were allowed to heal. The lower second bicuspid has a conical root and a large crown; however, the crown-root ratio is good and the space is short. Bridges were built.

D, Radiograph shows good alveolar bone and crown-root ratio around upper second bicuspid and cuspid and lower second molar and bicuspid. Upper molar was considered unfavorable for abutment, because of tipping and pocket. It was retained until extraction was necessary.

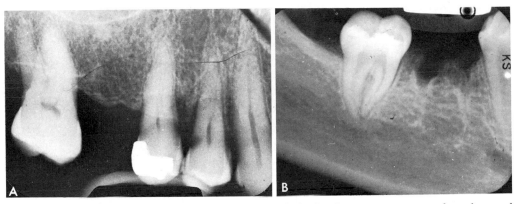

FIGURE 2-6. *A,* Radiograph showing receded alveolar support around molar and bicuspids. Long-axis relationship good. Using three abutments would distribute load and probably would extend service of first bicuspid.

B, Radiograph showing molar with converging conical roots. Used with two anterior abutments this tooth would support fixed replacement for many years.

tion; (3) when there is pocketing that would not respond to treatment (Fig. 2-9); (4) when there is an involvement of the bifurcation; (5) when there is an apical area to be treated by a root-end resection that would adversely alter the crown-root ratio; and (6) when the supporting alveolus around roots that are excessively curved and that have received pressure along their sides when force was exerted in the direction of the long axis already shows evidence of a reaction. If it is thought that a bridge will stabilize the proposed abutment (Fig. 2-10), the end result might be favorable.

Diagnostic Casts

Diagnostic casts (often referred to as "study casts") are positive reproductions of the maxillary arch and hard palate and of the mandibular arch, mounted in accurate relationship on an articulator capable of lateral and protrusive movements similar to those that commonly take place in the

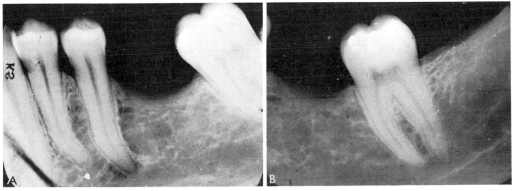

FIGURE 2-7. *A,* Radiograph showing good alveolar support, crown-root ratio, and root form.

B, The molar has a mesial tip, but it can be prepared without obvious risk. Bridge indicated.

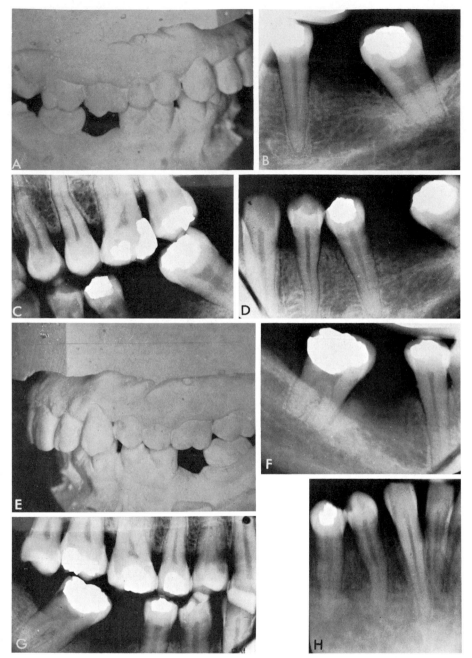

FIGURE 2–8. *A*, Articulated casts (right side), mandibular molar having been extracted for a long time, and second molar unsupported mesially. Maxillary first molar extruded in an arc, with distal cusps extending into space.

B, Radiograph of mandibular second molar. Crown-root ratio 1½:1. Root fused. Apical thickening of periodontal membrane. Second bicuspid shows evidence of abnormal occlusion.

C, Maxillary first molar restored in distal half, making it possible to recontour occluding surface, without probability of sensitivity or shock.

D, Mandibular bicuspids have all requisites for abutments.

E, Articulated casts (left side). *(Continued)*

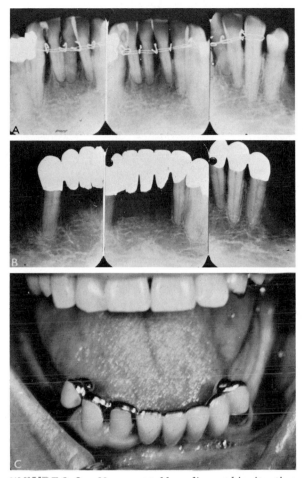

FIGURE 2–9. *Nonacceptable radiographic situation.*

A, Radiographically, situation is not acceptable. Did not respond to periodontal treatment. Incisors and one cuspid removed.

B, Radiograph of bridge constructed with four abutments.

C, Bridge shown in *B*. The three splinted abutments will stabilize the single bicuspid on the left side of the arch. It has good bony support and will receive bilateral bracing from removable partial denture.

FIGURE 2–8. *(Continued)*

F, Radiograph of left mandibular second molar and second bicuspid. Crown-root ratio about the same as on right side but roots are not fused, making situation better for bridge support.

G, Extruded maxillary third molar should be extracted and distal of first molar shortened to coincide with occlusal plane.

H, Left mandibular bicuspids. Second bicuspid effective abutment.

Despite bone loss around lower second molars and their acquired mesial inclinations, fixed partial dentures are indicated. Including the first bicuspids for anterior support might be considered; however, the length of the bicuspid clinical crowns is not suitable for splinting, and there is no other reason for reducing the height of the gingiva.

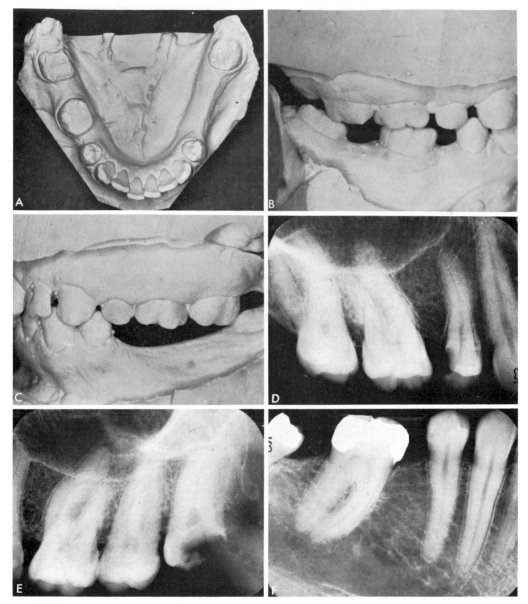

FIGURE 2-10.   *A*, Occlusal view of mandibular cast.

B, Right lateral view of articulated diagnostic casts. Mandibular third molar occludes only on mesial half.

C, Left lateral view of diagnostic casts. Maxillary second molar slips below lower occlusal plane.

D and *E*, Radiographs of maxillary molars. Carious left third was extracted.

F and *G*, Radiographs of right mandibular molars. Third inclined mesially. All force against this tooth absorbed by flat mesial surface of root. No evidence of adverse reaction.

H and *I*, Radiographs of left mandibular molar and bicuspid. Indications are that lower right posteriors could support any type and extent of load. Treatment plan suggested included a bridge from right first molar to first bicuspid and a Class III, Mod. I, partial denture. The third molar and right first molar were to have crowns with supporting circumferential ledges, with the clasps rebuilding the teeth to contour. The left bicuspid would be treated the same way on the lingual, but with a retentive clasp arm on the buccal.

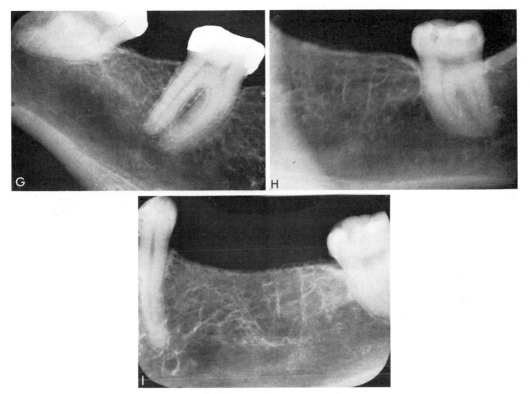

FIGURE 2-10   (*Continued*)

mouth. *Casts of the arches cannot be termed "diagnostic casts" until they have been so mounted and so related.*

Construction of Diagnostic Casts.   A perforated commercial alginate tray should be used. For the maxilla it should extend apically beyond the gingival line and distally to the terminal molars or the tuberosities, and it should clear the buccal and labial surfaces by not less than 3.0 mm. It usually is necessary to increase the height of the palatal area to adapt and support the impression material.

After the tray has been checked in the mouth, the patient is asked to rinse. Alginate, sufficiently precise for diagnostic casts, is used for the impression because of its simple and convenient technique and working qualities. Mixing should follow the manufacturer's directions as to relative quantities and spatulation time.

A bit of alginate is placed to the distals of the terminal teeth and also rubbed on the occlusals, using the finger as an instrument. This precludes voids and bubbles. The tray is filled and, with the patient in an upright position, is placed in the mouth. A saliva ejector will help to keep the patient comfortable unless an excess of alginate has been inadvertently forced back into the throat. Gelation time will be approximately 4 minutes. As a rule, downward pressure on the tray handle will remove the impression, although occasionally it will be necessary to use finger pressure in the area of the tuberosity.

After the impression has been washed, stone is mixed, using 22 to 25 ml.

of water and 100 gm. of stone.* (See Figure 2–11.) It is spatulated until it will mound without slumping and is vibrated into the impression in small increments, starting at the posterior on one side and pulling the stone around the arch. Bulk is added until the impression is overfilled. Stone is then mounded on a glass slab and the inverted impression is pushed into the stone, which is adapted to the borders of the impression with a spatula. The stone should set for a minimum of 1 hour.

The lower impression tray should extend distally to the terminal teeth or over the retromolar pad. It should go no more than 3.0 or 4.0 mm. below the lingual gingival line, it should not deform the mucobuccal fold posteriorly, and it should not depress either frenum. Again using the finger as an instrument, impression material should be placed distally to the terminal teeth and along the labial surfaces and cervically to the anteriors. An impression tray should always be held in position by the operator until setting has occurred.

The lower impression is poured in the same way as the upper, but in order to make final trimming less arduous, any stone that rises above the lingual borders of the impression should be removed with a spatula (Fig. 2-12). The casts should be trimmed symmetrically and short enough in the posterior so there will be no interference in occluding them.

Registration.   A face-bow registration is a requisite. A bite fork is covered with three thicknesses of pink baseplate wax and the patient is asked to close so that the upper teeth indent the wax 2.0 mm. The bow is positioned on the face, adjusted to center on the condyle regions, locked (Fig. 2-13), and transferred to the articulator. The upper cast is mounted.

The patient should be assisted or guided in practicing closing the mandible. A wax registration is then made without allowing the teeth to touch if the objective is to appraise the occlusion. A Kerr Bite Frame and Kerr's Bite Registration Paste are excellent for this purpose if the existing centric occlusion is being accepted. The lower cast is mounted and the preliminary diagnostic casts are now ready for examination and study (Fig. 2-14).

Prior to taking impressions, the occlusion should have been checked closely and equilibrated. After mounting, if other occlusion factors must be corrected, this should be done both on the casts and in the mouth. The extent of changes will determine the necessity for making and occluding new casts.

Value of Diagnostic Casts

Diagnostic casts are essential in the planning of a bridge (Fig. 2-15). They enable the operator (1) to evaluate the forces that will act against the bridge; (2) to decide whether any grinding or rebuilding of teeth will be obligatory so that a suitable or improved opposing occlusal plane can be formed; (3) by use of the surveyor, to locate the path of insertion and outline

---

*Vel-Mix, Kerr Mfg. Company, Romulus, Mich.   (Text continues on page 35)

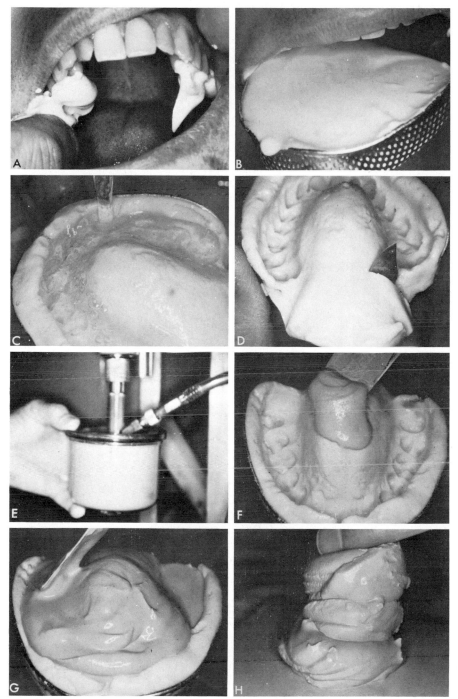

FIGURE 2-11.   *A*, Alginate placed to distal of terminal teeth and on occlusals of posteriors.

B, Tray filled.

C and *D*, Washing and trimming impression.

E, Mixing stone in vacuum.

F, First increment of stone. It flows under vibration. Thin film will enter teeth without forming bubbles.

G, Impression filled.

H, Mound of stone onto which inverted and filled impression will be placed.

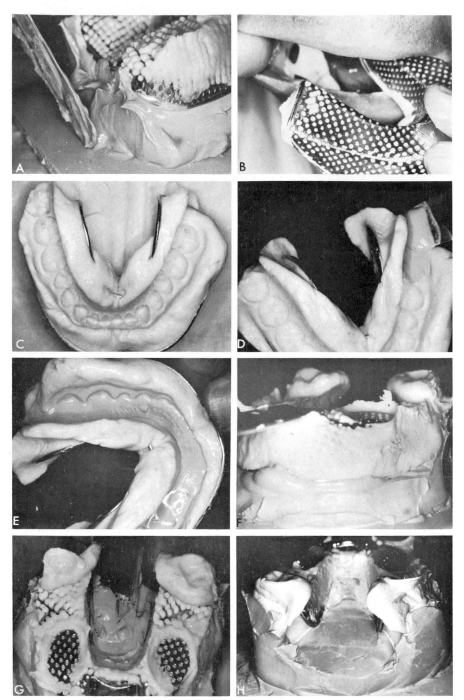

FIGURE 2–12. *A*, Adapting stone to borders of impression.

B, Placing lower tray in mouth with rotating motion. Tray displaces one corner of mouth while fingers of other hand open and widen orifice. No alginate should be left on lower lip.

C, Lower impression.

D, Stone is added at one end and, using vibration, is pulled in thin layer around to opposite end.

E, Occlusals filled. There should be no bubbles in cusp tips.

F, Inverted impression placed on mound of stone.

G, Adapting stone to lingual border and removing excess.

H, No excess stone around lingual border.

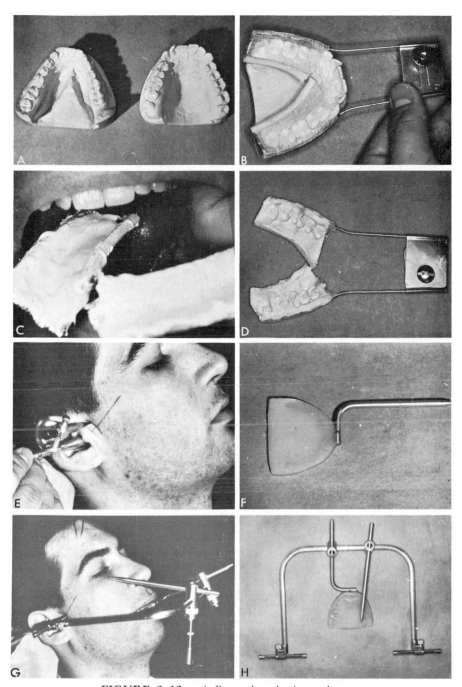

FIGURE 2–13. *A*, Poured and trimmed casts.
B, Fitting Kerr Bite Frame.
C, Placing Bite Frame, with paste, in mouth.
D, Registration.
E, Arbitrary point for positioning face-bow.
F, Bite fork covered with wax.
G, Face-bow adjusted to patient.
H, Face-bow locked and removed from patient.

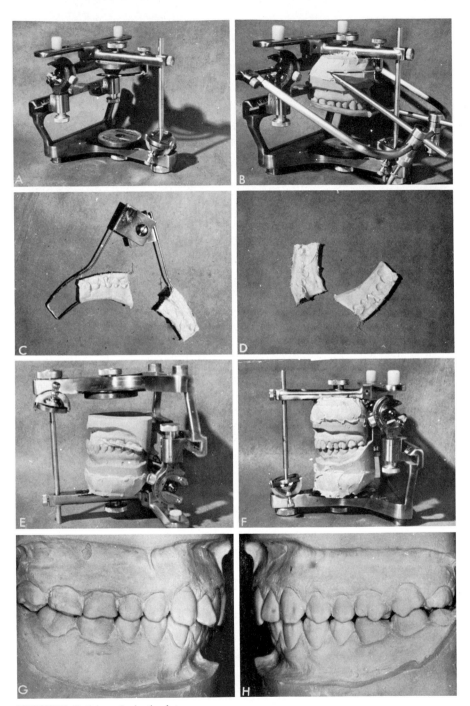

FIGURE 2–14.   *A*, Articulator.
B, Upper cast mounted to face-bow setting.
C and *D*, Registration for relating lower cast.
E, Articulator reversed. Lower cast related to upper with Bite Frame registration.
F, Both casts mounted.
G and *H*, Right and left occlusion.

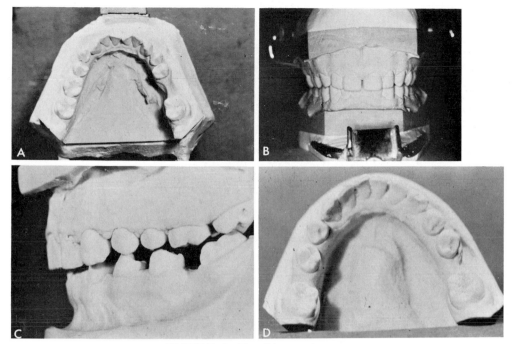

FIGURE 2–15.   *Diagnostic casts.*

A, Mandibular first molar space; normal mesiodistal width; abrasion on occluding surfaces; square teeth; path of insertion satisfactory on two abutments.

B, Diagnostic casts articulated correctly.

C and *D,* Teeth have drifted following extraction of first molars, creating handicaps of reduced space, rotated abutments, slightly extruded upper first molars, and the problems of re-establishing occlusal plane and occlusion.

the reduction necessary to make the abutment preparations parallel and to arrive at a design for maximal esthetics; (4) to visualize the directions in which force will be applied to the finished restoration and to plan reduction in the size or changes in the form of the opposing cusps, if such actions are warranted; (5) to select, contour, and position the facings and to use them as guides in preparing the abutments; and (6) to resolve the plan of procedure for the entire mouth.

"Plan of procedure" refers to a determination of the sequence of restorations. For instance, in order to develop the occlusal plane of the bridge more competently, it might be logical to restore opposing teeth first. Again, sometimes there is a likelihood that a bridge will function more effectively and with less chance for trauma if its construction is delayed until occlusal balance is achieved by grinding, by placing a crown or some other restoration on the opposite side, or by a combination of both.

Mouth Examination and Consultation with the Patient

Mouth examination provides an opportunity for studying tissue conditions, the quality of the surface tooth structure, the movements of the teeth under pressure or the excessive mobility of teeth by finger manipulation, and the oral hygiene and tolerance of mouth tissues to previous restorations. Mouth mirrors, explorers, dental floss or tape, water, and air are used for this type of examination.

Consultation with the patient should be conversational, rather than limited to direct questions and answers, because such an approach will often expose the patient's misgivings and hopes. Of course, in order to gain specific information, conversation must be augmented by some questioning. It is advisable to tell the patient frankly the anticipated nature of the operation, the extent of preparations to be made on the teeth, the need for anesthesia, the type of discomfort, fatigue, and inconvenience that may be experienced, and the amount of time to be spent. Absolute co-operation, respect, and trust from the patient must prevail from the beginning. These intangible but vital requisites make the technical work more facile and pleasant for both the patient and dentist.

The initial consultation is not the time for a discussion of fees. This should take place after all phases of the examination have been completed and findings co-ordinated, and the patient has been told what method and type of treatment will give him the most comfort and the longest period of useful, nondestructive service. "The size of the patient's purse should not alter the dental truth. He has the right to be well-advised and to be given time to consider that advice. Then, and only then, should the fee be quoted and the method of payment, sequence of operations, and appointments arranged."[11]

Exploration of Abutments and Associated Teeth

Exploration of abutments and associated teeth differs from *examination* in that it encompasses the removal of caries or old and doubtful restorations in order to ascertain the proportion of the remaining tooth substance and the probability of pulp exposure. Usually radiographs and oral examination will contribute ample information, but if there is any suspicion regarding the residuum of tooth structure, an exhaustive exploration of the abutment tooth must be made before planning continues. If any other tooth, the loss of which might affect the proposed prosthesis, has a carious lesion or a dubious restoration it too should be explored before the treatment plan is formulated.

Consideration of Periodontal Factors

The occlusion should be equilibrated, a prophylaxis given, and any required surgical treatment, such as a gingivectomy or reduction of the ridge, instituted before abutment preparations are planned. The gingiva, the periodontal membrane, and the alveolar process should be brought to the highest level of health attainable before abutments are prepared. Although one of the purposes in placing a bridge is to promote the well-being of the oral structure, an optimal state must be established beforehand. When this is apparent to the patient, he will comply with suggestions regarding his part in maintaining oral hygiene.

For the surest measure of success there should be no more recession than would be normal for the age of the patient, but variation is to be expected, inasmuch as this is governed to some extent by occlusal wear. If the alveolar process has receded without undue irregularity and if this recession has not resulted in pocketing or the bifurcation has not been implicated, the tooth may be used as a single or a splinted abutment. If the bony support is weak, all facets of the case should be scanned before such a tooth is used as an abutment, applying Ante's law in estimating the support (Fig. 2–16).

Both on the diagnostic casts and in the mouth, the *form*, the *distribution*, and the *position* of the opposing teeth must be heeded, and the plan of

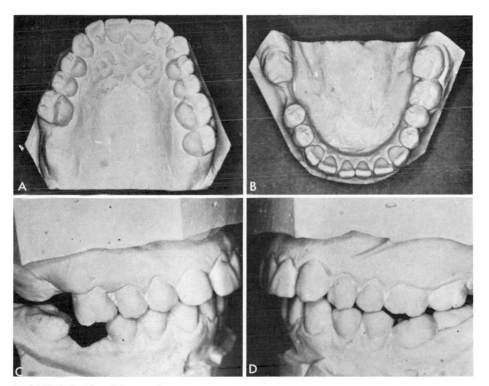

FIGURE 2–16. *Diagnostic casts.*

A and *B*, Upper and lower casts, occlusal view.

C, Right lateral view. Lower bridge will occlude only on anterior half, placing an added load on the bicuspid abutment and retainer. Two crowns should be considered; also the possible need for splinting the upper molar and second bicuspid to prevent distal movement of the molar.

D, Left lateral view. Upper first molar must be recontoured, making distal half shorter and mesial longer. Lower second molar, now in first molar position, must be built into occlusion, which will necessitate reshaping the distal half of the second bicuspid.

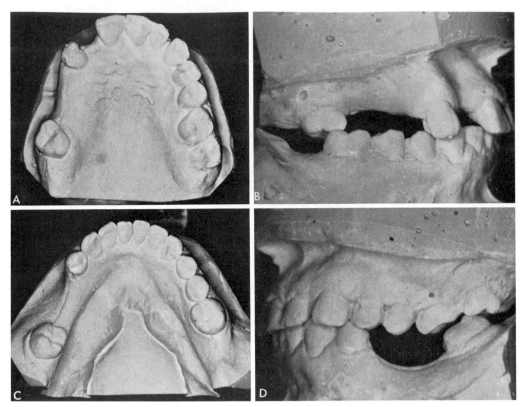

FIGURE 2-17. *A* and *B*, Diagnostic casts viewed from occlusal and right. Lateral incisor, first and second bicuspids, and first molar lost. Posterior space long for a bridge unless construction is sturdy. Occlusion on molar not completely favorable to cantilevering lateral incisor pontic. Long-axis relationship of three abutments good.

   C and *D*, Lower left space long for fixed prosthesis unless two abutments are used anteriorly.

construction and the esthetic concept deferred to these factors (Fig. 2-17). The form or length of an opposing tooth can be altered a little by grinding and to a major degree by the construction of a crown or an inlay, or by splinting two teeth (Fig. 2-18). Distribution may be revamped by extraction or multiple abutments.

When mandibular bicuspids occlude buccally to opposing teeth, a greater amount of metal may be displayed unless drastic changes are made in the preparations. Not infrequently, also, when an abutment is unopposed, with no teeth posterior to it, the treatment plan must include a greater number of supporting teeth at the anterior end of the prosthesis to offset the increased leverage on the anterior abutment.

Orthodontic Positioning of Abutment or Opposing Teeth

Distribution and position of abutment teeth can often be improved by orthodontics. Minor and uncomplicated treatment can be done by general

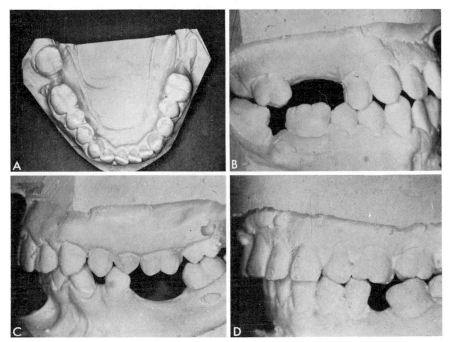

FIGURE 2-18. *A*, Occlusal view of diagnostic cast. Third molar has moved mesially. Both second molars missing.

B, Lateral view of occluded diagnostic casts. Bicuspid and molar lost. Principal force of occlusion will be on pontics. To prepare opposing arch prior to building upper bridge, lower first molar and third molar should be connected by a small pontic, with both joints and molar soldered. First molar must be recontoured to occlusal plane. Maxillary bridge will be more comfortable and will serve longer if it has continuous occlusion. Also, mastication will be improved.

C and *D*, Maxillary first molars have extruded in an arc and must be "leveled" before occluding prostheses are built.

practitioners, thus decreasing the difficulties in preparation and construction and adding materially to the life of the restoration (Fig. 2-19). This phase of the restorative procedure deserves more attention than it normally receives (Fig. 2-20). (See Chapter 29.)

Planning Appointments

Arranging appointments is an individual office matter. In this respect, however, in every office it should be emphasized that preparations on vital teeth should be completed in one visit and it must be remembered always that *abutment teeth should be left unrestored for the shortest possible period of time to prevent movement, sensitivity, and annoyance to the patient.*

THE FOUNDATION

The preferred clinical crown for an abutment is one of average length or longer, of square form, and of more than average bulk. Nevertheless,

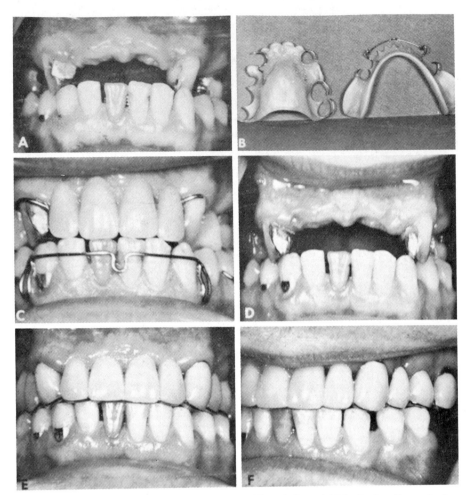

FIGURE 2–19. *A*, Labial view showing maxillary left cuspid locked to lingual of mandibular teeth.

B, Working retainers that were used to improve tooth position. The upper left cuspid clasp is free of acrylic resin over most of its length so that it can be activated to cause labial movement of the tooth. The labial wire on the lower will be used to move the incisors lingually and together.

C, Appliances in the mouth. The mandibular posterior supplied teeth are set high to increase the vertical dimension so that the left cuspid will be free to move into proper position.

D, Left cuspid has moved to position. Teeth have temporary amalgam restorations.

E and *F*, Bridge cemented.

short teeth may be used when the preparations are altered to develop resistance to displacement. Frail teeth may be employed also, provided the spaces to be filled are correspondingly narrow and the opposing forces are relative. Tapered or ovoid teeth may be prepared as abutments if the pulps have receded enough to allow safe and sufficient reduction of tooth structure. This will have occurred in most instances.

The length of the root segment supported by the alveolar process should be one and one-half times that of the crown of the abutment. The root

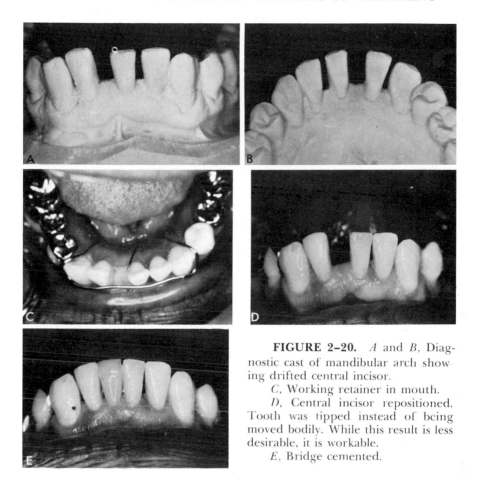

FIGURE 2–20. *A* and *B*, Diagnostic cast of mandibular arch showing drifted central incisor.

C, Working retainer in mouth.

D, Central incisor repositioned. Tooth was tipped instead of being moved bodily. While this result is less desirable, it is workable.

E, Bridge cemented.

should not be conical, but need not be straight. When the apical segment of the root is curved to create an area that might bruise the periodontal membrane under masticating force, the previous load or types and strength of forces should be assessed. If the reaction is adjudged healthy, roots of this type will afford excellent support for fixed prostheses.

The abutment teeth should have a near-parallel relationship with each other and a normal long-axis relationship to the opposing teeth, although there may be many digressions from this requirement.[12] Teeth that are tipped mesially or distally can be used as abutments without apprehension if the inclination is not so great as to interfere with preparation. Teeth that are tipped buccally or lingually are less qualified abutments because, when such teeth are used, rotation or torque can damage supporting structure or cause retainers to become loose.

A tooth free of caries is likely to have a pulp less prone to future pathologic reactions; also, it permits the most nearly perfect type of preparation, since minimal coronal reduction is possible. Still, teeth that have caries involving areas not usually included in the preparations may be used as abutments provided the caries is removed, the pulp is protected against thermal shock, and the tooth is restored to "prepared form"* by a gold casting or amalgam. In a few circumstances, if the carious area does not approach the margin of the preparation and if the retainer will be supported by tooth structure, cement or resin may be used instead of metal. When caries is extensive and little dentin remains in the crown area, extraordinary care must be used during the preparation to conserve tooth structure.

If the tooth is pulpless, it may be rebuilt with a crown and used as an abutment if there is no apical rarefaction or root resorption and if the root canal can be enlarged to receive a post for the support of a cast or amalgam core. This post must be of a length equal to or greater than that of the crown or retainer. Because the remaining coronal structure of a pulpless tooth is brittle, it is seldom capable of supporting the restoration without one or more posts being extended into the root area.[13]

Splinting

An abutment tooth usually is required at each end of the space to be restored, but if the construction of a bridge were to create a lever arm of some length, additional terminal abutment teeth, splinted, would be in order (Figs. 2–21 and 2–22). (Other exceptions are discussed in Chapter 26, Bridge Patterns.)

The term *splinting* denotes the rigid joining of two or more approximating teeth (Fig. 2–23). In bridge construction splinted abutments are called *multiple abutments.* This practice is employed when the supporting structure is weak around one or more of the terminal abutment teeth, or when the space is long or curved or embraces the corner of the mouth in such a way that extra abutments are needed to offset the destructive rotating force generated from the tip of the lever arm. This situation occurs in the maxillary arch, particularly when replacing a cuspid, a cuspid and a lateral, or a cuspid and a first bicuspid.

A lever arm is seen in every upper anterior bridge, but the line of force directed against maxillary anterior fixed restorations comes from the lingual, as a rule, and therefore the lever arm is not such a serious factor. Shorter ones are found in the anterior segment of the mandibular arch and occur frequently with the construction of bridges supplying the bicuspids. Here punctilious planning is essential in the design of the pontics and in the retentive characteristics incorporated in the abutment preparations.

Splinting is a procedure demanding ingenuity, scrupulous attention to details in the preparation of the teeth, modification of the form of abutment castings, and precision in the placement and dimension of solder joints. Unless kept to appropriate size, the joints diminish embrasure space and

---

*"Prepared form" is the shape of the reduced tooth when it is completed to receive the specific type of retainer or restoration planned. It must provide maximal retention and resistance to caries and fracture, and encourage biologic acceptance of the treatment as a whole.

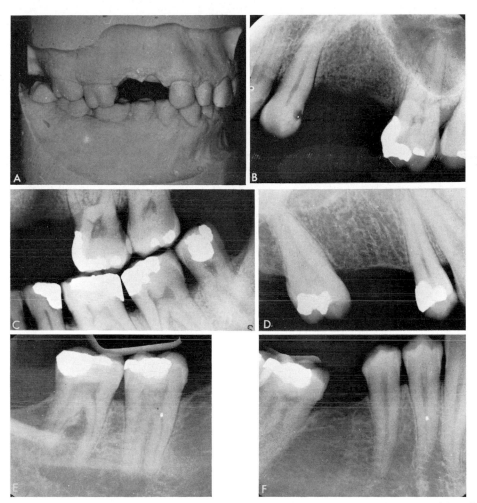

FIGURE 2-21. *A*, Diagnostic casts showing contour of gingival tissue resulting from unsupported removable prosthesis. Partial denture must not be worn, because tissue should be allowed to recontour prior to the construction of a bridge. Mandibular third molar should be extracted to protect distal of second molar from pocketing, even though it has abraded and is integrated with incisal guidance.

B and *C*, Radiographs of arches shown in *A*. Periodontal treatment needed before and after bridge is constructed.

D, A molar inclined mesially, but this is an excellent situation for a bridge.

E and *F*, Second molar and second bicuspid are good abutments. Plus contact on mesial of bicuspid retainer should move first bicuspid into contact with cuspid. Bridge cemented following this treatment and necessary equilibration.

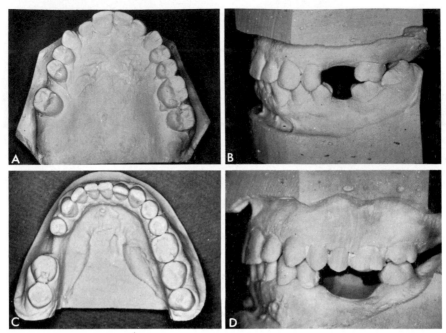

FIGURE 2–22. *A*, Maxillary diagnostic cast. First molar missing, with second molar moved mesially. Space less than bicuspid width. A bridge may be needed to support molar or second bicuspid and to aid mastication. Hygiene frequently difficult in such cases.

B, Mandibular third molar should be extracted and spaces restored with bridges.

C, Bridge indicated, but space between bicuspid and cuspid should be kept the same. Food packing will be no problem unless bicuspid retainer is overcontoured on mesial.

D, Maxillary first molar must be recontoured. Bicuspid abutment must be carefully evaluated. Many of these bridges fail unless cuspid is also included.

cause stagnation of underlying soft tissue owing to lack of stimulation from the massage of food particles. (See Chapter 27, Splinting Teeth.)

THE PATH OF INSERTION

The path of insertion is that line or direction in which the prosthesis may be seated simultaneously on all the abutments without causing lateral force or torsion on any one of them. Any semblance of an undercut or a convergence must be eliminated if the bridge is to be seated. The presence of any undercut may be disclosed by taking an impression, pouring a plaster cast, and checking it with the surveyor.

Several circumstances control or influence the path of insertion. The most important are the long-axis relationship of the abutment teeth and the long-axis relationship of the abutment teeth with those adjacent. Malaligned teeth approximating abutments sometimes interfere with the proposed path of insertion, making it necessary to change the path slightly or to alter the form of the offending approximating tooth by grinding or by placement of a restoration.

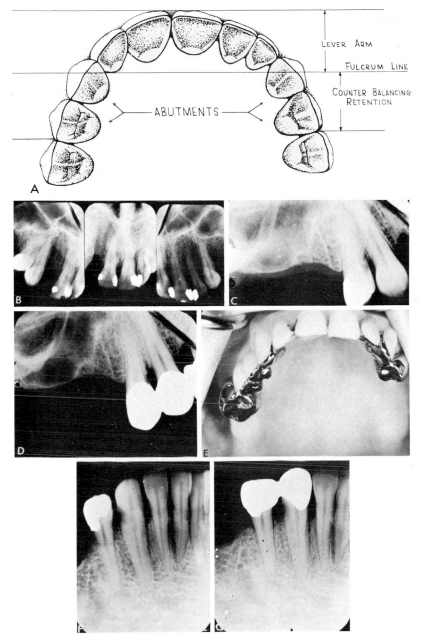

FIGURE 2-23. *Splinting.*

A, Cuspid and bicuspid retainers splinted to form "multiple abutments."

B and *C*, Good alveolar process and crown-root ratio on cuspid and first bicuspid. Lateral incisor space.

D, Splinted cuspid and bicuspid abutments; cantilever lateral incisor pontic.

E, The three-unit bridge.

F, Reduced support around first bicuspid; too weak for partial denture abutment.

G, Splinted first bicuspid and cuspid; now a strong abutment.

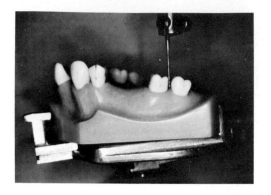

FIGURE 2–24. Path of insertion marked on bicuspid abutment. Distal of molar prepared to same angle.

The logical path of insertion can be confirmed on the diagnostic cast with the analyzing rod of the surveyor checking the long-axis relationship of the crowns (Fig. 2-24). It should assume a direction most compatible with the long axes of all the involved crowns, and one that will necessitate minimal cutting on all the surfaces to be included in the preparations. When more than two teeth are to be used as abutments, one, not necessarily a terminal abutment, serves as the norm and the others are prepared parallel to it.

With this survey marked on the teeth and with radiographic information of root direction and periodontal membrane condition in mind, a calculation should be made concerning the amount of cutting indicated on the other abutment teeth in order that this designated direction may be used as the path of insertion. If esthetic considerations are to be emphasized and exaggerated cutting avoided, generally some departure from the most retentive preparation will be compulsory on one or more abutments whose long-axis directions are not parallel to the guiding tooth.

Except for the young patient, selection of a path of insertion on tipped teeth is a simple matter, since pulp recession ordinarily will assure safety in the reduction of the crown. Many times this is obvious to the experienced operator during the oral examination, after the size and location of the pulp horns have been verified by radiographs. Nevertheless, with few exceptions, cuts for parallelism should be traced on the diagnostic cast by a surveyor.

SPACE LENGTHS

The length of the space has a definitive bearing on the type of construction. The ideal space is that of only one missing tooth, unless the third molar is involved. Before the acceptance of this tooth as an abutment, it should be judged as to fitness in regard to long-axis relationship, crown-root ratio, relationship of the crown to the surrounding soft tissue, shape of the root (conical or curved), and type of occlusion.

The wisdom of constructing a bridge supplying three approximating missing posterior teeth may be debatable in the majority of instances, especially in the mandibular arch (Fig. 2-25). To prevent a springing reaction in

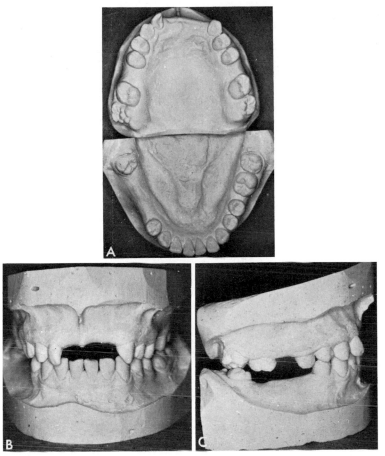

FIGURE 2-25. *A*, Maxillary and mandibular casts. All edentulous areas in upper arch can be filled with bridges. The cuspids and the lateral incisor will give good support for a six-unit prosthesis; however, if there is doubt, the left bicuspid should be included. The third molars are of questionable value, but need not be condemned unless hygiene or periodontal considerations dictate removal. Lower right space is very long, and inclination of molar abutment must be considered. Space on left may be used for clasping.

B, Vertical overlap favorable for bridge construction.

C, Upper bicuspid abutment must be shortened and lower molar "leveled" and recontoured for clasping. Space is too long and abutments are too short for a bridge to be successful.

the center of the span, the bridge must be bulky and solder joints large; thus the embrasure areas will be reduced in size, with a resultant lack of stimulating massage of food on the underlying tissue. Also, it is hard to satisfy Ante's law under such conditions. In the maxillary arch, however, many bridges, constructed from cuspid to second molar, have provided long periods of clinical service. It has not been proved that any type of removable bridge would have served to better advantage.

ABUTMENTS IN ABNORMAL POSITIONS

Abutment teeth, even in short spaces, must be examined critically for rotation, tipping, and recession. If the rotated tooth has erupted in that position, the supporting structure probably has not been seriously impaired, but if the rotation has occurred because of the loss of an approximating tooth or the extrusion of an opposing tooth, the rotated abutment may be much less desirable. Sometimes the crown form must be changed considerably when constructing a retainer for a rotated tooth. On the other hand, if the abnormal position of a rotated tooth is mechanically and esthetically satisfactory and if retention can be secured by restoring the tooth as it is, minimal change in form should be contemplated.

The rotation of an abutment can either reduce or increase the normal space length. The problem of constructing a pontic of abnormal size should be recognized in advance, as a slight decrease or increase in the mesiodistal width of the abutment teeth can be embodied in the construction of the retainers so that the pontic may be more nearly normal in size.

Tipping mesially or distally usually will reduce space lengths; consequently, there must be some alteration in crown form when the retainer is carved, and also a more careful analysis of the occlusion, connectors, and embrasures when constructing the pontic. Inordinate tipping can preclude the use of the tooth as an abutment. The force of occlusion, the degree to which the tooth may be stabilized, the capacity of the supporting structure, and pocketing must be considered, as well as the willingness of the patient to accept the actual and ensuing state of affairs.

When an abutment is inclined buccally or lingually, the space length is not perceptibly affected, but the position of the connector will be altered. The resistance to forces directed against a bridge supported by one or more such teeth will be less substantial than when the abutments are in normal position. The ability of the supporting structure to withstand these abnormal forces should be reviewed. When a tooth is tipped to the buccal or the lingual, the path of insertion on all the teeth to be used may be a compromise. The solution can be aided appreciably by surveying the diagnostic casts.

PREPARATION OF OPPOSING ARCH

To facilitate making a bridge, it is often mandatory to change slightly the length and occlusal form of opposing teeth. Retainers may then be constructed to direct the forces as desired, pontics may be placed in more normal positions with better form, and the teeth may occlude with minimal interference.

Occasionally a tooth will have extruded into a space to such a degree that reduction of length and alteration in shape become impossible. The interfering tooth must be removed in such an instance, even if this should entail building another bridge.

If one of the opposing teeth has been lost, resulting in enough drifting or tipping to nullify the continuity of the opposing occlusal plane, those teeth that remain should be restored with crowns, inlays, or a splint, prior to construction of the bridge. If restorations already in place are effectual in terms of margins and preservation of the teeth, but are lacking in occlusal or embrasure form, they should be reshaped.

*   *   *   *   *   *

The student should realize that all these complex factors cannot be readily defined or positioned in order of their significance. Relative importance will change with individual mouths. In fact, each succeeding case presents new problems and new difficulties to the novice. These principles will be applied to the examples cited throughout the text so that in planning a bridge the student or dentist will learn to make use of such diagnostic aids automatically. Gregory's[14] observation that "after years of practice, each new case is a variation of one previously handled" should become a slogan in the profession.

Rules of procedure included here, if followed diligently, will result in gratification for patient and dentist alike. Experience will modify thinking and technique and will broaden judgment, but to avert chaos for the beginner, one method should be mastered before versatility is attempted. It is to be hoped that the contents of this chapter and those that follow will equip the student with a firm foundation for progress.

REFERENCES

1. Dykema, R. W.: Fixed partial prosthodontics. J. Tennessee D. A., *42*:309, Oct. 1962.
2. Tylman, S. D.: Theory and Practice of Crown and Fixed Partial Prosthodontics (Bridge). St. Louis, The C. V. Mosby Company, 1970.
3. Myers, G. E.: Textbook of Crown and Bridge Prosthodontics. St. Louis, The C. V. Mosby Company, 1969.
4. Greeley, J. H.: Planning for fixed prosthesis. J. Pros. Den., *20*:412, Nov. 1968.
5. Meadows, T. W.: Diagnosis and treatment: crown and bridge prosthodontics. J. Tennessee D. A., *45*:425, Oct. 1965.
6. Raper, H.: Personal communication.
7. Smith, G. P.: Factors affecting the choice of partial prosthesis — fixed or removable. D. Clin. N. Amer., March, 1959, p. 3.
8. Lakermance, J., and Laudenbach, P.: Indications and contraindications for fixed prosthesis. Rev. Stomat., *63*:46, Jan.-Feb. 1962.
9. Tylman, S. D.: Fixed partial denture prosthodontics. Internat. D. J., *10*:58, March 1961.
10. Contino, R. M., and Stallard, H.: Instruments essential for obtaining data needed in making a functional diagnosis of the human mouth. J. Pros. Den., *7*:66, Jan. 1957.
11. Adams, J. W.: Lecture, Postgraduate course, Indiana University School of Dentistry, April 1958.
12. Schweitzer, J. M.: Oral Rehabilitation. St. Louis, The C. V. Mosby Company, 1951.
13. Markley, M. R.: Pin reinforcement and retention of amalgam foundations and restorations. J.A.D.A., *56*:675, May 1958.
14. Gregory, G. T.: Personal communication.

Abramson, I.: Role of endodontics in crown and bridge prosthesis. J. Maryland D. A., *1*:28, No. 1, 1958.
Ante, I. H.: The fundamental principles of fixed and removable bridge prosthesis. Dominion D. J., *42*:109, 1930.
Bastian, D. C.: Consideration of some of the clinical problems of crown and bridgework. W. Virginia D. J., *17*:120, Jan. 1943.

Coelho, D. H.: Ultimate goal in fixed bridge procedures. J. Pros. Den., *4*:667, Sept. 1954.

Ewing, J. E.: Surgical crown and bridge prosthodontics. J. Pros. Den., *4*:523, July 1954.

Granger, E. R.: Occlusion in temporomandibular joint pain. J.A.D.A., *56*:659, May 1958.

Grubb, H. D.: Fixed bridgework. J. Pros. Den., *3*:121, Jan. 1953.

Landa, J. S.: An analysis of current practices in mouth rehabilitation. J. Pros. Den., *5*:527, July 1955.

McCall, J. O.: The periodontal element in prosthodontics. J. Pros. Den., *16*:585, May–June 1966.

Miller, S. C.: Periodontics and restorative dentistry. J.A.D.A., *47*:282, Sept. 1953.

Mitchell, D. F., Standish, S. M., and Fast, T. B.: Oral Diagnosis/Oral Medicine. Philadelphia, Lea & Febiger, 1969.

Nuttall, E. B.: Diagnosis and correction of occlusal disharmonies in preparation for fixed restorations. J.A.D.A., *44*:399, April 1952.

Nuttall, E. B.: Development of basic prosthodontic principles of crown and bridge. Pennsylvania D. J., *21*:6, May 1954.

Pruden, W. H., II: Today's approach to fixed denture prosthesis. J. New Jersey D. Soc., *32*:11, Sept. 1960.

Shooshan, E. D.: Adequate operative dentistry and its significance in maintaining oral health. J. Pros. Den., *6*:710, Sept. 1956.

Tylman, S. D.: To what degree can the partially edentulous patient be rehabilitated biologically and mechanically by means of crowns and fixed bridges? J. Ontario D. A., *30*:255, Aug. and Oct. 1953.

Tylman, S. D.: Discussion of the biologic factors involved in the fixed partial denture. J. Canad. D. A., *23*:67, Feb. 1957.

chapter 3

TOOTH REDUCTION

The building of retainers or individual crowns must be achieved without enlarging tooth dimensions and adding further to the load that abutments and supporting structures must withstand. Sound enamel and dentin must be cut away to produce space and retentive form for such restorations. The one method of reduction that has been universally adopted makes use of rotating cutting or abrading instruments, such as carbide or carbon steel burs, diamond or carborundum stones and disks, and abrasive-coated paper disks.

LUBRICATION AND COOLING OF TOOTH STRUCTURE

In any grinding operation on teeth, especially those involving stones or accelerated speeds, consideration for the pulp cannot be overemphasized. The dentin and the pulp are subjected to a series of insults, such as caries, instrumentation, placement of restorative materials, and thermal and traumatic shock. One of the most active irritants can be the heat generated by the high-speed cutting tools used in modern cavity preparation. If the preparation is deep, the heat must be controlled and dissipated or severe pulpal reaction may occur. Lubrication and cooling are essential.[1] Air, which can dehydrate the tooth substance, is NOT an adequate coolant.[2, 3]

The authors have seen excellent results from the washed field technique, but have had less experience and have been less favorably impressed with air cooling. Data on clinical cases coming from a cross section of practicing dentists do imply that with *any technique* caution cannot be thrown to the winds, that respect for living tissue must be paramount, and that in those cases treated most carefully, postoperative sensitivity in teeth is infrequent.

51

EFFECT OF SPEED AND CUTTING ON
PULP AND TOOTH STRUCTURES

It is thought by the authors and numerous clinicians and investigators with whom the subject has been discussed that overly rapid cutting can bring about changes within the pulp, which will cause the tooth to be sensitive after restorative operations are completed, and that lubrication and coolants contribute a great deal to the comfort of the patient during and probably following the operation. Davila Alonso et al.[4] maintain that there will be little permanent change in the pulp unless it is *directly* traumatized. Kasloff[5, 6, 7] has demonstrated that some instruments will cause more checking (at least microscopically) in the enamel than others, although he does not attribute distinctive clinical significance to this.

Using ultra high-speed rotary cutting, most preparations can be made in less time with less effort and trauma. An extended observation of preparations executed in what must have been the absolute minimal time would seem to indicate a larger percentage of such teeth exhibiting sensitivity following cementation of bridges,[8, 9] and an increase in the eventual number of candidates for endodontic therapy. There is no apparent advantage in striving for a routine that will eliminate from 30 seconds to 2 minutes in the preparation of a tooth. If, in order to make a preparation with finesse, an additional 5 minutes must be used and more instrument changes must be made, and if there is evidence that because of this extra attention the preparation will be less traumatic for the tooth, the surrounding tissue, and the patient, the authors insist that *more time should be taken.* The authors believe also that the suggestion that all prepared teeth be coated with a cavity varnish, such as Copalite,* immediately following the taking of an elastic impression and before the seating of temporary coverings, is worthy of reflection. However, if a liner is used under temporary coverings, the anodyne effect of eugenol in the luting material is lost.

Ultra high speed with all its virtues is not a panacea. There are a few hazards that must be checked and diminished. A goodly number say that it is mandatory that water be applied as a water spray or air-water spray in ultra high-speed cutting to prevent excessive pulpal response histologically. Conversely, some contend that the water never really reaches the cutting area of the instrument and because of this is not effective as a coolant. Besides, it is claimed that the pulpal response is reversible and consequently physiologic rather than pathologic.

More research must be done in this area. Until disproof can be presented, ultra high-speed cutting should be done in a wet field. If nothing more, it will help to lessen odor and remove debris. While visibility is affected adversely by water, this is not to a degree that instrumentation is impossible. Lukewarm water, in either a stream or a spray, must be used with a diamond stone, not only as a coolant, but also as a cleanser to keep the

---

*Harry J. Bosworth Co., Chicago, Ill.

surface of the stone free of debris so that it may work with maximal capability.

PRECAUTIONS NEEDED WHEN CUTTING TEETH

Certain precautions must be taken during the preparation of a tooth. A disk that is being used to cut through and remove a portion of a mesial or distal surface must be guided and steadied so that it will not bind and as a result jump out of control, cutting or harming the gingiva, tongue, cheek, lip, or another tooth. Instruments must be handled on the buccal and lingual surfaces so that gingival tissue will not be injured to a point that precludes healing and return to original form. With the speedy technique of tooth reduction, the operator is more prone to mar the approximating tooth. There must be no contact of the cutting instrument with any tooth not included in the treatment plan. Mobile tissue may be retracted and shielded by the fingers, mirrors, tongue blades, or mechanical devices, such as disk-guards. Sometimes an assistant must help.

Beginning students should proceed warily when first operating in the oral cavity. Increased rotational speeds are recommended for many procedures only when the operator has become highly trained, with an accurate concept of what the finished preparation should be, and with the ability or willingness to concentrate and avoid overreduction of teeth.

With the evolution of rotating cutting instruments so that they may be used beneficially with augmented speeds,[10, 11] the trauma from many preparations, notably in the fixed partial denture field, has been dramatically reduced. Faster cutting speeds, and superior cutting tools recently developed, enable the dentist markedly to reduce operating time and discomfort to the patient. This statement does not imply that teeth may be cut painlessly without the use of local anesthetics. It does mean that there will be less force required and less vibration with these mechanical advances. While there are those who proclaim that every phase of most preparations can be realized satisfactorily and safely with the faster techniques of instrumentation, it is generally accepted that the so-called high-speed reduction of tooth structure is only a preliminary procedure in the correct preparation of a tooth. It should be used for competent gross preparation only. Finishing and refinement of all preparations should be done at slower speeds and with hand instruments.

INSTRUMENTATION IN PREPARATIONS

Instrumentation is simplified and reduced at ultra high speeds. Fewer rotary instruments are used. Gross reduction of most surfaces can be made with one bur. For example, in the preparation of a posterior tooth for a full

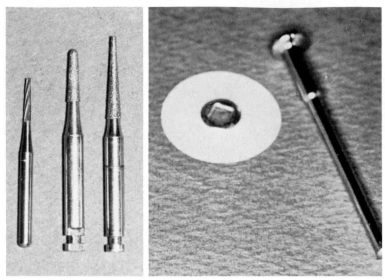

FIGURE 3-1.   **FIGURE 3-2.**

FIGURE 3-1.   Left to right: 169L-FG carbide bur (S.S.W.); 1D-T latch tapered diamond stone (Densco); ¼D-L latch tapered diamond stone (Densco).

FIGURE 3-2.   Moore's disk and mandrel.

veneer crown, only two rotary instruments need be employed, with perhaps a third if the interproximal space is very narrow. The *169L* (S.S.W.)*, the *69L* (Densco)†, or the *699L* (Densco) *carbide tapered fissure bur*‡ is the one essential instrument with ultra high speed, and the *1D-TL diamond* (Densco) for slow speed. The ¼ *D-L diamond* (Densco) may be used if the interproximal space is restricted (Fig. 3 − 1). Other brands of similar design, and other lengths if teeth are short, are also suitable. (See Figures 3–17 to 3–21.)

At slow speeds, in addition to diamond and carborundum stones and metal burs, paper disks coated with grits of several kinds and finenesses can be used for a number of the steps in the preparations to be described later. One brand of disk, utilizing a snap-on mandrel§, is illustrated (Fig. 3–2), but other disks are equally efficient. With few exceptions, stones, burs, and disks are made for both the straight and the contra-angle handpiece.

CONCEPTS OF TECHNIQUE AND PREPARED FORM MODIFIED

Procedural techniques and concepts of form have been modified somewhat since the advent of accelerated speeds in tooth reduction, without altering the requirements of retention and stability of restorations and pros-

*The S. S. White Dental Mfg. Co., Philadelphia, Pa.
†Teledyne Densco, Denver, Colo.
‡Current Clinical Dental Terminology uses "tapered," but some manufacturers use "taper."
§E. C. Moore Company, Dearborn, Mich.

theses. These will not change even if some contours in prepared form are altered slightly to make new instruments and techniques more manageable. Comprehension and acceptance of such changes or advances are inevitable.

The extracoronal reduction of teeth in the forming of preparations to receive cast retainers may be divided into basic steps. Each will have variations, depending on the position of the tooth in the mouth, its length, contour, angle of eruption, rotation, and the kind or type of retainer planned. Regardless of variation or tooth, the fundamental approach, procedures, and accomplishments are the same.

STEPS IN TOOTH REDUCTION

With any form of instrumentation used to prepare a tooth for a crown, a sequence must be followed. Each phase of reduction has a purpose that is vital to the longevity of the restoring retainer.

The steps in reduction may be classified as follows, but the order may be changed:

(1) proximal slices;

(2) shortening the occlusal surface or

(3) incisal edge;

(4) preparing convex lingual, labial, or buccal surfaces and concave lingual surfaces;

(5) rounding corners and completing the cervical finishing line (Fig. 3-3);

(6) making shoulders to include labial or buccal and proximal, or all axial surfaces (Fig. 3-4); and

(7) cutting grooves, ledges, or pinholes, or a combination of these.

The Proximal Slice

The objectives of the proximal slice (or reduction) are to parallel or adjust the mesial or distal surfaces (or both) to the path of insertion for retention, to remove the surface bulge that would prohibit making and seating a casting adapted to the cervical region of the tooth, to create space for a thickness of metal in the casting that will be sufficient for strength and restoration of tooth form, to afford access for rounding corners or cutting grooves or retentive boxes, and to extend the proximal cervical margins into areas immune to caries (Figs. 3-5 and 3-6). There is some danger of overtapering the preparation with a loss of retention.

With the occasional exception of the inlay, all abutment preparations can include proximal slices. A bur on a disk is used for this step. With a bur (high speed), reduction begins lingually or buccally (see Fig. 3-3H) and proceeds toward the opposite side; with a disk (slow speed), cutting begins at the incisal edge or occlusal surface, ending at or just under the gingival crest

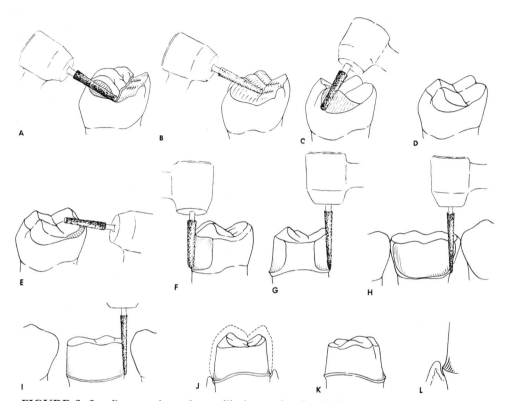

FIGURE 3–3.   Preparation of mandibular molar for full veneer gold crown. (Dr. Lundeen has altered the sequence of basic steps without change in final result.)

A and *B*, Reduction of occlusal surface using stone with square-cutting end. General contour of surface maintained.

C and *D*, Reduction of occluding portion of buccal surface.

E, Reducing lingual portion of lingual cusps.

F, Cutting down buccal surface. Stone has a round tip.

G, Lingual reduction. Stone has curved tip, less round than on buccal surface.

H and *I*, Cutting through proximal surfaces and establishing cervical margin.

J, Outline of structure cut away.

K and *L*, Chamfered finishing line.

(These drawings are based on the syllabus written and used by Dr. Harry Lundeen, School of Dentistry, University of Kentucky.)

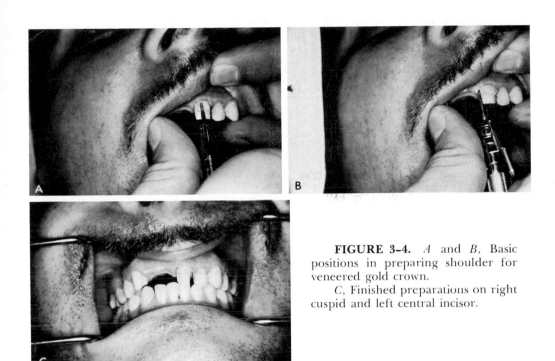

FIGURE 3-4. *A* and *B*, Basic positions in preparing shoulder for veneered gold crown.

C, Finished preparations on right cuspid and left central incisor.

FIGURE 3-5. Disk is in position to make proximal slice. Second and third (hidden) fingers of right hand, resting on incisors, support handpiece. Thumb and first finger hold and control handpiece and second finger supports it. Lip and cheek are retracted by first and second fingers of left hand and by mirror held between thumb and first two fingers. Lower lip and tongue protected by mirror.

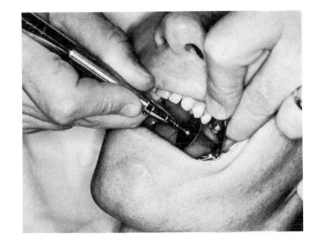

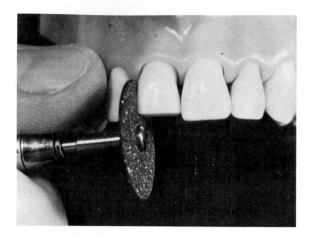

FIGURE 3-6. Proximal slice, maxillary central incisor. Cut, parallel to predetermined path of seating, started at reduced incisal edge and ended at gingival crest.

or cementoenamel junction. Essentially it will be parallel to the path of insertion, may follow the plane of the surface being reduced, and can have many relationships with the long axis of the tooth.

The cervical margin of a proximal cut will be completed in most cases using a round-end fine tapered stone in a contra-angle handpiece.

Reducing Occlusal Surfaces

Occlusal reduction opens a space for an irregular and strong metal plate that will connect and stabilize the circumferential segments of the retainer and protect the tooth against caries, irritation, or fracture. At the same time provision will be made for natural wear or future equilibration, and for recontoured occlusal surfaces that will re-establish occlusion or decrease leverage or stress on the supporting structure (Fig. 3–7). (See also Figure 3–3*A*, *B*, *C*, *D*, and *E*.)

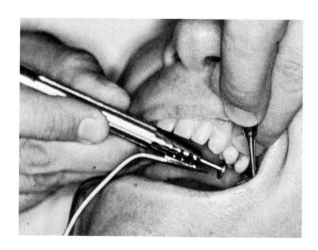

FIGURE 3-7. Handpiece with water spray attachment. Position of handpiece will be rotated so that occlusal surface may be reduced to conform to contour of cusp planes.

Occlusal reduction can be without complications when the tooth to be prepared has been worn so that the surface is relatively flat, and it may be involved when the tooth has sharp cusps, prominent ridges, and deep grooves and sulci. All occlusal surfaces should be prepared to reproduce roughly the contour of the uncut surface, or, if occlusal patterns are to be changed, the contours of the restoration. If the tooth is abraded, a small wheel stone with a square edge will suffice. If the occlusal surface is unworn, the groove pattern should be cut out with a tapered fissure bur to the depth desired, and with this as an indicator the whole occlusal surface should be reduced.

Areas of contact in centric occlusion and in masticatory excursions must be marked, observed, and prepared deeper than others to be certain that minimal clearance has been obtained and will remain. On teeth tipped so that one or more cusps or a marginal ridge may be out of occlusion, cutting should be done only in those areas that have remained in contact or, in any position, are within 1.0 mm. of the opposing teeth.

Reducing Incisal Edges

An incisal edge is shortened to forestall fracture of the labial enamel and gain space for connecting and strengthening metal that later may be adjusted for equilibrium, and for the bulk of material or materials wanted to restore the tooth to esthetic and functional form (Fig. 3–8).

Incisal edges may be shortened with any of a variety of wheel stones. This cut ideally should be at right angles to the line of force from the opposing teeth. Reduction of an upper incisal edge resembles that done on the lingual planes of buccal cusps of maxillary bicuspids and molars, while the shortening of the incisal edge on a mandibular anterior tooth can be compared with the same cutting operation on the buccal surfaces of buccal cusps of mandibular bicuspids and molars.

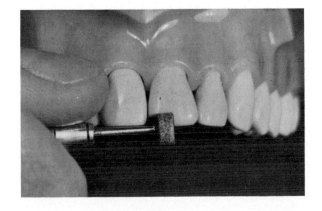

FIGURE 3–8. Position of stone when reducing incisal edge. Approach can be from lingual, labial, or proximal.

Preparing Convex Lingual, Labial, or Buccal Surfaces and Concave Lingual Surfaces

Reduction of the buccal surface of a mandibular posterior tooth or the lingual surface of either a maxillary anterior or posterior tooth gives room for the metal that will absorb and dissipate forces of occlusion and connect the retentive proximal sections of the retainer (Fig. 3–9). It also permits the rebuilt tooth to be normal, reduced, or recontoured in size and form, and enables an encircling band of metal to increase retention, strengthen and avert splitting of the tooth, and adds substance for later wear and adjustment. The lingual surface of a mandibular tooth is reduced so that retention may be increased, caries inhibited, and the tooth size either maintained or reduced.

On the lingual surface of a posterior tooth a cylindrical cutting instrument, held parallel to and rotating at right angles to the long axis, may be preferred if it is used so that no cervical undercut will be formed and so that the occlusal half of the surface will be prepared to conform to the natural lingual contour.

Labial and buccal surfaces are cut down so that the tooth may be contained within metal to increase retention, hinder the progress of caries, decrease the chances of breaking, and supply space for veneers that will be pleasing in appearance.

Although many types of burs or stones may be used on convex surfaces,

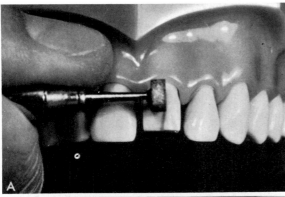

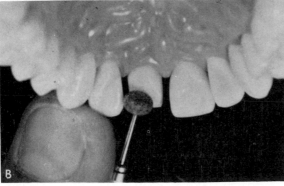

FIGURE 3–9. *A*, Reducing labial one-half at a time, using same stone that cut incisal.

B, Round-edge stone for lingual.

the choice on the concave surface is restricted to a small wheel stone with a round edge, or to a round stone, if the preparation is to be smooth and have a uniform depth.

Before any cutting is done on an occluding concave surface, the occlusion should be checked so that points of contact and excursive paths may be diagrammed. It will be beneficial if these areas are cut to a greater depth than the parts of the surface that never make contact. It is suggested, as it should be in the reduction of all surfaces, that the concave lingual be prepared one-half at a time so that equalized reduction and contour may be more readily produced. In a tooth with deep pits or grooves in the cervical third, either a fissure or a round bur should be used to explore these areas for assurance that no caries has penetrated beyond the enamel fold.

Forming the Cervical Margin

The phases of reduction discussed previously can leave the tooth angular at the line angles, the occlusal margin, and along the labioincisal, and extremely uneven at the cervical margin. Corners must be rounded in order that the thickness measurements of the casting will be similar and the cervical finishing line may be adjusted to the configuration of the gingival crest. (See Figure 3-10.) The cervical margin must be given chisel-edge or chamfer form, rather than an indefinite feather edge, so that the extension of the preparation and margins of the preparation in the impression may be checked, and so that it is possible for patterns to be carved on the die with exactness and castings finished precisely.

This is a critical aspect of the preparation. One of the primary points of axial reduction, necessitating concentration, is to achieve a prepared form that will make the cervical margin of the preparation the largest diameter of the prepared portion of the clinical crown, without undercuts and without the tooth being too tapered for maximal retention.

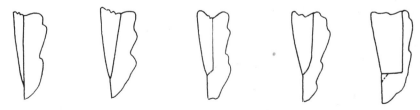

FIGURE 3-10. *Types of finishing lines on cervical margins.*

Left to right: The feather edge—to be avoided since it is indefinite and makes difficult exactness in carving patterns or finishing castings; the chisel edge—satisfactory and produced very often in lingual and proximal reduction; the bevel—used where shallow caries has made it necessary to cut deeper; the chamfer—the ideal finishing line to be developed when routine preparation does not produce a chisel edge; the shoulder—for areas to be veneered and for jacket crowns. (The shoulder can be beveled. Circumferential shoulders require excessive cutting of tooth structure.)

The axial line angles may be rounded and reduced with burs, diamond stones, or sandpaper disks. Sandpaper disks usually may be used with the straight handpiece, while burs and stones should be used with the contra-angle.

Rounding the corners and establishing the finishing line on the proximals should be completed with a round-end tapered stone in the contra-angle handpiece, one small enough in diameter to enter the space between the prepared tooth and the approximating tooth, and long enough to reach the cervical boundary of the preparation and still extend occlusally beyond the tooth. The cervical finishing line on the buccal and lingual surfaces may be formed with a cylindrical stone having a round tip or by one of the self-limiting diamonds or carbides.

Forming Shoulders

A shoulder preparation facilitates neither the taking of an impression nor the fitting and seating of a casting and sealing the tooth or polishing a seated restoration. The only aim of such extensive reduction should be to guarantee correct depth in the preparation to allow substantial thickness of porcelain or resin when constructing veneered and jacket crowns. Here the tooth structure incisally or occlusally to the shoulder must be reduced an extra amount pulpally, at least equal to the width of the shoulder. When cutting a shoulder, the handpiece must not be angled to cause an undercut at the cervical (Figs. 3-11 and 3-12).

Before a preparation is started, it is well to consider the material that will be used in the restoration, to note its requirements for strength and esthetic fulfillment, to study the radiograph for pulp size, and to calculate the width that will be needed in the shoulder and determine whether it can be secured under the existing conditions.

Customarily shoulders are outlined grossly with high-speed cutting, given definitive form with lesser speeds, and then honed and smoothed with hand instruments.

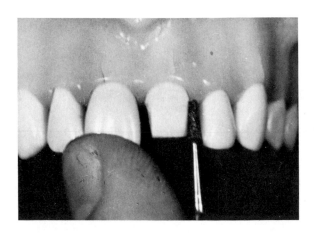

FIGURE 3-11. Rounding corners prior to taking tube impression and cutting shoulder.

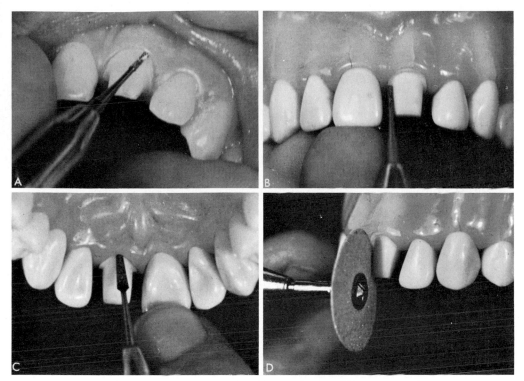

FIGURE 3–12. Cutting shoulder and smoothing preparation.

Shoulders may be formed with several types of stones or burs. At conventional speeds they may be cut on anterior teeth with a straight handpiece using small fissure burs or cylindrical stones. Wheel diamond stones, coated only on the edge and with smooth surfaces rotating against the tooth, may be used also. Shoulders invariably must be smoothed with hand instruments.

Posterior shoulders can be cut in the same way, but the contra-angle handpiece will be more convenient, although a little more difficult to manipulate.

Making Grooves

Grooves are used in preparations to increase resistance to displacement lingually, buccally, incisally, or occlusally, to add to the bulk of metal in the casting in such a way that it will have form to give it rigidity, and to add auxiliary paralleled surfaces for frictional retention. Axial grooves must be parallel to the path of insertion and to each other. They must have form, length, and depth that will give maximal retention, but at the same time enable the casting to seat without interference.

Grooves in anterior teeth may be made with tapered or straight fissure burs, then shaped labially or buccally with chisels, sandpaper disks, or files,

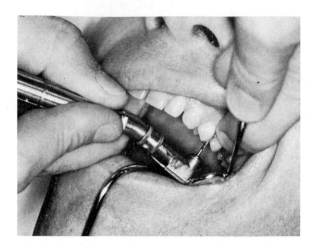

FIGURE 3–13. Support on incisors is obtained from third finger after second finger is placed at lingual of incisors for more versatile movement of stone or bur.

and lingually with smaller burs, stones, or files. They should terminate cervically in a flat, beveled, or chamfered seat. A groove running mesiodistally along the incisal edge of a partial veneer preparation in maxillary teeth must be cut so that the labial wall will be of *enamel and dentin* and about twice as wide as the lingual wall. The incisal treatment is different for mandibular anterior teeth.

Incisal grooves provide space for metal that may wear or be reduced to simulate wear, give extra protection to the labial enamel, connect the proximal struts, and stiffen the castings. They may be cut with inverted cone burs or stones and should be constant in width from one proximal surface to the other.

Auxiliary grooves in posterior teeth can be made with tapered or straight fissure burs or stones; they must be parallel to the path of insertion and end short of the cervical finishing line in an unbeveled, flat seat. (See Figure 3-13.) Such grooves, as a rule two or three in number, are of necessity short.

Making Ledges

Ledges, or steps, are cut to support castings under incising pressure, to create surfaces for pinholes, and to give irregularity and strength to thin castings. On the lingual surfaces of anterior teeth they should be approximately at right angles to the long axis of the tooth or path of insertion mesiodistally, rather than parallel to the incisal edge. The axial wall of a step should be parallel to the path of insertion or diverge labially from 2 to 5 degrees from the path. The ledge should be of a width commensurate to performing the services expected.

Ledges may be cut with cylindrical stones or fissure burs. A straight handpiece with few exceptions will have advantage in control and position.

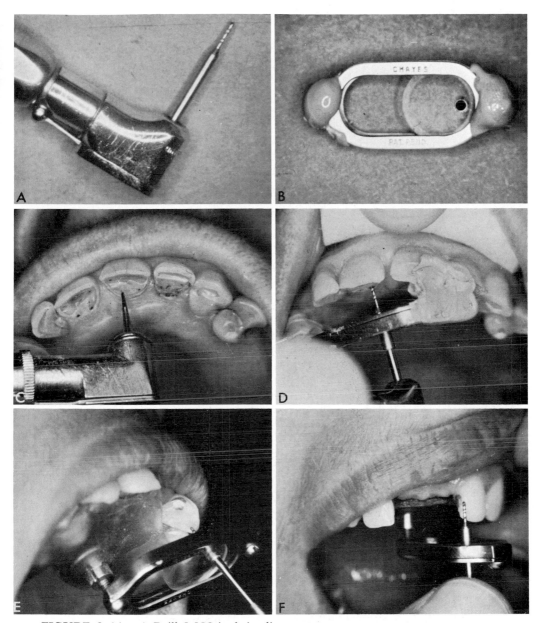

FIGURE 3-14. *A*, Drill 0.023 inch in diameter.

B, Loma Linda Parallelometer with modeling compound, ready to be attached to teeth for support. Disk in center, holding guiding sleeve, rotates and moves back and forth inside frame. A very effective instrument.

C, Countersinking points of entry for pinholes so that drill will not bounce, and to make the use of Parallelometer easier.

D, Drilling pinholes; lingual path of insertion.

E, Parallelometer attached to baseplate. Holes being drilled for incisal path of insertion.

F, Using Parallelometer and drill to make groove parallel to lingual pinholes. Equally effective in partial veneer preparations.

Making Pinholes

A pinhole is made to accommodate a pin that may make the third leg of a tripod to resist lingual displacement, lifting, torque, or rotation around the long axis. It may be a part of any abutment preparation. The walls of a pinhole are effective as "snubbing" surfaces; also they increase the area of frictional retention.

A pinhole must be parallel to the path of insertion (Fig. 3–14), and if all the retention for the casting accrues from the accumulated pinholes, its depth, and occasionally its diameter, must be increased. If it is being used in conjunction with grooves, the diameter should be large (the size of a No. 702 bur, if circumstances will permit), and from 1.0 to 2.0 mm. in depth. A pinhole for a cast pin may be made with either a tapered fissure bur or a drill with parallel sides, but a No. $1/2$ or 1 round bur will be suitable for a 24-gauge or 22-gauge wrought wire pin.[12, 13]

Drills for making holes for smaller and more numerous pins have parallel sides. A popular size is 0.023 inch in diameter, but they may be procured in larger diameters, such as 0.028 or 0.030 inch.

CONCEPTS OF INSTRUMENTATION SURVEYED

Many handpieces and contrivances have been designed to power rotating cutting instruments, and each lends itself to a given technique. When skill has been acquired, the equipment to be employed should be a personal matter. The instruments to be used for each abutment preparation, for shaping facings, and for polishing metal will be named and illustrated in the sections devoted to such operations (Figs. 3–15 and 3–16).

A survey conducted to ascertain the instrumentation for use for full crown, veneered crown, and partial veneer crown preparations showed a wide choice in instruments being used and considerable latitude in the sequence of their use. Predominating was a combination of conventional and accelerated speeds with both standard and very new rotating cutting instruments.

Included among the questions were requests for the following:

(1) sequence, name, and number of instruments used;

(2) accomplishment with each instrument; and

(3) speed at which each instrument was used.

Five of the returned questionnaires, depicting the stated instrumentation used in the offices of these operators, who are in full-time practice on the east coast, in the midwest, and in the far west regions of the United States, covered almost every routine and contingency.

Tables will be included in the chapters on The Full Veneer Gold Crown, The Partial Veneer Crown, and The Veneered Gold Crown. These techniques have been evolved by erudite and thinking practitioners who are con-

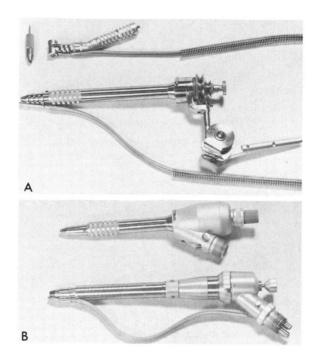

FIGURE 3-15. *A,* Densco belt-driven straight handpiece with ball bearings for high speed use. Contra-angle handpiece for friction grip instruments and wrench for instrument insertion and removal. Both handpieces may be used with spray attachments.

B, Top: Densco AFB slow speed air handpiece. Bottom: Midwest Tru-Torc slow speed air handpiece with spray attachment. (Midwest American, Melrose Park, Ill.)

vinced that everything must be done to safeguard living tissue and the comfort of the patient during the entire period of construction, delivery, and postcementation.

Each of these techniques has been used by the authors or their associates with end results almost identical to those of the dentists who developed them. It is not believed that they are always appropriate for use by the undergraduate student except in the final phases of instruction. This is particularly true if ultra speeds have not been used in the preclinical technique courses.

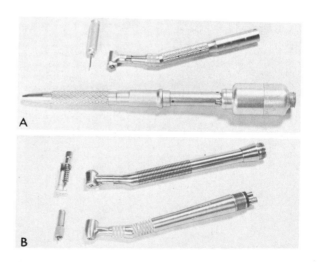

FIGURE 3-16. *A,* Kerr Electro-Torque slow speed electric handpiece, friction grip contra-angle handpiece, and bur removal instrument.

B, Top: Star Futura air rotor handpiece and chuck wrench. (Star Dental Mfg. Co., Inc., Philadelphia, Pa.) Bottom: Midwest Quiet-Air air rotor handpiece and chuck wrench.

FUNDAMENTALS OF RETENTION

The fundamentals of retentive form for a prepared abutment tooth include (1) walls within 5 to 7 degrees of parallel, and grooves or pinholes to resist displacement (except along the path of insertion) and to assure friction or binding between the casting and the tooth; (2) circumferential irregularity to forestall rotation around the long axis of the crown; and (3) reduction to admit a bulk of metal capable of withstanding deformation.

In short teeth, angulation at the occlusoaxial angles, as opposed to "rounding of corners," is indispensable. A factor not associated with preparation, but one that must be taken into account, is the height of the supporting structure of the abutments in case their long axes are not parallel. The less propitious the crown-root ratio, the more the abutment is prone to movement.[14, 15]

Grooves and pinholes, used to advance mechanical retention, must have both length and depth. Grooves should diverge cervically from the line of seating, and pinholes, if tapered, will ease insertion and withdrawal.

TOOTH FORM AND ITS INFLUENCE ON THE ABUTMENT PREPARATION

Tooth form often influences the selection of retainer and method of stabilization. For instance, on a short clinical crown there will not be competent frictional retention with a standard preparation; it must be supplemented by extra grooves and pinholes. A tooth with a long crown may be prepared with minimal grooving unless it is so positioned that approximate paralleling of the surfaces is impossible. A tooth that is excessively pyramidal or ovoid must be studied carefully so that the pulp will not be traumatized by reduction.[16] One that is small or frail, or one with a large pulp, many times requires extracoronal retention.

Other useful cutting instruments are illustrated in Figures 3–17, 3–18, 3–19, 3–20, 3–21, and 3–22.

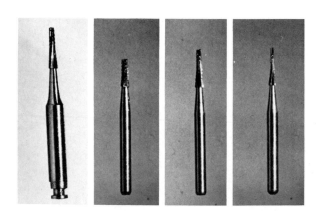

FIGURE 3–17. Densco carbide burs, 700L, 701, 701L, 699L.

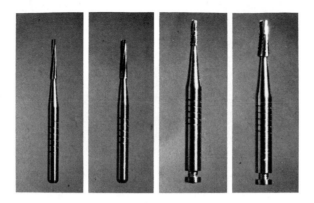

FIGURE 3-18. Premier "Ela" carbide burs. 70L, 71L, 701, 702. (Premier Dental Products Company, Philadelphia, Pa.)

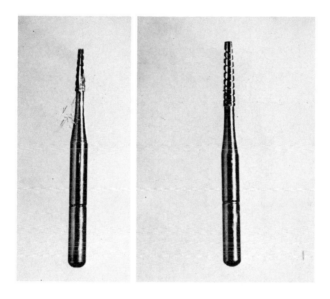

FIGURE 3-19. R&R carbide burs. 699, 700L. (The Ramsom & Randolph Co., Toledo, Ohio.)

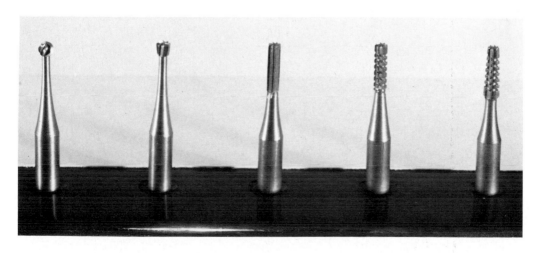

FIGURE 3-20. R&R carbide burs. 4, 37, 59, 558, 702.

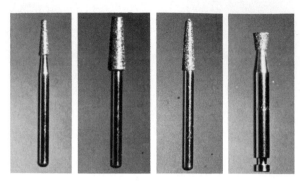

FIGURE 3-21.   Densco diamond stones. ½D, 2D, 1D-TF, 1K.

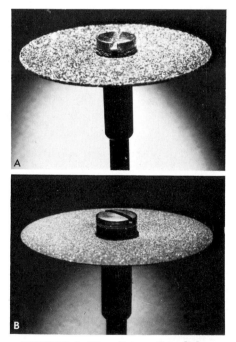

FIGURE 3-22.   *Separating disks.*

A, Carborundum disk. Useful in preparing teeth and cutting metal.

B, Steel disk. Used when proximal cuts must be very thin and extension labially held to minimum.

REFERENCES

1. Peyton, F. W.: Effectiveness of water coolants with rotary cutting instruments. J.A.D.A., 56:664, May 1958.
2. Weiss, M. C., Massler, M., and Spence, J. M.: Operative effects on adult dental pulp. D. Progress, 4:10, 1963.
3. Stanley, H., and Swerdlow, H.: Biological effects of various cutting methods in cavity preparations: The part pressure plays in pulpal response. J.A.D.A., 61:450, Oct. 1960.
4. Davila Alonso, H. M., Van Huysen, G., and Johnston, J. F.: Changes in pulp and periodontal tissues of teeth subjected to crown prosthesis. J. Pros. Den., 10:350, March-April 1960.
5. Kasloff, Z.: Cracks in tooth structure associated with rotary cutting instruments. J. D. Res., 40:769, July-Aug. 1961 (Abstract).
6. Kasloff, Z.: Continuing study of cracks in teeth associated with various rotary cutting instruments. J. Canad. D. A., 28:244, April 1962.
7. Kasloff, Z., Swartz, M. L., and Phillips, R. W.: In vitro method for demonstrating the effects of various cutting instruments on tooth structure. J. Pros. Den., 12:1166, Nov.-Dec. 1962.
8. Mosteller, J. H.: The prevention of postoperative thermal sensitivity. D. Clin. N. Amer., Nov. 1963, p. 881.
9. Wilson, H. D.: Hypersensitivity in tooth preparations. D. Survey, 36:36, Jan. 1960.
10. Kilpatrick, H. C.: Ultra-speed and auxiliary equipment in fixed partial denture construction. J. Pros. Den., 10:574, May-June 1960.
11. Kilpatrick, H. C.: Recent trends in the management of pain in dentistry—the role of ultra-speed and auxiliary equipment. J. D. Med., 18:113, April 1963.
12. Moffa, J. P., and Phillips, R. W.: Retentive properties of parallel pin restorations. J. Pros. Den., 17:4, April 1967, p. 387.
13. Moffa, J. P.: Razzano, M. R., and Doyle, M. G.: Pins—a comparison of their retentive properties. J.A.D.A., 78:3, March 1969, p. 529.
14. Pruden, K. C.: Abutments and attachments in fixed partial dentures. J. Pros. Den., 7:502, July 1957.
15. Adams, J. D.: Planning posterior bridges. J.A.D.A., 53:647, Dec. 1956.
16. Brotman, I. N.: The roentgenogram, as an aid in veneer crown preparation. J. Pros. Den., 4:349, May 1954.

Leff, A.: Evaluation of high-speed in full coverage preparations. J. Pros. Den., 10:314, March–April 1960.
Wheeler, R. C.: The implications of full coverage restorative procedures. J. Pros. Den., 5:848, Nov. 1955.

chapter 4

THE FULL VENEER
GOLD CROWN

The full veneer gold crown (see Fig. 1–1C and D) may be used as a single-unit restoration or as a retainer for a bridge. A retainer has been defined as the restoration that rebuilds the prepared abutment tooth and attaches the bridge to the abutment. In fixed partial denture construction the abutment must be reduced to accommodate the metal structure. This should be accomplished in such a way that the restored tooth will not be endangered later by disintegration of the pulp,[1] fracture, or caries. Both the single-unit restoration and the retainer must be biologically and esthetically acceptable. Function, comfort, and improvement or maintenance of the environment must be introduced or continued with the seating of all restorations.

INDICATIONS

The full veneer gold crown may be placed on any tooth that cannot be returned by other means to an effective working capacity and contour. It should be used as a bridge retainer[2, 3, 4] when the caries index, torque, leverage, or load contraindicates the partial veneer crown, the pinledge, or the inlay. In full mouth reconstruction, on teeth that must be splinted or that are to receive clasps or precision attachments for the support and retention of partial dentures, it can be the restoration of choice because of its strength, long life, resistance to displacement, protection against caries, and adaptability to changes in form and occlusion. When appearance is an issue, the gold crown with a veneer of porcelain or resin is indicated. It can be overcontoured to provide maximal masticating efficiency, or undercontoured to curtail stress or to distribute it more evenly over a prosthesis. The preparation, construction, and cementation, even if exacting, are not complicated procedures.[4, 5, 6, 7, 8]

CONTRAINDICATIONS

If the occlusion is adequate, the gold crown is contraindicated in mouths in which the caries index is low or in which the prosthesis need have less than maximal retention. These conditions make it feasible to use less extensive preparations and to save the labial or buccal enamel. The full veneer gold crown has some minor disadvantages, such as display of metal, the impossibility of testing vitality,[4] the call for added prophylactic measures to forestall tarnish or corrosion of the metal, and the adverse effect it sometimes has on tissue, even when contoured correctly and extended cautiously into the gingival crevice.

PREPARATION OF NONCARIOUS TEETH

The preparation for a full veneer gold crown should cause no harm to the pulp when it is properly done, but it can be a dangerous procedure if performed by a thoughtless or unconcerned operator. Rapid preparation may have grave consequences unless the tooth is lubricated and its temperature controlled. Gingival tissue can be insulted beyond the point of repair, not only during preparation and at the time of its displacement for taking impressions, but also under poorly designed and carelessly made temporary coverage.

If the crown to be constructed will serve as a bridge retainer, the diagnostic casts should be surveyed with the analyzing rod so that a path of insertion, compatible with all the abutment teeth, can be pictured. A full veneer crown preparation can deviate from the ideal more than other types and still retain the casting. Often, because of long-axis variables of the abutments, it will have walls that converge grossly.

The operator must be adroit when making this preparation so that construction and seating will not be jeopardized by an undercut, which may be formed in one of three ways. When the walls converge cervically toward the path of insertion, the retainer cannot be seated. If the long axis of the preparation diverges from the path of insertion, causing the cervical on the mesial or distal of the preparation to be in an undercut area, the fabricated prosthesis will not go into place even though the proximal walls are parallel or converge occlusally. A third type of undercut could be a depression in a wall surface of the preparation.

A prescribed sequence of steps and a predetermined goal for each step are beneficial in any operation. One method for the full veneer gold crown preparation will be presented at this time. Other plans, utilizing accelerated and slower speeds, are equally productive[3, 6, 7, 8] and will be outlined.

PREPARATION OF A MANDIBULAR MOLAR USING BOTH ULTRA HIGH AND SLOWER CUTTING SPEEDS

Only two rotary instruments are necessary in the preparation of any molar tooth for a full veneer crown, namely, the 169L or 699L carbide tapered fissure bur with high speed, and the 1D-T diamond stone for slow speed. The 1/4D-L diamond may be used in the interproximal space if it is narrow[9] (Fig. 4-1). (See also Figures 3-17 to 3-22.)

Following are the steps in the mandibular molar full veneer crown preparation.[9] With only minor variations this concept is applicable to all posterior teeth.

Proximal Reduction

If the tooth to be prepared is in contact, a steel matrix should be fitted around the adjacent tooth (Fig. 4–2*B*), which will help in avoiding abrasive contact with the approximating tooth. The proximal reductions should be started from the buccal or lingual, with the bur (169L)* within the circumference of the tooth to be prepared (Fig. 4-3*A* and *C*) and made parallel to the path of insertion. The tip of the bur should be at the level of the finishing line or at the crest of the interdental papilla, whichever is more occlusal. The bur should be "walked" slowly into and through the contact area by taking three "steps" forward and two backward. Cutting through the contact will allow further instrumentation.

---

*The 699L and 700L R&R and Densco, or 70L and 71L Premier, carbide burs are equally effective.

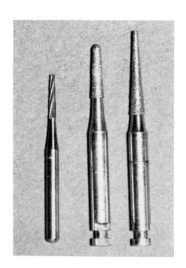

FIGURE 4-1. Cutting instruments for full veneer crown preparation on posterior tooth: 169L-FG carbide bur (S.S.W.); 1D-T latch tapered diamond stone (Densco); 1/4D-L latch tapered diamond stone (Densco).
Other makes and combinations are similarly good.

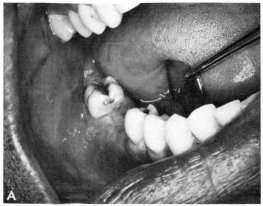
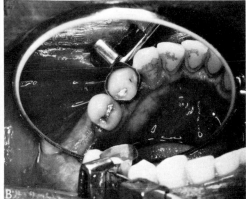
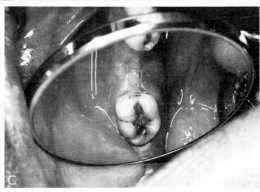

FIGURE 4-2. *A*, Right mandibular molar to be prepared for full veneer gold crown retainer.

B, Steel matrix band fitted around first bicuspid to protect it from possible mutilation when cutting mesioproximal of second bicuspid. Molar and bicuspid were prepared simultaneously, but procedures are shown separately.

C, Occlusal view of molar.

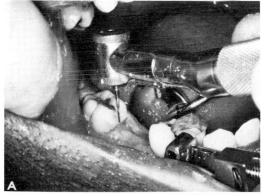
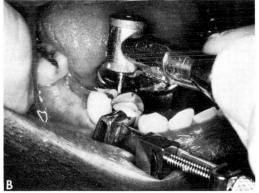
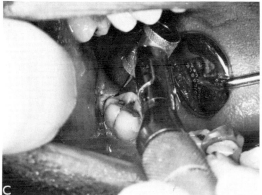

FIGURE 4-3. *A*, Making first proximal reduction on mesial of molar.

B, Making mesial proximal cut on bicuspid.

C, Starting distal proximal cut on molar.

Buccal and Lingual Reductions

The reductions should be made in two distinct planes occlusocervically and following tooth contour mesiodistally. It is helpful to groove the buccal and lingual surfaces in two planes (Fig. 4–4*A*, *B*, *C*, and *D*) before proceeding to reduce the surfaces. The occlusal one-third should be cut at about a 45-degree angle to the long axis of the tooth (Fig. 4–5*A*, *B*, and *C*), and the cervical two-thirds should be cut parallel to the path of insertion, eliminating undercuts (Fig. 4–5*D* and *E*). Mesiodistally the surfaces should be reduced one-half at a time, following tooth contour (Fig. 4–6*A* and *B*). This will show the amount of reduction being made and aid in making a preparation that will require a casting of uniform thickness. The buccal and lingual surface cutting is completed (Fig. 4-6*C*).

Occlusal Reduction

The central fossa, grooves, and marginal ridges frequently are areas where preparations are shallow and castings would be too thin. To obviate

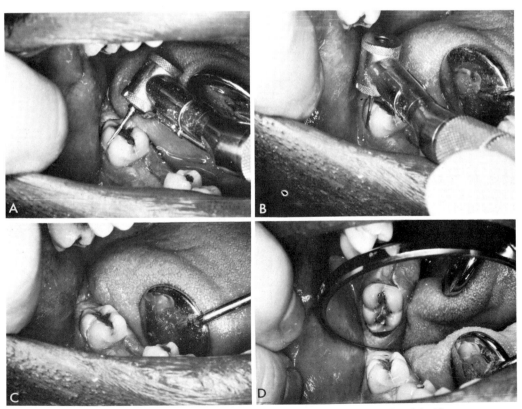

FIGURE 4-4.   *A*, Starting groove in buccal groove, occlusal half.
B, Cutting groove, buccal groove, cervical half.
C and *D*, Buccal and lingual grooves.

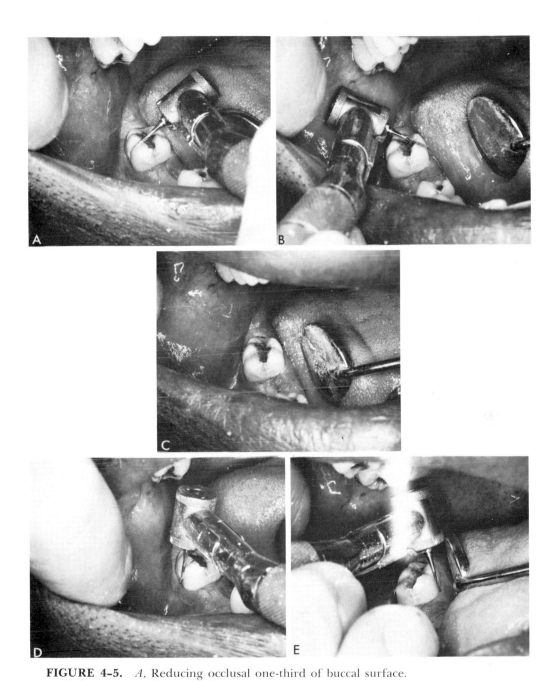

FIGURE 4–5. *A*, Reducing occlusal one-third of buccal surface.
B, Reducing occlusal one-third of lingual surface.
C, Only one-half of buccal and lingual surfaces prepared to check depth of cutting.
D and *E*, Preparing one-half of cervical two-thirds of buccal and lingual surfaces.

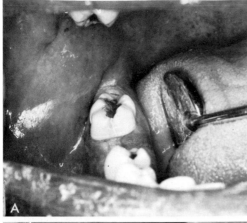
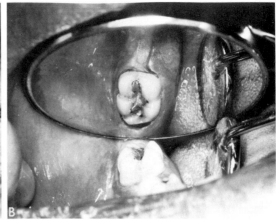
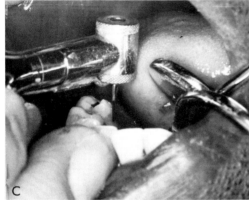

FIGURE 4–6. *A* and *B*, Mesial and occlusal views of reduction of first half of buccal and lingual surfaces.

C, Completing cutting on lingual surface.

this the major occlusal grooves and marginal ridges should be cut to a depth of 1.0 to 1.25 mm. to guide the operator in the occlusal reduction (Fig. 4–7*A* and *C*), and then the occlusal reduction should proceed, following the major planes (Figs. 4–7*B* and *D* and 4–8).

Proximal Line Angles

The proximal line angles should be rounded to join the proximal walls with the buccal and lingual walls and to develop a better (more even) contour for the cervical margin (Fig. 4–9). (See also Figure 3–3*J, K,* and *L*.)

From this point all instrumentation should be at slow speed using the 1D-TL diamond. The finishing line is made at its most protected or adaptable location (within the gingival crevice or at the cementoenamel line); the occlusal and proximal line angles are rounded and the preparation is smoothed. (See Figures 3–3*H* and *I,* 4–6*B,* 4–9*B,* and 4–10*B.*)

There is considerable controversy as to where the cervical margin of a full veneer crown should be placed. The authors believe and teach that usually the preparation should be extended approximately 0.5 mm. into the

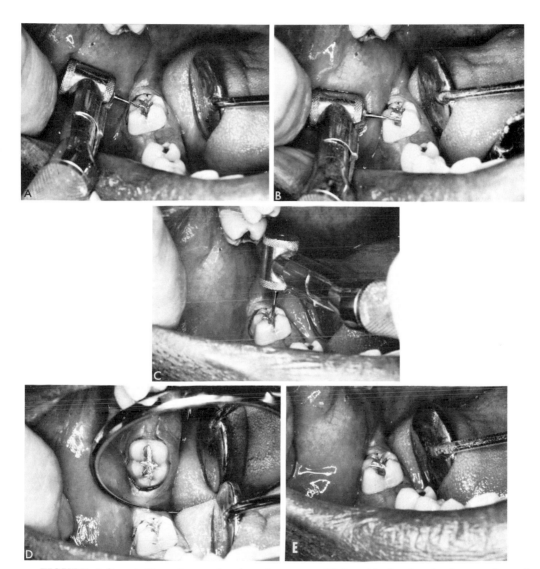

FIGURE 4-7. *A*, Grooving occlusal surface to establish guide for depth of cut on buccal half.

B, Reducing buccal half.

C, Establishing depth in occlusal groove pattern.

D and *E*, Occlusal reduced.

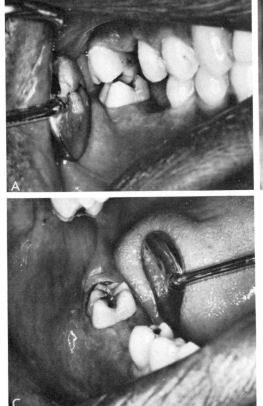

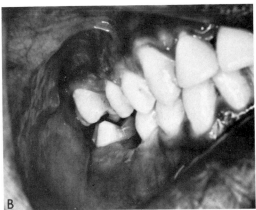

FIGURE 4-8. *A,* Checking occlusal reduction in closure. Deficient on lingual half.

B, Deficiency corrected.

C, Tooth ready for finishing and placing of cervical finishing line.

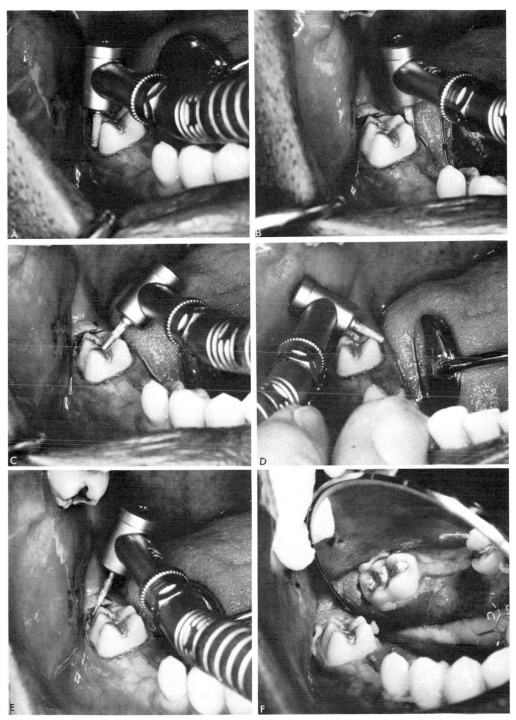

FIGURE 4–9. *A* and *B*, Smoothing axial surfaces and making chamfered cervical margin.

C, *D*, and *E*, Rounding and softening occlusal angles.

F, Finished preparation. All reductions except mesial and distal follow natural tooth contours. Mesial and distal prepared surfaces should be parallel to path of seating.

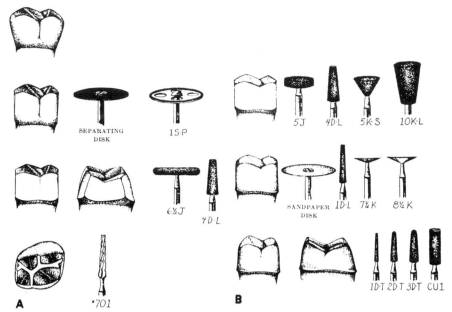

FIGURE 4–10.   *Preparation on a molar with cutting instruments suitable for each step. (Numbered stones are Densco diamonds.)*

A, Top to bottom: Uncut tooth; proximal slices; facial and lingual reduction; first phase of occlusal reduction.

B, Top to bottom: Occlusal reduction; rounded angles; chamfered finishing line and softened occlusal angles.

gingival crevice (see Fig. 3–3L). If there is gingival recession and the neck of the tooth is quite constricted, the cervical margin should parallel the cementoenamel line, but remain in enamel.

OTHER ROUTINES FOR PREPARATIONS AT ACCELERATED SPEEDS

There are many routines for preparing teeth for full veneer gold crowns that include accelerated speeds. Some of these, occasionally used by the authors, will be listed in table form.

PREPARATION OF A MANDIBULAR MOLAR USING SLOWER SPEEDS

There are still reasons for familiarity with the older so-called standard preparation. The routine is relevant to all techniques and the concepts by which this approach evolved remain valid.[6, 7, 8]

POSTERIOR TEETH

Table 4-1

INSTRUMENT	TO BE ACCOMPLISHED	R.P.M.
71L Premier "Ela" carbide	Complete axial and occlusal reduction. Location and contour of cervical margin.	150,000
70L Premier "Ela" carbide	(When there is an approximating tooth, a 70L premier "Ela" carbide is used to cut from either buccal or lingual to break the contact and simultaneously reduce the proximal surface.)	150,000
4D Densco diamond	Irregularities smoothed and sharp angles rounded.	8,000 to 10,000
Note: Round burs, steel fissure burs, spoon excavators, hatchets, chisels	Removal of caries, if present. Cement or amalgam smoothed if used to build tooth to prepared form.	Slow speeds

Table 4-2

INSTRUMENT	TO BE ACCOMPLISHED	R.P.M.
701L R&R carbide	Gross buccal, lingual, and occlusal reduction.	150,000
700L R&R carbide	Proximal surface reduction.	150,000
Safe-side disk (any brand)	Proximal surface reduction (when a 700L carbide cannot be used).	6,000
1D-T Densco diamond	Location and contour of cervical margin.	150,000
Sandpaper disks (any brand)	Irregularities smoothed and sharp angles rounded.	Slow speeds

Table 4-3

INSTRUMENT	TO BE ACCOMPLISHED	R.P.M.
2D Densco diamond	Complete axial reduction.	200,000 (approx.)
3/4D Densco diamond	(When there is an approximating tooth, a 3/4D Densco diamond is used to cut from either buccal or lingual to break the contact and simultaneously reduce the proximal surface.)	200,000
123 SSW diamond	Occlusal reduction.	200,000
116 SSW diamond	Location and contour of cervical margin.	200,000
1D-T Densco diamond (worn) or 44 SSW carborundum stone	Irregularities smoothed.	200,000 or 3,000

Table 4–4

INSTRUMENT	TO BE ACCOMPLISHED	R.P.M.
701 R&R carbide	Buccal, lingual, and occlusal reduction.	150,000
700 or 699 R&R carbide	Proximal surface reduction.	150,000
1D-T or 1D-C Densco diamond	Peripheral finish and location and contour of cervical margin.	150,000

Mesial and Distal Surfaces

Step 1 is the reduction of the mesial and distal surfaces. This can be done in a normal situation with diamond or carborundum disks in the straight handpiece. After the demands of the path of insertion have been weighed, these cuts will be started on or just inside the marginal ridges on the occlusal surface (Fig. 4–10A) and should extend in a direct line to the gingival crest without producing convexities or concavities in the walls. Although the preparation usually narrows about 5 degrees occlusally along the path of insertion, the long-axis inclination may suggest more convergence.

Facial and Lingual Surfaces

Step 2 is a reduction of the facial and lingual surfaces (Fig. 4–10A). On the buccal surface of both upper and lower teeth and on the lingual of uppers in accurate alignment, it should follow the surface convexities and on most teeth should be made 1.0 mm. deep. The preparation on the lingual surface of mandibular teeth must be congruous with the path of insertion. Buccal and lingual reductions continue to the gingival line, to the cervical line, or (preferably) cervically to Class V caries or restorations. Tooth position and type may hinder the cervical finishing line on the lingual surface of some lower posterior teeth from going into the gingival crevice.

Table 4–5

INSTRUMENT	TO BE ACCOMPLISHED	R.P.M.
701 or 701L Densco carbide	Complete axial and occlusal reduction. Location and preparation of cervical shoulder.	150,000 to 200,000
1D Densco diamond	Irregularities smoothed and shoulder finished.	150,000 to 200,000
Sandpaper disks (any brand)	Irregularities smoothed and sharp angles rounded.	500 to 1,000

Occlusal Surface

Steps 3 and 4: The first phase of occlusal reduction is done in the occlusal grooves with a No. 700 or 701 bur and is made 1.0 mm. deep (Fig. 4-10*A*). If caries has penetrated the enamel fold, it must be removed. The prepared grooves will regulate the depth of subsequent cutting on the occlusal surface and also will ensure room for sufficient metal in the central area (Fig. 4–10*B*). If the over-all reduction is 1.0 mm. deep and if it follows the contour of the cusp planes (Fig. 4-11), the casting will have greater security against movement because there will be broad, semiflat surfaces to oppose forces from many directions.

When the crowned tooth will support a clasp, the marginal ridge under the occlusal rest must be cut down enough to afford depth in the metal for the occlusal rest seat. The area of extra reduction should go about 1.4 mm. in all directions beyond the periphery of the rest seat (Fig. 4-12).

Cervical Margin

In step 5, the line angles are rounded until all angulation is removed. The four "corner triangular" cervical areas must be obliterated so that the gingival finishing line (Fig. 4–10*B*) is smoothly continuous and closely follows the configuration of the gingival crest. (See Figure 3–3*H*, *I*, *J*, *K*, and *L*.) This can be done with a coarse sandpaper disk or a long tapered diamond stone. With the special "push" and "pull" stones that have been designed for this step, there may be a tendency to overreduce the angles and thus make the preparation too conical.

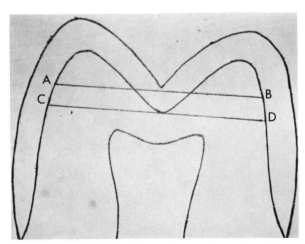

FIGURE 4–11. Proper reduction of buccal and lingual surfaces of a posterior tooth results in relatively parallel surfaces in the cervical one-third. When a preparation follows the anatomical form of the tooth on the occlusal, there will be greater length than can be obtained by making the surface flat. Reduction along line AB would make the preparation unnecessarily short around the periphery and too shallow in the central groove area. If the tooth were reduced to the line CD, the central groove and fossa would be correct in depth, but the over-all preparation would be even shorter and would encroach upon the pulp.

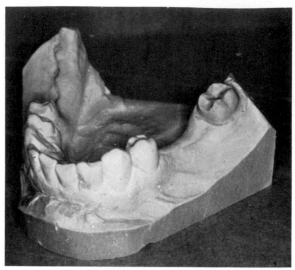

FIGURE 4–12.   Change in occlusal preparation to make space for rest seat.

A chamfer must be developed when a natural chisel-edge does not occur at the cervical finishing line. This concave bevel should be about 0.4 mm. in width and from 0.5 to 1.0 mm. under the gingival margin. It is advantageous if the finishing line can be very close to the height of contour on both the buccal and lingual surfaces of upper posterior teeth and the buccal surface of lowers. However, tooth position and contour, the occlusocervical length of the clinical crown, gingival recession, or cervical caries may compel a relocation of the cervical margin. The chamfer may be made quickly on the buccal and lingual and at the line angles with a No. 2D-T or 3D diamond stone, while on the proximal surfaces a No. 1D-T diamond stone may be used.

PREPARING TEETH WITH LONG, MEDIUM, OR SHORT CROWNS

In the preparation of teeth with long crowns, there is an inclination to form cervical undercuts on the distal surfaces. If the handpiece and the disk are not moved cervically simultaneously, the cutting edge of the disk will move in an arc, causing an inward deviation from the path of insertion in the cervical area. This error seldom can be rectified without inordinate reduction of the tooth in the middle and occlusal thirds. The resultant thickness of metal in the crown may provoke sensitivity. The angle at the junction of the occlusal and axial walls should be rounded, since there is no compulsion to provide stability for the casting.

On crowns of medium length, cuts can be visualized and executed, and line angles rounded easily. Here also the occlusoaxial should be softened to facilitate taking impressions, fitting and investing patterns, and seating castings, and to make room for more metal in an area susceptible to wear.

The crown of the short tooth is often conical and the preparation will taper occlusally so much that little mechanical retention can be obtained. The occlusoaxial angles should be left sharp on such a tooth (Fig. 4-13). Grooves must be cut on the buccal or lingual surface, parallel with the opposite surface or path of insertion. Using a No. 701 or 702 bur, pinholes 1.5 mm. deep can be placed in the occlusal surface immediately under the cusp tips, or a well can be prepared using the occlusal grooves as a pattern. This should be not less than 1.0 mm. deep and may be made with a No. 558, 559, or 702 bur.

PREPARING TEETH WITH GINGIVAL RECESSION

When the cementoenamel junction is exposed, the size and form of the neck of the tooth and the predisposition to cervical caries will determine whether the preparation should be moved onto the cementum and into the gingival crevice. This is salutary unless the tooth must be cut so much that the pulp is injured.

PREPARATION OF CARIOUS TEETH

When cervical caries is present, the involved structure should be replaced by gold or amalgam (Fig. 4-14). The final preparation should go cervically beyond the margin of such a restoration, but if this is not feasible, because of the eminent dipping of the cervical outline, the margin may rest on the metal.

When a filled or mutilated tooth is to be prepared to receive a full veneer gold crown, the series of steps will differ in some respects from that employed in preparing a sound tooth. All amalgam, gold, cement, and carious tissue should be removed, and the walls and occlusal surface that remain should be prepared in the same way and in the same order as for the noncarious tooth. The tooth is then built to prepared form with a gold casting or amalgam.[8, 10, 11]

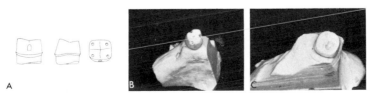

FIGURE 4-13. *Preparations on medium and short teeth.*
A, Occlusal pinholes and axial grooves.
B, Axial grooves.
C, Occlusal well used to increase retention and stability on short teeth.

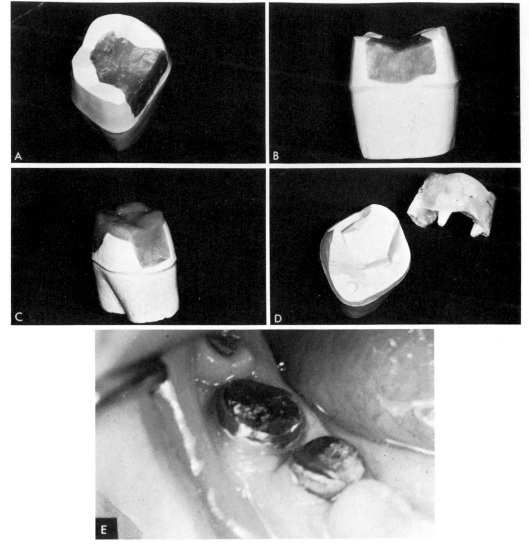

FIGURE 4-14.   *Preparations on carious teeth.*

A, Rebuilding tooth to prepared form with amalgam.

B, Preparation should extend, if possible, beyond junction of metal and tooth.

C, Rebuilding tooth to prepared form with gold casting.

D, Casting removed, showing two posts and proximal step.

E, Two teeth rebuilt to prepared form with castings. Remaining tooth structure was exposed by gingivectomy.

The Cast Core

If a casting is to be used, the margins of remaining walls are paralleled or undercuts are removed. Three, four, or five pinholes (1.5 or 2.0 mm. deep) are placed in the dentin with a tapered fissure bur or a drill. The pattern can be carved direct, using wax or plastic pins, or an indirect procedure may be used.

Every effort should be made to have the wax pattern free from distortion and the casting fit with the preciseness of an inlay. After it has been cemented, the cervical margin and all other details of the preparation should be perfected.

The Pin-retained Amalgam Core

Markley[10, 11] has devised a technique for reinforcing and retaining amalgam cores with threaded steel wire pins (Fig. 4–15), with results comparable to those of the cast core. By this means also, mutilated or extensively carious vital or pulpless teeth with good root structure can be built to prepared form for either single-unit restorations or bridge retainers. When caries has penetrated close to the pulp,[12] that area should be insulated against thermal shock with one of the calcium hydroxide-type base materials, a layer of cement, and routinely an application of Copalite cavity varnish.[13] Cement in bulk should be avoided.[14]

Drilling Pinholes.   Twist drills,* 0.027 or 0.024 inch in diameter, depending on the size of the tooth, are used in a contra-angle handpiece. The pinholes, carefully located (by viewing radiographs and by a knowledge of tooth anatomy) to avoid the pulp or the perforation of the outside root surface or bifurcation walls, are drilled from 2.0 to 4.0 mm. into the dentin. The holes need not be parallel; in fact, pins will be more retentive if they are not parallel. A speed of not more than 1000 r.p.m. is recommended, with a stream of air as a coolant. The drill should be removed from the hole repeatedly to clean out the debris (Fig. 4–16).

Preparing Pins.   Threaded stainless steel wire,** 0.025 to 0.022 inch in diameter, is used for the pins. The end of the wire is made square, the edge

---

*Star Dental Mfg. Co., Inc., Philadelphia, Pa.
**K and R Dental Products Co., Blue Island, Ill.

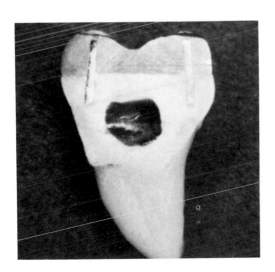

FIGURE 4–15.   Cross section of molar and two cemented steel pins. Two of eight pins that, through threading and irregular alignment, substantially support and retain alloy restoration.

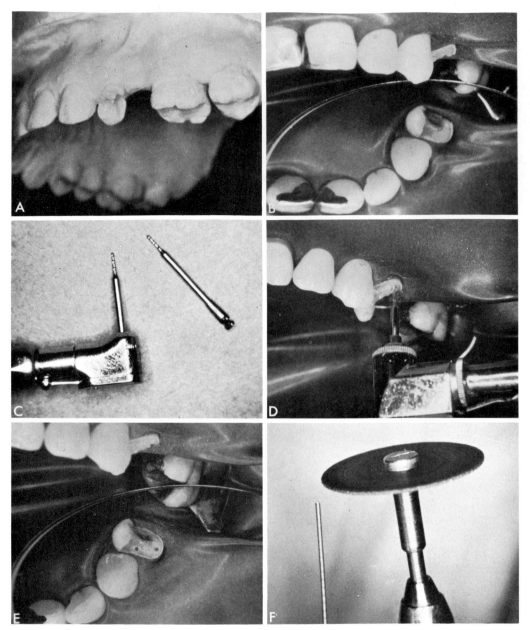

FIGURE 4–16. *A,* Fractured maxillary bicuspid to be built to prepared form for a veneered gold crown retainer.

   B, Tooth explored and caries removed.
   C, Twist drills 0.027 inch in diameter.
   D, Drilling holes using water and air as a lubricant. Heavy rubber dam in position.
   E, Tooth prepared for pins.
   F, Wire being squared on end. It was notched irregularly before being cut to length.

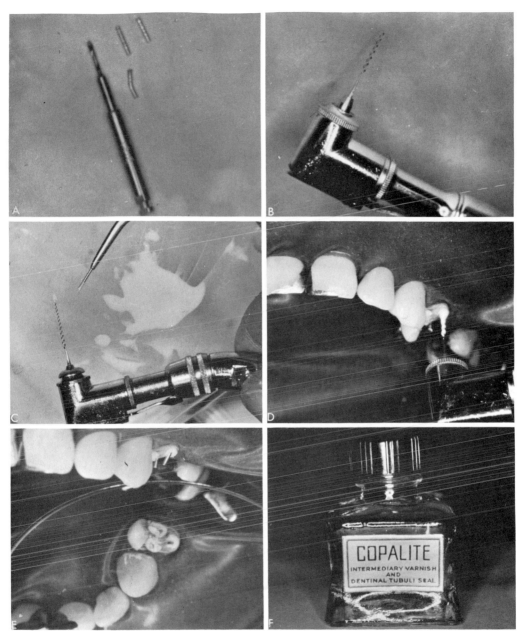

FIGURE 4-17. *A*, Drill, three cut pins. One is bent to make it conform to the peripheral outline of preparation. Pins protruding through the amalgam are not easily smoothed to surface of preparation.

B, Spiral for carrying cement into pinhole.

C, Spiral and pin, each carrying cement. Pin is held with grooved pliers.

D, Spinning cement into hole.

E, Pins cemented. Excess will be broken off.

F, Copalite varnish used on exposed dentin.

rounded, and the wire then is cut to correct length for the individual hole. When pins have been seated in all the holes (from 5 to 9), some must be bent to conform to the periphery of the prepared form anticipated. Cotton plier beaks may be grooved to promote handling.

Cementing Pins.   A shortened lentulo-spiral, for filling root canals with medicaments, should be used to carry cement into the pinholes (Fig. 4-17*B*). Mixing should be on a cold slab. One pin at a time is removed, and the cement is carried into the pinhole with the revolving spiral while an assistant coats the pin with cement. The pin, held by the grooved pliers, is repositioned in the hole. If air is trapped and the pin fails to seat, the process is repeated. Excess cement is removed after setting (Fig. 4-17*E*).

Threaded and gnarled pins (there are kits for seating them) may be substituted for the cemented smooth or threaded pins. Empirical data on their success are favorable (Fig. 4–18).

The Matrix.   A heavy rubber dam is placed on the tooth. The matrix may be a copper band or an adjusted steel band contoured to a snug fit around the cervical of the remaining tooth structure and competently supported by modeling compound (Fig. 4-19*B*).

Condensing the Amalgam.   Small condensers, 1.0 mm. or less in diameter, should be used to insert the amalgam. This phase must be done *thoroughly*, to eliminate any voids. Several mixes of amalgam will be required for bulk and consistency. After placing the alloy, the compound and matrix are removed (Fig. 4-19*C* and *D*).

Completing the Preparation.   The authors have found that final preparation of the tooth can be done with greater ease if the alloy is given time

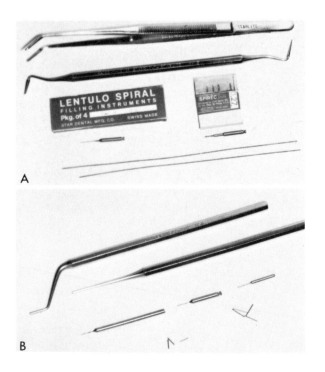

FIGURE 4–18. *Prepared kits for rebuilding teeth with pin-retained amalgam cores.*

A, Star pin kit. Top to bottom: Pin pliers; pin seating instrument and plugger; lentulo-spiral for carrying cement into pinholes; Spirec drills; threaded wire.

B, Unitek pin kit. (Unitek Corporation, Monrovia, Calif.) Top to bottom: Top two instruments used to tap pins into place. Three drills: straight handpiece, latch, and friction grip. Pins of various lengths.

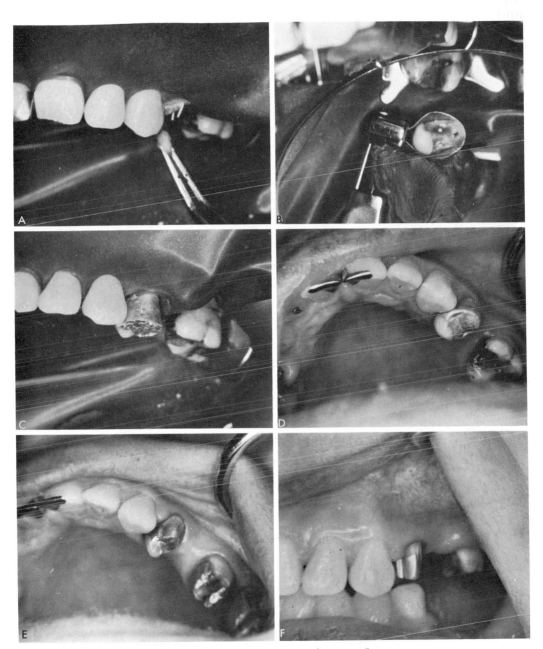

FIGURE 4–19. *A*, Applying Copalite to exposed cut surface.

B, Adapting band and supporting modeling compound. Steel band must be well stabilized.

C, Rebuilt tooth after matrix was removed.

D, Alloy trimmed.

E and *F*, Tooth prepared.

to set. Hardening may take place under any kind of temporary covering, which is positioned and trimmed to push away the gingival tissue so that there may be better access for establishing the cervical margin[15] and finishing the preparation with either diamonds, carbides, or disks (Fig. 4-19E and F). (See Figures 4-20 and 4-21.)

Smith[16] has designed a set of self-limiting diamond and carbide cutting instruments of excellent quality that make it possible to displace the gingival

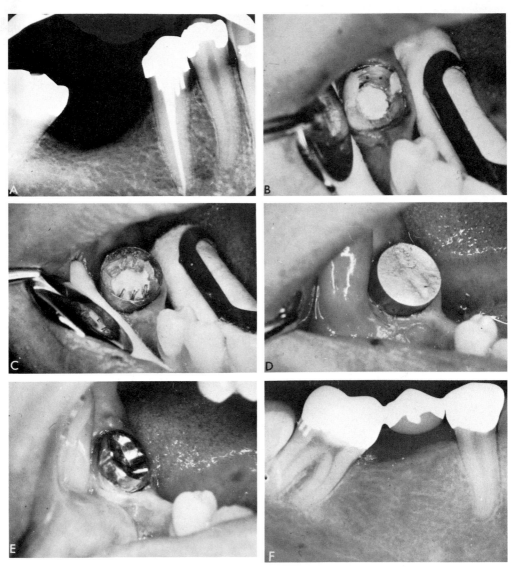

FIGURE 4-20. *A*, Radiograph of mandibular bicuspid showing pins.
B, Mandibular molar showing five pinholes.
C, Copper band fitted; rubber dam and modeling compound reinforcement were used.
D, Compound and dam removed. Band still in place.
E, Tooth prepared.
F, Radiograph of bridge.
(Illustrations *B, C, D, E,* and *F* through the courtesy of Dr. William Hohlt.)

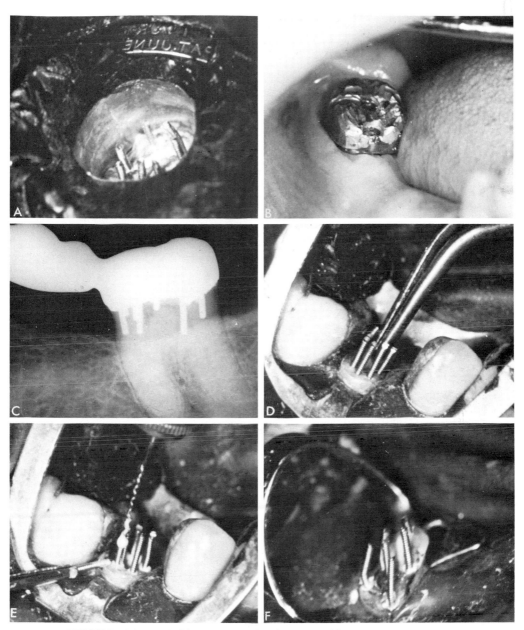

FIGURE 4-21. *A*, Pins cemented prior to packing.
B, Rebuilt tooth.
C, Radiograph of abutment.
D, Pins fitted prior to cementing.
E, Cementing pins.
F, Pins cemented and contoured to dimension of finished preparation.
(These illustrations through the courtesy of Drs. Markley and Going.)

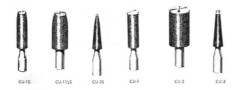

CU-1S CU-1½S CU-3S CU-1 CU-2 CU-3

FIGURE 4–22. Self-limiting diamond stones (Densco) designed by Dr. Gilbert Smith.

tissue and extend the full veneer gold crown preparation evenly into the gingival crevice. Stones are manufactured for either the chisel-edge or chamfer finishing line. (See CU series of Densco diamonds, Figure 4–22.)

Before the prepared teeth are covered, impressions for the working casts, a face-bow registration, and an occlusion registration may be taken, and cut surfaces should be coated with a cavity varnish. These are discussed in Chapter 9, The Working Cast.

TEMPORARY PROTECTION

A vital tooth that has been prepared for a full veneer gold crown must be shielded at all times. The temporary covering must keep it free from contact with saliva and food debris and must be contoured to block extrusion or lateral movement.[17]

Aluminum Shells and Resin Crown Forms

An aluminum shell, a little larger in circumference than the cervical of the preparation, should be trimmed to conform to the contour of the gingival margin and to rest on the occlusal surface of the preparation without displacement of, and about 0.5 mm. short of, the gingival tissue. Aluminum shells are pliable and can be manipulated or ground to integrate with the opposing teeth. When a resin crown form is in position, it should be in alignment without displacing the soft tissue (Fig. 4–23A and B).

Temporary stopping, when used inside either an aluminum shell or a resin crown form, serves well as a protective cover for a prepared tooth. The shell, filled with heated stopping, must be forced onto the tooth so that the preparation is covered and the occlusion is comfortable.

The shell is removed, and after the cervical excess of stopping has been trimmed so that no blanching of the soft tissue will occur, the temporary covering is replaced and the stopping going into the gingival crevice is smoothed and adapted to the tooth with a warm instrument. The crown is removed and the inside is cleaned, dried, and moistened with eugenol or a cavity varnish before being returned to the *isolated* and *dried* tooth. If the period of construction is not overlong, the temporary crown will safeguard the tooth and keep it in the same position. Zinc oxide and eugenol paste is used more often than stopping, but it does not displace tissue.

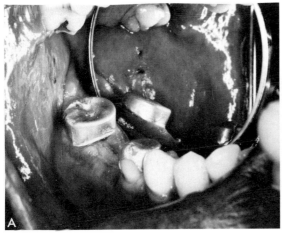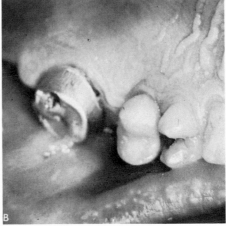

FIGURE 4-23. *A,* Trimmed aluminum shell crowns adapted to molar and bicuspid. Cervical of molar crown contoured just short of gingival crest. Buccal of bicuspid crown trimmed to height of contour on uncut surface.

B, Trimmed shell on molar. Resin covering on bicuspid. Was made with seated impression, but resin can be painted on dried isolated tooth, trimmed cervically and occlusally, and then polished. Latter method is speedy and will serve adequately for short periods. Is destroyed when removed.

Construction of a Temporary Resin Crown or Bridge

Temporary crowns suitable for all teeth, but for use particularly on bicuspids or anteriors, can also be constructed with a self-curing tooth-colored resin. They can be made over a stone die or on the prepared tooth. In each instance the stump should be lubricated. Before the preparation was made, an alginate or rubber impression (of the tooth, quadrant, or arch, as the case may be) should have been taken and stored in a humidifier. The areas in the impression covering the teeth that have been prepared are filled with self-curing resin, and the impression is reseated in the mouth or on the cast. Before the resin has polymerized beyond the semiplastic stage, the impression and resin must be taken from the mouth or cast and the resin lifted from the impression or removed from the teeth. The rough, temporary crown can then be trimmed, shaped, and adjusted for occlusion. Polishing can be done after seating with a temporary luting material. (See Figures 4-24 and 4-25.) Resin crowns may be sealed with zinc oxide and eugenol paste or cavity varnish. However, on teeth with limited retention, zinc phosphate cement can be more effective.

A temporary resin crown may be built in advance over a simulated preparation made on the stone diagnostic cast. Before seating it must be machined inside, trimmed, and, with added resin, readapted to fit and length.

For an edentulous space, wax pontics should be built on the diagnostic cast and an alginate impression taken over the stone and wax. The tempo-

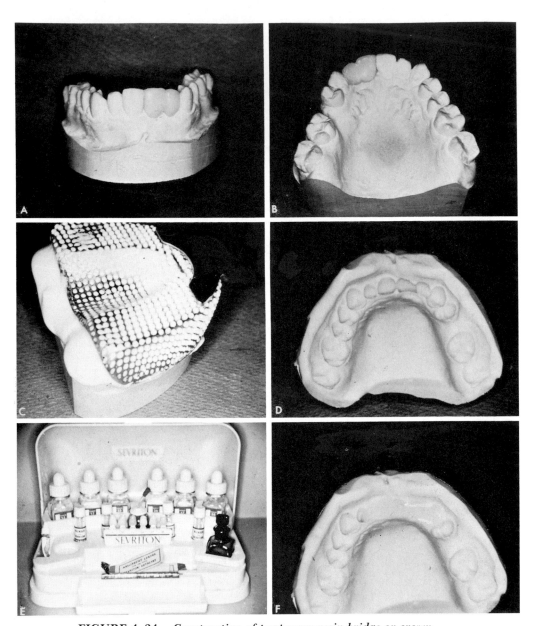

FIGURE 4–24. *Construction of temporary resin bridge or crown.*

A and *B*, Diagnostic cast with pontics in wax.
C and *D*, Impression of cast.
E, Material used for temporary bridge.
F, Resin placed in impression.

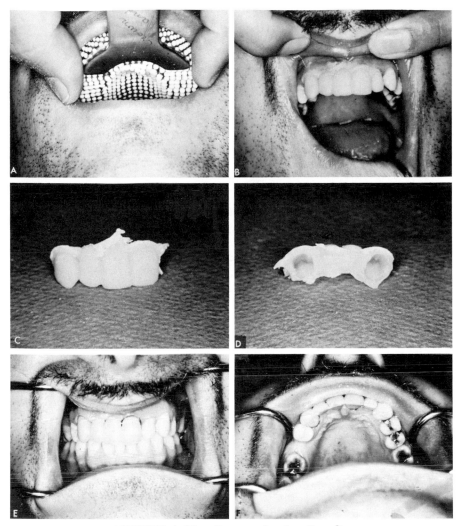

FIGURE 4–25. *Construction (continued).*

A, Filled impression seated in mouth. Abutments were lubricated. There is slightly more difficulty in correctly seating impression in mouth, but time is saved. Heat generated by most materials suitable for temporary bridges does not seem to overstimulate the pulp.

B, Before removal for trimming.

C and *D,* Bridge removed.

E and *F,* Temporary bridge trimmed and seated with temporary cement over lightly lubricated teeth.

rary bridge is then constructed by filling the prepared teeth and pontic areas with self-curing resin and seating the impression on a duplicate or simulated plaster cast of the prepared arch.[18, 19] Removal, trimming, and polishing follow the technique used for the temporary single unit.[20, 21]

THE WAX OCCLUSION REGISTRATION

Before placing the covering on the tooth, an occlusion registration is sometimes made by using softened inlay wax to cover the occlusal, mesial, and distal surfaces and partially to cover the buccal or lingual of the preparation. When this has been placed on the occlusal surface, the patient should be asked to close in centric occlusion and to open immediately. After compressing the wax against the occlusal, buccal, and lingual surfaces, the patient is instructed to close again and to hold this position until the wax has become rigid. The wax registration, which is made more advantageously on the working cast, will furnish a crude pattern on the die for occlusal carving and for thickness in the contact area between the preparation and the approximating tooth. Adding wax to the "bite" to build the pattern to contour must be done meticulously, else the finished casting may have flaws and potentially weak areas.

The die and working cast should be constructed by the methods described in Chapter 9, The Working Cast.

REFERENCES

1. Langeland, K.: Dentin and pulp reaction to cavity and crown preparation. Survey of literature. Amer. Inst. Oral Biol. and Med., 23:73, 1966.
2. Reynolds, J. M.: Abutment selection for fixed prosthodontics. J. Pros. Den., 19:483, May 1968.
3. Kafalias, M. C.: Abutment preparation in crown and bridge. Aust. D. J., 14:1, Feb. 1969.
4. Smith, G. P.: What is the place of the full crown in restorative dentistry? Am. J. Orthodont. & Oral Surg., 33:471, June 1947.
5. Wheeler, R. C.: The implications of full coverage restorative procedures. J. Pros. Den., 5:848, Nov. 1955.
6. Thom, L. W.: Principles of cavity preparation in crown and bridge prosthesis. I. The full crown. J.A.D.A., 41:284, Sept. 1950.
7. Barker, B. C. W.: Restoration of nonvital teeth with crowns. Aust. D. J., 8:191, June 1963.
8. Kuratli, J.: Restoration of broken-down vital teeth for fixed partial denture abutments. J. Pros. Den., 8:504, May 1958.
9. Maesaka, R. K.: Personal communication.
10. Markley, M. R.: Pin reinforcement and retention of amalgam foundations and restorations. J.A.D.A., 56:675, May 1958.
11. Markley, M. R.: Restorations of silver amalgam. J.A.D.A., 43:133, Aug. 1951.
12. Silberkweit, M., Massler, M., Schour, I., and Weinmann, J. P.: Effects of filling materials on the pulp. J. D. Res., 34:854, Dec. 1955.
13. Going, R. E., and Massler, M.: Influence of cavity liners under amalgam restorations on penetration by radioactive isotopes. J. Pros. Den., 11:298, March-April 1961.
14. Volland, R., et al.: Zinc phosphate cement. J.A.D.A., 22:1281, Aug. 1935.
15. Wheeler, R. C.: Complete crown form and the periodontium. J. Pros. Den., 11:722, July-Aug. 1961.
16. Smith, G. P.: The marginal fit of the full cast shoulderless crown. J. Pros. Den., 7:231, March 1957.
17. Johnston, J. F., Mumford, G., and Dykema, R. W.: Modern Practice in Dental Ceramics. Philadelphia, W. B. Saunders Company, 1967.
18. Freese, A. S.: Impressions for temporary acrylic resin jacket crowns. J. Pros. Den., 7:99, Jan. 1957.
19. Rubinstein, M. N.: Immediate acrylic temporary crown and bridge. D. Digest, 60:12, Jan. 1954.
20. Segat, L.: Protection of prepared abutments between appointments in crown and bridge prosthodontics. J. Michigan D. A., 44:32, Feb. 1962.
21. Taylor, A. G.: Temporary protection of prepared abutment teeth. Roy. Canad. D. Corps Quar., 2:8, Oct. 1961.

Behrend, D. A.: Temporary protective restorations in crown and bridgework. Aust. D. J., *12*:411, Oct. 1967.

Capland, J.: Maintenance of full coverage fixed-abutment bridges. J. Pros. Den., *5*:852, Nov. 1955.

Harrison, J. D.: Crown and bridge preparation, design, and use. D. Clin. N. Amer., March 1966, p. 185.

Hoffman, J. M.: Common problems in the construction of the full cast crown. J.A.D.A., *48*:272, March 1954.

Kilpatrick, H. C.: Ultra-speed and auxiliary equipment in fixed partial denture construction. J. Pros. Den., *10*:574, May-June 1960.

Knight, R. M.: Temporary restorations in restorative dentistry. J. Tennessee D. A., *47*:346, Oct. 1967.

Lyon, D. M.: Abutments in fixed prosthesis. Arkansas D. J., *24*:6, Dec. 1953.

McCabe, D. J., and Rinne, V. W.: Treatment of carious teeth. Disadvantages of full coverage. D. Clin. N. Amer., Nov. 1960, p. 639.

Murphy, E. J.: A method of protecting three quarter and full crown preparations. D. Digest, *72*:392, Sept. 1966.

Murto, C. B.: Modern bridge retainers. J. Ontario D. A., *33*:15, Feb. 1956.

Rose, H. P.: A simplified technique for temporary crowns. D. Digest, *73*:449, Oct. 1967.

Shooshan, E. D.: Full veneer cast crowns. J. South. California D. A., *23*:27, Sept. 1955.

Smith, G. P.: Full crown preparation. New York J. Den., *26*:307, Oct. 1956.

Stone, E.: Gingivectomy and crown preparation in occluso-rehabilitation. J. Pros. Den., *8*:640, July 1958.

Tanner, H.: Ideal and modified inlay and veneer crown preparations. Illinois D. J., *26*:240, April 1957.

chapter 5

THE PARTIAL VENEER
CROWN

The partial veneer (three-quarter) crown is used primarily as a bridge retainer, but may be used in combination with resin or silicate cement as a single-unit restoration on a fractured tooth. It ordinarily covers the proximal, lingual, and occlusal surfaces or incisal edge of the tooth, with the labial or buccal surface being untouched except along the labioincisal or bucco-occlusal margin. (See Figure 1-5.) When conditions permit minimal labial or buccal extensions, the impression created will be in accord with discriminating taste.[1, 2, 3, 4, 5]

INDICATIONS

This retainer, which demands far less cutting of the tooth than the veneered gold crown, will provide retention for the fixed prosthesis when the abutment tooth is well supported, when there is a good axial relationship to the path of insertion, when the clinical crown of the tooth is sturdy and of average length or longer, and when there is dentin connecting the tooth walls.

It is indicated particularly on maxillary centrals, cuspids, and bicuspids, and on mandibular second bicuspids of at least medium length. (See Chapter 26, Bridge Patterns.) Usually these teeth can be reduced enough to guarantee ample thickness in the casting to resist deformation from the occlusion and to have proximal surfaces that can be grooved to assure retention of the bridge. The metal over the reduced lingual surfaces will have irregular form and rigidity.

This retainer, when used on maxillary bicuspids, can support posterior bridges supplying one, two, or three teeth, and anterior bridges replacing the cuspid or the cuspid and lateral. When splinted, it may be used on longer anterior prostheses. It has merit, also, on intermediate abutments. The partial veneer crown may be placed on rotated or tipped bicuspids if the latter eccentricity is not too pronounced. It can be applied where the lingual cusp has been fractured or where most of the supporting dentin under the lingual cusp has been destroyed. If such teeth were prepared for veneered gold crowns, the remaining tooth structure would not stand up against the forces sometimes transmitted through a bridge.

The partial veneer crown may be used on the upper first molar when the mouth is relatively caries-free, when the crown is long occlusocervically, and when the mesiobuccal area of the tooth is exposed as the patient talks or smiles. Otherwise, because of its long marginal line and likely resultant vulnerability, and since the maxillary molar is rarely noticeable, it is contraindicated in favor of the full veneer gold crown.

Occasionally a broken-down vital upper cuspid or bicuspid may be restored to prepared form with a pin-retained casting, and, using another path of seating, a partial veneer crown may be placed over the reconstructed tooth. This infrequent preparation can be made after caries has occurred around and under some other kind of retainer, causing a weakened labial or buccal wall with too little bulk for a veneered gold crown.

Square tooth form is a requisite to the most satisfactory application of this retainer. Gold is most often seen when the partial veneer crown preparation is made on teeth that are ovoid, tapered, or conical, and on anterior teeth with proximal caries, but generally this can be avoided. Some patients do not object, but if there will be an unsightly exhibition of metal, the veneered gold crown should be substituted.

CONTRAINDICATIONS

Partial veneer crowns are contraindicated on (1) short teeth, teeth extensively carious, and (barring a few lower molars) those that have a poor long-axis relationship with the path of insertion; (2) upper cuspids that have long incisal arms, contact areas at the gingival margin, and very short mesial and distal surfaces (because grooves in such surfaces will not hold the prosthesis); (3) teeth too small or too thin for accurate positioning and cutting of the proximal grooves; (4) teeth in which there is extensive cervical caries, since the grooves would extend into partially disintegrated tooth structure; and (5), because of large areas of susceptibility, in mouths in which the caries index is high. The partial veneer crown cannot be used advantageously and with pleasing esthetic effects on many of the extreme forms of upper lateral incisors, because of the problem in making or paralleling grooves without either very deep linguoproximal reduction or a wide band on both the mesioproximal and distoproximal.

Brooks[6] says: "Where there is extensive loss of tooth structure, a large restoration with resultant weakened tooth walls, or multiple active carious areas in the abutment tooth, a full veneer crown should be considered rather than the partial veneer retainer."

The partial veneer crown is contraindicated on a short maxillary bicuspid when it is to be used alone on one end of a bridge, but it may serve efficiently on this type of tooth when used as a segment of a multiple retainer.

The partial veneer crown cannot routinely be adapted with unqualified success to lower incisors, cuspids, first bicuspids, and molars. Although some mandibular incisors have the bulk to accept this preparation, on many teeth the lingual surface of the retainer must be overcontoured. The crown forms and occlusions of mandibular cuspids and first bicuspids are in many instances unsuitable for preparations that will furnish retention without an obvious show of metal. It may be used on mandibular molars that, owing to malrelationship with the approximating teeth, are not receptive to the full veneer gold crown preparation.

PREPARATION OF ANTERIOR TEETH USING ULTRA-HIGH AND MODERATE SPEEDS AND HAND INSTRUMENTS

Partial veneer crown preparations on maxillary anterior teeth, which are gratifying esthetically, can be made effectively with a combination of ultra-fast instrumentation for gross cutting and with slower speeds and hand instruments for refinement. The initial reductions on the proximal surfaces, done with a long, small, tapered bur, start on the lingual, inside the tooth circumference, and are halted at a point just to the labial of the contact height of contour, which will leave all labial enamel and contour intact and under control. Later the anterior walls of these cuts are flattened and located with a hatchet or fine disk. Lingual and incisal reduction follows, and then the incisal and proximal grooves are placed and given definitive form. The cervical margin is established and all other areas of the preparation are finished. This includes softening the incisal point angles and the angular line joining the cingulum and lingual surface, and checking on the cervical bevel of the proximal grooves. The last step is to place the posthole in the cingulum. (See Figures 5–11, 5–12, and 5–13.)

Several rotary instruments are needed in the preparation of an anterior tooth for a partial veneer crown. They are the 169L-FG carbide bur (S.S.W.) for gross cutting at high speeds, the 110-P wheel diamond stone (Starlite)* for incisal and lingual reduction, and the ¼K, ¼D-T, and 1D-T diamond stones (Densco) and No. ½ and 700 steel burs for more detailed cutting and refinement at slower speeds (Fig. 5–1). Hand instruments should be used to plane the labial walls of the proximal grooves. Fine paper disks may be used supplementally.

The theoretical steps in these preparations, applicable to all anterior teeth, may be outlined in this order, but economical utilization of instruments may cause some change in sequence, without altering the end result:

*Star Dental Mfg. Co., Inc., Philadelphia, Pa.

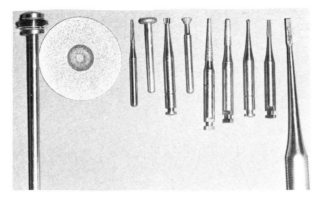

FIGURE 5–1. Left to right:
Mandrel for straight handpiece;
5/8 inch Horico* diamond disk;
169L-FG carbide bur (S.S.W.);
110P-FG wheel diamond stone (Starlite);
No. 37 inverted cone latch carbide bur (S.S.W.);
1/4K-FG inverted cone diamond stone (Densco);
1/4D-L latch tapered diamond stone (Densco);
1D-T latch tapered diamond stone (Densco);
No. 1/2 round latch steel bur;
No. 700 latch tapered fissure carbide bur (S.S.W.);
No. 10 straight Tarno chisel (S.S.W.).

*Pfingst and Company, Inc., New York, N. Y.

(1) proximal reduction;
(2) lingual reduction;
(3) incisal bevel;
(4) cingulum reduction;
(5) incisal groove;
(6) proximal grooves;
(7) cervical margin;
(8) labial and incisal margins, and angles; and
(9) cingulum posthole.

PREPARATION OF A MAXILLARY CUSPID USING HIGH SPEEDS FOR GROSS CUTTING AND SLOWER SPEEDS AND A CHISEL FOR DETAILS AND FINISHING

The instruments shown in Figure 5-1 include all those used for this procedure, and also a disk and bur to be used when only slow speeds are employed. When there is malalignment, the proximal contact areas will be removed with a disk as a preliminary step for each technique. For a tooth in normal relationship, a bur would be used with accelerated speeds. The inverted cone bur is excellent for cutting the incisal groove or for sharpening it following preparation with a diamond stone.

Proximal Surface Reduction (High Speed)

The proximal surface is reduced with the 169L carbide bur. Starting at the mesiolingual line angle, cutting proceeds toward the labial surface, guiding the bur into the tooth structure (Fig. 5-2B and C) until the mid-point of the contact area is reached, when the bur should be inside the cervical periphery of the tooth (Fig. 5-2D and E). Proximal cuts should parallel the path of seating or converge incisally less than 5 degrees, and labiolingually should converge a little more than the planes of the untouched proximal surfaces.

Proximal Grooves (High Speed 169L bur)

The first indentations for the proximal grooves are located just to the lingual of the centers of the contact areas (Fig. 5-3). They are made parallel to the path of insertion and ideally will be parallel to the plane of the incisal two-thirds of the labial surface. In depth the grooves at the cervical seats should equal the diameter of the bur. If the cervical margin of the preparation is to be placed within the gingival crevice, the groove should end at about the level of the gingival line or 0.5 to 0.6 mm. short of the margin of the preparation. (See Figure 5-4D.)

Cingulum Wall (High Speed 169L bur)

The cingulum wall seldom can be made parallel to the proximal grooves without forming an unwanted wide cervical shoulder. Usually this wall will incline toward the labioincisal after a chamfer has been made and 1.0 mm. of tooth substance has been removed. Reduction starts at either line angle and connects with the opposite surface, rounding the line angles so that there is a smooth, convex (nonangular), and even junction of surface cuts (Fig. 5-4).

Incisal Bevel

Ordinarily the incisal bevel is done at a slower speed with a diamond stone (Fig. 5-5). The space created must allow for a bulk of metal that will withstand deforming forces in all positions of the occluding teeth, even after future equilibration. The tooth structure removed is wedge-shaped, with the narrow side to the labial. On abraded teeth the cut cannot be the same width from side to side, but this should be approached as closely as possible. For the most part the maximal depth at the lingual margin is 1.1 mm.

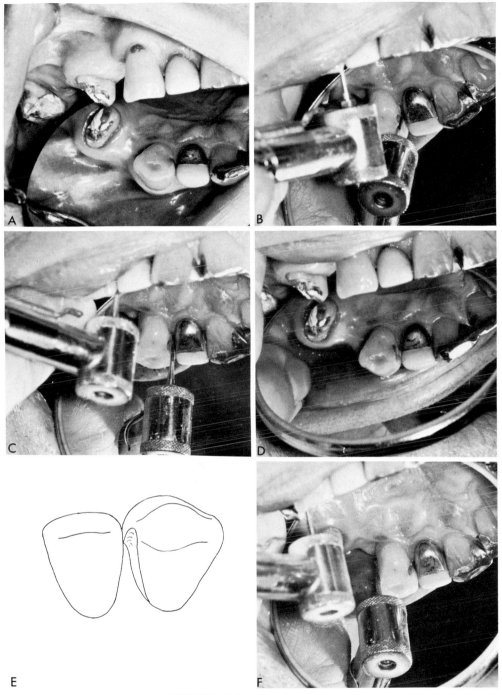

FIGURE 5–2. *Proximal cuts.*

A, Incisal view of maxillary cuspid to be prepared to receive a partial veneer crown. Note abraded wide incisal surface, abraded lingual surface and cingulum, and mesial caries. Cuspid will be anterior abutment for five-unit posterior bridge.

B, Start of mesial proximal cut.

C, Finish of mesial proximal cut at mid-point of contact area.

D, Incisal view of mesial proximal cut.

E, Diagram of proximal cut ending at mid-point of proximal area and inside cervical periphery of tooth.

F, Making distal proximal cut.

107

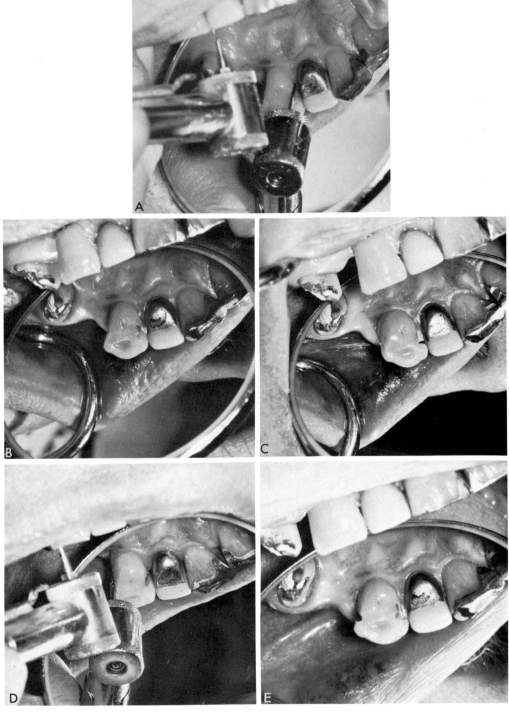

FIGURE 5-3. *Proximal grooves.*

A, Starting indentation for mesial proximal groove.
B and *C*, Mesial proximal groove.
D, Starting distal proximal groove.
E, Incisal view of started proximal grooves.

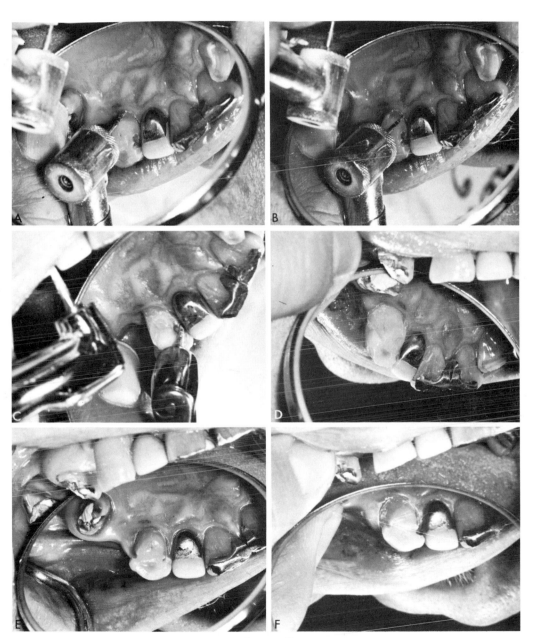

FIGURE 5-4. *Reducing cingulum wall.*

A and *B*, Gross cutting with 169L bur.

C, Increasing width of mesial groove lingually to obliterate carious area.

D, E, and *F,* Three views of reduced cingulum.

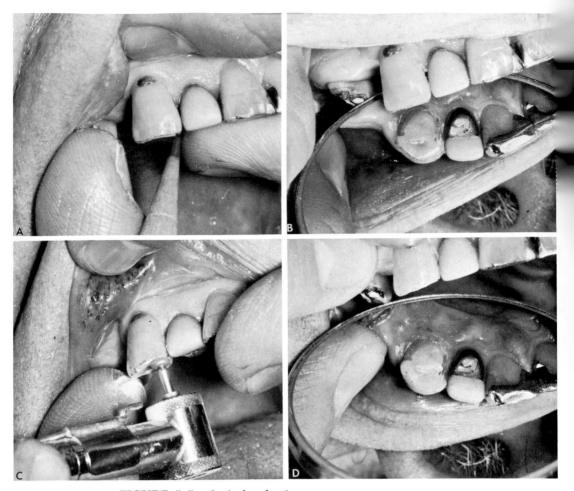

FIGURE 5–5. *Incisal reduction.*

A and *B*, Marking depth of labioincisal reduction.
C, Reducing incisal surface with flat side of diamond stone.
D, Incisal view of incisal cut.

Lingual Surface

Reduction of the lingual surface is accomplished at reduced speeds with a diamond stone (Fig. 5-6). The normal depth is 1.0 mm. except on paths of excursion, in which areas the depth measurement should be increased to 1.4 mm. These paths must be ascertained in advance with articulating paper and outlined on the diagnostic cast for reference.

Incisal Groove

The incisal groove, made at slow speed with either an inverted cone stone or bur, connects the proximal grooves. Its labial wall should be wider than the lingual wall, thus moving the crest of the angle a little to the lingual

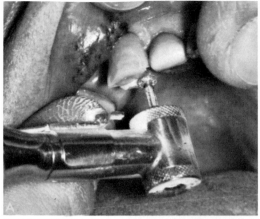
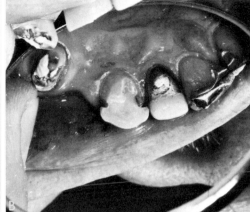
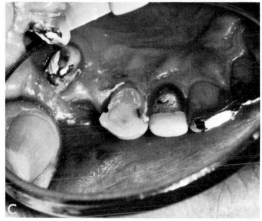

FIGURE 5–6. *Reducing lingual surface.*

A, Starting cut on lingual surface. Straight handpiece stones are equally effective.

B, Mesial half reduced. Notice wide mesial groove after extension to lingual of carious area.

C, Incisal view of lingual cut. Angle formed with lingual wall is sharp.

(Fig. 5–7). When there must be a heavier mass of metal to withstand occluding forces, the lingual wall may be cut to form a ledge at more than a 90-degree angle to the labial wall. In wide, abraded incisal surfaces, the labial wall of the groove, or step, can be flat. However, if the reflecting surface of the casting is close to right angles to the line of vision of an observer, this wall should be convex to break up the concentration of light rays that might be reflected through the tooth structure. The labial wall should be fashioned so that dentin remains behind the enamel.

Labial Walls of Proximal Grooves

The irregular labial margins left by the bur making the proximal cuts are planed and smoothed with a chisel or a fine sandpaper disk (Fig. 5–8). The proximal labial margins are established so that the junction of tooth and metal can be cleansed by brushing, but if the tooth structure is sound and intact they are kept in the lingual part of the curved line angle. These walls *must* be without undulations.

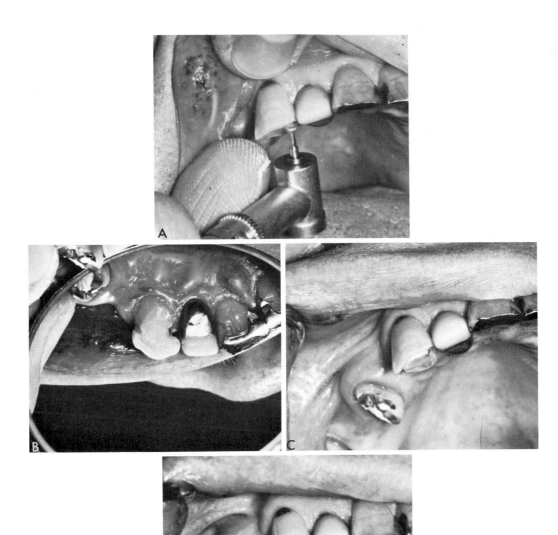

FIGURE 5-7. *Forming incisal groove.*

A, Initial cut with diamond stone.
B and *C*, Incisal and labioincisal views.
D, Incisal clearance in protrusion.

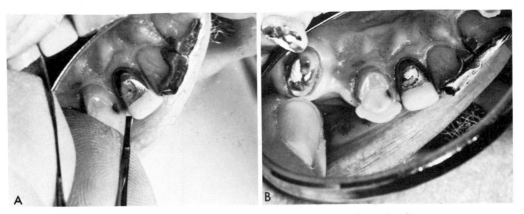

FIGURE 5–8. *Planing and establishing labial walls of proximal grooves.*

A, Cutting and planing enamel with chisel.

B, Incisal view.

Cervical Chamfer (Finishing Line)

A round-end tapered diamond stone is used to form the chamfered cervical margin (Fig. 5-9). The chamfer is a concave bevel and should be used whenever the required tooth reduction does not leave a chisel-edge margin. This finishing line extends from the mesial of one groove around the cingulum to the mesial of the other groove. It should be 0.3 to 0.4 mm. in depth and follow the outline of the gingival line inside the gingival crevice.

Relieving Angles

The incisal point angles and the angle formed by the cingulum wall and lingual surface should be rounded (Fig. 5-10). This seems to make easier the impression-taking, waxing, and seating of the casting, and to increase slightly the thickness of metal in areas that are under the most pressure and are first to deform. The smooth, flat end of an inverted cone diamond is used as an abrading surface.

Cingulum Posthole

The post extending into the cingulum area is a stabilizing and retentive device that greatly enhances the worth of an anterior partial veneer crown. It locks the retainer in place and nullifies forces of rotation. A ledge is cut into the lingual slope just to the incisal of the margin of the cingulum wall (Fig. 5-11*A*). This ledge is approximately two and one-half times as large as the hole to be cut. With a small round bur an indentation is made (Fig. 5-11*B*) to locate the hole, which is cut with a tapered bur (No. 700, 701, 702) to a

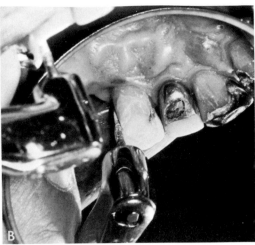

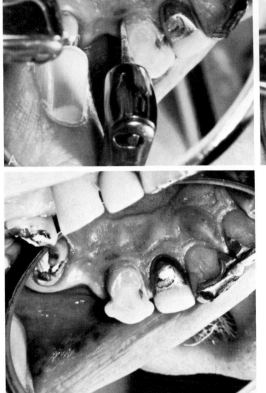

FIGURE 5-9.   *A* and *B*, Establishing chamfered cervical margin.
    C, Incisal view of lingual and distal cervical margin.

depth of 1.3 to 2.0 mm. (Fig. 5-11*C* and *D*). When tooth form suggests a pulp horn extending a short distance into an exaggerated cingulum, it can be advantageous to sink the hole off center.

Final Check of Preparation

When completed the preparation should be checked for (1) clearance in all movements, (2) marginal regularity and location, (3) parallel surfaces free of undercuts, (4) retention potential, and (5) esthetic potential. (See Figure 5-12.)

There should be no question about sufficient clearance in all positions of the opposing teeth. This must be checked scrutinously to preclude the necessity for overmuch adjusting of the cast retainer and the detrimental alterations on the occluding surfaces of pontics and the protective metal covering margins of porcelain facings.

Marginal regularity and correctness of form are essential for bulk in the casting and for facility in finishing the cemented retainer.

Almost always parallelism and freedom from undercuts can be found visually. If there is doubt, a rubber base tube impression poured in plaster of Paris will yield a die that can be checked with a Boley gauge. Many discerning operators do this quite often.

The retentive and esthetic potentials undoubtedly were planned as the preparation of the tooth progressed, but the sensitive clinician never fails to take one last look.

Temporary Coverage

A temporary crown for an anterior tooth can be made in a very short time by isolating and drying the tooth and applying self-curing resin. The patient is asked to close the jaws. When the resin has hardened, occlusion is equilibrated and margins are trimmed with knives, burs, and disks. The surfaces are smoothed. A covering of this kind will remain in place for several days. It fractures when removed. (See Chapter 4.)

An alginate impression of the unprepared arch, with resin placed in the prepared tooth, can be seated, covering the preparation with resin. When made by this process, the crown must be trimmed and luted to the tooth with a weak temporary cement. It can be removed and reseated.

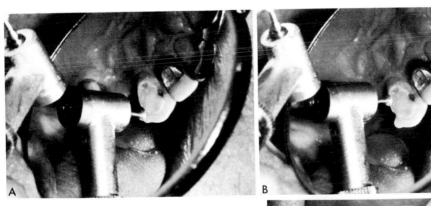

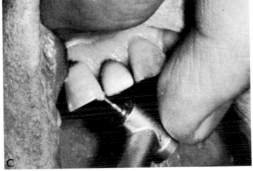

FIGURE 5–10. Rounding point and lingual angles.

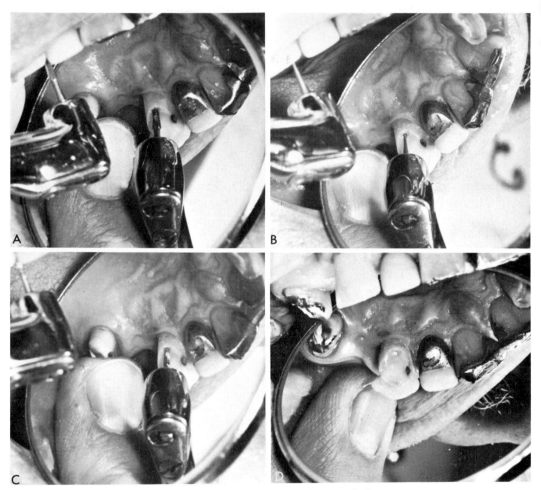

FIGURE 5-11. *Sinking cingulum posthole.*

A, Cutting ledge just to incisal of cingulum wall.
B, Indenting with round bur.
C, Cutting posthole.
D, Incisal view, lingual posthole.

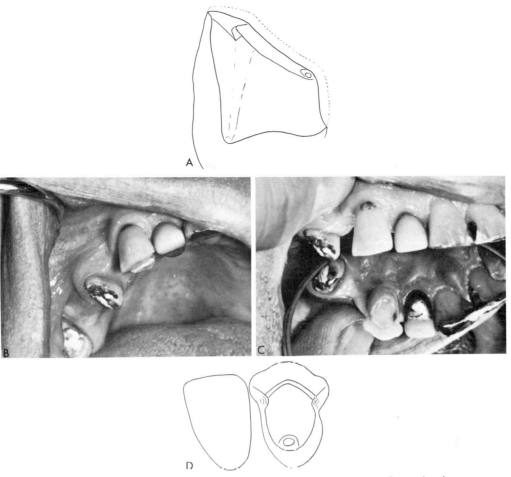

FIGURE 5-12. *A*, Diagram of lingual reduction and placement of proximal groove. *B* and *C*, Labioincisal and labial views of prepared tooth. *D*, Diagram of finished preparation.

If the interval of construction will be prolonged, it is wise to use a casting cemented with a temporary cement that is soft and can be fractured.

MODIFIED PREPARATION OF A MAXILLARY CENTRAL INCISOR

Willey[1] has described a variant to the original concept of the anterior partial veneer crown preparation. The basic differences are (1) less labial extension, especially on the mesioproximal; (2) more axial reduction of the cingulum, both proximally and lingually (the greater bulk of metal augments rigidity of the casting and minimizes any tendency to deformation at the cervical); (3) an incisal offset rather than a groove; (4) labial walls of proximal grooves and incisal offset convex instead of flat; and (5) no pinhole in the cingulum (Fig. 5-13).

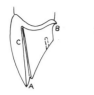

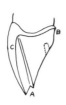

FIGURE 5–13. Figure on right shows proximal view of maxillary anterior PV preparation as taught by the authors. Figure on left shows concept of maxillary anterior PV preparation as advocated by Smith and Willey. Pinhole has been placed in cingulum because authors consider this one of the fundamentals of this preparation.

The labial extension is started from the lingual and brought labially only to the center of the contact area. A fine sandpaper disk or a chisel is used to bring the margin labially as far as is esthetically desirable, with a *slightly convex* rather than a flat surface. The finished proximal groove is less deep, but the casting is more bulky. If the facings were selected, contoured, and aligned on the diagnostic cast prior to preparing the teeth, they can be used to help to place the margin of the preparation (Fig. 5–14).

The form given to the cingulum will show a much heavier chamfer or shoulder on the lingual, and a wall parallel or almost parallel to the proximal grooves. The added bulk of metal increases the rigidity and stability of the casting and lessens the probability of deformation through extended use. In theory this supersedes using a pin in the cingulum. (See Figures 5-13, 5-17, 5–18, and 5–19.)

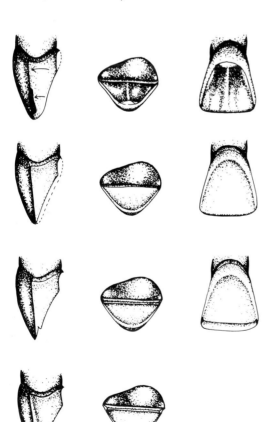

FIGURE 5–14. Top to bottom: Reduction of cingulum and proximals; reduction of lingual; incisal groove or offset; proximal grooves. (Smith and Willey.)

In form the incisal offset is more shallow than the incisal groove described earlier, going a little farther cervically onto the lingual surface. With increased bulk in the labial wall, it can be made convex, which is believed to throw back light rays in a favorable direction. This is an empirical assumption, but the end result, using this form, is indisputably good.

Because of the limited labial extension of this preparation, it is difficult if not impossible to reproduce with an elastic impression material. Direct wax pattern carving is imperative.

The castings should be fitted and equilibrated in the mouth. If the pontics are completed and aligned on the diagnostic cast and then transferred to the mouth on a baseplate, assembly of the bridge can be done without a working cast and the final two solder joints may be done singly, thus checking each step. There must be considerably more chair time reserved for such a procedure, but the possibilities for subtle pontic alignment and ridge adaptation make it worthwhile.

PREPARATION OF A MANDIBULAR INCISOR

The mandibular incisor is *not* well adapted to a partial veneer crown preparation, and use of this retainer should be limited. The long established routine, which begins with proximal slices, does not meet all esthetic demands, even though retention may be adequate.

For the most pleasing result, carbide burs should be used (Fig. 5–15) for both proximal and cingulum reduction, at a rotational speed best suited to the operator. Cutting should be started on the cingulum, with the instrument parallel to the intended path of insertion, and should proceed around the tooth and onto the proximal surface. Depth on the proximal must be enough to avoid contact with an approximating tooth. Reduction should stop

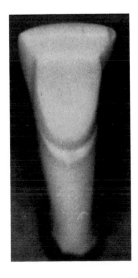

FIGURE 5–15. Preparation on mandibular incisor without cingulum pinhole. (Smith and Willey.)

just labially to the center of the contact area, but short of the labial line angle. Cervically, barring recession, the preparation on the proximals should be 0.25 mm. below the gingival crest. Lingually, gingival recession can make it impracticable to place the margin in the crevice.

The lingual surface is not reduced except where the linguoincisal offset, or groove, is cut from proximal surface to proximal surface. The offset is 1.0 to 1.5 mm. below the incisal edge. Its pulpal wall should be made convex and be extended just beyond the linguoincisal angle. The proximal grooves are made with a long, small carbide bur or with a No. 700 steel bur. As a rule, the direction is the same as for other anterior teeth, although the depth may be less. The labial walls of the proximal grooves, shaped with either disks or chisels, are also convex. A pinhole 1.0 mm. deep is placed in the cingulum. The preparation should be deep enough to create a discernible and helpful finishing line.

It can be troublesome to reproduce the partial veneer crown preparation on a mandibular incisor with an elastic impression unless it is made too deep and is overextended. The sharp labial margins and the direction of the grooves make withdrawal precarious and cause tearing or cutting of the impression material. Direct pattern carving is suggested.

PREPARATION OF A MANDIBULAR CUSPID

When the partial veneer crown is planned for the lower cuspid, there should be a comprehensive evaluation of the occlusion of the incisal third of the labial surface with the linguals and incisals of the opposing teeth. In many cases, the linguoincisal groove must be omitted, with a step across the labioincisal being substituted. The metal covering this area will curb lingual movement of the casting, will receive and dissipate the incising and masticating forces, and can be contoured to support occlusion and guide and control mandibular movement. When it is essential to eliminate any display of metal and the tooth is long, a lingual offset, sometimes as much as 2.0 mm. below the incisal edge, may be used. (In most cases a veneered crown would be preferred.) The proximal grooves should follow the plane of the labial surface, but can be made to parallel the long axis of the tooth (Fig. 5-16). Occasionally, before a pinhole can be made, a ledge or an indentation must be cut on the lingual surface at the cervical.

The partial veneer crown can be a competent retainer on the mandibular cuspid if (1) the preparation will control lingual displacement; (2) the reduction on the proximal surfaces and across the incisal can have depth for a strong, rigid casting; (3) the cervical pin is employed; (4) an adjacent tooth will not interfere with seating the bridge or it can be changed in form to nullify interference; (5) the long-axis relationship with the other abutment teeth is approximately parallel and will permit substantial proximal grooving; (6) the caries rate seems to be low; and (7) extra lingual pins are placed to supplement the retention from the proximal grooves when the labioincisal ledge is not used.

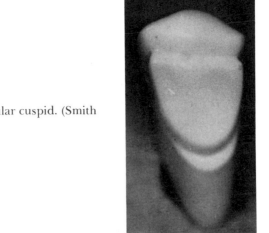

FIGURE 5–16. Preparation on mandibular cuspid. (Smith and Willey.)

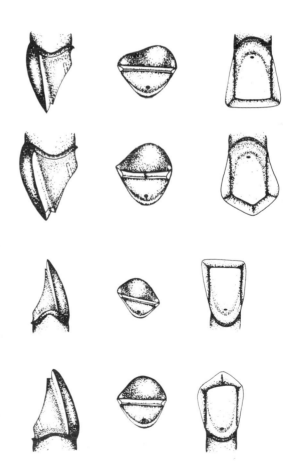

FIGURE 5–17. Top to bottom: Finished preparation, maxillary central; finished preparation, maxillary cuspid; finished preparation, mandibular incisor; finished preparation, mandibular cuspid. (Smith and Willey.)

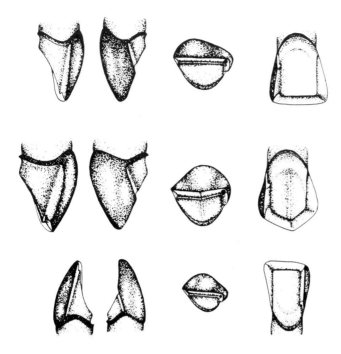

FIGURE 5–18. Preparations involving only one contact area: Top, maxillary central incisor; center, maxillary cuspid; bottom, mandibular incisor. (Smith and Willey.)

When the mouth is being prepared for a removable partial denture, the cingulum of the partial veneer crown can be shaped to support the denture, and on the distal and lingual it can be flattened to form a guiding plane and to receive the lingual arm of a clasp. It will retain a six-unit anterior bridge, and unilaterally, alone or splinted, a posterior bridge supplying one or two, and now and then three, teeth.

Other modified preparations are shown in Figures 5–17, 5–18, and 5–19.

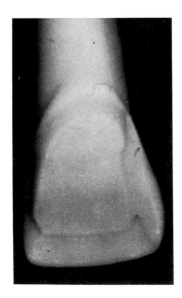

FIGURE 5–19. Maxillary central. Groove on proximal at right of cingulum prepared as usual. Short groove to lingual of contact on left. Preparation crosses left marginal ridge. Lingual reduced. Incisal groove ends in pinhole inside left marginal ridge. (Smith and Willey.)

OTHER SYSTEMS OF INSTRUMENTATION

The authors have used the following patterns of instrumentation with success. These were submitted by the same operators referred to in Chapter 4, The Full Veneer Gold Crown. The same "prepared form" can and should be obtained with them as with the standard continuity stated later in this chapter.

PREPARATION OF POSTERIOR TEETH USING ULTRA-HIGH AND MODERATE SPEED FOR TOOTH REDUCTION

Maxillary and mandibular posterior teeth may be prepared for partial veneer crowns using a 169L carbide bur for gross reduction at ultra-high speed and 1D-T and $\frac{1}{4}$D-L diamond stones for detail and finishing at slower speeds. Labial walls may be smoothed with chisels or hatchets.

The basic order of cutting operations, which may be changed to suit personal preference, is:

(1) proximal surfaces;
(2) lingual surface;
(3) occlusal groove pattern;
(4) occlusal surface;
(5) proximal grooves or boxes;
(6) cervical margin (finishing line);

ANTERIOR TEETH

Table 5–1

INSTRUMENT	TO BE ACCOMPLISHED	R.P.M.
⅞" steel "Lightning" separating disk	Proximal contact reduction.	3,000
70L Premier "Ela" carbide	Placement of proximal grooves. Reduction of periphery of cingulum. Location and contour of cervical margin.	150,000
3½J Densco diamond	Lingual surface reduction.	10,000
4D Densco diamond	Incisal beveled.	8,000
36 or 37 steel bur (any brand)	Placement of incisal groove.	500 to 1,000
701 or 702 steel bur (any brand)	Placement of cingulum pinhole.	1,000
Sandpaper disks (any brand)	Axial walls and cavo-surface angle smoothed.	500

(7) buccal bevel;

(8) distobuccal groove;

(9) softening of angles; and

(10) auxiliary postholes or grooves, if needed to supplement retention.

The ultimate forms for both maxillary and mandibular teeth are illustrated, as well as the step-by-step preparation of a mandibular second bicuspid.

Table 5–2

INSTRUMENT	TO BE ACCOMPLISHED	R.P.M.
701 R&R carbide	Incisal reduction.	150,000
700 R&R carbide	Proximal surface reduction.	150,000
5J-T Densco diamond	Lingual surface reduction.	6,000
701 R&R carbide	Reduction of cingulum periphery. Location and contour of cervical margin.	150,000
700 or 701 steel bur (any brand)	Placement of proximal grooves and cingulum pinhole.	6,000
35, 36, or 37 steel bur (any brand)	Placement of incisal groove.	1,000
Sandpaper disks (any brand)	Axial walls and cavo-surface angle smoothed.	500

Table 5–3

INSTRUMENT	TO BE ACCOMPLISHED	R.P.M.
1D Densco diamond or 7/8" steel "Lightning" separating disk or carborundum disk	Proximal surface reduction. (When there is an approximating tooth, a disk is used to open contact.)	200,000 6,000
123 SSW diamond	Lingual surface reduction.	200,000
1D Densco diamond	Reduction of cingulum periphery. Location and contour of cervical margin. Incisal reduction.	200,000
½ D Densco diamond	Proximal grooves started.	200,000
700 R&R steel bur	Proximal grooves finished.	3,000
37 SSW carbide	Placement of incisal groove.	200,000
701 R&R steel bur	Placement of cingulum pinhole.	3,000
Sandpaper disks (any brand)	Axial walls, grooves, and cavo-surface angle smoothed.	500

Table 5–4

INSTRUMENT	TO BE ACCOMPLISHED	R.P.M.
170 SSW carbide	Incisal reduction.	200,000
1D-C Densco diamond	Reduction of cingulum periphery.	200,000
2½ J Densco diamond	Lingual surface reduction.	200,000
170L SSW carbide	Proximal grooves started.	200,000
700 SSW steel bur	Proximal grooves finished. Interproximal cervical reduction.	5,000
35, 36, or 37 SSW steel bur	Placement of incisal groove.	5,000
1D-T Densco diamond	Location and contour of cervical margin. Preparation smoothed.	200,000
701 SSW steel bur	Placement of cingulum pinhole.	5,000

Table 5–5

INSTRUMENT	TO BE ACCOMPLISHED	R.P.M.
2T Densco diamond	Proximal surface reduction.	4,000
701L Densco carbide	Reduction of cingulum periphery. Placement of proximal grooves. Location and contour of cervical margin.	200,000
1½ J Densco diamond	Lingual surface and incisal reduction.	10,000
1K Densco diamond	Placement of incisal groove.	6,000
Sandpaper disks (any brand)	Axial walls and cavo-surface angle smoothed.	500

(See Figures 5–29, 5–31, 5–32, 5–33, and 5–35.)

BICUSPIDS

Table 5–6

INSTRUMENT	TO BE ACCOMPLISHED	R.P.M.
70L Premier "Ela" carbide	Complete axial and occlusal reduction. Placement of proximal boxes.	150,000
1D Densco diamond	Location and contour of cervical margin. Irregularities smoothed. Buccal cusp contrabeveled.	10,000
700 R&R steel bur	Refinement of proximal boxes.	5,000

Table 5–7

INSTRUMENT	TO BE ACCOMPLISHED	R.P.M.
7/8″ carborundum disk (any brand)	Proximal reduction.	6,000
701 R&R carbide	Lingual and occlusal reduction. Buccal cusp contrabeveled.	150,000
701 R&R carbide	Location and contour of cervical margin.	6,000
700 or 701 steel bur (any brand)	Placement of proximal boxes.	6,000
Cervical trimmers	Beveling of proximal box cervical margin.	Hand
Sandpaper disks (any brand)	Axial walls and cavo-surface angle smoothed.	1,000

Table 5–8

INSTRUMENT	TO BE ACCOMPLISHED	R.P.M.
1D Densco diamond	Complete axial and occlusal reduction. Buccal cusp contrabeveled. Location and contour of cervical margin.	200,000
1/2 D Densco diamond	Placement of proximal boxes.	200,000
1D-T Densco diamond (worn) or 44 SSW carborundum stone	Preparation smoothed.	200,000 3,000
701 R&R carbide	Cervical seat of boxes made square.	8,000
700 R&R steel bur	Refinement of proximal boxes.	3,000

Table 5–9

INSTRUMENT	TO BE ACCOMPLISHED	R.P.M.
701 R&R carbide or 701 SSW carbide	Occlusal and lingual reduction.	200,000
700 SSW carbide or 699 Densco carbide	Placement of proximal boxes.	200,000
700 SSW steel bur	Refinement of proximal boxes.	5,000
5/8″ Moore garnet disk	Finish and flare of proximal boxes.	5,000
F, 1D-T, or 1D-C Densco diamond	Completion of proximal reduction. Location and contour of cervical margin. Preparation smoothed.	200,000
170 SSW carbide	Buccal cusp contrabeveled.	200,000

Table 5-10

INSTRUMENT	TO BE ACCOMPLISHED	R.P.M.
701 or 701L Densco carbide	Complete axial and occlusal reduction. Placement of cervical shoulder. Placement of proximal boxes.	200,000
¾D Densco diamond	Irregularities smoothed. Refinement of cervical shoulder. Buccal cusp contrabeveled.	200,000
Sandpaper disks (any brand)	Axial walls and cavo-surface angle smoothed.	500

PREPARATION OF A MANDIBULAR BICUSPID FOR A MODIFIED PARTIAL VENEER CROWN

Proximals and Lingual

The steel matrix should be used when the tooth has proximal contact (Fig. 5-20A and B). The reduction should be made from the lingual, parallel to the path of insertion and extending to and including, but not beyond, the buccal aspect of the contact area. Cervically it extends to the gingival crest or the planned finishing line, whichever is more occlusal. The planes of the prepared mesial and distal surfaces should converge lingually.

The lingual reduction is made parallel to the path of seating or converging occlusally from 3 to 5 degrees. Mesiodistally it follows tooth contour. The surface should be grooved in the middle before gross cutting begins and reduced one-half at a time, as with the full veneer preparation (Fig. 5-20C).

Occlusal

The occlusal reduction is similar to the full veneer preparation. The groove pattern is cut to a depth of 1.0 mm. (Fig. 5-21A), and the remainder of the occlusal is reduced following the major occlusal planes (Fig. 5-21B and C).

Proximal Grooves

The proximal grooves should be made parallel to the path of insertion and as far buccally in the contact area as feasible without extending beyond the contact area. Pulpally at the cervical seat they should be the depth of the diameter of the 169L bur. Cervically they should extend to the finishing line (Fig. 5-22).

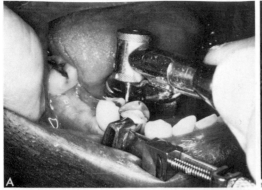

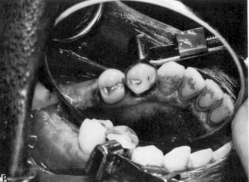

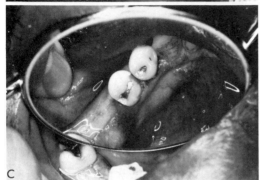

FIGURE 5-20. *Proximal and lingual cuts.*

A and *B*, Matrix band around approximating tooth to protect it against possibility of damaging abrasion.

C, Occlusal view showing mesioproximal and half of lingual reduced.

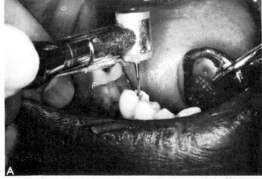

FIGURE 5-21. *Occlusal reduction.*

A, Cutting occlusal groove pattern to depth of 1.0 mm.

B and *C*, Reducing occlusal surface, following planes of occlusal surfaces of cusps.

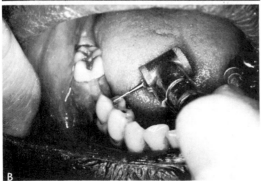

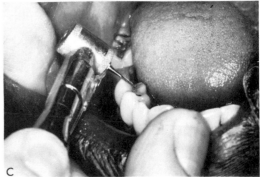

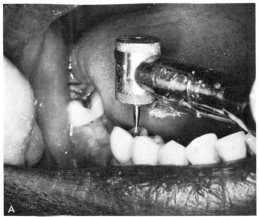
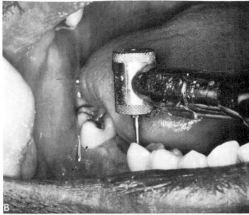

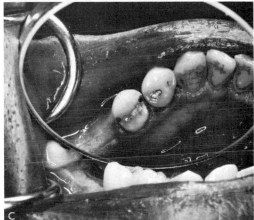

FIGURE 5-22. *Proximal grooves.*

A and *B,* Making initial indentations for mesial and distal proximal grooves.

C, Occlusal view showing proximal grooves and proximal, lingual, and occlusal reduction.

Distobuccal Groove

The distobuccal groove is made in the middle of the distobuccal half of the buccal surface and parallel to the path of insertion mesiodistally (Fig. 5-23*A* and *B*). Buccolingually it should be made in two planes, with the occlusal one-third of the groove at a 45-degree angle to the long axis and the cervical two-thirds parallel to the path of insertion. It should extend a little beyond the height of contour on the buccal surface and end in a knife edge. Then the area between the distal groove and the distobuccal groove is reduced in two planes occlusocervically around the distobuccal line angle (Fig. 5-23*C* and *D*).

Line Angles and Margins

The mesial groove is flared to the buccal with the ¼D-L diamond, just breaking contact buccally (Fig. 5-24*A*), and planed and smoothed with enamel hatchets (Fig. 5-24*B* and *C*) or sandpaper disks. The line angles are

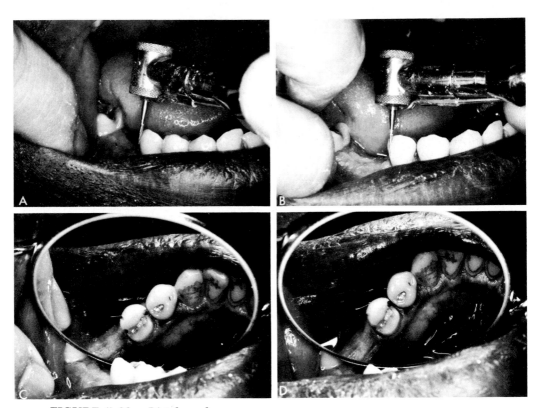

FIGURE 5-23. *Distobuccal groove.*

A and *B,* First cuts of distobuccal groove cut in two planes.
C, Occlusal view of preliminary groove.
D, Occlusal view showing removal of tooth structure around distobuccal angle.

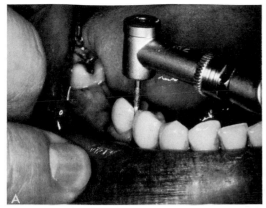

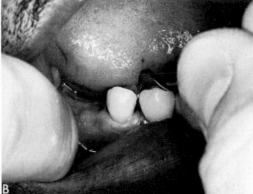

FIGURE 5-24. *Line angles and margins.*

A, Breaking mesial contact toward buccal.

B, Planing and forming mesiobuccal margin.

C, Occlusal view of completed grooves.

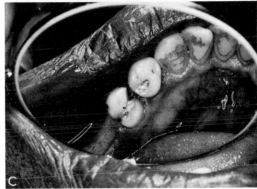

rounded to join the proximals with the lingual surface (Fig. 5-25*A* and *B*). The finishing line and the terminus of the distobuccal groove are given chamfer form (Fig. 5-25*B* and *C*). Finally, the contra-bevel is placed over the buccal cusp with the ¼D-L diamond (Fig. 5-25*D* and *E*).

The preparation is finished and made smooth with the ¼D-L diamond at slow speed.

TEMPORARY COVERAGE

Posterior partial veneer preparations can be covered temporarily with trimmed aluminum shells (Fig. 5-26), resin crowns, or with castings if the waiting period will be lengthy.

TEACHING CONCEPTS AND PROCEDURES

It is of paramount importance in the teaching of an undergraduate student that he acquire a respect for the preservation of tooth structure as well as a knowledge of esthetic form, and the verities of retention and

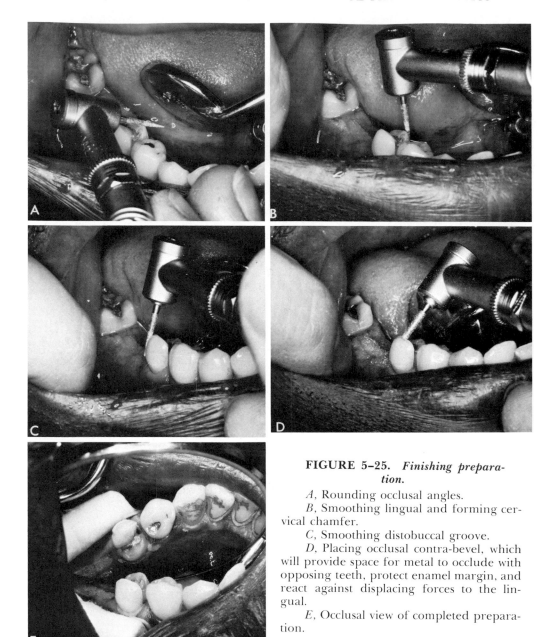

FIGURE 5-25. *Finishing preparation.*

A, Rounding occlusal angles.

B, Smoothing lingual and forming cervical chamfer.

C, Smoothing distobuccal groove.

D, Placing occlusal contra-bevel, which will provide space for metal to occlude with opposing teeth, protect enamel margin, and react against displacing forces to the lingual.

E, Occlusal view of completed preparation.

resistance to deformation. The authors feel that respect for these principles can be instilled by a rigid discipline and an adherence to a prescribed formula when the first preparations are made. Once the idea is fixed, the novice can be advanced to the speedier, but potentially more dangerous, cutting program. Because of this belief, step-by-step procedures for partial veneer crown preparations on maxillary and mandibular teeth are included in this chapter. The use of instruments and orders of procedure can be more slowly paced, which will make scrutinous supervision possible.

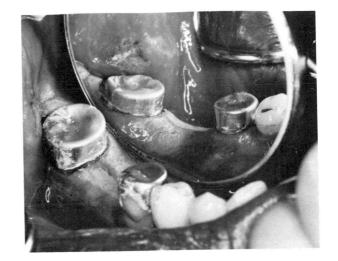

FIGURE 5-26. Temporary coverings are trimmed aluminum shells.

A preparation that affords greater capabilities and the expectation of fewer corrections can be accomplished in shorter time if the sequence of steps and the instrumentation are standardized. The rules and systems that will be described have been used for years and have been discussed by many authors.[7, 8, 9, 10, 11, 12, 13] Other designs and approaches to partial veneer preparations are equally meritorious and have primarily the same guides for retention and fixation.

PREPARATION OF A MAXILLARY CENTRAL INCISOR

After a survey of the diagnostic cast has determined the most logical path of insertion for the involved teeth, the labial outlines of the proximal cuts, paralleling the path of insertion, should be drawn on the central incisor of the cast. The exposure of metal on the labial surface will depend to some degree on the lingual convergence of the proximal surfaces, proximal caries if present, the contour of the labial surface, and the amount of metal necessary to avert deformation.

With this picture in mind, the tooth can be prepared in the following manner:

(1) reduction of the mesial and distal surfaces;
(2) reduction of the lingual surface from the middle of the cingulum to the incisal edge of the tooth;
(3) beveling the incisal edge and cutting the incisal groove;
(4) penciling the proximal grooves parallel to the previously planned path of insertion;
(5) cutting the proximal grooves;
(6) reduction of the cingulum area;
(7) beveling the labial walls of the proximal and incisal grooves;

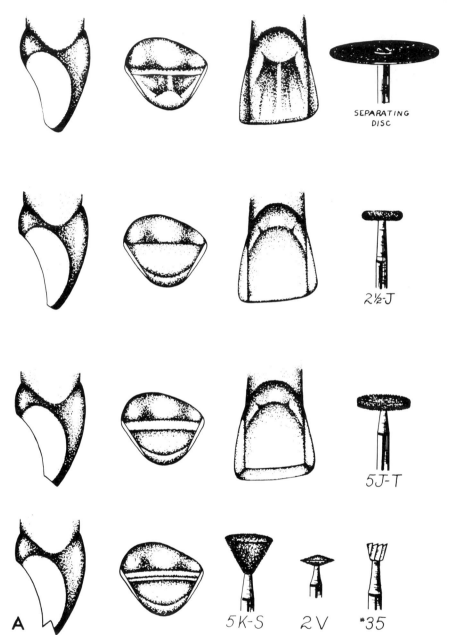

FIGURE 5–27. *Preparation on a maxillary central incisor with cutting instruments suitable for each step. (Numbered stones are Densco diamonds.)*

A, Top to bottom: Proximal slices; lingual surface; incisal bevel; incisal groove.

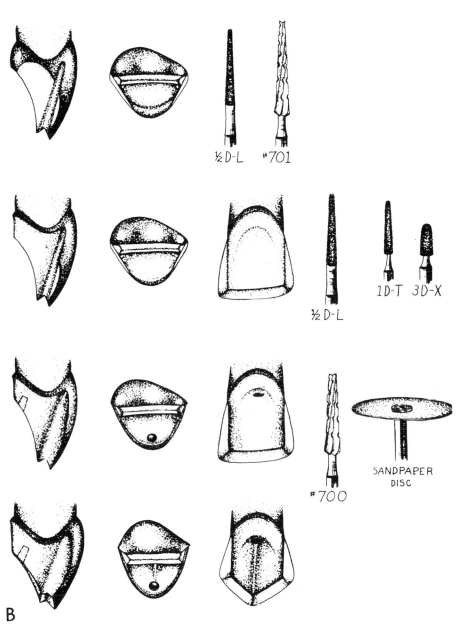

½D-L   #701

½D-L   1D-T 3D-X

#700   SANDPAPER
              DISC

B

B, Top to bottom: Proximal grooves; cingulum reduction; beveling labial walls of all grooves; cervical finishing line and pinhole in cingulum. Preparation on maxillary cuspid.

(8) rounding the lingual walls of the proximal grooves and finishing the cervical margin (finishing line); and

(9) sinking a pinhole in the cingulum, parallel to the proximal grooves.

Mesial and Distal Surfaces

The proximal cuts can be made using a disk in a straight handpiece (Fig. 5-27A). These should converge lingually a little more than the mesial and distal surfaces and should extend from the incisal edge to the gingival line unless the tooth is too angular or the gingiva has receded beyond the cementoenamel junction. The preparation should not continue beyond the line angles on the labial.* On any surface made more prominent through rotation, the labial margin must be kept to the lingual so that the finished casting will be inconspicuous. Often adjacent teeth must be separated and a thin steel disk used to prevent the labial surface from being cut beyond the desired point.

Lingual Surface

By using a No. 2½J diamond stone in the straight handpiece, the lingual surface should be reduced uniformly to a depth of 0.7 mm. from the crest of the cingulum to the incisal edge. Where contact is made with opposing teeth, in centric closure and along the paths of eccentric excursions, the depth should be at least 1.0 mm.

Incisal Bevel and Groove

The bevel on the incisal edge may be made with the same instrument used on the lingual or with a No. 5J-T flat-edge wheel. It should be approximately at right angles to the line of force against the linguoincisal of the tooth, the same width from mesial to distal, and have a clearance of 1.0 mm. at the lingual margin and 0.25 mm. at the labial margin of the bevel. The labial margin of the bevel should simulate the uncut incisal edge of the tooth.

The incisal groove can be cut using a No. 37 inverted cone bur in a straight handpiece. The labial wall should be twice as wide as the lingual wall in order to throw the apex of the groove toward the lingual surface of the tooth, leaving dentin to support the labial wall of enamel. This will ward off discoloration of the tooth when the casting is cemented. When the incisal edge has been abraded markedly, because of powerful thrusts from opposing teeth, a deeper groove is required.

---

*The labial "line angle" is assumed to be the junction of the labial and proximal surfaces. It is an imaginary line slightly to the labial of the contact area, following the height of convexity produced by the merging of the labial and proximal surfaces.

The incisal groove is an integral feature of this preparation. It makes room for metal that will add to the rigidity of the casting and impede its springing away from the proximals, and it furnishes gold for future incisal equilibration. In teeth with thin incisal thirds, a lingual step or offset may be substituted.

Proximal Grooves

The directional line of the parallel proximal grooves, co-ordinated with the plane of the incisal two-thirds of the labial surface, should be penciled on the tooth. In a majority of instances, the grooves can be so placed and thus can be longer, can terminate in cleansable areas, will institute more circumferential retention against lingual displacement, and will exact the least reduction of the labial enamel.

Using a No. 700 tapered fissure bur, an indentation is made in the proximal surface at the incisal groove. With this as a point of stabilization, the groove is cut along the pencil line to a depth matching the greatest diameter of the bur. There are numerous teeth in which it will be impossible for the groove to reach the gingival crevice without excessive cutting. Parallelism to the path of insertion will be expedited if the first groove is cut on the surface next to the edentulous area. (See Figure 5–27B.)

Cingulum

The cingulum must be decreased about 1.0 mm. by use of a cylindrical or tapered round-tip stone in the contra-angle handpiece. Theoretically the lingual wall should be parallel to the proximal grooves, but this creates a lingual shoulder, which should be avoided.

Bevel and Finishing Line

Using sandpaper disks in a straight handpiece, the labial wall of the incisal groove should be made smooth, being certain that the mesioincisal and distoincisal angles are beveled so that the casting will protect them. The labial walls of the proximal grooves should be projected on a flat plane from the deepest part of the groove to the buccal margin of the preparation, erasing all the proximal cut. The groove length should not be increased nor should the end of the groove be scarred at this time.

The cervical finishing line is made with a No. ½D-L, 1D-T, or 3D-X diamond stone in the contra-angle handpiece. In this step the critical portions are on the proximal surfaces between the mesial and distal grooves and the cingulum reduction. These sections can be prepared 0.5 mm. in depth at the same time that the finishing line is made and the linguals of the proximal grooves are rounded. Using a No. 56 bur, the grooves should be recut pulpally until they are at least 0.75 mm. deep.

Pinhole

A pinhole should be made in the cingulum with a No. 701 or 702 tapered fissure bur. It should be 1.25 mm. deep and parallel to the proximal grooves. It must be placed a little to the mesial or distal of the center of the cingulum so that any lingual pulp horn may be skirted. The pin of the casting will form a tripod with the struts in the proximal grooves, immobilizing the casting. Also, the frictional retention will be increased and there can be no movement except in reverse along the path of insertion. For these reasons, the pinhole is a fundamental part of the partial veneer preparation on any anterior tooth.

PREPARATION OF A MAXILLARY CUSPID

The partial veneer crown preparation on the upper cuspid is virtually the same as that on the central incisor. The chief difference is in the incisal groove, which may be divided and sharp-cornered, since it must follow the cusp arms. Frequently, too, the preparation must be deeper so that the casting may withstand greater torque. When the mesial and distal surfaces are short incisocervically, it will be mandatory to supplement the retention with two additional pinholes in the lingual surface, placed at points close to the mesial and distal margins and 0.7 mm. from the incisal groove. Either a No. 700 or 701 tapered fissure bur may be used to prepare these pinholes. This mode of auxiliary retention can be made a part of any anterior partial veneer preparation. (See Figure 5-27*B*.) If the incisal cusp arms end mesially and distally in contact areas that are on a level with the gingival crest, it may be unwise to use a partial veneer crown unless supplementary retention can be gained from lingual pins. There must be enough proximal surface showing for grooves to be formed and a solder joint to be placed. When the silhouette of such a tooth is re-formed with a partial veneer crown the restoration is unsightly.

Indications, other contraindications, steps of preparation, and instrumentation are the same as for a central incisor.

PREPARATION OF A MAXILLARY BICUSPID

The partial veneer crown preparation on the upper bicuspid might be termed a combination of the MOD inlay and full veneer gold crown preparations. All the occlusal surface must be covered with this retainer. The reduction of the lingual surface follows its contour and may have a chamfer finishing line. If the crown is long occlusocervically and if dentin remains buccally and lingually, the lingual margin may be short of the gingival crevice. The proximal surfaces are prepared in inlay form, although more shallow pulpally and more narrow buccolingually.[14]

The routine for this preparation is:

(1) reduction of the mesial and distal surfaces;
(2) reduction of the occlusal surface, and
(3) reduction of the lingual surface;
(4) cutting the proximal boxes;
(5) flaring the buccal walls of the proximal boxes;
(6) establishing the cervical finishing line; and
(7) beveling the bucco-occlusal margin.

When the diagnostic cast is surveyed, the path of insertion should be marked on the buccal surface to pilot the proximal slices and the buccal margins of the preparation. When the long-axis directions of the bicuspid and the other abutments are identical (Fig. 5-28), the proximal cuts can closely parallel the path of insertion. When there is a discrepancy in the long-axis relationship between the abutment teeth, the bicuspid partial veneer preparation should be near-classic in form and other abutments made to harmonize.

For example, if the bicuspid partial veneer crown is to be the anterior retainer, most of the deviations must be in the preparation of the molar tooth. With the bicuspid position upright and the molar tipped to the distal and the buccal, the mesial of the bicuspid and the distal and buccal of the molar must be made parallel or be so prepared that they approach each other slightly toward the occlusal. In this case, because of the long-axis relationship of these two teeth, the distal of the bicuspid and the mesial of the molar could not be paralleled, but would diverge occlusally. The major retention for this bridge would then come from the mesial of the bicuspid and the distal of the molar. Here the associated angulation of the walls could be calculated on the diagnostic cast with the analyzing rod of the surveyor. If

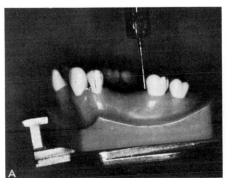 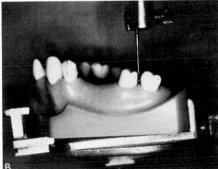

FIGURE 5-28. *Survey of diagnostic cast and check on preparation.*

A, Path of insertion drawn on buccal of bicuspid abutment; buccal extension of distal proximal slices on bicuspid and molar. Analyzing rod shows that minimal cutting will be needed on mesial of molar.

B, Teeth prepared to marked path of insertion, which is parallel to analyzing rod.

the bicuspid is the posterior abutment, the partial veneer crown probably could not be relied on if the long-axis relationship with the anterior abutment were distinctly abnormal.

Mesial and Distal Surfaces

The mesial and distal surfaces are flattened with a separating disk in the straight handpiece, starting on or inside the marginal ridge and ending at

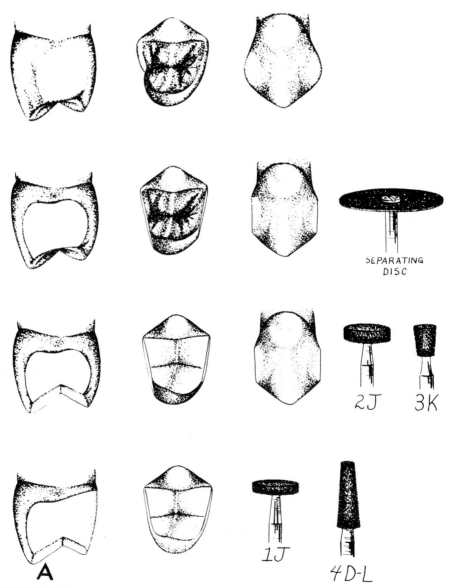

FIGURE 5–29. *A*, Top to bottom: Uncut tooth; proximal slices; occlusal reduction; lingual reduction.

the gingival line or the cementoenamel junction (Fig. 5-29A). One proximal cut must be parallel to the path of insertion or converge only a few degrees occlusally. The other proximal surface should be prepared, as nearly as conditions will permit, parallel to the first cut or barely inclined toward the center of the occlusal.

Buccolingually, the width of the lingual embrasures will be increased, in which case there will be access for the preparation of the cervical finishing line. On the distobuccal, the margin should stop at the line angle, and on the mesial, to enhance esthetics, it may be just to the buccal of the contact area.

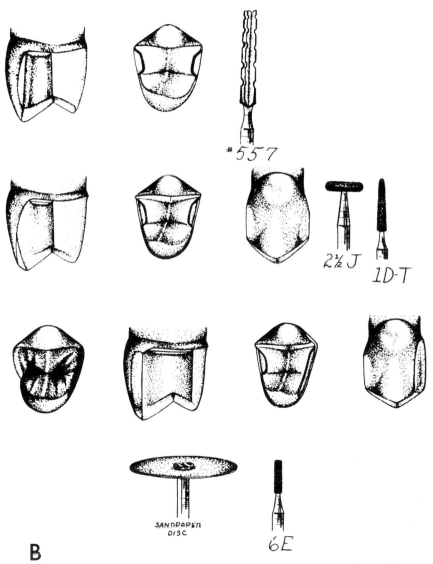

B

B, Top to bottom: Proximal boxes; buccal walls of boxes angled to buccal line angle and cervical finishing line; buccal chamfer on carious tooth.

Occlusal Surface

The groove pattern may be prepared with a bur in order that space for metal will be guaranteed. The occlusal is shortened 1.0 mm. in all other sections, using wheel-shaped and inverted cone stones. To check clearance, the patient should be asked to close on articulating paper (folded to eight thicknesses) and to move the mandible in lateral and protrusive excursions.

Occasionally there is a temptation to leave the labial portion of the buccal cusp of a maxillary bicuspid uncovered (Fig. 5–30). Although no line of gold will show, a retainer of this pattern is less stable and less protective. Full occlusal coverage is much safer and more productive of long life in the prosthesis.

Lingual Surface

The lingual preparation, following the normal contour from cusp tip to cervical, can be made with wheel-shaped and tapered round-end stones. If the tooth is in normal alignment, the depth should be approximately 1.0 mm. except in the occluding area. Here it should be somewhat deeper.

Boxes

The proximal boxes should parallel each other and the path of insertion (Fig. 5–29B). Best produced with a No. 557 or 556 bur, they should be in the buccal half of the tooth and twice as wide as the diameter of the bur used. In depth, pulpally, they should be one-half the diameter of the same bur. The beveled cervical margin of the box should be in the gingival crevice, but recession may make this infeasible.

The buccal walls of the proximal boxes should be angled from the pulpal wall to the buccal margin, obliterating the original cuts on the proximal surfaces. This can be effectuated with hand instruments or a sandpaper disk.

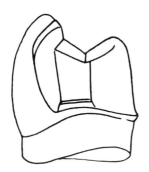 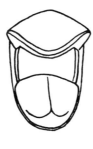

FIGURE 5–30. Preparation on maxillary bicuspid not covering all of buccal cusp is used only on teeth with long crowns when minimal display of gold is imperative. Teeth so prepared seem to be more susceptible to splitting; also, the retainers loosen more often.

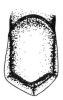

FIGURE 5-31. Modified PV preparation on maxillary bicuspid. (Smith and Willey.)

Finishing Line and Bevel

The cervical finishing line is begun by beveling the cervical seats of the proximal boxes with a cervical margin trimmer. The remainder of the cervical finishing line may be chamfered with a No. 1D-T tapered round-end stone in the contra-angle handpiece.

A bevel 0.5 mm. wide is placed on the buccal surface at the bucco-occlusal margin. It should be at such an angle that the seated casting will engage the buccal surface when forces on the casting are toward the lingual.

Willey[1] advocates proximal grooves instead of boxes, and he deepens the preparation on the lingual half of the tooth. (See Figure 5-31.) The greater bulk of metal increases the rigidity of the casting. He also recommends less extension at the buccoproximal and bucco-occlusal angles. However, the authors feel that the shorter the teeth, the more the indication for proximal boxes.

A modification of the maxillary bicuspid partial veneer preparation (Smith and Willey) is shown in Figure 5-31.

PREPARATION OF A MAXILLARY FIRST MOLAR

The preparation on the upper first molar differs from that on the bicuspid in two ways. To attain a circumferential hold on the tooth, its mesial

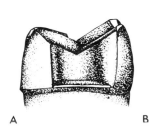
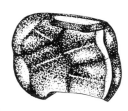
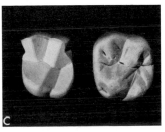

A   B   C

FIGURE 5-32. *Preparations on maxillary molar.*

A and *B*, With boxes. When molars are short and a partial veneer crown is indicated, boxes provide more stability.

C, With grooves.

and distal surfaces should converge buccally instead of lingually. Proximal retention is increased by cutting wide grooves, instead of boxes, in the buccal one-third. If the crown is long, the finishing line on the lingual surface can be placed 1.5 to 2.0 mm. occlusally to the gingival line.

The steps and the instruments used in this preparation are the same as for the bicuspid except that the proximal grooves are cut with a No. 702 tapered fissure bur (Fig. 5-32).

PREPARATION OF A MANDIBULAR BICUSPID

In numerous instances the partial veneer crown is contraindicated on the lower first bicuspid. The lingual slant of the crown and the extremely short lingual cusp often will make a retentive preparation doubtful unless the preparation can be extended so far cervically on the buccal surface that it

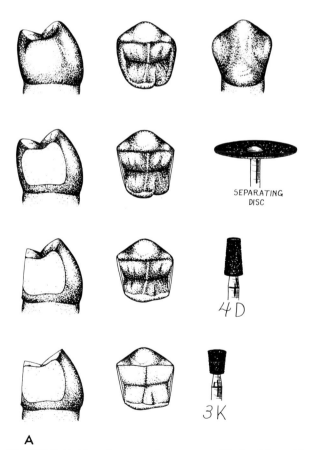

A

FIGURE 5-33. *Preparation on mandibular bicuspid.*

A, Top to bottom: Uncut tooth; proximal slices; lingual aligned to path of insertion; occlusal reduced.

shows as much metal as the full veneer gold crown. In such a case, its esthetic characteristics are negated. (See Figure 5-33A.)

The mandibular second bicuspid is better suited to this preparation,[15] because the crown has less lingual angulation and a longer lingual cusp, and is more nearly square when viewed from the occlusal. Much of the time it may be prepared in a manner corresponding to the maxillary bicuspid, except that proximal grooves are used instead of boxes, and by means of a bevel or a step the preparation covers the occluding portion of the buccal surface so that only the casting will contact the opposing teeth in all excursions.

Retention will be increased by a bevel 1.0 mm. wide on the buccal surface along the distobuccal margin. (See Figures 5-33B and 5-34.) Since it will not be parallel to the path of insertion, it should go as far cervically as the convexity of the tooth will tolerate. The bevel should be 0.7 mm. deep at the junction of the buccal surface and distal cut, and with a small cylindrical stone should be made concave, in the form of a chamfer. This concavity will

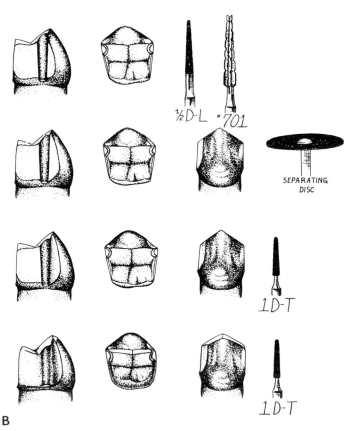

B, Top to bottom: Proximal grooves; buccal bevel; buccal chamfer; cervical finishing line; bucco-occlusal bevel.

FIGURE 5-34. Preparation on mandibular bicuspid. (Smith and Willey.)

improve the finishing line at the buccal margin of the bevel and also will increase the strength of the lip of metal coming around onto the distobuccal surface. Two pinholes, 1.0 mm. deep, may be placed in the occlusal surface at the tips of the cusps, to augment the stability and holding power of the retainer. They should be made with a No. 701 or 702 tapered fissure bur. The finishing line on the lower bicuspid may be a chamfer, but usually the mesial, distal, and lingual walls will end at a chisel-edge margin, which suffices (Fig. 5- 33*B*).

Partial veneer crowns on lower bicuspids are satisfactory when splinted to each other or to a retainer on the cuspid.

A modification of the preparation on a mandibular bicuspid (Smith and Willey) is shown in Figure 5-34.

PREPARATION OF A MANDIBULAR MOLAR

The partial veneer crown is not indicated on a lower molar except under one peculiar condition; when the molar is tipped mesially so much that the path of insertion cannot be accommodated to a distal approximating tooth, this retainer may function admirably. With the mesial contact area of the distal tooth anterior to the distal gingival line of the abutment, placement or removal could not be effected without radically altering the path of insertion, which may be impractical, or reshaping the mesial of the overhanging tooth with another restoration.

The preparation should be started by slicing off the mesial of the abutment along the plane of the path of insertion (Fig. 5–35*A*). The occlusal is then cut distally to the marginal ridge. From this line, grooves are made in the buccal and lingual surfaces, parallel to the path of insertion, and as far cervically as form and lingual inclination will allow. These two surfaces are then connected with the mesial reduction, after which the buccal and lingual grooves are made deeper to ensure a horseshoe grip on the tooth. Using a No. 702 tapered fissure bur, three pinholes, from 1.0 to 1.5 mm. deep and parallel to the path of insertion, are placed in the occlusal surface. One is near the disto-occlusal margin, midway between the buccal and lingual surfaces; the others are placed in the mesial cusps. The cervical finishing line will be either a chamfer or a chisel-edge, depending on tooth position and contour (Fig. 5–35*B*).

Text continued page 152.

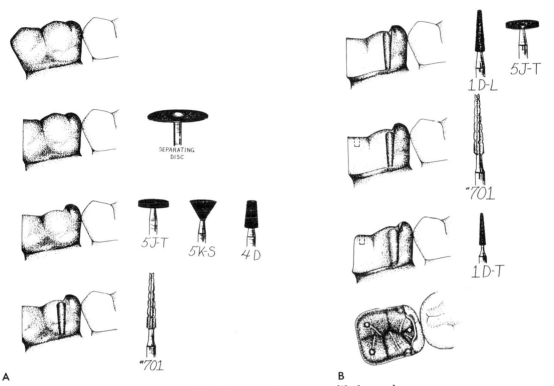

FIGURE 5-35. *Preparation on mandibular molar.*

A, Top to bottom: Uncut tipped tooth; proximal cut; occlusal reduced; buccal and lingual grooves.

B, Top to bottom: Grooves connected to proximal by reducing buccal and lingual; cervical finishing line and pinholes; occlusal view.

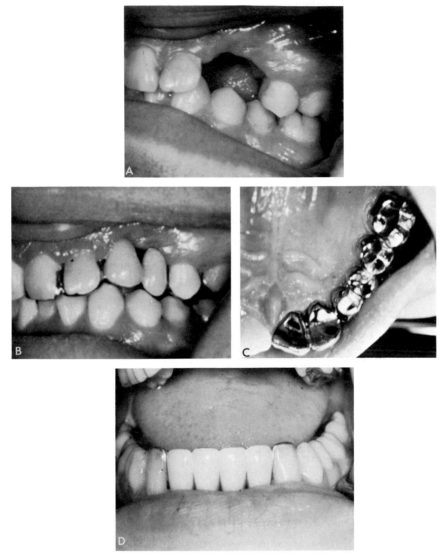

FIGURE 5–36. *A*, Edentulous area with cuspid and first bicuspid missing. The proposed abutment teeth are quite short. The vertical overlap is more than 50 per cent.

B and *C*, Six-unit bridge constructed to restore space (A). Four partial veneer crown retainers were used on the central and lateral incisors, second bicuspid, and first molar abutments. Short crowns and lever arm made this necessary.

D, Mandibular anterior bridge with partial veneer crown retainers on cuspid abutments.

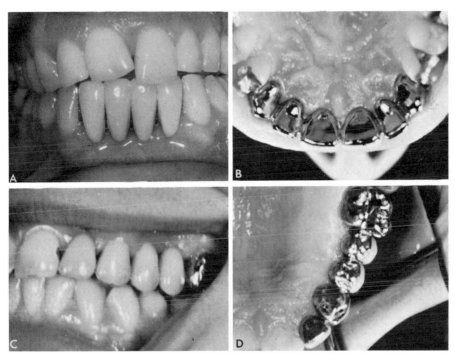

FIGURE 5-37. *A*, Lower six-unit bridge retained by partial veneer crowns on cuspids.
B, Lingual view of six-unit upper anterior bridge supported by partial veneer crown retainers on the cuspids and lateral incisors.

C and *D*, Five-unit upper posterior bridge with a cantilever lateral incisor pontic. Partial veneer crown retainer on the cuspid abutment.

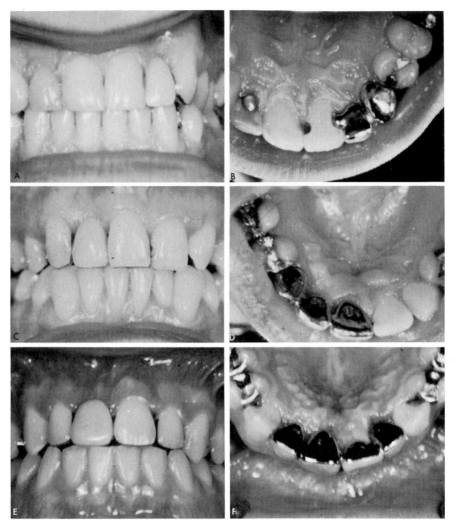

FIGURE 5–38.   *A* and *B*, Two-unit bridge replacing upper left lateral incisor. Partial veneer crown retainer on cuspid abutment with a lingual rest in rest seat prepared in gold foil restoration in distolingual of central incisor.

   C and *D*, Three-unit bridge replacing upper right lateral incisor. Two partial veneer crown retainers. Mesioincisal angle of cuspid preparation should have been rounded slightly.

   E and *F*, Three-unit bridge replacing upper right central incisor. Partial veneer crown retainers and a third partial veneer crown, a single-unit restoration, on left lateral. Lingual extension of pontic was reduced to a minimum because of chronic irritation of the palatal mucous membrane.

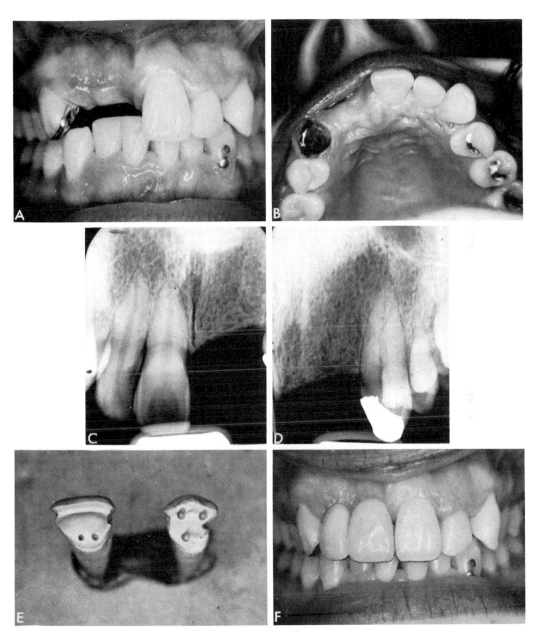

FIGURE 5–39. *A* and *B*, Maxillary anterior space.
C and *D*, Radiographs of abutments. Incisor very thin.
E, Dies of prepared abutments.
F, Cemented bridge.

This retainer should never be used if caries is active; instead, the abutment tooth should be prepared for a full veneer gold crown and the tooth to the distal recontoured and restored.

Mouths restored with fixed partial dentures with partial veneer crown retainers are shown in Figures 5-36, 5-37, 5-38, and 5-39.

REFERENCES

1. Willey, R. E.: Preparation of abutments for veneer retainers. J.A.D.A., *53*:141, Aug. 1956.
2. Maesaka, R. K.: Personal communication.
3. Borkowski, M. J.: Personal communication.
4. Grubb, H. D.: Fixed bridgework. J. Pros. Den., *3*:121, Jan. 1953.
5. Cowger, G. T.: Retention, resistance and esthetics of the anterior three-quarter crown. J.A.D.A., *62*:167, Feb. 1961.
6. Brooks, E. C.: A practical approach for crown and bridge construction. Paper read before Kentucky State D. A., April 1955.
7. Ante, I. H.: Abutments. J. Canad. D. A., *2*:249, 1936.
8. Tinker, H. A.: Three-quarter crowns in fixed bridgework. J. Canad. D. A., *16*:125, March 1950.
9. Thom, L. W.: Principles of cavity preparation in crown and bridge prosthesis. II. The three-quarter crown. J.A.D.A., *41*:443, Oct. 1950.
10. Guyer, S. E.: Partial veneer crowns: preparation alignment. Washington Univ. D. J., *26*:72, May 1960.
11. Paul, F. K.: Personal communication.
12. Scull, J. L.: Personal communication.
13. Oldham, P. R.: Personal communication.
14. Murto, C. B.: Modern bridge retainers. J. Ontario D. A., *33*:15, Feb. 1956.
15. Lyon, D. M.: Abutments in fixed prosthesis. Arkansas D. J., *24*:6, Dec. 1953.

Marcum, J. S.: The tissue response to different crown marginal depths. J. Kentucky D. A., *20*:21-8, April 1968.

Moulton, G. H.: Esthetics in anterior fixed bridge prosthodontics. J.A.D.A., *52*:36, Jan. 1956.

Simpson, D. H.: Considerations for abutments. J. Pros. Den., *5*:375, May 1955.

chapter 6

THE PINLEDGE
RETAINER

In the field of anterior fixed partial dentures, stability and esthetic quality deserve equal consideration. Stability can be obtained with partial veneer and veneered gold crowns and the MacBoyle retainer, even though constructed without finesse. However, to achieve a wholly satisfactory appearance with the partial veneer crown, alterations that might lessen both retention and stability may have to be made in the standard preparation.[1, 2, 3, 4] The veneered gold crown poses the problems of trauma, contour, masking, and shading.[5] The MacBoyle retainer usually leaves much to be desired esthetically.

Preservation of unblemished labial enamel is always an asset to appearance.[6] A correctly designed and well-made pinledge displays minimal metal, requires the least cutting of tooth structure of any of the anterior retainers, and has the expectancy of long life. It is unexcelled if used in mouths in which the caries index is low or in which it has been controlled, if used on caries-free teeth or those that have been restored with gold foil, and if used on teeth with some bulk in the incisal one-third. With meticulous application, when the occlusion is favorable, it can be placed on thin teeth; and if the patient and operator will co-operate in observing the mouth closely in the future, it can be placed over exposed proximal silicate or resin restorations.

There has been much progress during the past ten years in the indirect construction of the pinledge retainer. New techniques in preparation of the abutment tooth and methods of obtaining the die and casting have given the profession a retainer with esthetics equal to that produced by the direct technique heretofore used, and with retention or stability seemingly equal to the partial veneer crown and many of the veneered crowns that are built over the omnipresent tapered preparation.

The use of drills that are small in diameter has made it possible to place pinholes more strategically and thus to make them deeper without heightening the danger of pulpal trauma. The facts that these holes have parallel walls and the castings made to fit into them have closely fitting parallel sides are all-important in augmenting resistance to displacement.[7] The cast pins are small enough to enable them to be covered by a layer of dentin behind the

153

labial enamel. There may be an occasional exception when the 24-gauge wire pin would be more acceptable esthetically, but such a situation is very rare.

A great majority of operators can prepare teeth for the pinledge, provided that a paralleling device is employed while drilling the pinholes. Several such instruments are available.*[8, 9]

It is highly recommended that a diagnostic cast of the arch to receive the fixed prosthesis be mounted on a surveying table, so that by using an analyzing rod the most logical mechanical path of insertion may be determined, although information from radiographs may suggest some modification.

There must be no stress on the teeth when seating a pinledge bridge. It must fit precisely and it must slip into place without interference, or the bridge must be reassembled. In an end-to-end occlusion the casting must provide incisal protection or the path of insertion must be from the lingual. Even here incisal coverage is safer. All joints must be rigid.

INDICATIONS

Formerly the pinledge bridge was used only where moderate torque would be generated and where the lever arm was short or broken by intermediate abutments. Now retention has been greatly increased and seems to compare favorably with more extensive retainers. When used on multiple splinted abutments, resistance to displacement is notable.[10, 11]

Maxillary Arch

In the maxillary arch the pinledge can be used in the following circumstances:
   (1) on the central and lateral incisors when replacing a central;
   (2) on the cuspid and central when the lateral is missing;
   (3) on the central and cuspid when replacing an approximating central and lateral;
   (4) for older persons, on the lateral incisor, or on both the lateral and central, with an inlay or partial veneer crown on the first bicuspid when the cuspid has been lost;
   (5) if cusp angles are flat, on the cuspid, with an inlay or partial veneer crown on the second bicuspid, when the first bicuspid space is to be filled; and
   (6) on the cuspid, central, and lateral when replacing the left lateral and right central.[12]

---

*Loma Linda Parallelometer, Chayes Dental Instrument Corp., Danbury. Conn.
Pontistructor, J. F. Jelenko & Co., Inc., New Rochelle, N. Y.
Jermyn Parallaid, Williams Gold Refining Co., Inc., Buffalo, N. Y.

On maxillary cuspids with long mesioincisal and distoincisal arms and short mesial and distal surfaces, the pinledge, when made with cast pins, has more retention than a partial veneer crown. It is an efficient splinting restoration on upper anteriors, and it may be used to recontour lingual occluding surfaces in oral reconstruction.

Mandibular Arch

In the mandibular arch, when the abutments are caries-free, the pinledge is the retainer of choice when one or two central incisors or one lateral must be inserted. By using a partial veneer crown or pinledge on the cuspid, and pinledges on the central and lateral abutments, a bridge replacing an approximating central and lateral will cause a minimum of mutilation to the abutments. It makes an ideal splinting attachment for slightly mobile mandibular anteriors, and it may be used to recontour lingual surfaces of cuspids or incisors for the support and retention of partial dentures.[13]

PREPARATION

A pinledge preparation is best done at moderate speeds and with a variety of stones and burs (Figs. 6-1 and 6-2). It is a delicate preparation and must be planned from surveyed diagnostic casts and bite-wing radiographs so that the pinholes can be placed to the mesial, distal, and lingual of the pulp without danger of injury.

The operation on a maxillary central incisor may proceed in the following sequence of steps, but this can be altered to suit the convenience of the operator:

    (1) reduction of the marginal ridge and contact area adjacent to the space, and

    (2) reduction of the lingual surface;

    (3) locating and placing ledges;

    (4) making indentations;

    (5) sinking pinholes;

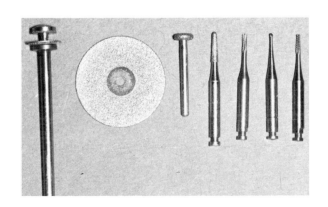

FIGURE 6-1. Left to right:
Mandrel for straight handpiece;
⅝ inch Horico diamond disk;
110P-FG wheel diamond stone (Starlite);
1D-T latch tapered diamond stone (Densco);
No. 556 latch carbide fissure bur (S.S.W.);
No. ½ round latch steel bur;
No. 700 latch carbide tapered fissure bur (S.S.W.).

(6) creating the finishing line; and

(7) beveling the prepared incisal edge and incisal angle.

Proximal Surface.   The marginal ridge (Fig. 6-2*A*) is reduced with a disk in the straight handpiece. This cut, compatible with the path of insertion, extends from midway on the cingulum to the incisal edge, covers the contact area, and reaches the labial surface at this point only. It is made at an angle of 45 degrees from the plane of the lingual surface and may or may not go through the enamel.

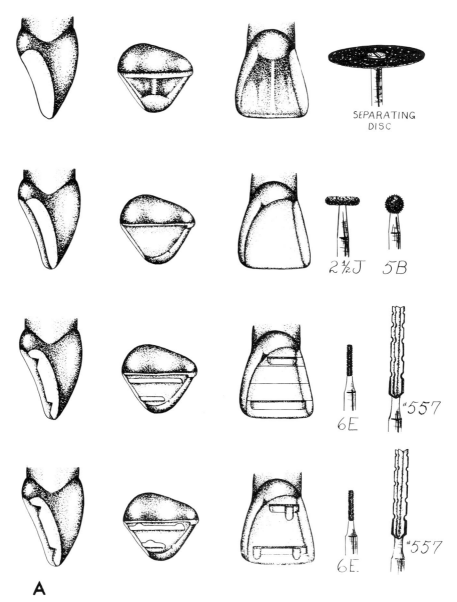

FIGURE 6-2. *Preparation on a maxillary central incisor.*

A, Top to bottom: Reduction of marginal ridge and contact area; reduction of lingual surface; ledges cut; indentations prepared.

Lingual Surface. Using a small wheel stone with a round edge, the lingual surface is reduced evenly to a depth of 0.5 mm., starting from the original cut and extending to and frequently onto the remaining marginal ridge. On teeth with incisal edges without abrasion, the preparation should extend labially just past the crest of the labiolingual curve of the incisal. When the incisal has been abraded to form a surface, the preparation must cover all the occluding area. Almost always a line of metal will border the labioincisal. It need not be wide or unsightly. When the maxillary teeth are

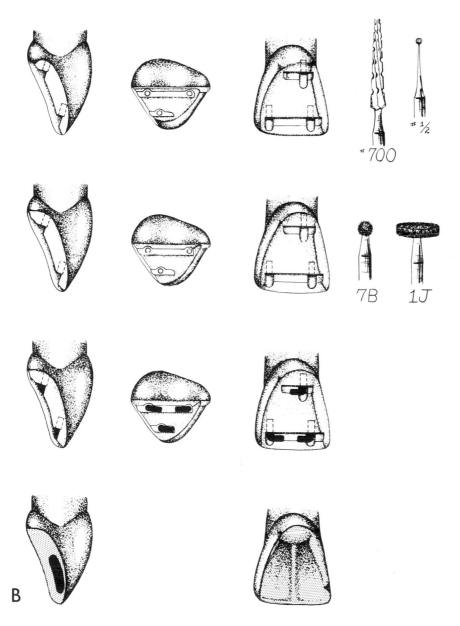

B, Top to bottom: Pinholes: chamfered finishing line and incisal and corner bevel on lingual; pins in position; usual area of solder joint (left) and notch cut to facilitate seating in a plaster impression, in event a direct technique is being used.

thin, with a long vertical overlap and little overjet, a compromise in depth may be necessary, with some space being procured by grinding the incisal edges and upper labial surfaces of the mandibular teeth. On an upper, when the bite is open, and on a lower incisor, less cutting should be done on the lingual, even though the casting will increase the over-all thickness of the tooth, but a discernible finishing line must be produced.

Ledges and Indentations.   Two supporting ledges, as a rule perpendicular to the long axis of the tooth, must be cut on the lingual surface. Exceptions are the maxillary cuspid or an abraded incisor, when the incisal ledge can conform to the outline of the incisal edge of the tooth. The prepared portion of the lingual surface is divided into fourths, and one ledge is made on the line between the incisal and second sections. The other is cut on a new line made by bisecting the prepared cervical fourth incisocervically.

These ledges must completely cross the prepared lingual surface. Linguolabially they should be uniformly as wide as half the diameter of the bur used, with the pulpal wall being parallel to the path of insertion. They should be made with a No. 557 or 57 bur, or a small cylindrical stone. If the tooth is thin, a No. 556 or 56 bur may be substituted. A straight handpiece is advised for upper preparations, a contra-angle for lowers.

Before making the indentations, bite-wing or apical radiographs should be re-examined to verify the exact position of the pulp and the proximal dentinoenamel junctions. The incisal indentations must be *just inside* the marginal ridges between the dentinoenamel junctions and the pulp horns, and the one at the cervical *slightly off center* toward the space. The wider their triangular spread, the greater is the stability of the casting. Using either a No. 557 or 56 bur, the indentations are cut as deep as half of the diameter of the bur and should be parallel to the path of insertion.

Pinholes.   Pinholes may be made with No. 700 or 701 tapered fissure burs, with a No. 1/2 round bur, or with 0.023 inch drills. This phase of the preparation may be done freehand with a straight handpiece on upper teeth and a contra-angle on lowers. (See Figure 6–2B.) The holes must be parallel to the path of insertion, 2.0 to 2.25 mm. deep, and should start from the center of the indentation. When using No. 700 or 701 burs or drills, a pilot hole may be made first with a No. 1/2 round bur, then enlarged with the tapered bur.

When made with drills (see Figs. 6–3 and 6–5), it is recommended that a paralleling device be used, either stabilized on the teeth with modeling compound or held in position by a baseplate.

A self-curing resin baseplate is adapted to the diagnostic cast (Figs. 6–4 and 6–5) so that it covers all the occlusal surfaces of the posterior teeth and leaves uncovered the lingual surfaces of the teeth to be prepared. With the cast still mounted on the surveyor, the paralleling instrument is slipped onto a special analyzing rod (made from a bur to fit exactly the bur guiding sleeve) and is mounted on the baseplate with self-curing resin so that the sleeve is parallel to the predetermined path of insertion.

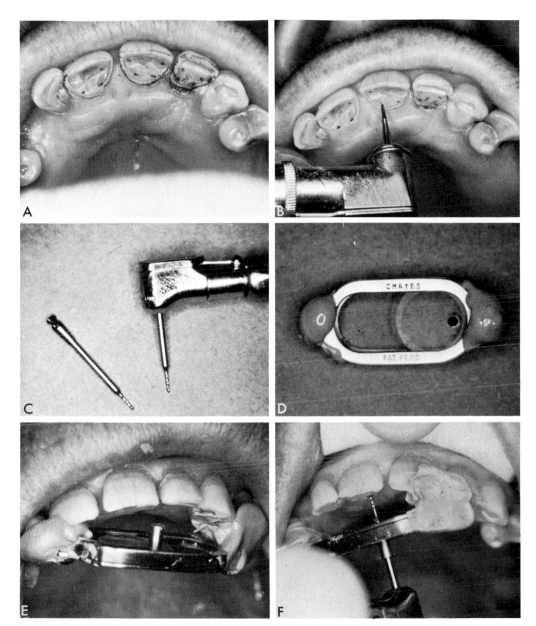

FIGURE 6–3. *A*, Lingual surfaces of three maxillary incisors with preparations outlined and finishing lines prepared. Locations of pinholes marked. Vertical dimension will be increased.

B, Countersinking points of entry for pinholes.

C, Drills 0.023 inch in diameter.

D, Loma Linda Parallelometer with modeling compound on ends. Disk rotates and moves in frame. Sleeve guides bur to make all holes parallel.

E, Parallelometer secured to arch and aligned for preparation of left lateral incisor.

F, Parallelometer set for lingual path of insertion on right central incisor.

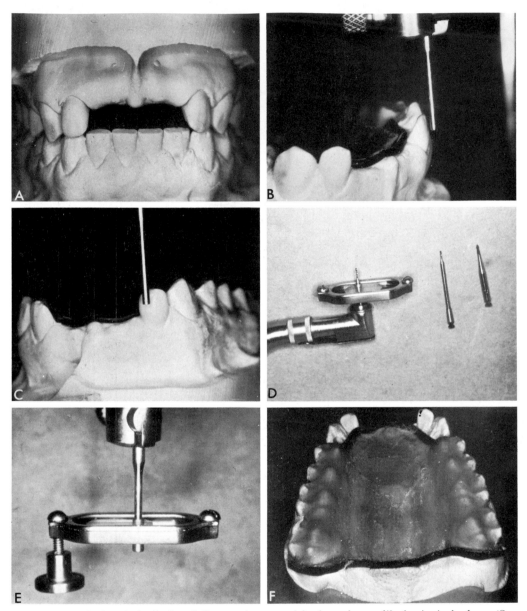

FIGURE 6–4. *A*, Articulated diagnostic casts with altered mandibular incisal edges. (See case history in Chapter 36.)

B and *C*, Using surveyor to help determine path of insertion.

D, Loma Linda Parallelometer and 0.023 inch drill.

E, Parallelometer placed on analyzing rod of surveyor. Attachment for baseplate has been added.

F, Resin base free of abutments, but covering all other occluding surfaces.

The baseplate is removed from the cast and taken to the mouth, where it can be held in position. The pinholes, when drilled, will be parallel to each other, regardless of the number.

In Figures 6-4 and 6-5 four teeth (both laterals and both cuspids) are involved. Before attempting to drill the pinholes, all other phases of the preparation were completed and a carbide bit was used to indent the enamel at the points on the ledges where the pinholes should start. These pinholes were cut 2.0 to 2.25 mm. deep and were made parallel to the normal path of insertion, although had there been reason for it, with the paralleling device the path of insertion could have been angled more to the lingual. Under some circumstances, particularly when using pinledges for splinting teeth, the holes may be made at right angles to the plane of the lingual surfaces, in which event ledges need not be cut on the lingual surfaces. There also may be some advantage to this linguolabial path of insertion when abutment teeth have diverging or converging long axes and incisal seating could endanger a pulp. When the lingual approach is being used on an individual tooth, the paralleler may be stabilized on supporting teeth with modeling compound.

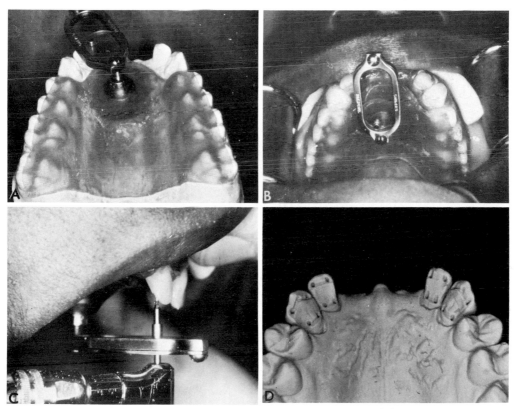

FIGURE 6-5. *A,* Parallelometer secured to acrylic resin palatal plate with sleeve parallel to predetermined path of insertion.

B, Device transferred to maxillary arch.

C, Four abutments have been prepared up to sinking pinholes. Points of entry have been indented with No. ½ round bur. The sixteen pinholes—four in each tooth—will be parallel.

D, Cast of prepared teeth.

On a very thin tooth the holes in the incisal one-third, suitable for pins of bent wire (24-gauge PGP wire*), can be made with a No. 1/2 round bur. With such pins, owing to the color of the wire, there possibly is less chance that a shadow will show through the labial enamel. However, cast posts or pins will serve the purpose in almost every case and under almost all conditions. For example, in mandibular incisors, regardless of bulk, the closer-fitting, even though shorter (1.3 to 1.5 mm.), cast pins give a snug fit that is impossible on these teeth with bent wire pins. On a maxillary lateral or central, when the cingulum is deeply indented, a pin 1.25 mm. long and the size of a No. 702 or 703 bur may be used. With the Pinwaxer† these can be waxed directly or indirectly, without flaws.

Should the operator prefer to use a direct waxing technique, the pin-holes can be made with No. 700 or 701 tapered fissure burs if the pin patterns will be resin or wax, or with drills or No. 1/2 round burs if nylon bristles or wire will be used in the holes.

The Finishing Line and Incisal Bevel.   The finishing line for a pin-ledge is in three sections. The lingual surface segment is a chamfer and is accentuated by using a small round stone from the incisal edge to the point where the proximal cut and cingulum reduction join. The proximal cut has produced a chisel-edge margin on that surface admirably suited for a finishing line. The incisal edge and angle must be beveled, although not drastically. This phase of the finishing line is the final step in this preparation.

TEMPORARY COVERINGS

A pinledge preparation may be covered with temporary stopping or resin. Stopping must be applied to a dry tooth, must be very warm and pliant, and must have minimal contact with the occluding teeth. If the patient is careful about incising, it will stay in place for some time. Fragments that remain in the holes after the covering is taken off can be removed easily with a No. 1/2 round bur rotated in the fingers.

A resin covering can be constructed by drying the tooth surface, packing the pinholes with waxed thread, and, using the brush technique, applying a filling resin. To obtain mechanical retention the resin is extended beyond the margins into undercut areas, because the moisture in the mouth will break down the adhesion of the resin to the tooth structure. Occlusion is adjusted and margins are finished. Removal will be without difficulty.

An indirect technique[14] may be employed for a single unit or a bridge, utilizing the diagnostic and working casts and an alginate impression. (See Figure 6-6.)

Figures 6-7 through 6-12 show the clinical applications of the pin retainer.

---

*The J. M. Ney Company, Bloomfield, Conn.
†The S. S. White Dental Mfg. Co., Philadelphia, Pa. (Designed by E. E. and L. L. Kraus, Milwaukee, Wis.)

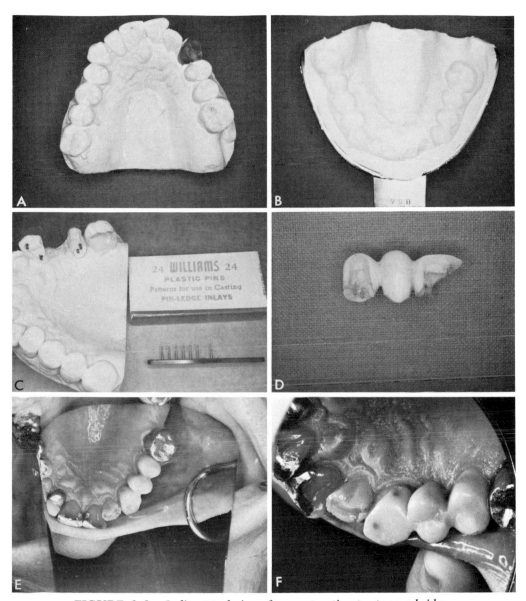

FIGURE 6-6. *Indirect technique for constructing temporary bridge.*

A, Diagnostic cast before extraction of maxillary first bicuspid. Cuspid abutment has been rebuilt to desired form with wax.

B, Alginate impression of prepared diagnostic cast. Impression stored in humidifier at 100 per cent humidity until needed. Abutment and pontic areas will be filled with acrylic filling resin and the impression seated on prepared working cast shown in C.

C, Preformed plastic pins placed in duplicate master cast of preparations.

D, The temporary bridge trimmed and polished.

E, and *F,* Two views of cemented temporary bridge. Cementing material should be soft temporary cement easily fractured. (See Chapter 4.)

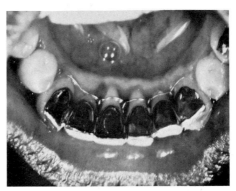

FIGURE 6–7.   Mandibular anterior splint made by Parallelometer technique.

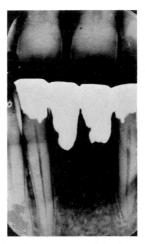

FIGURE 6–8.   Replacing lower central incisors. Pinledges on laterals.

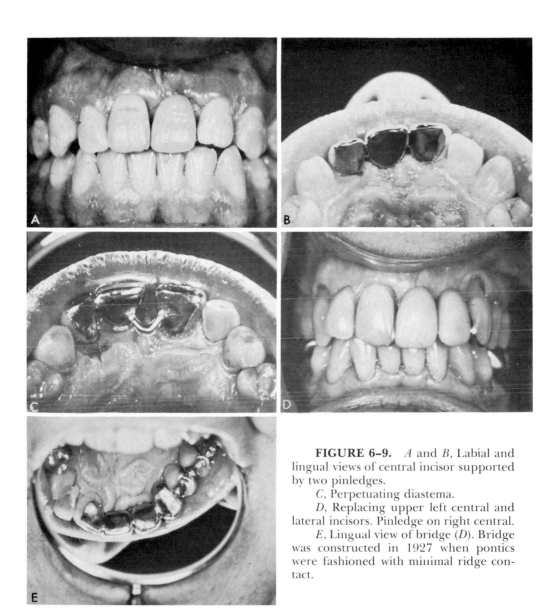

FIGURE 6–9. *A* and *B*, Labial and lingual views of central incisor supported by two pinledges.

C, Perpetuating diastema.

D, Replacing upper left central and lateral incisors. Pinledge on right central.

E, Lingual view of bridge (*D*). Bridge was constructed in 1927 when pontics were fashioned with minimal ridge contact.

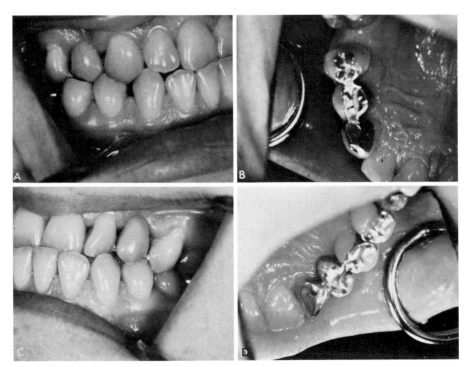

FIGURE 6-10.   *Fixed partial dentures retained by pinledges.*

A and *B*, First bicuspid pontic retained by pinledge on cuspid and inlay in second bicuspid.

C and *D*, Replacing upper cuspid. Pinledge on lateral incisor abutment; inlay in first bicuspid.

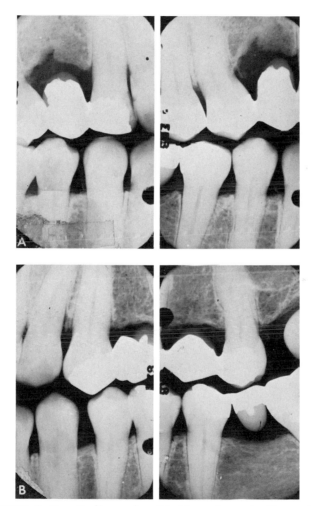

FIGURE 6–11. Radiographs of bridges shown in Figure 6-10.

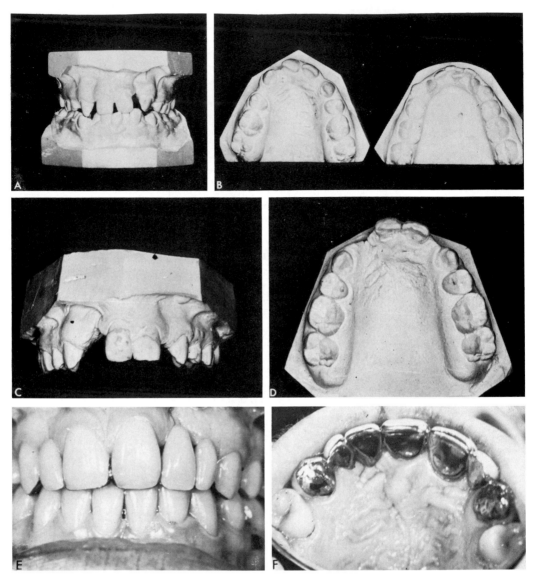

FIGURE 6–12.   Replacing maxillary lateral incisors; repaired cleft between right cuspid and central incisor. Seven-unit maxillary anterior bridge with four pinledge retainers and three lateral incisor pontics. Because of cleft, right lateral space is wide after orthodontic treatment. Each retainer has two wire incisal and two cast cervical pins. Wire was used in the incisal because a smaller hole could be drilled.

A and *B*, Casts of mouth before orthodontic treatment.

C and *D*, Upper arch after orthodontic treatment. The left lateral space is normal in width; on the right it is approximately two-thirds wider than the left. The cuspids have no proximal surfaces. The left central is normal; the right is ultraconcave on the lingual. The right ridge is abnormal, owing to closed cleft.

E, Fixed partial denture retained by four pinledges, each with two incisal wire pins and two cast pins in the cingulum.

F, Lingual view of bridge; three lateral incisor pontics.

REFERENCES

1. Grubb, H. D.: Fixed bridgework. J. Pros. Den., *3*:121, Jan. 1953.
2. Vedder, F. B.: Paper read before Crown and Bridge Symposium. Indiana University School of Dentistry, April 1956.
3. Willey, R. E.: Preparation of abutments for veneer retainers. J.A.D.A., *53*:141, Aug. 1956.
4. Cowger, G. T.: Retention, resistance and esthetics of the anterior three-quarter crown. J.A.D.A., *62*:167, Feb. 1961.
5. Barker, B. C., et al.: The crowning of vital anterior teeth. Aust. D. J., *10*:449, Dec. 1965.
6. Pruden, K. C.: A hydrocolloid technique for pinledge bridge abutments. J. Pros. Den., *6*:65, Jan. 1956.
7. Moffa, J. P., and Phillips, R. W.: Retentive properties of parallel pin restorations. J. Pros. Den., *17*:4, April 1967, p. 387.
8. Baum, L.: Progress report on intraoral precision drilling techniques. J. South. California D. A., *27*:134, April 1959.
9. Baum, L.: Technics for utilizing intraoral aligning devices for achieving parallelism in cavity preparations. J. D. Res., *39*:768, July-Aug. 1960 (Abstract).
10. Baum, L.: New cast gold restorations for anterior teeth. J.A.D.A., *61*:1, July 1960.
11. Curtis, G. H., and Baum, L.: New concepts in splinting the mandibular anterior teeth. J. Periodont., *31*:393, Oct. 1960.
12. Johnston, J. F.: The application and construction of the pinledge retainer. J. Pros. Den., *3*:559, July 1953.
13. Alpert, C. C.: Anterior pinledge abutment. J. Dist. Columbia D. Soc., *34*:11, Feb. 1959.
14. Johnston, J. F., Mumford, G., and Dykema, R. W.: Modern Practice in Dental Ceramics. Philadelphia, W. B. Saunders Company, 1967.

Pinkerton, R. G.: Anterior fixed bridge prosthesis. J.A.D.A., *44*:393, April 1952.
Pruden, K. C.: Abutments and attachments in fixed partial dentures. J. Pros. Den., *7*:502, July 1957.
Sanell, C., Mann, A. W., and Courtade, G.: The use of pins in restorative dentistry. Part I. Parallel pin retention obtained without using paralleling devices. J. Pros. Den., *15*:3, May-June 1965, p. 502.
Mann, A. W., Courtade, G., and Sanell, C.: The use of pins in restorative dentistry. Part II. Paralleling instruments. J. Pros. Dent., *15*:4, July-Aug. 1965, p. 691.

chapter 7

THE INLAY RETAINER

The inlay is a retainer that should be employed only under the most favorable conditions and when workmanship is of the highest order.[1] When an inlay-retained bridge is constructed by one who understands its limitations and does not exceed its potentialities, the prosthesis will have a surprisingly long life. When its use can be justified, minimal tooth surface is covered by metal.

INDICATIONS

For the inlay to be used successfully as a bridge retainer, the span must be short, preferably no wider than one tooth; the mouth must be relatively caries-free or must have entered into a caries-free period; and the clinical crown must be of average length and, in functional occlusion, must not be subjected to undue leverage. The tooth should be vital, with dentin lining all cavity walls. Theoretically only one joint should be soldered, and it should approximate the stronger of the two abutment teeth. With rugged teeth, there can be frequent exceptions to this rule. An inlay may be used to support the free end of a broken-stress bridge, since little or no stress will be transferred from the bridge.[2]

Inlays are being used in increasing numbers in the mouths of the young-age group because of the mounting evidence that crowns for adolescents cause considerable gingival irritation on the buccal and lingual surfaces, especially the lingual. While pulp size and crown length may make it necessary that the cavity preparations be shallow, pins can add to retention. In these cases, both joints are soldered.

CONTRAINDICATIONS

An inlay retainer is contraindicated for a tooth that is rotated, extensively carious, short (except in the very young), extruded, or pulpless, or that has a large cervical restoration. A cavity prepared in a rotated tooth will give substantial retention only when supplemented by two or more pinholes; even

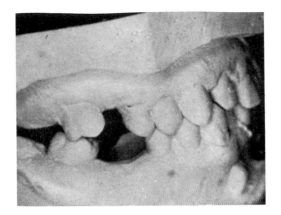

FIGURE 7-1. Mandibular molar has mesial tilt. Tooth should not be built up to occlusion on mesial with inlay retainer. Maxillary space suitable for inlay retainers.

then the inlay may not offer an area receptive to the solder joint. Usually an inlay cavity in a broken-down or short tooth is not retentive. When one abutment is extruded beyond the occlusal plane, the load will be unorthodox and excessive for the surrounding tooth walls. A pulpless tooth is brittle and often the retainer must be supported by cement. When there is cervical caries or a cervical restoration, the walls may be incapable of resisting the force transmitted through the inlay.

An inlay should not be used to build up one section of the occlusal surface of a tipped tooth, because leverage from the protruding casting may overcome stability (Fig. 7-1). It is contraindicated in an older patient, whose teeth may be severely abraded, because the lateral walls probably will be checked or cracked and unequal to the strain induced by mastication. Thus, in order to cover the occlusal surface, the tooth must be shortened so much that the proximal surfaces cannot control displacement.

The inlay retainer should be either an MO or DO restoration. If the abutment is a first molar, it may have steps into the buccal and lingual surfaces.[3] An MOD inlay is contraindicated as the major support for a bridge, because the cavity walls will be unduly weakened by the preparation without there being an increase in holding power. A partial veneer or full veneer gold crown should be substituted.

CAVITY PREPARATION

When compared with a single-unit preparation, the cavity walls for an inlay retainer must be more nearly parallel, there must be added depth and width, and the cavity outline should be extended into the auxiliary grooves (Fig. 7-2).[4] In width, the proximal step should include the buccal and lingual line angles, or go beyond one of them if the tooth is rotated. The occlusal margin should have a wider and heavier bevel so that the walls will have more protection during lateral excursions.

In a molar preparation a pinhole should be placed in the occlusal floor,[5] 1.0 to 2.0 mm. from the remaining marginal ridge. In a bicuspid it should be

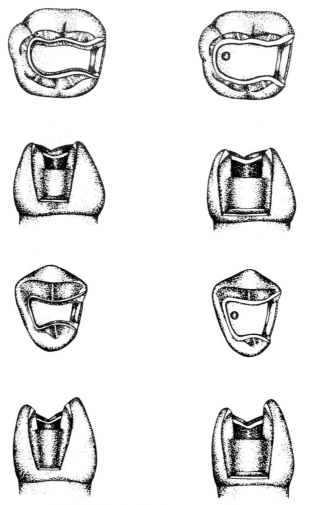

FIGURE 7–2. *Cavity preparations.*

Top to bottom: Occlusal and proximal views of MO preparations in mandibular molar and bicuspid. Left: For single-unit restoration; right: for retainer.

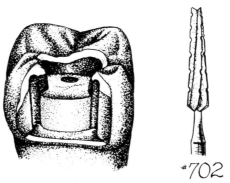

FIGURE 7–3.   MO preparation for maxillary first molar.

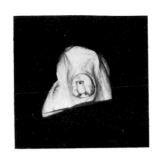

FIGURE 7–4. Preparation with three pinholes in mandibular molar.

adjacent to the marginal ridge. Occlusal pinholes should be 1.5 mm. deep and should be made with a No. 701 or 702 tapered fissure bur. Larger sizes are desirable occasionally. Location and depth are dictated by pulp position, form, and size. In the cervical seat of the cavity, pinholes should be made 1.0 mm. deep with a No. 700 bur and should be a continuation of grooved axial line angles. Pinholes must be in dentin, *not* in cement.

When an MO inlay is to be used in a maxillary first molar, the occlusal seat of the cavity need not cross the transverse ridge unless there is undermining caries in the distal pit or on the distal surface. It should be deeper than the conventional preparation, and the pinhole, to be made with a No. 702 tapered fissure bur, should be against the ridge and 1.5 mm. deep. The axial angles should be grooved with a No. 56 bur, and two pinholes should be made in the cervical seat (Fig. 7–3).

Retention in all inlay retainer cavities is effected not only through the parallel walls and width of the cavity floor, but also by the parallel relationship of the pin in the occlusal pinhole with the casting fitting against the axial walls. An accurately fitting occlusal pin will limit forces against the buccal and lingual walls of the tooth, while pins in the cervical seat of the cavity will transmit any stress to the entire tooth rather than one specific area (Figs. 7–4 and 7–5). In an indirect technique, pinholes should be a little larger in diameter and more shallow.

The instruments and instrumentation are the same as for any inlay preparation (Fig. 7–6).

FIGURE 7–5. Preparation advocated by Markley for either maxillary or mandibular molars.

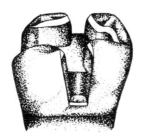
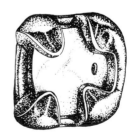

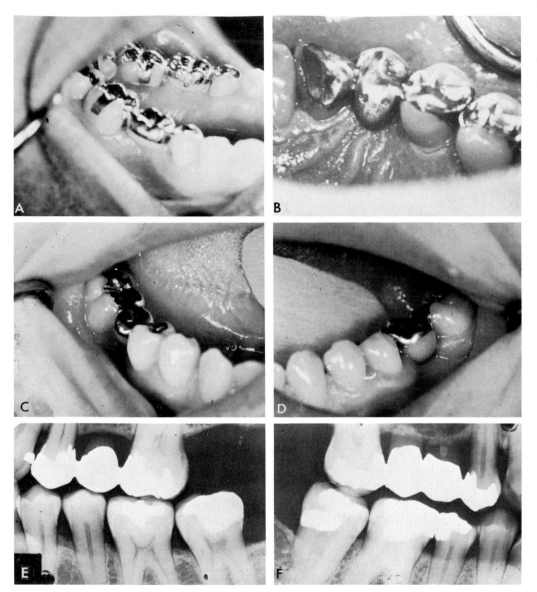

FIGURE 7–6. *Inlay-retained bridges.*

A, Replacing mandibular right first molar. Markley-type inlay retainer in second molar; DO inlay in second bicuspid; distal joint soldered; mesial connector a subocclusal rest.

B, Inlay-pinledge bridge supplying maxillary cuspid.

C and *D*, Inlay-retained bridges in same arch. MO inlays in second molars; DO inlays in second bicuspids; anterior connectors are subocclusal rests.

E, Replacing upper second bicuspid. DO inlay in first molar (note pins) and MOD inlay in second bicuspid (note pin); two solder joints.

F, Four-unit bridge retained by two two-surface inlays. This technique (and also E) is recommended only for an operator who has exceptional skill and judgment. (See Figures 6–10 and 6–11.)

REFERENCES

1. Pruden, K. C.: Abutments and attachments in fixed partial dentures. J. Pros. Den., 7:502, July 1957.
2. Markley, M. R.: The practical application of sound principles to the field of restorative dentistry. J. Pros. Den., 3:96, Jan. 1953.
3. Markley, M. R.: Broken-stress principle and design in fixed bridge prosthesis. J. Pros. Den., 1:416, July 1951.
4. Thom, L. W.: Principles of cavity preparation in crown and bridge prosthesis. III. The inlay abutment. J.A.D.A., 41:541, Nov. 1950.
5. Ante, I. H.: Abutments. J. Canad. D. A., 2:249, 1936.

Gilmore, H. W.: Textbook of Operative Dentistry. St. Louis, The C. V. Mosby Company, 1967.

chapter 8

THE MACBOYLE
RETAINER

The MacBoyle retainer, like the inlay, will be a serviceable retainer if meticulously designed and constructed. Its application is limited, but in a few instances it supersedes all other retainers.

INDICATIONS

The MacBoyle retainer may be used on mandibular central and lateral and maxillary lateral incisors, even though these teeth have proximal caries or large pulps. It is akin to the partial veneer crown, but the preparation is not so deep and the retention is derived from grooves at the labial line angles instead of on the proximal surfaces. It is indicated particularly for adolescents, but it will be satisfactory for any patient who does not object to a display of metal. It should be considered primarily as a retainer for temporary bridges.

PREPARATION

The steps in the preparation are as follows:
(1) reduction of the mesial and distal surfaces,
(2) reduction of the lingual surface from the crest of the cingulum to the incisal edge, and
(3) reduction of the incisal edge;
(4) beveling the mesiolabial and distolabial line angles;
(5) grooving the mesiolabial and distolabial bevels;
(6) reduction of the cingulum and establishing the cervical finishing line; and
(7) placing a pinhole in the cingulum.
The mesial and distal cuts, made with a disk in a straight handpiece, should be parallel to the path of insertion. Labially they can extend beyond

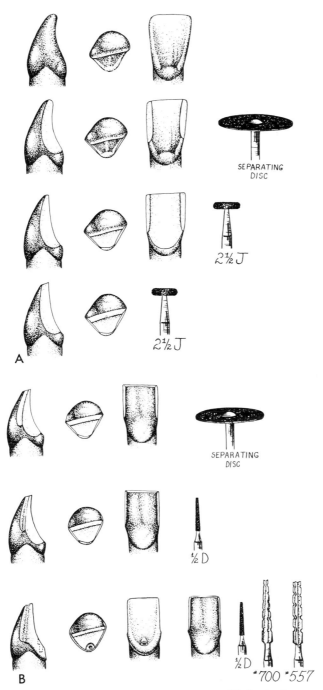

FIGURE 8–1. *Preparation on a mandibular incisor.*

A, Top to bottom: Uncut tooth; proximal slices; lingual reduction; incisal bevel.

B, Top to bottom: Labial line angles beveled; labial chamfer; finishing line, lingual pinhole, and rounded angles at labioincisal.

the line angles, but should converge lingually less than the proximal cuts for the anterior partial veneer crown (Fig. 8-1A).

The lingual surface may be prepared 0.5 mm. deep, with a round-edge wheel stone of appropriate size. This cut, starting on the cingulum, must include the incisal edge. Here the reduction is made at an angle similar to the abrasion, or indicated abrasion, on this surface. Using a disk or stone, the labial line angles can be beveled from 0.3 to 0.5 mm. onto the labial surface and as far cervically as the contour of the tooth will permit, which usually is three-fifths or two-thirds of the length of the surface (Fig. 8-1B). A small cylindrical or tapered stone is used to make the bevels concave, but not so deep that their axial margins are at right angles to the labial enamel surface (Fig. 8-2).

The cingulum is shaped the same as for a partial veneer crown. The cervical finishing line is continued onto the proximal surface and may go into the gingival crevice, although this is not a requisite.

A No. 700 or 701 tapered fissure bur is used to make a pinhole in the cingulum, 1.0 mm. deep and parallel to the path of insertion. The labial margin at the incisal edge is beveled only enough to protect the enamel rods.

When accelerated speeds are used for this preparation, the proximal surfaces should be reduced with a disk to avoid an exaggerated display of metal at the labial line angles. Otherwise, instrumentation closely follows the initial steps for a partial veneer crown.

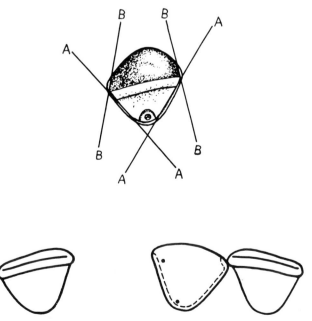

FIGURE 8-2. Schematic explanation of MacBoyle preparation, showing retentive grasp on labial. MacBoyle preparation combined with pinledge on rotated tooth. Lines A-A designate the direction of the proximal cuts; lines B-B show the labial convergence of the labial bevels, which provides resistance to lingual displacement.

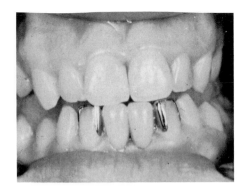

FIGURE 8-3. Lower anterior bridge constructed for adolescent. Pulps large, deep proximal caries. New bridge, with veneered crown retainers, was built after pulps had receded sufficiently to permit adequate preparations.

Direct wax patterns may be carved using the same technique advocated for the maxillary anterior partial veneer crown.

The sprue should be attached outside the mouth and in the same manner as for a pinledge retainer.

Figure 8-3 shows the clinical application of the MacBoyle retainer.

chapter 9

THE WORKING CAST

Many types and combinations of impression materials have been used for the fabrication of the fixed partial prosthesis, each having advantages and disadvantages. The two most popular kinds are the rubber base materials and the reversible hydrocolloids. The use of rubber base impression materials has become widespread since their introduction, often displacing hydrocolloid.

RUBBER BASE IMPRESSION MATERIALS

The rubber base materials fall into two broad classifications: the polysulfide rubbers and the silicones, of which there are several brands now on the market. Among the ways in which they are superior to hydrocolloid may be listed (1) the ability to pour two stone casts in one impression; (2) the possibility of seating metalized dies in a full arch impression and making a working cast with removable units; (3) the capacity to withdraw plastic pins and nylon bristles and thus reproduce all sizes and lengths of pinholes in the stone cast; (4) slightly lengthened working time; and (5) a more varied application in many offices.

Selection of a material probably will be based on office routine, mastery of the material, and objective handling characteristics. Discussion of the manipulation of some of these materials follows.

Polysulfide Rubber Impressions

The polysulfide rubber is prepared by combining two pastes. One tube, usually labeled "base material," contains a mercaptan, a compound having extremely reactive −SH terminals on the molecule.[1, 2] The other tube, labeled "accelerator," in most instances contains lead peroxide and small amounts of sulfur; such agents as zinc oxide, stearic acid, and calcium sulfate are added to regulate certain properties. Polymerization, and hence curing of the paste in the mouth to an elastic impression, is accomplished by mixing the second paste with the first. The basic compositions of these synthetic rubbers have now been well established, and shelf life and quality fluctuations among batches are no longer problems.

The individual tubes of the base material and the accelerator are marked with the particular lot number of the batch. The composition of the tubes is carefully balanced for each batch to insure the expected setting time and viscosity. Contents of partially used tubes of either the base material or the accelerator should *not* be mixed with a newly purchased tube of the other paste *unless* they have the same lot number.

The polysulfide rubber materials generally are brown in color and have a pungent odor (less noticeable to the patient than to the operator), are sticky, and for the inept can be messy to use. Clothing must be protected.

As with hydrocolloid, the manipulation of each of these materials must be punctiliously standardized. The variables that affect precision and sharpness of detail are common to both.

Construction of the Tray. In contrast to hydrocolloid, a lesser bulk of material is desirable in making a rubber base impression. Dimensionally true dies and casts cannot be produced regularly when ordinary stock impression trays are used. Since research has shown that precision of the rubber base impression is in part dependent on a thin, uniform layer of material, with an optimal thickness of 2.0 to 3.0 mm., a tray must be built to assure an even, minimal thickness of impression material around the preparations and working area in order to construct well-fitting, complicated restorations such as bridges.[3] It must be emphasized that a stiff tray, adherence of the rubber to the tray, and careful control of bulk are all essential to accuracy.

Divers satisfactory self-curing resin tray materials are available, and techniques for their use are basically the same. One layer of baseplate wax, or a layer of asbestos instead, is adapted over a diagnostic cast to create the space needed for the rubber (Fig. 9-1). This space is maintained in the oral cavity by stops that make contact with teeth or ridge tissue and preclude further seating of the tray. Stops are made by removing wax from the occlusal surfaces or incisal edges of three or more teeth that will not be used as abutments. These supporting teeth should be widely separated to form a tripod that will allow the tray to be held without movement during setting of the impression material. If the remaining teeth are insufficient to stabilize the tray, then one or two of the stops should be in contact with the ridge tissue, but definitely not in areas associated with the prosthesis.

Tin foil is burnished over the wax to keep it from contaminating the inside of the tray, and to prevent the impression material from pulling away and being permanently deformed when removed from the mouth. The tray resin is mixed in accordance with the manufacturer's directions, and pressed over the prepared cast; it should fill the spaces cut out for the stops. The tray should include enough of the soft tissue area so that pontics can be aligned, but should not reach so far apically that deep tissue undercuts are involved needlessly. To do so would make removal from the mouth difficult and might cause deformation of the impression material. If an extensive

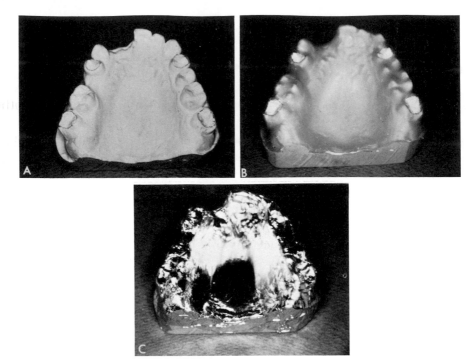

FIGURE 9–1.   *A*, Diagnostic cast with tray stops outlined on four teeth.

B, Wax over diagnostic cast to provide space for impression material. Stop areas cut through wax.

C, Wax tin-foiled to prevent contamination of tray resin.

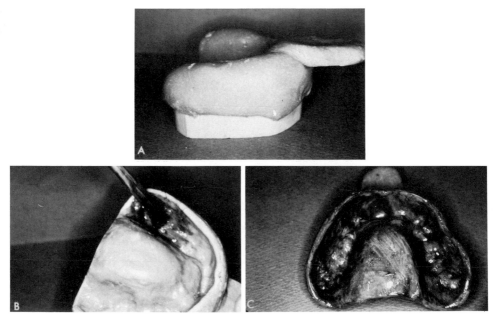

FIGURE 9–2.   *A*, Resin applied to waxed and foiled diagnostic cast.
B and *C*, Tray being coated with adhesive to secure rubber impression.

undercut must be included, it should be blocked out with wax before covering the cast with the single sheet of baseplate wax (Fig. 9-2).

After the material has set, the tray is removed from the cast, the tin foil and wax are stripped from its inner surface, and the borders are trimmed with an acrylic bur or stone.

Preparation of the Tray or Band. The rubber impression material must be held tenaciously to the sides of a rigid* tray or band for an impression of a single tooth. If it pulls away during removal from the mouth, irreparable distortion will result. To forestall this situation, the manufacturer supplies a rubber cement to coat the tray and thereby provide adhesion between the impression material and the tray. The cement is applied approximately 8 minutes before the tray or band is to be filled with the impression material, and it works very well if the surface of the vehicle is clean and sparingly coated. There must be more than one coat, as the acrylic resin tends to absorb the cement.

The Gingival Crevice. Before preparation of the abutment teeth the gingival crevice should be explored (Fig. 9-3). In the young patient it will be shallow and the gum will be more troublesome to retract. In the adult patient the depth is customarily more than 1.0 mm., giving room not only to place the cervical margin where, theoretically, it will be shielded against both recurrent caries and recession, but also to displace the tissue for an elastic impression. If extension of the preparation into this crevice is impracticable, the type of the cervical finishing line and its outline must be determined by the preference and judgment of the operator.

Mouth Preparation. Elastic impression materials will not significantly displace tissue, saliva, blood, mucus, or debris, and contact with any one of these, excepting tissue, will ruin an impression. Therefore, the most urgent aspects of mouth preparation are the lateral movement of the gingival tissue to uncover the cervical margin, or removal of a narrow wedge of the soft tissue to attain the same end, and cleaning and drying of the total area to be included in the impression.

---

*A pliable matrix will invariably distort when taken from the mouth.

FIGURE 9-3. Types of gingival crevices. Left to right: adolescent; adult; slight recession. (Courtesy of J. F. Jelenko & Co., Inc.)

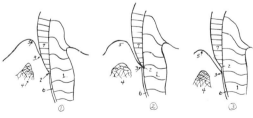

1 Dentin
2 Cemento-Enamel Junction
3 Gingival Attachment
4 Alveolar Process
5 Gingival Crest
6 Cementum
7 Enamel
8 3-5 = Depth of Crevice

Methods of Tissue Displacement.   Displacement of tissue, or exposing the margin of the preparation, may be done by mechanical pressure alone, which is slow and at times uncomfortable, or by mechanical pressure and drugs that will relax the soft tissue and inhibit the seepage of blood or serum (Fig. 9-4).[4] Surgical removal of gingival tissue demands a perfected technique, which will be discussed and illustrated in a limited way.

MECHANICAL DISPLACEMENT.   The mechanical method is applied most successfully to full veneer gold crown preparations or when surgical intervention is not warranted to alter an irregular or high gingival outline. An aid to, rather than a means of, marginal exposure, it is done with an aluminum shell that has been trimmed to conform to the gingival contour and *to rest on the occlusal surface* of the prepared tooth **without impinging** at any point on the tissue. The patient should be asked to close and contour the occlusal surface of the shell, after which occlusal irregularities must be smoothed and the cervical margin-gingival tissue relationship rechecked. This shell, coated at the cervical margin or partially filled with a soft temporary stopping that has been heated until flexible, is replaced in its predetermined position on the tooth. The stopping will be extruded, displacing the gingiva.

Outside the mouth, the cervical of the temporary stopping must be trimmed so that the tissue will be displaced laterally without blanching. A drop of cavity varnish or of zinc oxide and eugenol paste is placed inside the temporary crown, which is returned to the dried tooth for at least 12 hours. The stopping in the gingival crevice should be smoothed with a warm instrument.

This mode of coverage and displacement is acceptable if preparations

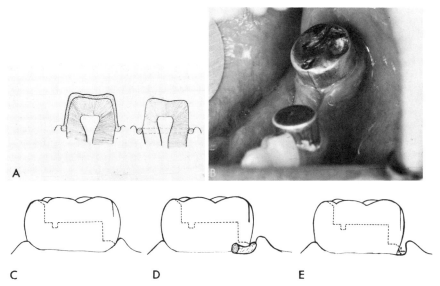

FIGURE 9-4.   *A*, Two methods of tissue displacement.
B, Mechanical displacement of tissue.
C and *D*, Displacing gingival tissue with cord and astringent liquids.
E, Correct type of displacement.

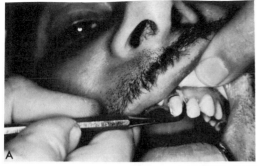
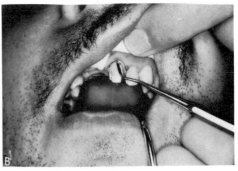
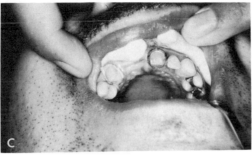

FIGURE 9-5. *A* and *B*, Packing gingival crevice with cotton fibers saturated with an alum solution.

C, Packing in position around each tooth. Alum was activated by an application of Hemodent. Displacement was lateral.

and impressions cannot be made at the same sitting. It is also suitable on posterior teeth prepared for partial veneer crowns.

WARNING: Displacement of tissue, if sustained for the entire construction period, may cause prolonged or even lasting recession. The resultant uncovered neck of the abutment may be sensitive and susceptible to caries.

COTTON FIBERS, COTTON CORD, ALUM, AND HEMODENT FOR TISSUE DISPLACEMENT. Gingival tissue can be displaced without risk with alum saturated fibers* and Hemodent Hemostatic Solution.† Other cords, equally efficacious, are Gingi-Pak,‡ Hemodent,† and Pascord.§

Injury to tissue is negligible, and packing may be repeated at once if desirable. The area should be dried and *kept dry* throughout the procedure, and the impregnated fibers or cord should be packed into the crevice in all areas where the preparation is below or at the gingival crest. More than one layer of cotton may be placed if the crevice is deep. Hemodent or Orostat,‡ carried between the beaks of cotton pliers, may be used to dampen, but not flood, the string (Fig. 9-5).

After 10 minutes, the crevice should be examined for displacement of tissue. If too little has been effected, or if hemorrhage or tissue seepage

*Westwood Dental Mfg. Co., Inc., Van Nuys, Calif.
†Premier Dental Products Co., Philadelphia, Pa.
‡Surgident Ltd., Los Angeles, Calif.
§Pascal Company, Seattle, Wash.

persists, the area must be repacked with fresh material for an additional 5 minutes.

Cotton, twisted into a loose string, is a very good pack and is easily used. Cord in various sizes may be soaked in a saturated solution of alum, dried, stored, and cut off as called for, but a kit now on the market is convenient and well stocked.†

The packing should push the gingival tissue laterally and expose the tooth surface 0.35 to 0.5 mm. past the cervical margin. If the impression material is hydrocolloid, after the mouth is rinsed, a clean, unimpregnated No. 8 thread may be tamped into the crevice to protract displacement in order that two impressions may be taken.

There are cogent reasons for using Hemodent rather than Orostat. It has none of the side effects of epinephrine, while Orostat is stronger than the maximal dosage recommended by quite a number of authorities. Hemodent does cause a granular residue in the presence of blood, but this can be removed.

Harrison[5] has shown conclusively that zinc chloride drastically affects the soft tissue and that healing following its use takes up to 60 days. It will effectively displace tissue, but lasting damage can be inflicted if it is mishandled, although some operators who are still using hydrocolloid still advocate its use.

EXPOSING CERVICAL MARGIN BY ELECTROSURGERY.   The cervical finishing line on a prepared abutment can be uncovered very satisfactorily by electrosurgical procedures[6] instead of by gingival displacement. The authors believe that the technique should be discussed thoroughly, demonstrated, and supervised critically. A detailed exposition is not feasible here.

It should be used only where the gingival tissue is healthy. Any periodontal problem should be eradicated before preparation of the tooth and excision of tissue. Cutting is done under local anesthesia (Figs. 9-6 and 9-7), the area is flushed with a 3 per cent solution of hydrogen peroxide (Fig. 9-8), and the impression is taken immediately. The type of cut is shown in Figure 9-9.

Healing should be uneventful and require no gingival packing. The tissue should recover to its original form (Fig. 9-10).

Mixing Impression Material.   A stiff yet slightly flexible spatula should be used to manipulate the material (Fig. 9-11). Paper mixing pads are commonly used, but glass slabs are advantageous since they can be cooled and in this way afford a longer setting time if wanted. Regardless of the kind of slab used, it should have a large surface area so that the pastes may be spread out widely during mixing. The manufacturer's directions for proportions must be methodically followed, as even seemingly trivial digressions may cause erratic setting.[7] Increased room temperature or high humidity does hasten the setting. In some climates, an air-conditioned operating room is indispensable to institute an atmosphere that will guarantee ample working time.

---

†Westwood Dental Mfg. Co., Inc., Van Nuys, Calif.

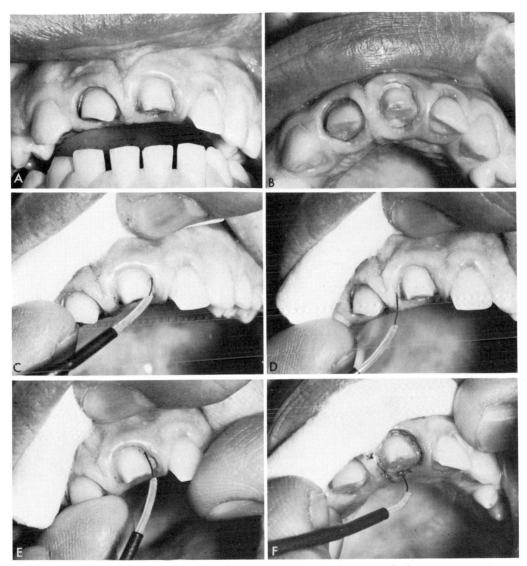

FIGURE 9-6. *Electrosurgical excision of tissue around prepared abutment or teeth prepared for single-unit restorations.*

A and *B*, Maxillary central incisors prepared for porcelain veneered gold crowns. Soft tissue is healthy. Patient had been on drug therapy.

C, D, E, and *F,* Beginning and continuing stages of electrosurgical removal of tissue to uncover cervical finishing line (margin) of preparation.

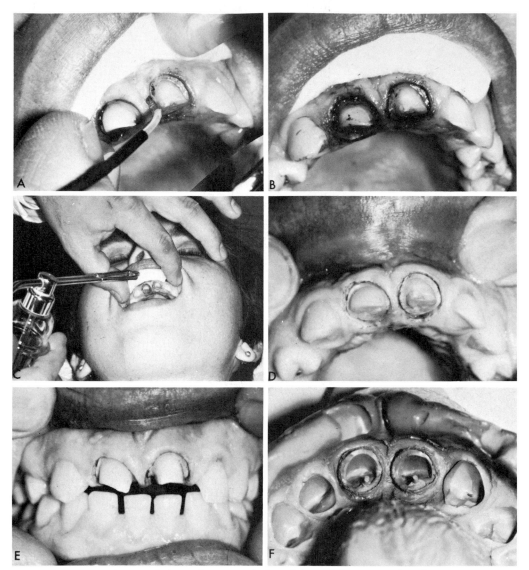

FIGURE 9–7. *Electrosurgical excision of tissue (continued).*
A and *B*, Completion of tissue removal.
C, Preparing to flush area of excision with solution of hydrogen peroxide.
D and *E*, Incisal and labial views of operated gingival margins.
F, Impression of maxillary arch.

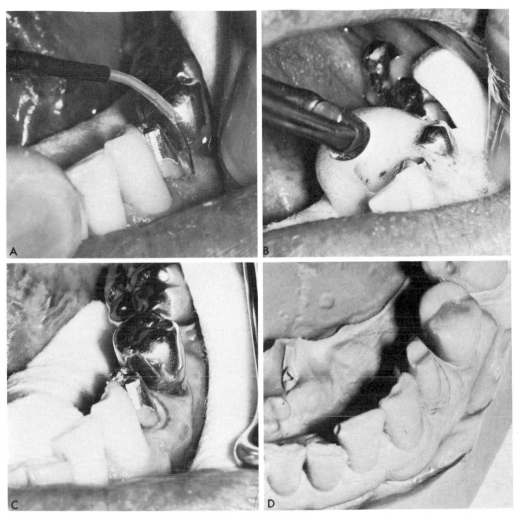

FIGURE 9–8. *Electrosurgical excision of tissue around mandibular bicuspid.*

A, Excision of tissue around buccal margin.
B, Flushing area with 3 per cent solution of hydrogen peroxide.
C, Crevice created by electrosurgical removal of tissue.
D, Cast showing crevice. Margin can be waxed without interference.

Most of the materials are furnished in at least two consistencies that are very similar to the syringe and tray hydrocolloids. One is thin, to be used for injecting into the cavity preparation, and the other is heavy-bodied, for filling the tray. A double-mix technique will minimize trapping of bubbles. Better adaptation and fewer chances for error will result from watchful injection followed by pressure from the less resilient rubber in the tray.

The syringe material is mixed until all streaks are gone (approximately 1 minute), and is then transferred to a Dappen dish. A proper mix of a polysulfide rubber impression material is shown in Figure 9–14C. The open end of the syringe barrel is placed into the mixture, a sufficient quantity is

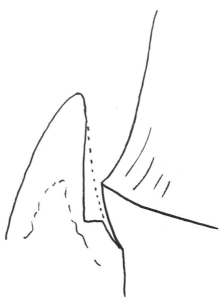

FIGURE 9–9.   Schematic drawing of ideal crevice created by electrosurgical removal of tissue.

drawn into the barrel, the excess is wiped off the outside, and the nozzle assembly is screwed on. (Wiping off the excess should be done with care or the syringe may be hard to disassemble and clean.) The heavy-bodied material is mixed and the tray loaded.

Zinc oxide-eugenol cement frequently is used as a temporary filling material or as a luting agent in the cementation of temporary crowns. Since eugenol curbs the set of the rubber impression materials, whenever such a cement has been employed the teeth should be meticulously cleansed before taking the impression.

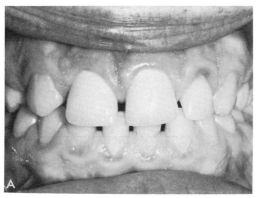
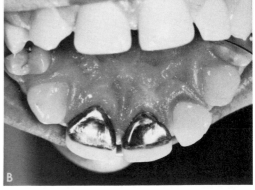

FIGURE 9–10.   *A* and *B*, Labial and lingual views of tissue repair of excised areas shown in Figures 9-6 and 9-7.

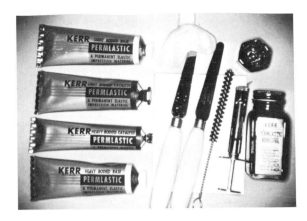

FIGURE 9-11. Material and equipment needed for the impression.

Injecting and Seating the Tray. The use of a syringe for injecting polysulfide rubber impression material is very helpful and will facilitate flow into the intricacies of the preparation and lessen the possibility of trapping bubbles (Fig. 9-12).[8, 9] Several types are available (Fig. 9-13). One that can be loaded by drawing the material into the barrel seems to be best (Fig. 9-14).

The syringe tip is placed in one of the cervical angles of the preparation, very near the tooth surface. These are the areas to be filled first, the syringe being handled so that the gingival crevice is filled under light but positive pressure (Fig. 9-15). The syringe tip is moved up to and across the occlusal. If the tooth has an MOD or PV preparation, the syringe is placed in the other cervical area, again very close to the tooth surface, and this area is filled as the syringe is moved toward the occlusal (Fig. 9-16). The occlusal surfaces of the approximating teeth and all surfaces of the abutments are covered. For a full crown, the gingival crevice is filled first; then with the syringe tip against the tooth and working with a circular motion around the tooth toward the occlusal, this surface is covered last. (See Figures 9-15 and 9-17.)

When pinholes have been made with tapered fissure burs, they will accept the small size syringe tip and may be injected and duplicated with polysulfide or silicone rubber. Immediately following injection with the syringe, the tray is filled with heavier material (Fig. 9-17), seated in the mouth, and held immobile.

FIGURE 9-12. Cross section of two polysulfide rubber impressions. One at left was single mix and shows more and larger internal bubbles than one at right, which was taken with a double-mix procedure. These bubbles are dangerous, since their collapse results in distortion.

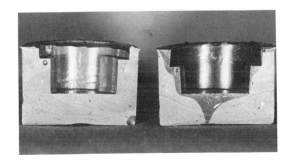

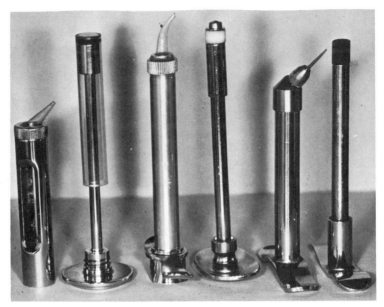

FIGURE 9-13.   Three different syringes available for polysulfide rubbers.

Clinical Manipulation.   One of the commonest causes for failure is premature removal of the impression. Curing continues for some time, and adequate polymerization must take place before it is taken from the mouth. The shortest possible length of time from the start of the first mix until the impression is removed is 10 minutes, during which time the tray is seated in the mouth approximately 7 or 8 minutes. Whatever the brand of rubber impression material being used, any reduction in this time will encourage distortion.

The impression is dislodged with a snap, removed, washed, and inspected. If free of menacing flaws, the impression is either poured in stone or electroplated.

Occasionally small voids or deficiencies may be detected. In such a case it is often advocated that these areas be filled with a mix of the syringe material and the impression reseated—a so-called wash technique. The stress generated and inability to reseat the impression exactly *contraindicate the use of such a procedure.* A new impression must be taken.

Storing Impression.   One of the publicized arguments for the use of the rubbers is their excellent dimensional stability, which supposedly will permit safe storage of the impression indefinitely. These claims are *not* based on fact.[10] There is no doubt that some dimensional change does occur with time and that these changes are due to further polymerization and to the release of internal stress. Distortion, particularly on preparations involving long and parallel walls, can be detected readily in a matter of hours (Fig. 9-18). In regard to storage of rubbers there probably is greater leeway than with hydrocolloid; nevertheless, it is advisable to pour the rubber base impression within the first hour, especially if the first cast poured is to be

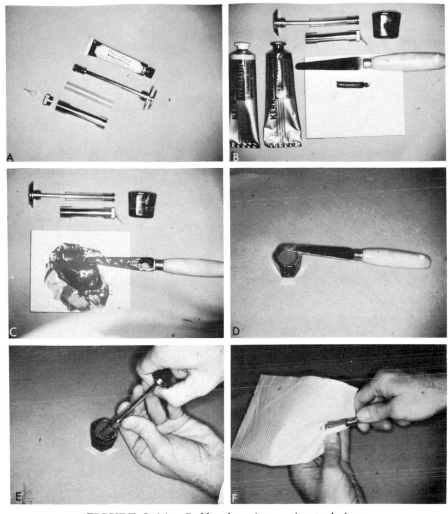

FIGURE 9–14. *Rubber base impression technique.*

    A, Syringe.
    B, Armamentarium assembled.
    C, Rubber mixed.
    D, Transferred to dish.
    E, Filling syringe.
    F, Cleaning syringe.

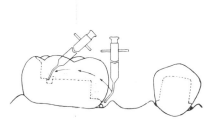

FIGURE 9–15. Syringe should be placed first at cervical margin and moved toward occlusal extremity of the preparation. (Courtesy of J. F. Jelenko & Co., Inc.)

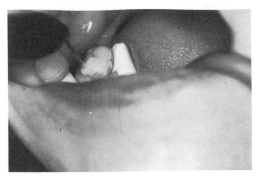

FIGURE 9-16.   Covering all surfaces of tooth with rubber base injected from syringe.

removed after 1 hour and sectioned for dies (Fig. 9-19). The second, or working, cast would then be poured not more than 3 hours after removal from the mouth. The range of certainty beyond this interval is questionable.

The Die.   Several stones for constructing the dies are on the market, e.g., Vel-Mix and Duroc.* Compared with the older stones[11] these newer materials (Class II stones) are harder and have a low (approximately 0.06 per cent) setting expansion. Differences in the physical properties of the brands are of no consequence, and selection may be governed by color and contrast to the wax pattern.[12]

The cast must be poured attentively, since a chalklike surface, nodules, or other imperfections may necessitate another appointment and impression. The manufacturer's directions should be followed in regard to the water-powder ratio for each stone, because variation influences surface smoothness as well as strength and setting expansion. Mechanical spatulation, which in this case is best done under vacuum, is valuable in assuring a compact, smooth surface. The stone is added in small increments and is mechanically vibrated into the mold, using *mild* agitation. The tendency is to use too much vibration, which results in holes in the die.[13] While the stone is setting, the poured impression is placed back in the humidifier in an atmosphere of 100 per cent humidity. The stone gains its strength slowly; therefore, the die should not be removed from the impression in less than 30 minutes, and preferably an hour. (See Figure 9-42.) Premature separation will cause a rough surface. Although it is desirable to separate the die within 2 or 3 hours, generally no harm will be done by waiting longer (even overnight) if the impression was treated in the potassium sulfate solution. No attempt should be made to fabricate the wax pattern until the stone has fully hardened, about 24 hours later.

Various solutions are now available that are added as a partial substitute for the water in order to yield a little harder stone. Unfortunately, such "gypsum hardeners" increase the setting expansion. It is doubtful that the

---

*The Ransom & Randolph Co., Toledo, Ohio.

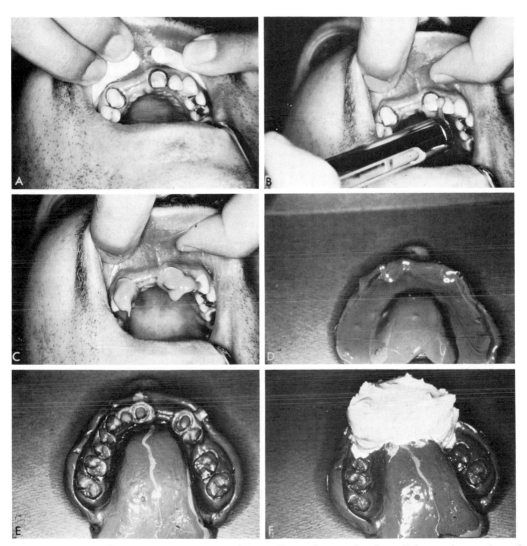

FIGURE 9–17. *A,* Tissue displaced laterally and to a depth well beyond margins of preparations. Area is isolated so that field may be kept dry during injection and seating of tray.

B, Starting the injection in interproximal area has a tendency to help force rubber into crevice. Syringe may be moved either to labial or lingual, but crevice and cervical margin must be covered first; then, with a circular motion, crown is covered, finishing at incisal.

C, Abutments and adjacent teeth covered with syringe material.

D, Tray filled with heavy-bodied material.

E, Impression removed and washed.

F, Area of abutments poured with stone.

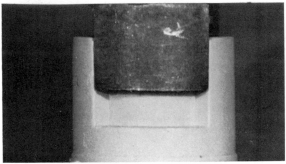

FIGURE 9-18. Gross distortion resulting in a silicone impression poured at 2 days. Casting was made on original die and will fit stone cast if impression is poured at once.

increase in surface hardness justifies the sacrifice in the accuracy of the die. Resin, sometimes reinforced with particles of metal, is also used as a die material. In this case, the polymerization shrinkage of the resin results in an undersize die.

It is apparent that there is no special advantage in using a material other than stone for the construction of the working die.

The experienced technician or dentist should be able to pour the impression without trapping air voids. Should there be a problem, a wetting agent may be used; the impression may be soaked for a minute in a detergent solution, the surface dried, and the stone poured with less turbulent vibration.

The cast to be sectioned for dies should be trimmed and a fine jeweler's saw used to cut it from the ridge through to within 3.0 mm. of the base. Pressure at either end will fracture the sections. If those sections that contain the reproductions of the abutments are trimmed so that the cervical margin of the preparation will have the greatest circumference on the die, there will be room for carving, and any tooth contour cervical to the margin of the preparation will be visible.

In another method for die construction, one impression may be poured to 2.5 mm. above the cervical margins of the teeth (Fig. 9-20).[14] Just after the stone is poured, dowel pins, flat on one side, should be set into the abutments almost parallel to the long axes of those teeth. Wire loops are placed to engage the second pouring of stone. Centering and paralleling of the dowel pins in the impression also can be done mechanically.[14]

After the stone has set in a humidifier, the stone surface is dried and lubricated with either petrolatum or shellac, and the ends of the dowel pins are covered with small balls of wax. The remainder of the impression is then filled, covering the wax on the ends of the dowel pins. As a guide to sectioning, the added stone should differ in color from the original.

With the use of a jeweler's saw, the abutment teeth are sectioned through the initial pouring of stone. The die can be detached by cutting out the wax at the end of the dowel pins and tapping the pins with a metal instrument.

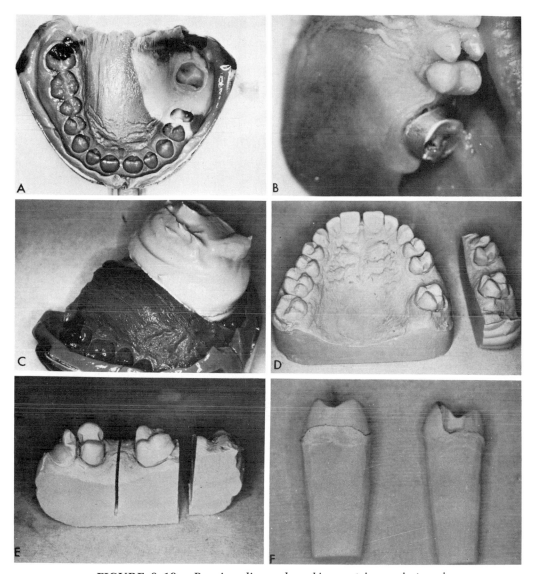

FIGURE 9–19. *Pouring dies and working cast in one impression.*

A, The impression.

B, Prepared teeth covered with aluminum shell filled with temporary stopping, and resin PV crown.

C, Prepared teeth poured for dies.

D, Casts trimmed for mounting and sectioning.

E, Sectioned die cast.

F, Dies trimmed.

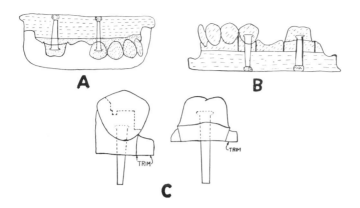

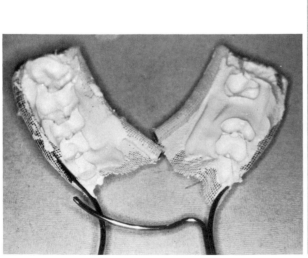

Figure 9–20. *Method for pouring impression in sections to produce removable dies*

A, Two mixes of contrasting colored stone are used.

B, Dies are sectioned through first pouring.

C, Dies trimmed.

(Courtesy of J. F. Jelenko & Co., Inc.)

The stone must be trimmed from the cervical margin to give access for carving the wax pattern.

The Opposing Cast. The impression for the opposing cast may be made with polysulfide rubber or alginate and poured with stone. If the operator chooses to work against a metal cast, a plaster of Paris or rubber impression may be taken. The occluding cast must be made from an impression just as precise as that taken for the working cast and should be poured soon enough to avoid distortion. The casts must be articulated and mounted with the maximal degree of accuracy that the equipment will allow.

The Registration. The registration is made, using a Kerr Bite Frame (Fig. 9–21) with a zinc oxide and eugenol impression paste that sets hard. The impression material is applied to both sides of the gauze bib on the Bite Frame, which is then placed over the prepared teeth and two or more

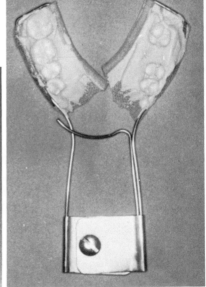

FIGURE 9–21. Kerr Bite Frame and registration.

posterior teeth in the adjoining quadrant. The patient is instructed to close in centric occlusion and to hold this position. After the paste has hardened the registration is put aside along with the locked face-bow for safekeeping.

MOUNTING THE CAST

After being trimmed, the maxillary cast must be mounted on an articulator that can simulate the movements dictated by the occluding surfaces of the opposing teeth. The mandibular cast can be related to it, using the registration procured with the Kerr Bite Frame, and can be fastened to the instrument.

Casts should be mounted, using a face-bow (Figs. 9-22 and 9-23). The technique to be described accepts the existing orientation even though it be an eccentric jaw relation. Hundreds of thousands of bridges and other restorations that have given many years of comfortable, efficient, nondestructive service have been built in this way. The authors are not opposed to reconstructing mouths using the hinge axis mounting, but are presenting a plea for sanity in the approach to the making of the requisite small fixed partial prosthesis.

Many prosthodontists believe that it is not necessary to mount casts with a face-bow registration. This may be true for the construction of complete dentures. However, bridges, constructed over casts that have been mounted on an adjustable articulator with the assistance of a face-bow, have better alignment and require less equilibration when placed in the mouth.

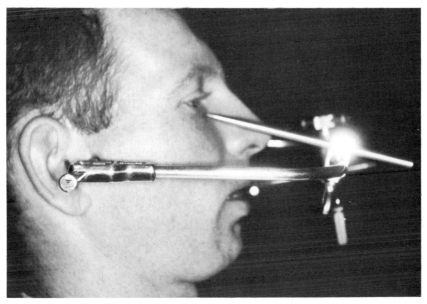

FIGURE 9–22.   Making face-bow registration.

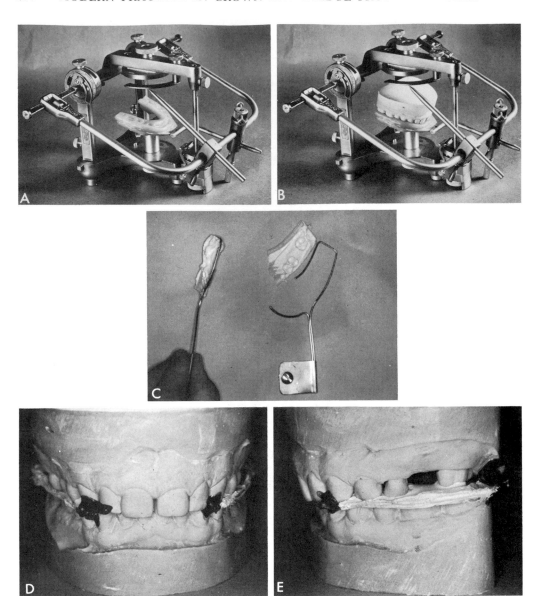

FIGURE 9-23.   *A*, Face-bow registration transferred to articulator.
B, Upper cast oriented for mounting.
C, Kerr Bite Frame and registration; left section removed from frame.
D and *E*, Lower cast articulated with and luted to upper cast, which has been attached to articulator.

The condyle should be located on each side of the face. The fork, covered above and below with two thicknesses of medium-soft baseplate wax, should be placed in the mouth and the patient instructed to close with force commensurate to indent the wax approximately 2.0 mm. The face-bow is adjusted and locked and the assembly is transferred to the articulator. The maxillary cast, whether it be the opposing or working cast, is secured to the fork and then attached to the articulator with plaster of Paris. Using the

Kerr Bite Frame registration for position, the opposing cast should be luted to the upper cast and fixed on the articulator.

The plaster of Paris must be trimmed and smoothed so that no crumbs will break off and interfere with carving the wax patterns. The condyle slots of the articulator should be set to accommodate the lateral and protrusive movements of the articulating surfaces. (See Figure 9-24.)

Any articulator used in constructing a bridge should be capable of reproducing in an over-all way the centric, lateral, and protrusive positions of the mandible. The dictatorial introduction of exceedingly complex mechanical armamentarium into the offices of all dentists who should be making bridges replacing one or two teeth will result only in bridges not being built. Prosthodontics need not be so spectacular. Small crown and bridge articulators may be adequate when short posterior replacements are being constructed by the direct technique, but larger, more versatile instruments and

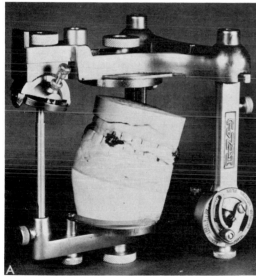
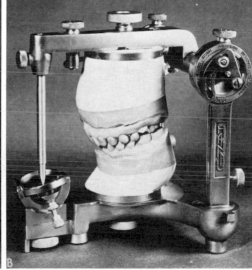
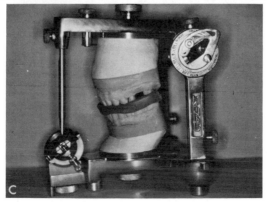

FIGURE 9-24. *A,* Articulator in position for mounting lower cast.
B, Mounted working cast.
C, Wax registration for setting protrusive or lateral position.

full arch casts should be considered mandatory for either direct or indirect construction of longer or anterior prostheses.

Dies Separate from the Working Cast.   When a pattern for a casting is made by an indirect technique, stated preliminary requirements must be met. The die must be constructed so that it can be removed from the articulated working cast, or it may be entirely separate if made from the same impression or from the same type of elastic impression. The correct-

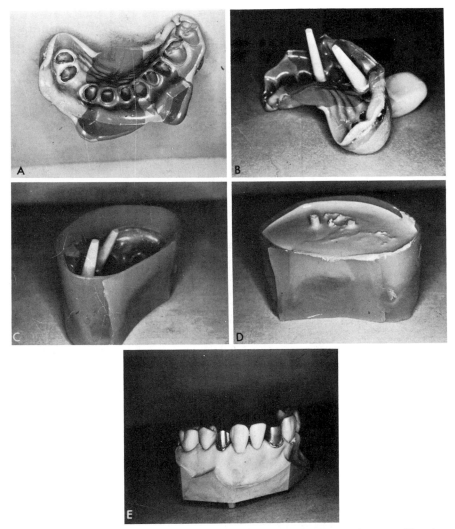

FIGURE 9–25.   *Constructing working cast from polysulfide or silicone rubber impression and metalized dies.*

A, Impression.
B, Dies seated and waxed to impression at gingival line. Stone roots have been lubricated with petrolatum.
C, Impression boxed.
D, Cast poured.
E, Cast separated.

ness of the die or the method for making the die must be proved. If the die was made by metalizing a copper band-modeling compound impression, a cast transfer can be made. If this casting fits the die, seats on the tooth, and fits the preparation, the die can be used. If a synthetic rubber or hydrocolloid impression was used to pour the die, accuracy may be taken for granted, provided the fundamentals of impression-taking have not been violated.

The pattern can be carved, polished, and invested with the expectation that the casting will fit the prepared tooth the same as the pattern fitted the die and that adjustments in occlusion will be minimal.

It is certainly advantageous to be able to pour two usable casts from a single rubber base impression. Separate dies and working casts may be made in this way without the expenditure of additional time and materials. The first cast, poured in the washed and dried impression, should include only the prepared teeth, and the die stone should be mixed sufficiently stiff so that its flow can be controlled. After the stone has set (1 hour), the dies are removed readily. By this procedure the possibility of distortion of the impression is also minimized. The working cast is poured in the same material, this time pouring the complete arch.

Metalized dies may be seated and luted in rubber impressions (Fig. 9-25). The working cast constructed here will have detached dies. Their stone roots should be lubricated with petrolatum to facilitate removal.

Rubber Impressions of Pinledge Preparations

With the use of the small orifice syringe tips now manufactured, complete polysulfide or silicone rubber impressions may be obtained of pinholes made with No. 700 or 701 burs (Fig. 9–26). This most likely is the technique of choice.

An alternate and very good indirect technique for use with tapered pinholes made with a No. 700 or 701 bur combines polysulfide or silicone rubber impressions with tapered plastic pins* inserted in the pinholes (Fig.

*Williams Gold Refining Co., Inc., Buffalo, N.Y.

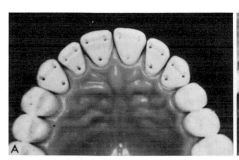 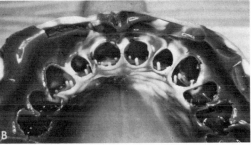

FIGURE 9–26. *A,* Model, with six pinledge preparations, which was used for both hydrocolloid and rubber impressions.

B, Impression of cast in *A* showing pinholes copied by injecting.

9-27). If the holes are too long for the pins, sections of the base may be included and the ends given a cylindrical form. For shorter holes the pins are broken off the plastic base. Retentive tack-type heads are made on each by pressing the ends of the pins vertically with a warm spatula until the plastic flows. The heads should be wide and must extend laterally in all directions from the pins to prevent their breaking out of the rubber. The head of the pin should extend 1.0 mm. beyond the tooth surface to admit a bulk of impression material. The pins should be lightly coated with petrolatum before being placed in the tooth. This will hold them in position and also make removal easy (Fig. 9-28).

When applying impression material with a syringe, it must be ejected in line with the pins, or they must be held in place so that the flow will not displace them.

With polysulfide rubber, as with silicone, the tray must be removed following the long axis of the pins. This makes building an individual tray inevitable, and it must be so constructed that the undercuts will be blocked out and the labial flange of the tray must be shortened even with the gingival line.

When bridges retained by tapered pins are constructed by indirect methods, hydrocolloid impressions can be recommended also, on condition that the material can be forced to the bottoms of the pinholes.

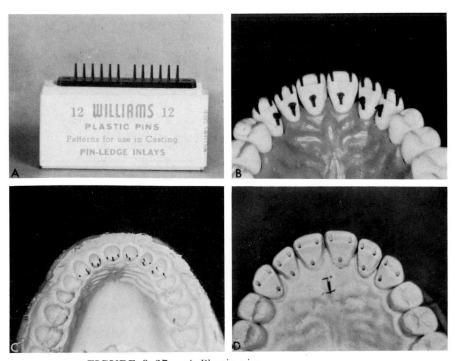

FIGURE 9-27. *A*, Plastic pins.
B, Plastic pins in position.
C, Rubber base impression showing pins removed.
D, Cast with impression and pins removed.

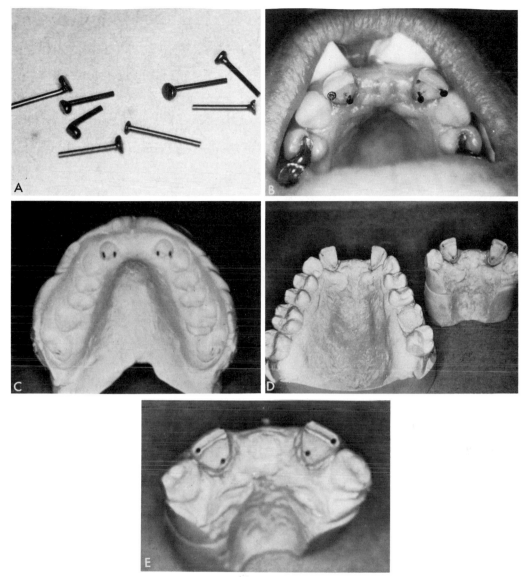

FIGURE 9-28. *Impression and cast from nylon bristles and elastic impression.*

A, Nylon bristles cut and headed.
B, Bristles in preparation pinholes.
C, Full arch rubber or silicone impression.
D, Two casts poured in same impression.
E, Cast to be sectioned for dies.

When the pinholes have been made with drills, they will be too small for injecting. Customarily only 0.023 inch in size, nylon bristles of 0.022 inch in diameter, with tack-type heads, are cut to protrude 2.0 mm. from the pinholes when fully seated. A special pair of cotton tweezers, which has been grooved to hold the pins, is used to place them in the holes. Lubrication is not a requisite.

A rubber base or silicone impression is taken and removed on a line parallel to the path of insertion. The area of the prepared teeth is poured in stone and left to set for approximately 1 hour. This block of stone is removed to be sectioned for dies. The full arch impression is then poured and this cast will be used for an intact working cast.

Silicone Rubber Impressions

The silicone impression materials have made great gains in popularity. They are cleaner to handle, have no offensive odor, can be colored as wished, and compared to the polysulfide polymers have superior esthetic characteristics. Notwithstanding that the shelf life of dental silicone impression materials is now improved, it remains limited. If undue time elapses between the manufacture and usage of the material, deviations in normal setting time may be encountered. For this reason, they should be purchased in small quantities and stored in a refrigerator. Storage at a low temperature provides maximal protection against deterioration. Because of the distortion that may occur, the silicone impression should not be electroplated.

The principal ingredient of the base is a poly (dimethyl siloxane). The polymerization is achieved by a reaction with an accelerator, usually an organo-metallic compound. The accelerator is chiefly in liquid form.

A custom-built tray is used, and the mixing technique for silicone duplicates that for polysulfide rubber. Because one ingredient is a liquid, thorough mixing of silicones is more simple than with polysulfide rubber. Since, as a rule, the mix sets more rapidly than the polysulfide polymers, the tray should be seated promptly. Elapsed time from beginning the mix until removal from the mouth should be at least 10 minutes.

A special adhesive is supplied for silicone rubber and it must be used in the tray. Silicone rubber flows somewhat better than polysulfide rubber, and for this reason it is preferred as a material for duplicating small pinholes.

REVERSIBLE HYDROCOLLOID IMPRESSIONS

Since it was presented to the profession, reversible hydrocolloid, because of its inherently worthy properties, has had widespread use. Its accuracy and ease of handling have made possible actual duplication of cavity or abutment preparations and their relationships, with less effort and time expended by both dentist and patient.

As with all dental materials, ultimate success with the hydrocolloid technique is dependent on a working knowledge and careful control of all variables. If appropriate equipment is at hand, if office or clinic routine is organized, and if strict attention is given to all steps, authentic reproduction of the involved areas can be expected. The technique is unexcelled for the indirect construction of restorations for individual teeth and partially edentulous mouths.

To appreciate fully the importance of certain manipulative variables, the composition and mechanics of gelation must be understood. Hydrocolloids may be classified as reversible or irreversible.[11] They are suspensions of aggregates of molecules in a dispersing medium of water.

The base of reversible hydrocolloid is agar (a seaweed), which at elevated temperatures forms a colloidal fluid sol and may be safely injected into the prepared cavity. By means of water-cooled trays, the sol material is converted into a firm yet elastic gel. Agar forms a complete gel at a temperature of approximately 102° F. This process of gelation is essentially a physical change only and is thermally reversible. In dentistry these materials ordinarily are referred to merely as hydrocolloids. The hydrocolloid is mostly supplied in tubes for filling the tray, and in jars of small cartridges for syringe injection into the cavity preparation. These slender sticks have a higher water content and therefore increased fluidity, and they spread into all areas without hesitation.

Preparation of the Hydrocolloid. The first step is the proper liquefying of the gelled material furnished by the manufacturer. The gel latticework must be broken down into a fluid sol that will precisely reproduce the cavity preparations. This is primary, since all succeeding phases of the technique rely on the right preparation of the hydrocolloid.

The tubes and loaded syringes are placed in the boiling compartment of the conditioner, which is basic apparatus (Fig. 9–29). Most agars will go into a complete sol at temperatures above 206° F. if the temperature is held sufficiently long. Boiling water is a convenient medium for liquefying the material, giving assurance that the minimal temperature has been attained.

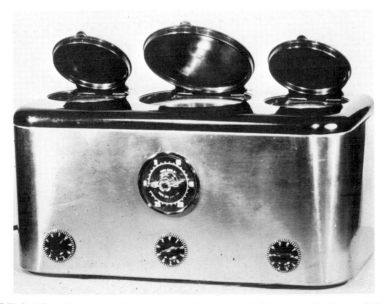

FIGURE 9–29. Example of one type of commercial hydrocolloid conditioner. Bath at left is for boiling, middle compartment for storage, while tempering of tray material is carried out in bath at right. Equipment of this type is essential to the technique.

No less than 10 minutes of boiling time is imperative in order that the hydrocolloid will change to a smoothly flowing and nongrainy substance. The real danger in preparing the material, and a frequent cause of disappointment and failure, is inadequate heating. There are no serious developments from prolonged boiling. If it is allowed to re-gel, approximately 3 minutes should be added *each* time the material is reboiled in order to bring the gel into a sol condition.

The hydrocolloid, when thoroughly liquefied, can be stored until needed (Fig. 9–30). With efficient equipment it may be boiled at the beginning of the day and maintained in a workable state for at least 8 hours. This fluid material must be stored at a temperature that will block any appreciable gelation, because as gelation proceeds, fluidity decreases, and the material will not flow into all fine lines of the cavity.

Since gelation of hydrocolloid is a function of both time and temperature, it will progress at any temperature if the material is held long enough. However, at 150° F. the gelation is retarded, and storage at that temperature will give the operator a usable material throughout the working day. Storage at temperatures below 150° F. may produce a stiff, granular mass that will be incapable of injection into the less accessible areas of the preparation. There is no risk of injury to the pulp by injection of the material at 150° F., or even 155° F., because as the hydrocolloid passes through the needle and onto the relatively cool tooth surface the temperature drops quickly.[15] Checking the temperature control indicators of the conditioning unit for erroneous readings should become a daily phase of this procedure.

The hydrocolloid in the syringe is now ready to be injected into the

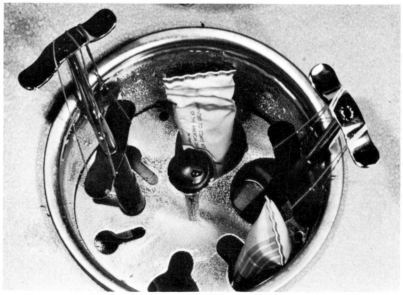

FIGURE 9–30. Tubes of hydrocolloid and syringes in storage compartment (145 to 155° F.). Material may be kept fluid all day at this temperature.

cavity preparation directly from the storage bath, but the material in the
tube, which will be used to fill the tray, must be cooled to below 150° F.
"Tempering" must be done to induce some gelation and to diminish the
temperature so that the large bulk of hydrocolloid will be neither uncomfortable to the patient nor difficult to contain in the tray. Likewise, the thermal
contraction will be lessened, leading to better reproduction of cavity angles
and contours.

The degree of gelation of the agar and the speed of its formation will be
controlled by the temperature of the tempering bath and the length of time
it remains in the bath at that temperature (Fig. 9-31). Various combinations
have been suggested. Naturally the cooler the tempering bath the faster will
be the drop of the temperature of the impression material in the tray, with
an accompanying decrease in the time required to secure ample gelation for
insertion into the oral cavity. If the tempering temperature is low, then the
period that the tray is stored in the tempering bath is quite important. A few
extra minutes at a low temperature, say 103° F., will lead to excessive
gelation and unusable hydrocolloid. Accordingly, a slower gelation carried
out at a little higher tempering temperature is more conducive to a favorable
outcome.

Although the time-temperature ratio may hinge on the consistency most
suited to the operator's preference, the suggested method is to temper at
115° F. for approximately 10 minutes.[16] Other procedures are applicable but
more demanding (Table 9-1). Different materials, and even different
batches of the same brand of hydrocolloid, may necessitate a slight alteration
in the proposed tempering time. The tray material can be tempered during

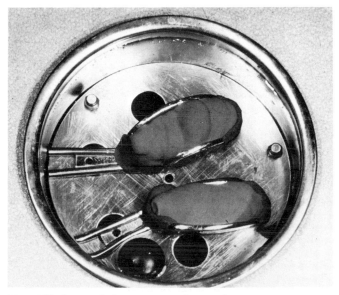

FIGURE 9-31.   Filled trays being tempered to reduce temperature and produce some
gelation.

Table 9–1.   TIME-TEMPERATURE COMBINATIONS FOR TEMPERING
HYDROCOLLOID

TEMPERATURE	TIME
115° F.*	10 minutes
110° F.	5–10 minutes
105° F.	5 minutes
102° F.	2 minutes

*Recommended method.

the final moments of tissue displacement and while the teeth are being prepared for injection of the syringe material.

Abutment Preparations for Hydrocolloid Bridges.   With an indirect impression technique, standard preparations should be made on the abutment teeth. If pinholes are to be placed in the abutment, it is helpful if they have greater diameter and less depth. For example, a pinhole in the occlusal of an inlay preparation, in the cusp tip of a partial veneer preparation, or in the cingulum area of a partial veneer preparation ordinarily would be made 2.0 mm. deep with a No. 701 bur (Fig. 9–32). To reproduce readily with hydrocolloid, the pinhole should be made with a No. 701 or 702 bur and reduced in depth to 1.5 mm. With the use of extra pressure and a special needle on the syringe, a pinhole made with a No. 700 bur may be copied. The cervical finishing line must be distinct.

For *Gingival Displacement*, see page 185.

Selection of Trays.   In an indirect technique, full arch impressions are indispensable for working *and* opposing casts. There are no articulated retainers to assist in relating the casts or to pilot their movements, and so the occlusion of the unprepared teeth is essential.

The tray must be selected with this in mind. It should extend distally past all teeth, be fitted with tubes for cooling (Fig. 9–33), and have room for 3.0 mm. of material around the teeth occlusally and laterally. Black tray compound is the best material for the "stops" that will guide the tray into position over the teeth. (Red and green compound and wax become too pliable in the tempering bath.) A black compound dam (Fig. 9–34) is built in the metal tray beyond the most distal abutment tooth, even though it may be supported by soft tissue, and trimmed so that it will not contact an abutment during gelation. A second stop should be located mesially to the most

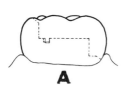
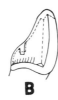

A   **B**

FIGURE 9–32. Pinholes should be changed in size for hydrocolloid technique.

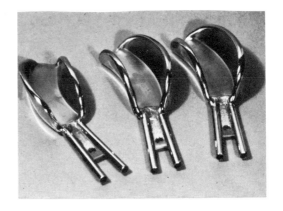

FIGURE 9-33. Trays fitted with flanges and tubes for retention and cooling of impression material. A complete arch impression should be made for the working cast.

anterior prepared tooth, and a third one in the approximating quadrant. They will form a tripod for positioning the tray. The compound in the tray is molded by pressure over the occlusal surfaces of the teeth or over the retromolar pad. Trays should be prepared before tissue displacement is begun, but filling the trays with liquefied impression material and tempering should be done during displacement (Fig. 9-35). If the trays are without perforations or rim locks, compound must be added to the inner borders to stabilize the impression material during removal.

The hollow point, or needle, on the syringe should be no larger than is needed to permit a free flow of hydrocolloid. The smaller the stream of impression material, the less apt will be the trapping of air. On the other hand, if there is resistance to pushing the hydrocolloid through the needle, there may be some uncontrolled movement of the needle point, with a chance of bubbles, or abrasion of the tissue, and hemorrhage.

Preimpression Steps. After the gingival crevice has been examined, it is washed and dried and may be repacked with a single strand of No. 8 thread (Fig. 9-36), which will not attach to the impression.[4] The field must be isolated by placing cotton rolls to the buccal and the lingual of the teeth. Warm air should be used cautiously to rid the surface of moisture or debris; otherwise, the gingival tissue may hemorrhage. The surface now should cause no discrepancies in the impression.

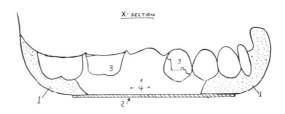

FIGURE 9-34. Cross section of compound stops for seating tray. (Courtesy of J. F. Jelenko & Co., Inc.)

X-SECTION

1. Compound
2. Tray
3. Preparations
4. Space for Hydrocolloid

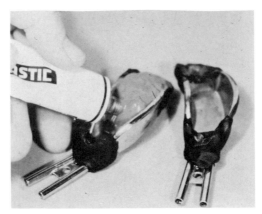

FIGURE 9–35.   Filling tray.

Use of the Syringe.   The syringe is taken from the storage bath and ½ inch or more of the material is ejected as waste, inasmuch as the hydrocolloid in the syringe tip may have been contaminated by water or air during conditioning. Air pockets must be avoided, because even the smallest nodule on a critical margin or in the angle of the cavity will render the die useless. The tip of the syringe must be confined to or dragged along the tooth surface.

Taking the Impression.   During the period of injection the assistant will have removed the tray from the conditioning bath and attached the hose for circulation of water. Some operators just blot the surface of hydrocolloid with a towel, but a much wiser practice is to scrape off the layer that has been in contact with the water in the conditioning bath (Fig. 9–37). Neglecting to remove this outer surface may hinder union between the tray material and the hydrocolloid that has been injected around the prepared tooth. The tray is now forced over the teeth until the compound stops are in position. Although haste is needless, if too much time elapses between injection and seating the tray, there will be a poor bonding between the syringe and tray materials.

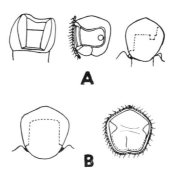

FIGURE 9–36.   Gingival crevice packed with No. 8 thread. This will prolong displacement of tissue in order that two impressions may be made. (Courtesy of J. F. Jelenko & Co., Inc.)

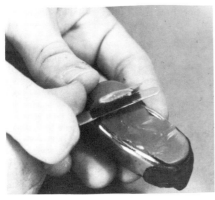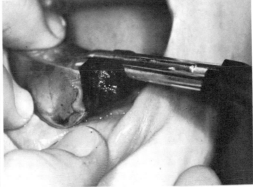

FIGURE 9-37. Surface of conditioned hydrocolloid should be scraped. Seated tray must be motionless for at least 5 minutes.

The tray is held passively for at least 5 minutes, which will result in a strong gel able to resist deformation or fracture. If the tray is withdrawn before 5 minutes have passed, the gel that has formed will not have strength to withstand the applied stresses. Premature removal is a common cause for inaccuracy.

Any movement of the tray will cause a distortion of the hydrocolloid, and because of this the dentist should stabilize the impression during the entire time it is in the mouth. Sometimes the dentist will hold the tray for a minute or two and then ask the dental assistant to hold it for the remainder of the time. The switching of hands can bring about movement of the tray and thus distortion.

The temperature of the circulating water should be approximately 60 to 70° F. Ice water should not be used, since it is annoying to some patients and may cause undue stress in the impression.[17] Cold water for the last 2 minutes probably has no deleterious effect, but must not be used during the first 3 minutes. If the water in the unit is too cool during the winter months, the temperature of the tray can be regulated by turning the water on at short intervals only, instead of using an uninterrupted stream.

The tray is removed with a quick thrust, parallel if possible to the long axis of the tooth or preparation (Fig. 9-38). It must not be teased or rocked from the cavity preparation. Contrary to prevalent opinion, this type of material will deform or rupture much less readily when subjected to a sudden movement rather than to a constant pressure.

Treating the Impression. After the impression is removed, it is washed and inspected. For most combinations of hydrocolloid and stone, it is beneficial to place the impression in a 2 per cent solution of potassium sulfate for about 5 minutes while the mix of stone is being prepared (Fig. 9-39). The purpose of the potassium sulfate bath is not to preserve dimensional stability, but to give a superior surface to the stone die. As mentioned previously, the commercial dental hydrocolloids contain borax as a filler. As the impression stands, even if for only a few minutes, a thin film of water forms on the surface. This water exudate contains borax that has leached

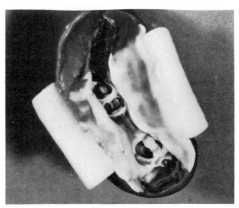

FIGURE 9–38.   Impression removed. Cotton should be left, as its removal could tear impression.

from the hydrocolloid. When the stone is poured against this surface, the set is retarded by the borax. In such a case, the stone may be contaminated by this watery film before it sets, and an inferior surface results.

If the impression is stored in a 2 per cent potassium sulfate solution, the sulfate ion is absorbed onto the surface where it acts as an accelerator for the stone, in essence counteracting the retarding effect of the borax. Even with this treatment there is still some softening of the stone by the hydrocolloid; for instance, as compared to stone poured against glass or a rubber impression material. The potassium sulfate treatment minimizes this interaction between the hydrocolloid and stone, providing a stone die of maximal hardness and sharpness of detail. Since distortion of the reversible hydrocolloid begins almost at once, the immersion time should not exceed 5 minutes.

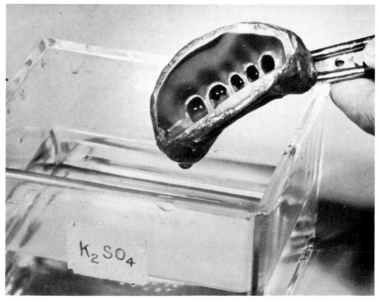

FIGURE 9–39.   Placing clean impression in potassium sulfate bath. This step, carried on while mix of stone is prepared, improves surface of stone cast.

An error often made is to wash the impression diligently after removing it from the potassium sulfate bath. This destroys the whole purpose of this treatment. The excess droplets of the potassium sulfate solution should be cautiously blown from the mold, with care being taken not to dehydrate the impression. The surface should always remain moist.

The final impression is essentially a suspension of water held in the micelles of the agar and it constitutes approximately 75 to 85 per cent of the composition. These materials will tend to lose water (syneresis) or gain water (imbibition), processes that result in dimensional change and distortion within the impression.[17, 18, 19] Also, there is a residual stress pattern in the impression, which will be relieved upon storage and cause distortion.

Pouring the Cast. Unfortunately, no chemical solution or storage environment that will maintain an equilibrium within the impression has yet been developed for use in the dental office. One of the recognized limitations of the hydrocolloid technique is the absolute necessity for pouring the cast without delay. This is true with most impression materials, but particularly with the hydrocolloids. Nevertheless, many operators continue to indulge in the bad habit of letting the impression stand for varying periods of time before pouring the cast. Undoubtedly, this is one of the most

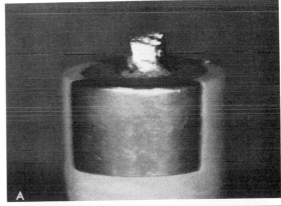

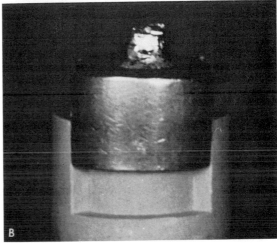

FIGURE 9-40. Master casting was made on original steel die. When tried back on stone die poured immediately (*A*) into hydrocolloid impression, no inaccuracy is apparent. However, the fit on a stone die poured in an impression allowed to stand 1 hour in air (*B*) readily demonstrates the distortion that occurred.

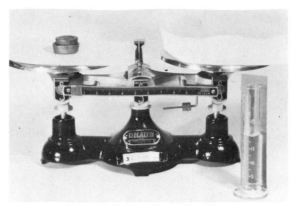

FIGURE 9-41.   Balance for weighing stone.

frequent reasons for distortion and imperfection. It has been shown that, on some types of preparations, distortion is evidenced within 30 minutes after removal from the mouth (Fig. 9-40). It bears repeating that a cardinal rule, which must be followed if the exactness of the impression is to be kept, is to *pour the cast within 15 minutes* after the impression is taken from the mouth. (See Figures 9-41, 9-42, and 9-43.)

Construction of the Die.   To assure a continuous correct relationship between the abutment teeth, bridges should be constructed and assembled

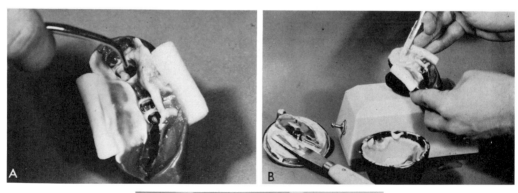

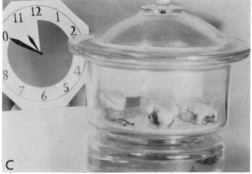

FIGURE 9-42.   *A*, Removing excess potassium sulfate solution before pouring cast.
B, Pouring cast.
C, Setting stone is stored in humidifier.

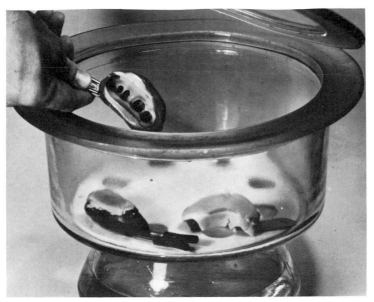

FIGURE 9-43. If storage is necessary, the best storage environment for hydrocolloid is an arrangement such as that shown. Water in bottom and tightly fitting lid provide atmosphere of approximately 100 per cent humidity.

on solid, complete arch casts from which no portion may be removed. Therefore, two impressions of the prepared area must be taken. The cast that appears to have the better reproduction of the abutments will be partitioned for the dies. The other may be articulated and used as the working cast. After the impressions have been taken for the dies and the working and opposing casts, a registration should be made with the Kerr Bite Frame.[20]

If, in an emergency, this policy of pouring the cast at once cannot be followed, what is the most reliable storage environment? This will change with the brand of material. The safest medium, one more dependable than either air or water, is an atmosphere of 100 per cent humidity—that is, a humidifier. (See Figures 9–42 and 9–43.) In view of the questionable behavior in any environment, storage is an unpredictable variable that can be— and certainly should be—eliminated from the technique.

Excess droplets of the potassium sulfate solution should be gently blown from the impression, being mindful not to dehydrate and subsequently distort the hydrocolloid. The surface of the impression should have a slightly wet appearance.

IRREVERSIBLE HYDROCOLLOID (ALGINATE) IMPRESSIONS

The irreversible hydrocolloids, commonly called alginates, gel by means of a specific chemical reaction. Alginates are used by many clinicians for indirect restorations, bridges, or removable partial dentures, because their use is somewhat less complicated. However, at present the reversible hydrocolloid still offers superior characteristics, such as greater accuracy on a long span, a better surface on the working die, and sharper detail.

Stock, perforated trays are used with alginate. These are procurable in many sizes, but for an extra large arch it may be necessary to add wax to the posterior border to give extra length. Wax may be vital in the center of an upper tray to push and hold the impression material against the palatal surface.

Alginate should be proportioned and mixed according to the directions furnished by the manufacturer. Setting time in the mouth is 2 minutes after it becomes obvious that gelation has begun. The impression should be washed and the cast poured at once. The effects of storage time and storage environments are identical to those discussed for reversible hydrocolloids in the section on pouring the die. The procedures that were outlined should be followed with the alginates as well.

PLASTER OF PARIS IMPRESSIONS

The use of a plaster of Paris impression to produce a working cast minimizes variables, reduces armamentarium, and requires only that the plaster impression for the working cast be taken and reassembled precisely. Many times small pieces of the impression are lost or cannot be reassembled and, as a consequence, details inherent in a cast made from an elastic impression are missing. The setting and removal of the impression material are quite distasteful to some patients.

In the construction of the small bridge, the jaws, hinged as they are at the temporomandibular joint, make a suitable preliminary articulator for establishing the relationship of the retainers to opposing teeth, but there is the disadvantage of extra appointments for the patient. For a long bridge (more than three units) the working cast must duplicate the entire arch.

After the castings have been polished, washed, adjusted for occlusion and contact, and reseated on the abutment teeth, a registration is made, using the Kerr Bite Frame.

Selection of the Tray. The tray should invariably extend distally beyond the most posterior abutment and across the median line to include two or more occluding posterior teeth on the opposite side (Fig. 9-44). There may be an exception for a bridge supplying only one tooth. A shorter working cast will suffice if the occlusion is well defined, since during pontic construction lateral movements will be guided by the already equilibrated occlusal surfaces of the retainers and the uncut teeth in that segment.

The tray must clear the teeth buccally, lingually, and occlusally by 3.0 mm. and must not impinge on the lingual gingival tissue. The tray need not be oiled or greased before taking a plaster of Paris impression, but it *must* be clean.

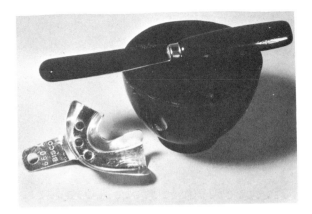

FIGURE 9-44. Plaster bowl, spatula and tray.

The Impression. Impression plasters differ from model plasters primarily in setting time and greatly reduced strength. Mixing plaster of Paris for taking impressions calls for more understanding and intuition than technical skill. Snowwhite No. 2* is an impression plaster that will harden quickly and break cleanly. Enough cool water to fill the impression tray one and one-half times is placed in a bowl. The plaster is slowly sifted into the water, using a sieve or a spatula, and the liquid is stirred after each addition of plaster until the mix is creamy but thin. Spatulation is continued until just before setting begins, a point the operator will learn to recognize only by experience. The plaster is transferred to the impression tray and the tray is positioned in the mouth so that there is an equal thickness of plaster over the buccal, lingual, and occlusal surfaces. It is held until the plaster has set. Setting can be gauged by testing small pieces of the plaster left in the mixing bowl. When it cannot be crushed between the thumb and finger, begins to feel warm, and breaks sharply, the impression is ready for removal. This should be done speedily before the plaster becomes excessively hard and hot.

Removal of the Impression. The tray is removed and laid to one side. Beginning at either end, a finger is placed under the buccal edge of the impression and pressure is exerted with some force labially and occlusally. As a rule, this will induce fracture and a section can be lifted out and placed in its relative position on a tray or napkin. This procedure is repeated until the outside wall of the impression has been disengaged (Fig. 9–45).

If the occlusal and lingual portion cannot be lifted out intact, a groove must be cut at the most advantageous point, generally at the lingual of a cuspid, so that pressure on the ends of the impression and toward the center of the mouth will split the remaining section. A knife or chisel may be helpful, but their indiscriminate use may induce so much fragmentation that reassembly of the impression will be impossible.

When all parts of the impression have been collected, the patient should be permitted to rinse with a flavored wash. (See Figure 9–45.)

---

*Kerr Mfg. Company, Romulus, Mich.

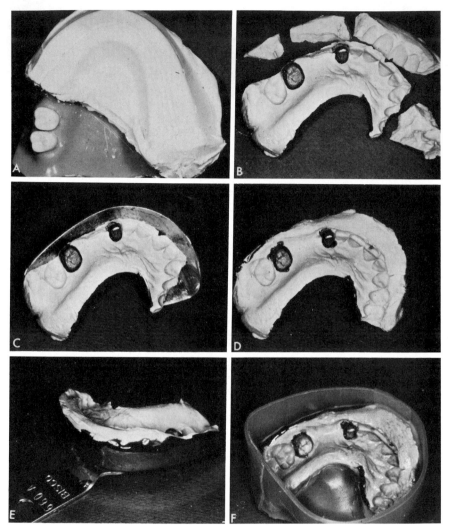

FIGURE 9–45.   *A,* Tray removed and impression scored to provide guide lines for fracturing.

   B, Sections of impression arranged on removal from mouth.

   C, Largest piece cleaned and seated in tray. It may be necessary to lift or remove this segment in order to adapt buccal parts to area of fracture.

   D, Retainers seated in the assembled impression and secured with wax.

   E, Impression luted to tray.

   F, Impression coated with separating medium and boxed for pouring.

Reassembly of the Impression. Only after all minute chips have been brushed from each surface of the impression, the retainers, and the tray, is it possible to reassemble and stabilize the impression and the retainers in the tray. Irregularities and inaccuracies are inevitable if the sections are joined outside the tray.

The retainers, if movable, are fixed to the impression with beeswax. The plaster should be coated with a separating medium, of which many are available. After this has dried, the impression is placed in water for a few minutes and then poured.

Pouring the Cast. Stone, commonly called hydrocal, is used because of its strength. The alginate impression for the opposing cast can be poured at the same time and with the same mix. It is never a good policy to pour a working cast with soldering investment, inasmuch as it breaks and abrades readily.

After the stone has hardened for a minimum of 1 hour, the alginate impression is removed and discarded. The plaster of Paris impression must be taken off one piece at a time, being watchful in the application of force not to break an abutment tooth. No working cast, fractured in an area directly connected with the construction of the bridge, can be mended so that the parts will be joined without error; a new cast must be made. If instructions have been followed, any plaster of Paris impression should separate with no difficulty (Fig. 9–46).

Technique for Constructing a Cast Transfer. A transfer is a nonanatomic cover for a tooth, which may be removed in an impression and used as a receptacle for dies to assure their correct relationship in the poured working cast. It may be made of resin, low-fusing metal, or cast gold alloy, which is preferable. A cast transfer may be used as a coping, to become an integral part of the finished restoration. If it fits both the die and the tooth, correctness of the die may be accepted. Fit of the retainer castings may be judged in advance, owing to the hardness of the gold.[21]

When the pattern is waxed on the die, it must contact all surfaces and be carved to marginal fit. The wax should be only as thick as required to make possible a complete casting. Anatomic form is not essential except at the

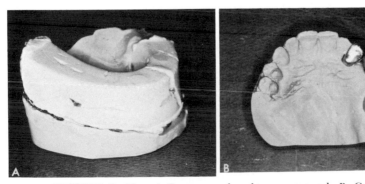

FIGURE 9–46. *A,* Cast poured and tray removed. *B,* Cast.

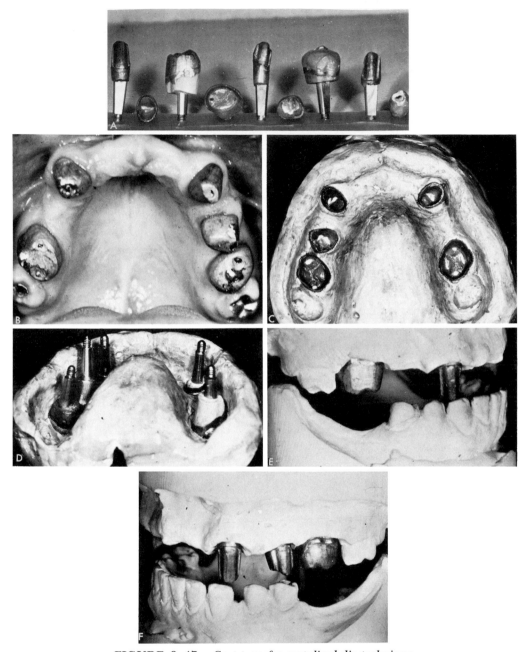

FIGURE 9–47. *Cast transfer–metalized die technique.*

A, Dies and cast transfers for the five abutments of a 12-unit upper bridge.

B, The transfers on the abutments. The windows make it possible to check seating.

C, The transfers removed in a plaster impression.

D, The dies seated in the transfers. Threaded and tapped dowel pins were used for greater accuracy in replacing the dies in the cast.

E and F, The working cast.

cervical periphery. The final step in building the pattern is the removal of several square millimeters of wax down to the surface of the die, from a buccal cusp or incisal edge, without disturbing the adaptation of the wax. This opening will ensure a means of checking the seating of the casting (Fig. 9-47*A* and *B*).

The pattern is sprued at the same angle and invested with the same amount of expansion that would be needed for a permanent restoration. The casting may be made with any dental gold, or if the coping technique is being followed, with the alloy to be used for the second casting. The sprue is cut off, leaving a stump of 1.0 to 2.0 mm. This stump and the window will orient the casting in the plaster of Paris impression. Cervical fit and occlusal or incisal adaptation should be checked on the die before the transfer is taken to the mouth.

THE WORKING CAST.   With the transfers on the teeth, a full arch plaster of Paris impression is made and reassembled with the castings seated in the impression. The plaster is luted to the tray, and the dies are placed in the transfers and supported in position by wax or rods. After separating medium has been applied and let dry, the impression is soaked for a short time and poured in stone (Fig. 9-47*B,C,D,E,* and *F*).

A mechanical vibrator should not be used unless the hand is placed between the impression tray and the instrument to reduce the agitation to a minimum; otherwise, the dies will loosen and the cast will be worthless. Model stone will flow into all recesses of the impression if the impression tray is tapped lightly against a rubber block or bench top. The casts are trimmed and mounted on an adjustable articulator with a face-bow.

Cast transfers may also be seated in rubber or alginate impressions, especially if a plaster core was placed over the occlusal surfaces of the teeth before the elastic impression was taken.

REFERENCES

1. Roydhouse, R. H.: Elastic impression materials. New Zealand D. J., *52*:187, Oct. 1956.
2. Fettes, E. M., and Jorezak, J. S.: Polysulfide polymers. Indust. & Engin. Chem., *42*:2217, Nov. 1950.
3. Bailey, L. R.: Acrylic resin tray for rubber base impression materials. J. Pros. Den., *5*:658, Sept. 1955.
4. Jelenko, J. F. & Co., Inc.: Crown and Bridge Construction Using Hydrocolloid Impressions. 2nd ed. The company, 1956.
5. Harrison, J. D.: Effect of retraction materials on the gingival sulcus epithelium. J. Pros. Den., *11*:514, May-June 1961.
6. Oringer, M. J.: Electrosurgery in Dentistry. Philadelphia, W. B. Saunders Company, 1962.
7. Skinner, E. W.: The properties and manipulation of mercaptan base and silicone base impression materials. D. Clin. N. Amer., Nov. 1958, p. 685.
8. Sturdevant, C. M.: Mercaptan rubber impression technique for single and multiple restorations. D. Clin. N. Amer., Nov. 1958, p. 699.
9. Myers, G. E.: Rubber base impression technics for operative dentistry. J. Michigan D. A., *39*:251, Oct. 1957.

10. Schnell, R. J., and Phillips, R. W.: Dimensional stability of rubber base impressions and certain other factors affecting accuracy. J.A.D.A., *57*:39, July 1958.
11. Skinner, E. W., and Phillips, R. W.: The Science of Dental Materials. 6th ed. Philadelphia, W. B. Saunders Company, 1967.
12. Peyton, F. A., Liebold, J. P., and Ridgley, G. V.: Surface hardness, compressive strength, and abrasion resistance of indirect die stones. J. Pros. Den., *2*:381, May 1952.
13. Phillips, R. W., and Ito, B. Y.: Factors affecting the surface of stone dies poured in hydrocolloid impressions. J. Pros. Den., *2*:390, May 1952.
14. Jelenko, J. F. & Co., Inc.: Crown and Bridge Construction. A Handbook of Dental Laboratory Procedures. 5th ed. The company, 1964.
15. Phillips, R. W.: Physical properties and manipulation of reversible and irreversible hydrocolloid. J.A.D.A., *51*:566, Nov. 1955.
16. Thompson, M. J.: Standardized indirect technic for reversible hydrocolloid. J.A.D.A., *46*:1, Jan. 1953.
17. Phillips, R. W., and Ito, B. Y.: Factors influencing the accuracy of reversible hydrocolloid impressions. J.A.D.A., *43*:1, July 1951.
18. James, A. G.: Maintenance of equilibrium in reversible hydrocolloid impressions. J. D. Res., *28*:108, 119, 447, April and Oct. 1949.
19. Skinner, E. W., Cooper, E. N., and Beck, F. W.: Reversible and irreversible hydrocolloid impression materials. J.A.D.A., *40*:196, Feb. 1950.
20. Emmert, J. H.: A method for registering occlusion in semiedentulous mouths. J. Pros. Den., *8*:94, Jan. 1958.
21. Schweitzer, J. M.: Oral Rehabilitation. St. Louis, The C. V. Mosby Company, 1951, p. 946.

chapter 10

INDIVIDUAL DIES CONSTRUCTED FROM TUBE IMPRESSIONS

This chapter will discuss making a die, or reproduction, of a single prepared tooth. It can then be placed in an impression to become a removable part of a working cast or it can be used as a detached unit for freehand carving. It must be done precisely.

Polysulfide rubber base materials and impression compound have specific advantages and disadvantages for making impressions. Silver-plated or copper-plated surfaces, stone, resin, and amalgam, for producing the die, have their proponents. (Impressions of polysulfide and silicone rubber and hydrocolloid for quadrant and complete arch casts and dies are discussed in Chapter 9.)

FITTING THE BAND

A copper band, stiff or annealed, depending on the impression material being used, should be selected as soon as the peripheral dimension of the preparation has been established, because when judging it for size and marking it for contour, manipulation on the tooth is far easier if one does not have to contend with a shoulder or a prominent finishing line. For elastic materials a *stiff* band must be used and have at least 0.35 mm. clearance at all points. For impression compound the *annealed* band should fit the cervical margin snugly. For either material the band should be about twice the length of the prepared clinical crown.

The band should conform to the silhouette of the preparation as seen from the occlusal. Its cervical outline must follow the configuration of the gingival tissue surrounding the tooth. If the preparation has been extended 0.5 mm. into the gingival crevice, then the band must be trimmed and contoured to extend evenly 0.3 mm. beyond the cervical margin of the preparation. While still uncut on the end, it can be placed over the tooth until it touches the gingiva, and these points of contact marked with a sharp instrument. Other marks should be made to indicate the distance of the labial and lingual edges from the tissue.

The band is removed and trimmed with shears or a stone to duplicate the cervical contour of the preparation, the edge is smoothed with a fine stone, the labial surface is identified, and it is put aside until the preparation is completed (Fig. 10-1).

Guide Lines

Before filling the band, it should be placed on the tooth in the position it must occupy in order to secure a satisfactory impression. If there are approximating teeth, perpendicular guide lines can be placed on both the mesial and distal of the band. A horizontal line to show cervical positioning can be

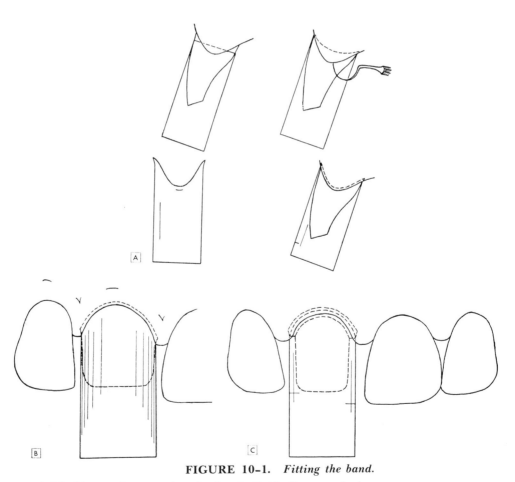

FIGURE 10-1. *Fitting the band.*

A, Marking and contouring the band. Guide lines marked.
B, Band on partially prepared tooth.
C, Band on prepared tooth, showing how guide lines help in positioning band.

made at any point where it will have a related object. If there are no adjacent teeth, seating the band will offer no problem.

TAKING THE IMPRESSION

Polysulfide Rubber Technique

When polysulfide rubber is used in taking a tube impression, the incisal end of the ordinary copper band must be plugged with impression compound (Fig. 10-2). It should come within 2.0 to 3.0 mm. of the incisal of the prepared tooth, further to reinforce the band against deformation upon removal of the impression and to control the thickness of the material. This will force all the excess to flow out at the cervical, presumably carrying away any bubbles of air that may have been trapped on the tooth surface as the band was seated. A selection of closed-end copper bands, which do not require the use of impression compound, is available.*

The inner surface of the band and compound is painted with a thin coat of the tray adhesive that accompanies the impression material. This is allowed to dry for at least 6 or 7 minutes. The band is filled completely with heavy base or regular tray polysulfide rubber, seated over the prepared tooth, and held without movement for 10 minutes (Fig. 10–3).

This technique seems to be somewhat less exacting than that needed to obtain an accurate compound impression. Also, the elastic material can be withdrawn from cervical undercuts without deformation or fracture of the impression.

Impression Compound Technique

The compound should be softened, preferably in boiling water; if dry heat is used, the surface that will contact the tooth must be tempered in hot

*Blue Island Specialty Co., Inc., Blue Island, Ill.

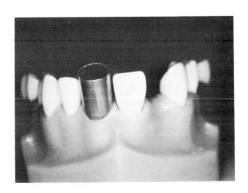

FIGURE 10-2. Copper band plugged with impression compound to confine and limit the amount of polysulfide rubber.

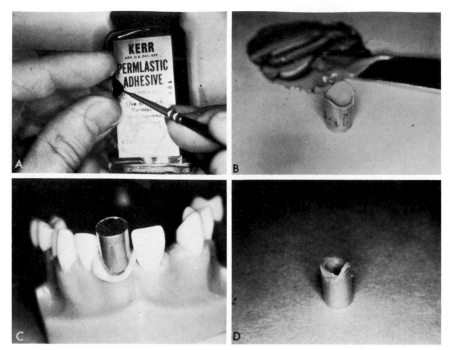

FIGURE 10–3. *Impression technique.*

A, Painting band.
B, Band filled.
C, Band seated.
D, Impression.

water. The opening of the band must not be closed with the finger tip while trying to seat the band and compound; instead, a little compound should be forced out at the cervical, and the band should be guided into position before putting pressure on the impression material (Fig. 10–4).

The impression should be chilled with cold water and pulled incisally from the tooth with a steady vertical pressure. It must *not* be rocked or rotated during removal. Grasping the band with a dry napkin, a fine sandpaper strip, or a pointed clamp will give traction.

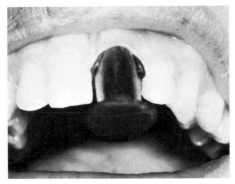

FIGURE 10–4.   Compound impression.

Every effort must be made to avoid taking the same impression repeatedly, as this may cause excessive thermal shock to the tooth, or it can traumatize the soft tissue, cut the periodontal membrane attachment, and stimulate gingival recession.

DIES

The Silver-plated Die

One of the virtues of the polysulfide rubber impression is the ease with which it can be plated with silver. Hydrocolloid, alginate, or silicone impressions cannot be electroplated suitably without some change in form.[1, 2]

After the impression has been washed with tap water and dried, a fine silver powder* is burnished into all areas with a soft brush. The powder should contact the copper band, the excess being blown out. The copper band is wrapped with masking tape or wax, extending 2.0 to 5.0 mm. (the same distance at all points) beyond the open end of the impression. The band is waxed onto the cathode holder and all conducting surfaces not to be plated are covered with wax. Other metalizing agents, such as bronze or graphite, may be employed, but silver powder gives a superior surface (Fig. 10–5).

A silver cyanide bath,* which must not be polluted with acid or other chemicals, is used for plating. To escape trapping air bubbles, the metalized impression is meticulously filled with the solution and is then lowered into the electrolyte. The upper end of the cathode is attached to the negative D. C. source. The silver anode is placed about 4 inches away and is attached to the positive D. C. terminal. Plating is carried out for approximately 12 hours at 10 milliamperes for each square centimeter of surface. If, on examination during the first half hour, some areas are not plating, the impression should be washed, dried, and remetalized with silver powder.

Forming the Root. Stone, low-fusing metal, or self-curing resin may be used to form the root, which should be tapered and without irregularities. Stone will expand very slightly when setting, whereas metal and resin contract. For this reason and because of its uncomplicated working properties, stone is recommended for the support and root section of a metalized die.

The Copper-plated Die

For a copper band—compound impression to be plated with copper, the inside, or preparation surface, must be metalized. The best reproduction of the surface and the sharpest marginal detail will result when metalizing is

---

*Kerr Mfg. Company, Romulus, Mich.

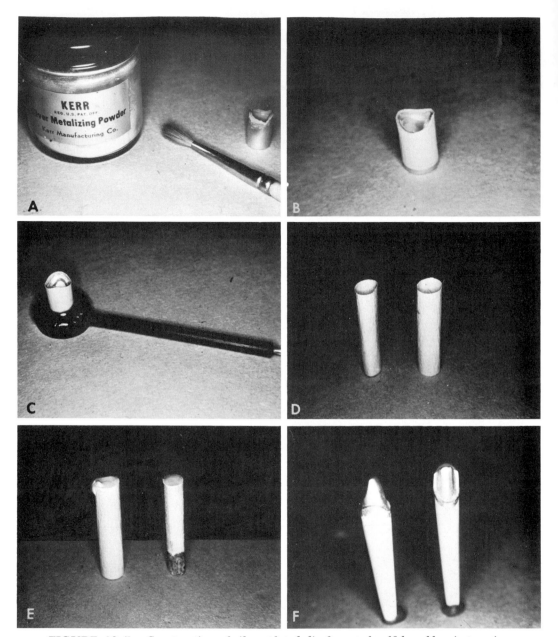

FIGURE 10–5. *Construction of silver-plated die from polysulfide rubber impression.*

A, Impression and metalizing powder.
B, Impression metalized.
C, Impression protected by tape and waxed to cathode holder.
D, Plated dies wrapped for pouring roots.
E, Roots poured.
F, Completed dies with roots tapered.

accomplished through the chemical reduction of silver nitrate. From this reaction, a film of pure silver 2 millionths of an inch thick is deposited on the surface of the impression.[3] Dietrich's* compound or wax impressions may be metalized by the same method.

Solutions.   Three solutions are needed. All must be handled carefully because they produce dark stains on almost all substances, including the skin and porcelain lavatories.

The sensitizing solution is made from

Stannous chloride	1.0 gm.
Hydrochloric acid	1.5 cc.
Distilled water	100.0 cc.

After the stannous chloride has dissolved, the clear liquid is poured off and bottled. The remains are discarded.

The silver nitrate solution requires

Silver nitrate	2.1 gm.
Distilled water	45.0 cc.

The reducing solution is made of

Pyrogallic acid	0.5 gm.
Citric acid	0.1 gm.
Distilled water	15.0 cc.

The sensitizing solution may be prepared in quantity and stored for a time in a brown glass bottle. The chemicals for the other solutions should be weighed and the designated amounts kept in capsules, to be emptied individually as wanted.

Metalizing.   The impression must be placed in the sensitizing solution for 3 to 5 minutes, with all surfaces in contact with the liquid. During this period the silver nitrate and reducing solutions may be mixed separately. The impression must be rinsed, placed in a cup, and the silver nitrate solution poured over the impression, moving the cup to assure complete wetting. After the liquid reducing reagent is added to the silver nitrate, the solution in the cup should be agitated, then allowed to set for 5 or more minutes. The impression is removed, rinsed, dried, and examined. If there are voids in the silver film, the process must be repeated. Paper drinking cups make suitable receptacles for the metalizing chemicals.

Plating.   After metalizing, the bottom of the impression band must be scraped clean in order to make good contact with the cathode holder. It is then waxed to the holder, covering all surfaces not to be plated. A collar of 32-gauge wax or masking tape is placed around the impression band to extend evenly from 2.0 to 3.0 mm. beyond the open end. If an eye dropper is used to fill the impression with the copper solution before attaching it to the plating apparatus, there will be less chance of trapping an air bubble and having an area unplated. The impression is attached to the negative pole, the copper anode to the positive pole. The distance between the anode and cathode is not critical, but a maximal distance up to 8 inches is desirable. The

---

*The Hygienic Dental Mfg. Co., Akron, Ohio.

amount of current will depend on the number of impressions being plated, roughly 20 milliamperes per average impression.

After approximately 20 minutes, the cathode should be removed, rinsed, and examined. If coverage is complete, plating may be continued. If there is an unplated area with a definitely circumscribed border, a bubble of air was trapped. Again completely filling the impression with solution, plating is continued for at least 5 hours. When the impression has been plated to an adequate thickness, it should be removed and rinsed with water and a sodium bicarbonate bath to eliminate all traces of acid. After plating, the impression is filled with a core of stone or resin and a root is formed.

The Stone Die

If the die is to be poured in stone, the band must be wrapped with a wax collar or masking tape extending about 10.0 mm. beyond the cervical margin. (See Figure 10–5D.) The stone mix, using the recommended water-powder ratio, should be vacuumed. Vibration, if used very sparingly, will cause the stone to flow into the impression without forming voids at the incisal angles. Vibration must not be excessive. Also, introducing very small increments of stone along one side of the impression and tapping the band vigorously on the bench will condense the material and give a good surface.

A die poured of stone will be as accurate as the impression and may be used for waxing a pattern for the indirect-direct technique or for a cast transfer. If carefully handled, a platinum matrix may be swaged over such a die; however, owing to abrasion and chipping, the end result is unpredictable and the silver-plated die may be preferable.

Dies formed from epoxy or acrylic resins are invariably undersize as a result of the polymerization shrinkage of the resin. Dies made from amalgam are erratic in dimension and can contaminate castings. Resin and amalgam are not used by the authors. Metal roots, poured into metalized impressions, shrink, and under swaging or burnishing there can be deformation of the die surface. Gypsum hardeners in the mixing solution increase setting expansion.

There seems to be no advantage in utilizing a material for the working die other than stone mixed with the highest possible powder-water ratio.

Quadrant Plating

A wax collar is not necessary when a quadrant or full mouth impression is to be plated. The cathode holder can be an insulated silver or copper wire, contacting the impression at some noncritical spot. Only the areas that are to be plated should be metalized, with silver-powdered wax strips leading to the wire cathode. When the impression is examined after 30 minutes, if the deposits are found to be satisfactory, these "leads" can be waxed over so that plating will not be continued in those areas.

REFERENCES

1. Phillips, R. W., and Schnell, R. J.: Electroformed dies from Thiokol and silicone impressions. J. Pros. Den., *8*:992, Nov.-Dec. 1958.
2. Hudson, W. C.: Clinical uses of rubber impression materials and electroforming of casts and dies in pure silver. J. Pros. Den., *8*:107, Jan. 1958.
3. Phillips, R. W., and Dettman, F. J.: A study of some variables associated with copper-plating of dental impressions. J. Pros. Den., *6*:101, Jan. 1956.

Eastman, R. F.: Individual copper band rubber base impressions for inlays and crowns. J.A.D.A., *59*:966, Nov. 1959.

Hoffman, J. M.: Common problems in the construction of the full cast crown. J.A.D.A., *48*:272, March 1954.

Schnell, R. J., and Phillips, R. W.: Dimensional stability of rubber base impressions and certain other factors affecting accuracy. J.A.D.A., *57*:39, July 1958.

chapter 11

WAX PATTERNS

Wax patterns for individual restorations or cast retainers may be fabricated in two ways: (1) by carving the pattern on a die expected to be devoid of dimensional imperfections (indirect), then making the casting; or (2) by carving the pattern to completion on the prepared tooth (direct), then making the casting.

The *indirect* technique is suggested whenever reproductions of the preparations can be made, because much of the procedure can be delegated to a technician, time will be saved, and almost always the restoration will be superior in contour, adaptation, and marginal fit.

The *direct* method for carving wax patterns (forming them in the mouth on the prepared teeth) should be restricted to anterior partial veneer crowns, pinledge retainers, and inlays. Wax must be applied to the tooth in such a way that all fine lines of the preparation are copied, so that there is ample material to permit carving to form, rather than building to form by the addition of wax, and so that the closed relationship of the teeth may be registered with the wax continuously confined to the tooth surface. Although the ability to produce patterns by this means is rapidly becoming a lost art, some of the more conservative and esthetically preferable partial veneer and inlay preparations demand that it be used. Also, total construction time can be lessened in many cases.

The *indirect-direct* procedure is *not recommended*. This approach to pattern-making is fraught with errors in obtaining proper fit. In addition, tiny fractures, which may occur and result in a weakened casting, as a rule are not detected.

SPECIFICATIONS FOR WAXES

The American Dental Association Specification now provides for two types of waxes, depending on the principal usage for which the wax is intended. In direct techniques, a Type I wax is used, whereas for indirect techniques a Type II wax is employed, the principal difference being in the amount of flow obtained at certain temperatures. A Type I wax, for example, must be very plastic at a temperature only slightly above that of the tooth so that it will flow readily into the details of the cavity preparation. At the same time this type of wax should have minimal flow at mouth temperature in order that the pattern will not distort when removed from the preparation. For indirect techniques, a lower solidification temperature is desired, since the wax is adapted to the die at room temperature. Thus the appropriate type of wax is selected for the technique being used.

Provided it is on the list of certified materials, the choice of the brand is a matter of personal preference with regard to facility in carving and other objective characteristics.

STRESS AND DISTORTION IN WAX PATTERNS

Any wax pattern contains some internal stress, due to carving, molding of the wax, spot heating, or the natural tendency of wax to contract on cooling. Stress can be reduced in any pattern by avoiding undue patching and pooling of the wax and by forming the pattern at as high a temperature as possible.[1] It is true that a pattern fabricated by flowing wax on the die, as in the indirect method, has minimal stress; nevertheless, some exists in any pattern.[2] However, if the pattern is invested immediately after it has been removed from the cavity preparation or die, this stress probably is insignificant.

The two factors exerting the greatest influence on the degree of distortion in the wax pattern before investing are the length of time between the removal and investing of the pattern and the temperature at which it is stored. Even though the storage temperature remains constant, the stress will be relieved over a period of time. Some types of patterns will distort enough in only 30 minutes to prevent critical fitting of the casting (Fig. 11-1). The degree of distortion will increase as the storage temperature is raised, because the lowered yield point and increased flow allow the internal stress to be liberated more easily.

The direct pattern should be placed in a refrigerator if it must be stored overnight, since any change in form is minimized at lower temperatures. Storage in a cup of water does *not* avert warpage. The bad habit of leaving patterns off the preparations, as in a direct technique, to accumulate throughout the day, is a familiar cause for distortion and failure. Also, investing multiple patterns on a single sprue former is contraindicated because of the danger of distortion through uneven expansion.

Patterns should be free of inner surface defects or creases. Outer surfaces should be smooth, polished, and without pits or blemishes. Grooves and sulci should not be scratched or retain small, almost-detached crumbs of wax. Margins should be definite, regular, with a little more bulk, and have substance to resist deformation.

An overwhelming majority of castings are made from patterns carved

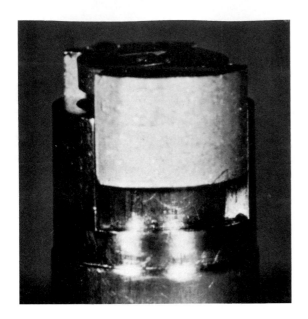

FIGURE 11–1. Wax pattern was stored away from the die for 24 hours and then casting was made. Distortion is result of release of internal stress.

on dies that reproduce teeth prepared so that the surfaces are covered with minute ridges and grooves. If the cut surfaces have been smoothed with fine carborundum stones or paper disks, or if the walls converge occlusally, removal of the carved pattern can be easy. If the tooth or die shows bur or stone marks, the inner surface of the pattern may be made of a thin layer of softer wax, and removal must be confirmed before it takes final form.

With the indirect technique, it is imperative that all margins be checked just before investing. Even on a stone die, the wax may distort some during the interval between fabrication and investing. Once the pattern has been surrounded by set investment, it may be cast when convenient.

INDIRECT WAX PATTERNS

Although the expert or the persevering can carve highly satisfactory direct wax patterns for anterior partial veneer crowns, pinledge retainers, and inlays, routinely the best patterns are made in the laboratory on dies made from elastic impressions. This is because of freedom from interferences found in the oral cavity, lack of tension associated with a "helpful" and uncomfortable patient, better access, and the use of auxiliary personnel unconcerned with other problems.

The die and working cast must be lubricated before the die is dipped into molten wax to assure a thin, contracting film next to all the prepared surfaces (Fig. 11–2). In this way there will be no creases in the internal surface. Regular inlay or Kerr's blue sprue wax may be used. The latter lessens the problem of removing the built-up wax, usually flowed on top of the dipped layer, from some dies; but before the cervical margin is perfected, this softer wax should be cut away 0.5 mm. short of the finishing line and a more rigid wax added. Marginal contour can be developed more quickly and precisely with harder wax.

Using a No. 39 or 40 inverted cone bur, a circumferential groove may be cut around the die about 0.3 mm. below the margin of the preparation to act "as a guide in carving the wax pattern, in checking the seating of the crown on the die and in finishing the crown to the margin."[3] This is an

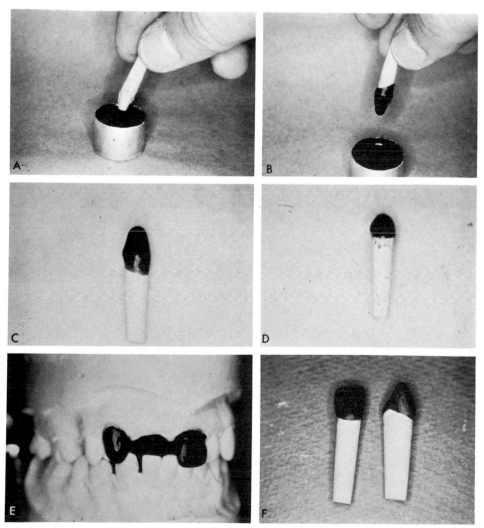

FIGURE 11-2. *A,* Dipping lubricated die into molten wax.

B and *C,* First application of wax at the beginning of formation of wax pattern for retainer casting.

D, Wax trimmed to margin of preparation.

E, Patterns, roughly contoured, transferred to working cast to establish occlusion, length, contacts and width, and to help in forming labial contour.

F, Wax patterns returned to dies for refinement of margins and completion of veneering areas.

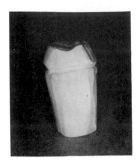

FIGURE 11–3. Prepared die.

excellent method for finishing crowns constructed by an indirect technique (Fig. 11-3). (See Chapter 9, The Working Cast.)

When waxing patterns on stone dies made from elastic impressions, a warm, blunt instrument, rather than one that is sharp, should be used to carve the margins. Otherwise, scarring the stone may lead to a discrepancy in the casting. The pattern can be tried on the working cast to position and gauge the strength of the contacts and to study occlusal carving and alignment (Figs. 11-4 and 11-5). It is then returned to the die, the margins are corrected, and the pattern is polished. It may be wise to examine all margins with a magnifying glass or loupe so that patterns will be more carefully waxed (Fig. 11-6).

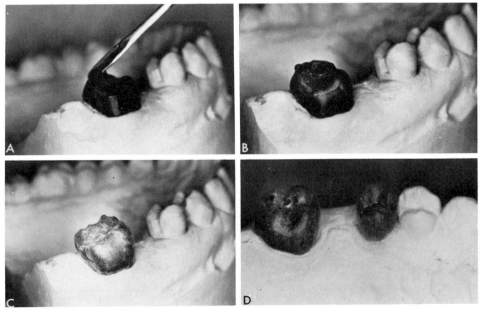

FIGURE 11–4. *The wax pattern.*

A, Wax being applied to lubricated working cast.

B and *C,* Occlusal height and pattern registered by closing articulated casts.

D, Patterns checked for occlusion in lateral and given final form. High spots were carved to a form that contacted but did not interfere with opposing tooth.

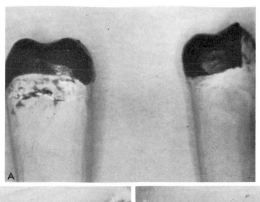

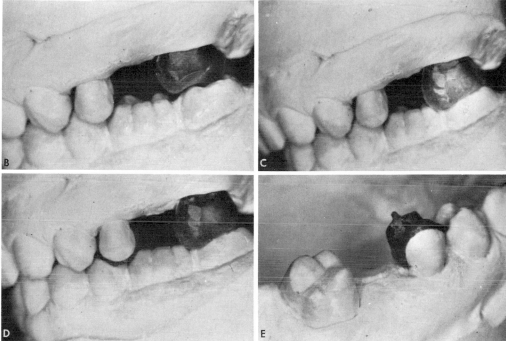

FIGURE 11-5. *Forming the wax pattern.*

A, Wax is flowed on the lubricated die, or the die may be dipped in molten wax if all surfaces of the tooth have been included in the preparation.

B and *C*, Crudely formed pattern is transferred to the lubricated working cast to establish occlusal pattern.

D, Giving occlusal form to second wax pattern.

E, Occlusal pattern formed on bicuspid.

The full veneer gold crown, partial veneer crown, pinledge, and inlay will be included here, but the veneered gold crown will be discussed later.

The Full Veneer Gold Crown

The diagnostic cast, taken before preparation of the tooth, will show the form to be given to the carving. Close attention should be paid to the

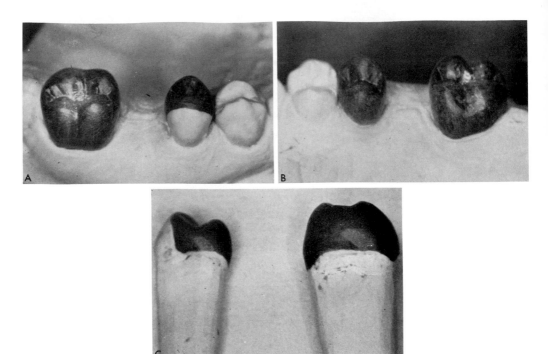

FIGURE 11-6. *Forming the wax pattern (continued).*

A and *B*, Patterns carved and refined.

C, Patterns returned to dies for refinement of cervical margins.

location of the contact areas, the height of contour on both buccal and lingual, the area between the cusp tips, the relation of the cusp tips to the anatomic center of the tooth as determined from the height of contour viewed from the occlusal, the relative size of the cusps, and the relation of the cusps to the marginal ridges. The wax pattern should represent exactly the form of the finished restoration that will be placed in the mouth.

The beginning student and the less apt technician should make some allowances at the cervical margin of a full veneer gold crown pattern. The pattern must not extend cervically beyond the preparation, but it should have just a little extra bulk in that area, possibly an added thickness of 0.3 mm., so that the casting can be polished without causing the margin to be short of the finishing line of the preparation, a common fault. Marginal fit requires adaptation to the prepared surface, with the pattern extending just to the finishing line, and in respect to convexities and concavities, a reproduction or continuation of the tooth form at the junction line. The pattern can be polished with wet cotton.

SPRUING.   The sprue should be attached to a thick area of the pattern and pointed toward the opposite margin. Established contact areas and portions of the pattern carved to functional occlusion need not be disturbed. (See Chapter 12, Spruing, Investing, and Casting.)

The Partial Veneer Crown and MacBoyle Retainer

The pattern for a partial veneer crown or for a MacBoyle retainer may be made by dipping, adding wax, and carving, or by fitting a band, filling it with softened wax, pressing it on the tooth, and carving.

SPRUING. This sprue, like that for a molar pattern, is attached to a heavy part of the pattern (just to the lingual of a contact) and directed toward the opposite margin. (See Chapter 12 on Spruing, Investing, and Casting.)

The Pinledge Retainer

The pattern for a pinledge retainer may be all wax or may utilize plastic pins or nylon bristles in the pinholes with wax flowed around and securely holding them.

Pruden[4] says: "The wax pattern is made by melting inlay wax over the well-lubricated stone cast, and driving it into the pinholes with a very hot pointed instrument, such as an old explorer point. The trapped air will

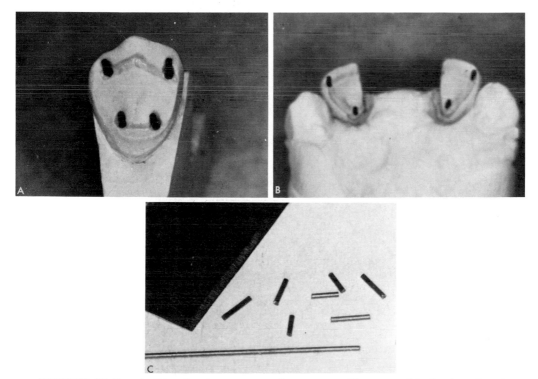

FIGURE 11–7. *A*, Die showing preparation on maxillary cuspid. Surface has been lubricated. Bristles are in place.

B, Die of maxillary lateral incisors ready for application of wax.

C, Cut bristles.

bubble through the melted wax, and a dense smooth wax pattern can be removed from the stone cast with surprisingly little difficulty."

This technique is good when the pinholes have been prepared with tapered fissure burs and the impression made using tapered plastic pins. However, even here plastic pins are an aid in pattern construction.

When the holes in this preparation were made with drills, nylon bristles, slightly smaller in diameter, are cut, headed, and placed in the lubricated

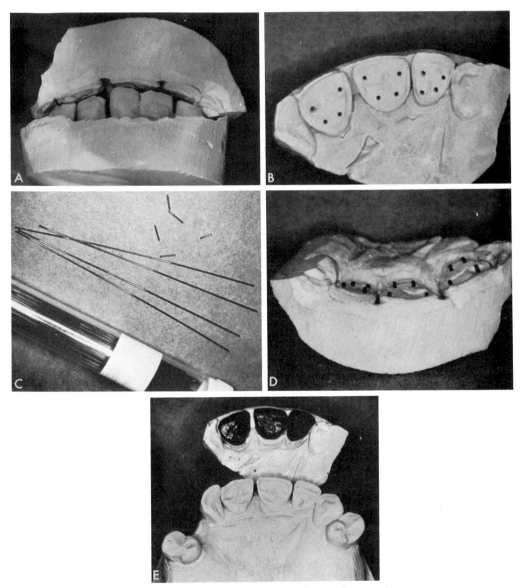

FIGURE 11–8. *A,* Articulated working and opposing casts.
B, Reproduction of three preparations.
C, Nylon bristles for patterns.
D, Bristles in place on lubricated cast.
E, Patterns carved to new vertical dimension.

die. Wax is flowed onto the cut surface and held in position with a finger until cool (Fig. 11–7). This precludes curling and pulling pins out of position (Fig. 11–8).

SPRUING. After the pattern has been carved and polished and the margins checked, a very small round mound of wax is placed in the center of the lingual surface to supply an attachment for the 18-gauge sprue pin. Spruing is done best off the die, with the pattern resting in the palm of the hand. The pin should be at right angles to the plane of the lingual surface. If the pattern is sprued on the die, the added wax must be closer to the incisal and the pin *must* be in line with the path of removal.

The pinledge pattern is the only one attached to the sprue pin so that molten metal enters the mold and strikes a flat or concave surface at a 90-degree angle. The 18-gauge pin is also the smallest used.

The Inlay Retainer

When making a pattern for an inlay, wax may be flowed into the lubricated die or be confined and forced to place with an adjusted matrix band. Carving and removal may be done routinely.

SPRUING. The sprue pin is attached to the contact area and pointed so that the flow of the molten gold in the investment will be divided.

DIRECT CARVING OF WAX PATTERNS

Carving an Anterior Partial Veneer Pattern by the Direct Technique

When it is desirable to carve an anterior partial veneer pattern directly on the prepared tooth, a circular matrix is so shaped that there will be at least 1.0 mm. clearance in the areas of the lingual line angles. The cervical of the band is trimmed to conform to the cervical outline of the preparation and the linguoincisal portion is cut away so that the teeth can be occluded. The inside of the band is coated with Microfilm,* the band is filled with soft wax, the cavity surface is resoftened, and the band is held in position against the labial surface and forced to place on the tooth with the finger being held over the top of the band. In this way wax is forced ahead of the band to insure an excess of wax around the margins of the preparation. When the band is partially seated, or when it appears that the preparation is filled and covered with wax, the finger is removed and the band is completely seated. The patient is asked to close so that the posterior teeth are in full contact, and then to open. Light pressure with the finger is applied to the lingual surface to readapt the wax in the incisal area.

*Kerr Mfg. Company, Romulus, Mich.

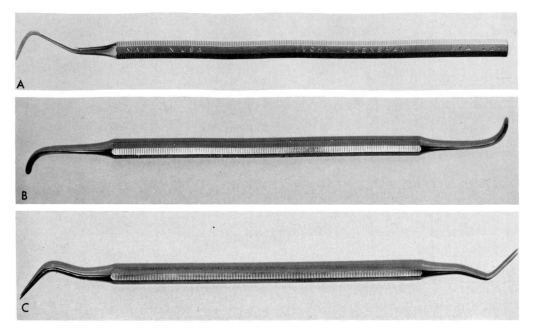

FIGURE 11-9. *A*, Crenshaw scaler.
B, Ash instrument.
C, Wagner instrument.

A heated root canal plugger or a Pinwaxer is inserted into the cingulum pinhole. This process is repeated, and the wax is permitted to solidify without chilling with cold water. The excess around the lingual and cervical of the band is trimmed off and the band is removed while the wax is held in position on the tooth. The pattern must be held on the tooth *at all times* while carving, and preferably all cutting strokes should be toward or along a margin. Trimming may be done and form produced with a variety of instruments, such as the Tarno No. 4 or 5 plastic instrument,† a discoid excavator, a Wagner instrument,‡ a No. 12 Crenshaw scaler,§ an Ash instrument†† (Fig. 11-9), and S. S. White Nos. 5 and 23 explorers.

Spruing. The sprue pin must not be attached in the mouth and used as a handle for removal of the pattern. Although proponents of this technique state that no pattern distortion results, in the hands of the authors and their students, many margins in the incisal area nearest to the point where the pin was attached have been distorted by this method.

Carving a Pinledge Retainer Pattern by the Direct Technique

If the operator elects to use a direct waxing technique for the pinledge pattern, the pinholes can be made with No. 700 or 701 tapered fissure burs,

---

†The S. S. White Dental Mfg. Co., Philadephia, Pa.
‡Dr. Wagner's Dental Specialties, Ellison Bay, Wis.
§J. W. Ivory, Inc., Philadelphia, Pa.
††Claudius Ash, Sons & Co., Inc., Niagara Falls, N. Y.

with drills, or with No. $\frac{1}{2}$ round burs. The pins can be waxed in holes made with tapered burs by using a Pinwaxer or a No. 23 explorer. Wax is pressed against the preparation and partly carved. The Pinwaxer or a blunted No. 23 explorer point is heated, seated in the pinhole, and slowly withdrawn. Molten wax will flow in behind it. Tapered plastic pins, 1.0 mm. longer than the depth of the hole, can be fitted into the pinholes. The wax pattern is readily adapted around that portion that extends beyond the surface of the tooth. Nylon bristles of appropriate size or 24-gauge PGP wire should be used when the pinholes have been made with a drill or a No. $\frac{1}{2}$ round bur.

When using tapered plastic pins, soft wax is pressed against the prepared lingual and proximal surfaces. It is held firmly in position while being carved to approximate form and dimensions. Carving strokes should be toward the cervical or a margin. The wax is pooled over the pins and pressed lightly with a finger in order to fill all indentations or voids. Carving is completed. A small nodule of wax is placed in the center of the lingual surface, and with a No. 5 explorer point engaging the excess wax the pattern is removed.

Direct Waxing with Nylon Bristles. Wax pressed against a lingual surface when nylon bristles are in place in the pinholes must be very soft and the pressure applied must be minimal. As quickly as possible the wax over the bristles must be pooled to enable the nylon to become straight. This will effect loss of tension and let the bristle stay in correct position and relationship to the other bristles and the path of seating.

Direct Waxing with Wire Pins. Each wire pin (24-gauge PGP wire) must be cut long enough to protrude 0.5 mm. from the orifice of the hole. The PGP wire must also have a horizontal extension of not less than 1.0 mm. It is imperative that this arm be bent sharply; otherwise, the pins may not be held tightly in the wax pattern on withdrawal, and the casting will not seat (Fig. 11–10).

After the preparation has been moistened with saliva, the wire pins, grasped by cotton pliers with the arm pointed into the mouth, can be placed in the holes without difficulty. They will be held there by the saliva and friction.

THE WAX PATTERN. With the pins flat against the tooth surface, a softened piece of inlay wax is pressed to place against both the lingual and the proximal surfaces. It must be held against the tooth from the lingual while the incisal and proximal are being carved. The lingual wax is then pared almost to tooth form. The wax is pooled over each pin with a heated canal plugger, and the pins are turned perpendicular to the lingual surface. The wax is resoftened and the arms are rotated into their original positions against the tooth, thereby assuring that wax completely surrounds the wire pins.

Just before the carving is completed, the pattern must be disengaged. If it cannot be removed with a No. 5 explorer point thrust into the lingual surface, the instrument is placed on the proximal and gentle pressure is applied toward the lingual. Minute movement will break the adhesion. It is

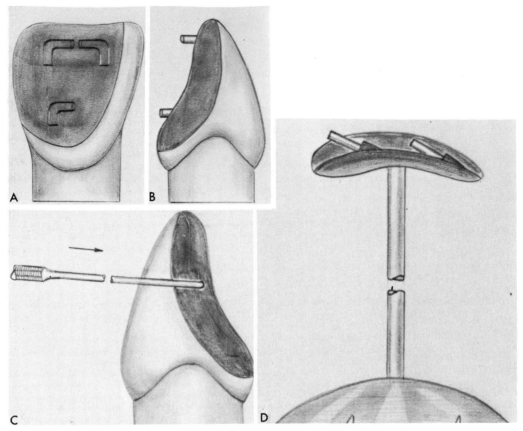

FIGURE 11-10. *A*, Direct wax pattern showing outline and position of pins.
B, Setting pins in wax.
C, Disengaging pattern.
D, Spruing pattern.

then reseated, margins are readapted, carving is finished, and the wax is polished, leaving a little excess on the incisal only.

Spruing. A small bead of wax is added in the center of the lingual surface to facilitate the attachment of the sprue pin. The pattern is removed and sprued as described in the indirect technique. (See Figure 11-10*D*).

(See Chapter 9, The Working Cast, for polysulfide rubber impressions of pinledge preparations. See Chapter 12 for Spruing, Investing, and Casting.)

Carving an Inlay Retainer Pattern by the Direct Technique

When carving an inlay pattern direct, a circular matrix band is fitted loosely around the tooth, the band being trimmed both occlusally and cervically to accommodate the opposing cusps and to avoid cutting the soft tissue. The inner surface of the band is coated with Microfilm and filled with softened inlay wax; then the surface to be applied to the cavity is warmed until the wax is quite soft, after which the band and wax are forced to place on the prepared tooth. The patient is asked to close and to hold this position with no lateral movement until the wax has solidified.

The excess wax is trimmed from the occlusal and cervical of the band, using a suitable wax carver or a warm No. 23 explorer point. A warmed canal plugger or blunted explorer should be used to force the wax into any occlusal or cervical postholes. The band is loosened and removed from the tooth, with the wax being held in position in the tooth either by the finger or by a pellet of damp cotton held by pliers.

At no time during direct carving should the carving stroke be in a direction that will remove the pattern from the tooth, unless it is maintained in its contact position under pressure.

Gross carving can be done with a Wagner or an Ash instrument, a No. 12 Crenshaw scaler, or any instrument most conveniently handled by the operator.

Final proximal carving is best done with the No. 23 explorer, or the tapered end of the Wagner, finishing at the cervical with the Tarno Nos. 1 and 2 wax burnishers. The No. 2 can be used with a lateral "push" or "pull" stroke.

The occlusal surface can be carved with the instrument of choice; either the flat end of the Wagner instrument or the No. 5 explorer is most efficient. If a margin is uncovered, small amounts of wax may be added to the pattern, making sure that no saliva is incorporated and that a union between the added wax and the pattern is consummated.

Contours compatible with the tooth being restored and with the occlusal pattern must be formed. If the tooth has abraded surfaces on the proximal or occlusal, such surfaces must be copied. If the patient is young, with normal convexities and grooves, then such form must appear in the carving.

There can be no overextended margins, occlusally, proximally, or cervically. Checking the wax pattern *before it is removed from the tooth* will disclose any such discrepancy. After the occlusal is polished with wet cotton and the proximal surface with smooth-edged seam binding tape, the pattern can be removed from the tooth, using an explorer on the proximal, or two explorers if the pattern is an MOD.

Spruing. With the pattern resting in the palm of the hand, the sprue pin should be attached at once. It must be invested immediately.

The Cone Waxing Technique will be discussed in Chapter 34.

REFERENCES

1. Lasater, R. L.: Control of wax distortion by manipulation. J.A.D.A., 27:518, April 1940.
2. Phillips, R. W., and Biggs, D. H.: Distortion of wax pattern as influenced by storage time,

storage temperature, and temperature of wax manipulation. J.A.D.A., *41*:28, July 1950.

3. Smith, G. P.: The marginal fit of the full cast shoulderless crown. J. Pros. Den., *7*:231, March 1957.

4. Pruden, K. C.: A hydrocolloid technique for pinledge bridge abutments. J. Pros. Den., *6*:65, Jan. 1956.

Hollenback, G. M.: Brief history of the cast restoration. J. South. California D. A., *30*:8, Jan. 1962.

Kasloff, Z.: Recent advances in casting techniques and their evaluation. Internat. D. J., *13*:331, June 1963.

chapter 12

SPRUING, INVESTING, AND CASTING*

The objective in any casting technique is to produce from a wax pattern a casting that will fit snugly on the preparation and be free of porosity. Success of an inlay or crown depends on minute accuracy and maintenance of the high physical properties of the alloy necessary to resist deformation and corrosion. Probably the most trying problem facing the dentist or technician is to obtain the vital over-all adaptation of metal to tooth surface and to margins.

Although it is true that the perfect casting has never been made, dental casting procedures have progressed to a point where failure, which has become the exception, usually can be traced to a lack of respect for the basic principles associated with a sound technique. The process of fabricating a dense small casting that fits cannot be a haphazard one, and short cuts inevitably lead to failure. Each operator must adjust his own technique to the fundamentals, inasmuch as fundamentals cannot be altered to accommodate every empirical method of investing or casting.

No single investing technique will satisfy all individuals. The one selected should be the method that best meets the desired standards and offers maximal reproducibility in the hands of the user. The choice should become established only after making test castings on machined cavity preparations, such as the Bureau of Standards steel dies, and comparing the capability of accurate copying. When the clinician is content with the results, the procedure should not be changed.

Zinc phosphate cement, the common luting medium, is soluble in oral fluids,[1] particularly the weak organic acids[2] that may be present for limited periods at the critical marginal areas. The less exact the fit of the gold restoration, the wider the band of cement that will be exposed and the sooner this margin will deteriorate, owing to dissolution of cement. A magnifying lens will show quickly that even the best inlay or crown attainable fits none too well. In fact, it is very difficult to determine the precise fit of a

*Investing and casting for *bonded porcelain veneers* is discussed in Chapter 21.

casting in the oral cavity. Many cemented restorations do not fit as well as clinical examination might indicate. In one clinical study ten experienced dentists were asked to evaluate the marginal adaptation of a group of inlays by means of a sharp and delicate explorer and roentgenograms. These marginal areas were then measured microscopically. Restorations classified as "acceptable" had marginal openings as great as 120 microns at certain areas such as the gingival, where visibility is restricted. It cannot be disputed that minor marginal seepage of fluids occurs with any gold restoration, as well as other restorative materials.[3, 4] Longevity of the crown or bridge rests to a notable extent on minimizing such leakage. If the casting is well adapted, disintegration of the thin layer of cement is of secondary importance.

A smooth surface and density are other requisites of the gold casting. Any porosity will result in pits or voids that drastically lower the physical properties and thus increase the possibility of distortion or fracture during mastication. Corrosion and discoloration will occur also, but the prevailing causes for corrosion are surface roughness or contamination of the alloy.

The finished casting can be no better than the original wax pattern; therefore, it follows that extreme care must be taken to assure maximal reproduction of the cavity preparation for the sake of stability, anatomical contour for function, and freedom from distortion to enhance seating.

SPRUING

Cleanliness must be pre-eminent in the investing process. Any separating medium, saliva, blood, or crumbs of wax must be removed from the pattern by gently brushing it with a soft brush, soap, and room-temperature water. Similarly the sprue base must be free of any particles of old investment that will leave a frayed or rough surface after separation.

KINDS OF SPRUES. Either wax or metal sprues may be used. If metal is employed, it should be rust resistant to prevent contamination of the mold. When joining a metal sprue pin to the pattern, the pin must not be overheated or it will melt or distort the adjacent area on the pattern, and as the wax resolidifies it will contract and perhaps draw away from the margins. A drop of wax may be added where the pin is to be attached, and the pin can be inserted without disturbing the body of the pattern. Hollow rather than solid metal sprues* (e.g., orthodontic tubing) are more desirable as they hold less heat.

SIZES OF SPRUES. The size of the sprue will be a determinant of the density of the casting.[5] If it is too small, the gold will freeze in the sprue first, and as it contracts will pull metal from the casting itself. (See Figure 12–1.) The ensuing porosity is termed "shrinkage porosity" and most often is found at the point of sprue pin attachment (Fig. 12–2). For the average size or large pattern, the sprue pin must be not less than 1.7 mm. (14-gauge),

---

*Whip–Mix Corporation (Louisville, Ky.) now supplies hollow sprues of four gauge sizes.

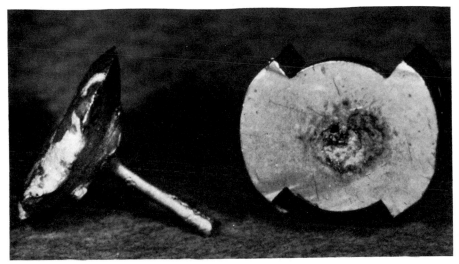

FIGURE 12-1. Example of shrinkage porosity resulting from use of a sprue that was too small.

preferably 2.5 mm. (10-gauge). When the pattern is very small or thin, an 18-gauge sprue pin should be used to avoid distortion of the wax. Reservoirs are recommended as an aid in eliminating any inclination toward shrinkage porosity, but they are superfluous if the sprue is of appropriate size.

ATTACHING SPRUES. The sprue pin should be placed at the bulkiest part of the pattern, but not at a place where it will obliterate carving designed to promote function in lateral excursions or in centric closing, with the inside or open area of the pattern toward the top of the ring. Fixing the pin at an angle, rather than vertically to a flat area, will lessen considerably the chance of gold "turbulence" and subsequent porosity.[6] (See Figure 12-3.)

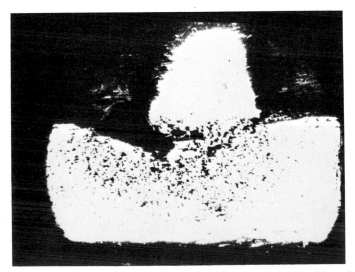

FIGURE 12-2. Shrinkage porosity as shown by metallographic picture. Porosity extends deeply into casting.

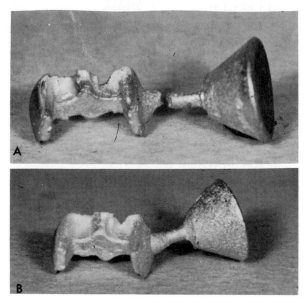

FIGURE 12-3.   Improper position of sprue (*A*) causes gold turbulence and porosity. Sprue should be placed at angle to proximal wall (*B*).

In most instances a mandibular full veneer gold crown pattern can be sprued on the lingual surface of a lingual cusp or on the surface approximating an edentulous area. A maxillary crown pattern will not be damaged if the sprue pin is placed on the buccal surface of a buccal cusp. A partial veneer pattern can have a reduced contact restored by spruing to it, but if the contact has been carved and adjusted, the pin should be placed either on the opposite proximal surface or lingually to the cusp tip (Fig. 12-4). An inlay pattern seldom can be sprued advantageously other than on the contact area. A pinledge or a MacBoyle pattern should be joined to the sprue pin in

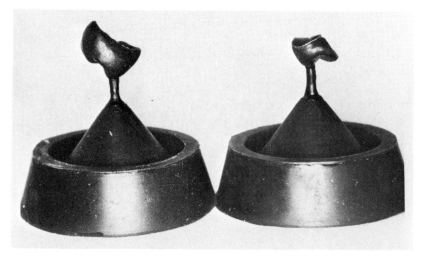

FIGURE 12-4.   Points and angles of attachment for attaching sprue pins to upper posterior patterns.

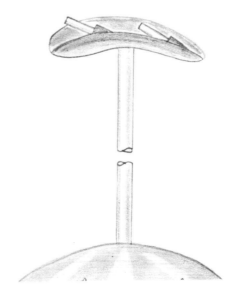

FIGURE 12–5. Spruing pinledge pattern.

the center of the lingual surface, perpendicular to the plane of that surface (see Figure 12-5); still, a MacBoyle pattern occasionally can be sprued in the same way as a partial veneer. Pins should be attached to pontics to cause the molten metal to flow along, rather than directly against, metal backings.

DOUBLE SPRUES.   Double sprues are not essential as a rule for the crown and bridge casting, but when an occlusal or a surface to be veneered is shallow in comparison with the proximal walls, a double sprue or vent must be used or the metal will tend to freeze first in the thinner area and lead to porosity or an incomplete casting.[7] (See Chapter 21, The Veneered Gold Crown.)

Location of a Pattern in the Ring

The location of a pattern in the ring is another variable that markedly affects the density of the casting. After the wax has been burned out, gases remain in the evacuated mold, and as the gold is forced into this space these gases must filter through the investment and out the end of the ring. If they are not expelled the gold cannot fill the pattern area, and, owing to the backward thrust of the gases that are still present, "back pressure" porosity results.[8] Many times wrongly diagnosed, this is one of the most frequent types of porosity seen in dental castings. It is prevalent especially in the full cast crown, in which the large inner core of investment slows the gas escape from the occlusal area. (See Figure 12–6.) The porosity pattern is inconstant and may be evidenced in various ways, such as rounded margins, general porosity, or a hole in the casting. The sprue pin should have the length to place the end of the pattern within ¼ inch of the end of the ring (Figs. 12-7 and 12-8). In this position the gases can be readily

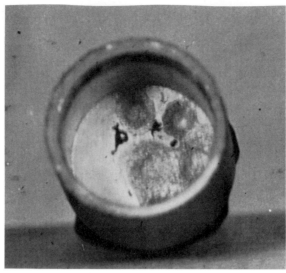

FIGURE 12-6. Example of back-pressure porosity caused by gases not being completely forced out of the mold. This type of porosity can be evidenced in many other ways.

expelled through the investment. If the diameter of the sprue pin is adequate, the length may be safely increased in order to locate the pattern close to the end of the ring.

Because of the density of the investments used in constructing the porcelain fused to metal restoration (Chapter 21), the mold itself may be vented. This is accomplished by attaching an auxiliary sprue from an external tip of the pattern up to the periphery of the crucible end of the ring, as

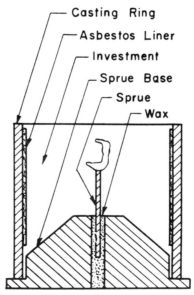

Casting Ring
Asbestos Liner
Investment
Sprue Base
Sprue
Wax

FIGURE 12-7. Schematic drawing to show proper location of pattern in ring and the various components that are used in making a dental casting.

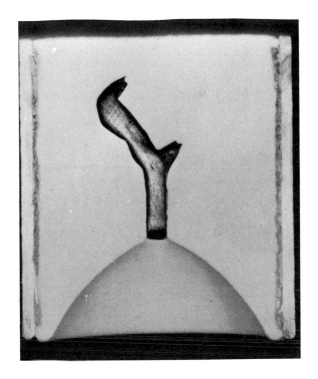

FIGURE 12-8. Section cut
through an invested pattern to show
the location in ring.

illustrated in Figure 12-9. Venting is not needed with the gypsum type
investments that are to be discussed in this chapter.

A further factor in this phenomenon of back pressure is the casting
pressure. It must be sufficient to force the gases out. Within reasonable
limits, little danger exists from too much pressure. At least four turns of the
casting arm are suggested with a centrifugal machine; a minimum of 15
pounds should be used in air pressure casting. Some of the newer casting
machines make use of vacuum, either wholly or in conjunction with centrifugal force or air pressure. Properly used, all these devices bring comparable
results.

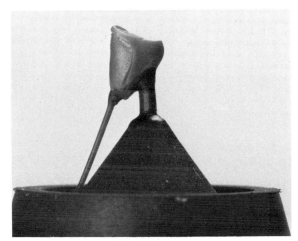

FIGURE 12-9. Vented pattern.

THEORY OF COMPENSATION

One of the perplexities associated with the casting process is the change in dimension of the casting, owing to the contraction of the gold alloy when it solidifies. The true figure for this shrinkage remains unknown, but values have been published ranging from 1.1 to as high as 2.1 per cent.[9, 10] A value of 1.4 ± 0.2 per cent is considered satisfactory for the practical dental casting.

Various methods to compensate for this contraction of the alloy are employed in different casting techniques. All, to some extent, make use of the three types of expansion that occur in dental investments; these are (1) the normal setting of the investment as it hardens, (2) thermal expansion as the investment is heated, and (3) hygroscopic expansion from water if it is brought into contact with the investment during setting.[11] Assuming that the wax pattern meets expectations, the investment mold is enlarged via these three mechanisms to adjust for the shrinkage of the alloy.

There has been extensive theorizing that one realm of expansion cannot be used for all types of restorations made in dental practice. For example, the investment expansion required for a full cast crown involving long and parallel walls might not be the same as that for a three-quarter crown having short and tapering walls. It has been generally accepted that the investing technique has to be modified for the particular type of casting to be made.

In principle this concept is still factual, and in certain situations it is necessary to vary the expansion, as will be discussed. However, with today's investments and a keener appreciation of the circumstances that control the dimensions of the mold, a single technique can be used for *most* of the usual types of cavity preparations encountered clinically. Apparently with an accepted technique as described in this chapter, the total investment expansion closely approximates the contraction of the gold alloy, providing expansion for the extracoronal castings to seat fully, yet expansion not so great that the intracoronal casting is kept from seating.

INVESTMENTS AND INVESTING TECHNIQUES

Thermal Expansion

The basic ingredients of dental inlay investments used with conventional gold alloys are dental stone, some form of silica, and divers modifiers that include reducing agents, accelerators, and retarders. The stone furnishes the refractory binder, while the silica is used principally to cause the thermal expansion of the mold.

Two physical forms of silica are found in dental investments, and investments may be classified on the basis of whether they contain predominantly the *quartz* or *cristobalite* type. These two allotropic forms of silica undergo a transition in their particle size as they are heated. They differ in the amount of the thermal expansion that is reached during this transition and the temperature range at which it occurs.

Characteristic thermal expansion curves for investments containing quartz and cristobalite are shown in Figure 12-10. It can be seen that the ultimate thermal expansion of the cristobalite investment (Curve A) is greater than that of the quartz investment (Curve B). Likewise the maximal expansion takes place over the rather narrow temperature range of 450 to 700° F., then levels off to a comparatively flat plateau.

If the investment is permitted to cool, the contraction follows essentially the same curve, and so the plateau of a cristobalite investment affords quite a bit of latitude during the casting procedure. For instance, if the casting ring were taken out of the furnace at 1200° F. and several minutes were taken to melt the alloy and make the casting, the temperature drop in the investment would not bring about a significant contraction in the mold.

Because of the rapid expansion of a cristobalite investment over a somewhat narrow temperature range, heating must be slow during the burnout of the wax pattern so that the mold will not crack. If the investment is heated too fast, the outer portion of the investment that is next to the metal ring may be much hotter than the inner portion. The difference in the rate of expansion between the two areas can produce cracks in the investment.

The utmost thermal expansion of a quartz investment is less than that of a cristobalite investment and it expands more gradually. Maximal expansion is not reached until approximately 1100° F., and because of this, the plateau of the thermal expansion curve is not so long as for a cristobalite investment. Consequently whenever a quartz investment is used a burnout temperature

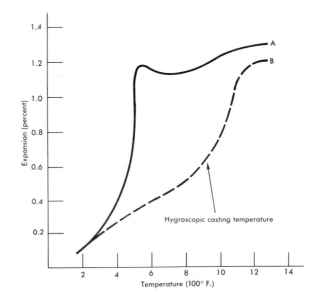

FIGURE 12-10. Thermal expansion of a typical cristobalite (*A*) investment and a quartz (*B*) investment. The amount of expansion that occurs in a quartz investment at the wax burnout temperature when the hygroscopic investing technique is used is also noted. (After R. Neiman, Whip-Mix Corp.)

of 1250° F. is vital to preclude an undue contraction of the mold during the time the gold alloy is melted and the casting is made.

Since the thermal expansion of a quartz investment occurs over a much broader range of temperature than a cristobalite investment, there is a little greater leeway in the rapidity with which the ring may be heated. It should be heated slowly, though, regardless of the composition of the investment.

Setting Expansion

The mold is enlarged to a lesser extent by the setting expansion of the investment as it hardens. The normal *unrestricted* setting expansion is approximately 0.3 per cent (Curve A, Fig. 12-11), but this amount of expansion may not take place when the investment is confined by the metal ring that is used to contain the pattern and the investment. The setting expansion that actually does contribute to an enlargement of the mold is called the "effective" setting expansion.

Part of this effective setting expansion is the result of the thermal expansion of the wax pattern stemming from the heat liberated during the setting of the investment. In addition, as the investment hardens it eventually gains enough strength so that it can effect a movement in the wax pattern. To exemplify, during the setting expansion the inner core of investment within an MOD wax pattern reaches a strength that will impel the proximal walls slightly outward.

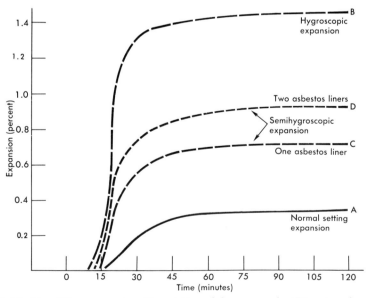

FIGURE 12-11. The normal setting (A) and hygroscopic (B) expansion of an investment are compared to the somewhat restricted expansion that occurs in a metal inlay ring, which is lined with one (C) and two (D) asbestos liners. (After R. Neiman, Whip-Mix Corp.)

The configuration of the individual pattern has some influence on the amount of effective expansion that occurs. If the walls are thin, the expansion will be greater than in the case of a pattern with thick walls. The investment can move the thinner walls outward more easily; moreover, the proximal walls of an MOD may be propelled outward with less force than those of a full cast crown with continuous walls that offer more resistance to the expansion of the investment. Thus, for certain types of patterns, additional thermal or hygroscopic expansion may be required because of the lower effective setting expansion that really does take place in the ring, and vice versa.

Hygroscopic Expansion

The hygroscopic expansion investing technique evolved because it was believed that if the wax elimination were carried out at a temperature of approximately 1250° F., the gypsum in the investment would break down and the surface of the resultant casting would be rough. It was rationalized that if the wax burnout was made at a lower temperature, such as 900° F., then the gold casting would have a smoother surface. There is no evidence that a mold heated to 900° F. yields a smoother casting than one that has been rightly heated to 1250° F. Nevertheless this theory has led to the development of the modern hygroscopic investing procedures.

Curve B in Figure 12-10 shows that if the casting is made at a temperature of 900° F., the full benefit of the thermal expansion of a quartz investment is not realized. This temperature is at the midpoint of the thermal expansion curve. By casting at the lower temperature, the thermal expansion that would occur between 900 and 1200° F. is sacrificed.

To secure the additional expansion necessary to compensate for the loss in the thermal expansion, hygroscopic expansion techniques were developed. The most common method is to expose the investment to an unlimited amount of water by placing the ring immediately after investing in a 100° F. water bath for approximately 30 minutes. A noteworthy amount of expansion takes place under such conditions (Curve B, Fig. 12-11).*

Another way for providing hygroscopic expansion is by the addition of a limited amount of water to the setting investment, usually referred to as the "controlled water added" technique.[12] The degree of hygroscopic expansion is regulated to some extent by the amount of water that is added to the surface of the setting investment.

Whatever the investing technique, since the metal ring is ordinarily lined with a layer of wet asbestos, semihygroscopic expansion invariably occurs. The water in the liner causes a hygroscopic expansion of the investment in the area where it is in contact with the wet liner. The additional expansion induced by one asbestos liner is shown in Curve C in Figure 12-11; with two

---

*The reader is referred to accepted texts in the science of dental materials for a discussion of the theory of hygroscopic expansion.

liners there will be an even greater semihygroscopic expansion as shown in Curve D in Figure 12–11.

Selection of Investment

Equally satisfactory castings can be made with a number of techniques that make use of the thermal, setting, and hygroscopic expansion of the investment in order to enlarge the mold and compensate for the contraction of the gold alloy. Too much time is spent in defending one expansion technique against another.

Occasionally there may be reason to increase or decrease dimensions of the mold. A full cast crown, particularly if the walls are long and parallel, in the main calls for more investment expansion than a two-surface or a partially circumferential restoration. In the case of the crown, if the casting is a little undersize, friction between the casting and the walls of the preparation impedes seating the casting.

Short and converging retentive walls necessitate less compensation. There is little friction in the seating of such a crown, inasmuch as the casting does not touch the cavity walls until it is almost in place, and the configuration of the pattern may influence the amount of effective setting or hygroscopic expansion.

The degree of expansion required for each type of preparation is learned through experience, and the technique is changed accordingly to increase or decrease the compensation.

It must be remembered that stability in a seated casting is mandatory, resisting all forces that cause motion and, to a lesser degree, movement directed opposite to the path of insertion. The casting should fit closely on the preparation, but it should slip to place with finger pressure or very light tapping with a mallet and an orangewood stick or metal instrument.

The Asbestos Liner

One of the means by which the dimensions of the mold may be altered is by use of an asbestos liner to permit more freedom in the expansion of the investment, freedom that otherwise would be restricted by the ring.[13] In addition, the compressible property of the liner assists in offsetting the contraction of the more rapidly cooling ring after it has been removed from the furnace and while the gold alloy is being melted. Also, if a wet liner is used, the water in the liner affords some hygroscopic expansion (Fig. 12–11).

The distance between the end of the pattern and the unlined portion of the ring has been found to affect significantly the size of the castings. Both the pattern and the lining must have a specific position in the ring to eliminate this variable. It is recommended that the pattern be placed at a constant distance of 6.0 mm. from the open end of the ring. (See Figure 12-7.)

When expansion must be maximal, a liner flush with the open end (the end opposite from the sprue opening) of the ring should be used. A liner that is 3.0 or 6.0 mm. short of the open end of the ring will bring about a somewhat smaller casting; the greater the unlined portion of the ring, the greater will be the restrictive effect. The distance by which the liner is short should be carefully controlled, and the liner should be attached firmly to the ring by wax to prevent it from "riding up" during the investing procedure and inadvertently modifying the size of the casting. Increasing the number of liners will provide additional expansion.

Use of a liner that is flush with the end of the ring removes the need for measuring the distance of the liner from the open end of the ring and so may simplify the standardization of the procedure.

Practically all types of castings can be cast to an accurate fit with one sphere of expansion, at least at the level reached by several of the available investments (e.g., Luster Cast* and Beauty-cast†). There may be a few instances in which a casting that fits tighter may be sought or, conversely, in which a shade more of expansion is needed. Some latitude in expansion may be had by altering certain of the variables found in the investing procedure. Decreasing the powder-water ratio will reduce the setting expansion slightly, and vice versa. This should be done with discretion, since undue deviation from the suggested ratio may affect deleteriously the strength of the investment and the mold surface.

The orientation of the pattern in the ring also plays a role in this regard. If an MOD pattern is sprued on the occlusal surface, the mesial-distal expansion is reduced by the confining action of the ring. The expansion may be increased a bit by attaching the sprue on the proximal surface so that the mesial-distal expansion is in the direction of the open ends of the ring.

One manufacturer* supplies a specially prepared quartz investment, referred to as Control Powder, that has a thermal expansion of approximately 0.75 per cent.[14, 15] When this investment is mixed in varying proportions with a cristobalite-type investment, thermal expansion values between 0.75 and 1.3 per cent may be obtained. Experience will dictate modifications in technique.

Hand Investing

Wax patterns can be invested regularly by hand without nodules or imperfections on the gold casting,[16] although care and practical knowledge are invaluable in overcoming human inconsistencies.[17] Whether the pattern is to be invested by hand or by vacuum equipment, strict adherence to the powder-water ratio is a must. Deviations from the recommended ratio will have an effect not only on the setting and thermal expansion, but also, and of more consequence, on the surface smoothness of the casting. If the mix is too thick, the investment will flow sluggishly onto the surface of the pattern

---

*Kerr Mfg. Company, Romulus, Mich.
†Whip-Mix Corporation, Louisville, Ky.

and air bubbles may be formed. A thin mix will have a lower strength, increasing the possibility of fracture, particularly at the margins, during burnout or casting.

Nodules on the surface of a casting are due to air that was either incorporated in the investment itself or trapped during the investing process. If investment and water are blended with a mechanical spatulator, any large air bubbles will be broken up. A wetting agent, painted on the surface of the pattern before investing, will decrease the likelihood of enclosing air, but more than a very light coat will cause surface flaws on the casting; hence, any excess should be taken up with a dry camel's-hair brush. Vibration should be avoided when a wetting agent has been used, because the liquid tends to flow irregularly and to foam.

When the correct powder-water ratio has been used, the consistency of the mix will be such that a small portion of the investment, placed on an inside edge of the pattern, will flow onto the floor of the pattern as it is gently pushed with a brush (Fig. 12–12). It should be applied from only one spot, because bubbles can be trapped wherever two separate portions of investment join. After the pattern has been covered, the investment may be blown off the surface, leaving a thin film and disengaging any large bubbles. The pattern should be repainted, the inlay ring filled, and the invested pattern cautiously seated in the ring with an oscillating motion; or the ring may be placed over the painted pattern and the investment flowed in on one side until the ring is filled (Figs. 12–13 and 12–14). A mechanical vibrator

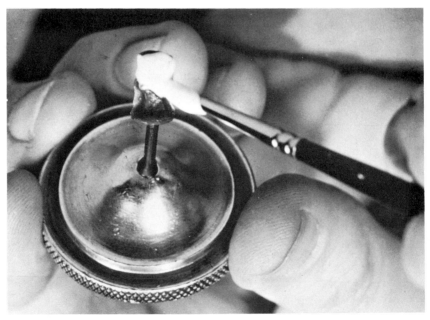

FIGURE 12–12.   Investment is gently flowed onto pattern with a small brush, applying from only one spot. Note clean surface on sprue base. If wetting agent is used, it must be a very thin coat.

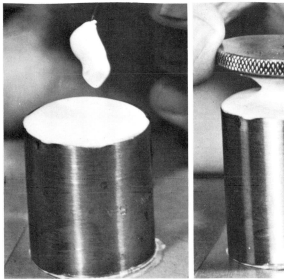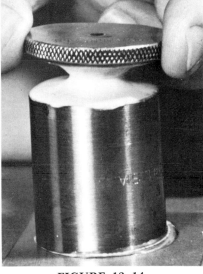

FIGURE 12-13   FIGURE 12-14

FIGURE 12-13.   Painted pattern is carefully vibrated into filled ring.

FIGURE 12-14.   Final step in seating pattern in ring. If proper powder-water ratio is used there is no danger in breaking off pattern.

should not be used, because any air remaining in the investment seems to collect around the pattern.

Vacuum Investing

Castings free of nodules can be secured routinely by either hand or vacuum investing, but if it is astutely handled, vacuum investing is certainly more nearly foolproof.[17] With it, reproduction of minute marginal detail is sharper and, because of a more compact mass of investment adjacent to the pattern, the surface density of the gold is greater.

Many kinds of vacuum equipment are at the disposal of the profession (Fig. 12-15). Perhaps the most satisfactory is one in which both the mixing and the investing are done under vacuum. Directions for using two types follow.*

Equipments and Their Use.   The mixing bowl, spatulator, and vacuum line must be free of investment. If the equipment has not been used recently, the pump should be operated (with the mixing bowl, spatulator, stainless steel casting ring, and rubber crucible former in place) to make sure that the vacuum will measure up to 26 to 28 pounds.

The ring designed for the investor being used is lined with one or more layers of asbestos of proper width. The wax pattern is sprued in the same manner as for hand investing. To resist pull from force of the vacuum, the

---

*Whip-Mix Corporation, Louisville, Ky.; Kerr Mfg. Company, Romulus, Mich.

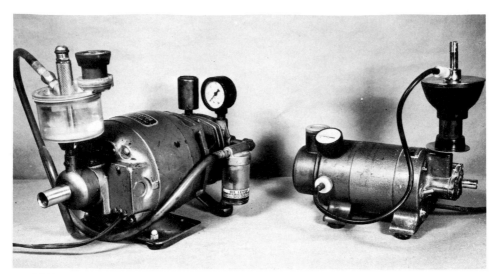

FIGURE 12–15. Various types of vacuum equipment for investing patterns are available.

pattern must be solidly attached to the sprue pin. The pattern is cleaned and, if desired, is painted with a very small quantity of wetting agent. Any excess should be removed with a dry brush.

The sprue pin is placed on the special rubber crucible former, which is fitted to the asbestos-lined casting ring. Room-temperature distilled water and investment powder (previously measured and weighed to meet specifications) are placed in the bowl and mixed with a plaster spatula.

The clean, dry spatulator is placed on the mixing bowl and the inlay ring inserted into the spatulator (Whip-Mix), or it is placed on the bottom of the rubber bowl (Kerr) after removing the plug. The motor operating the vacuum pump is turned on and the vacuum hose is connected to the spatulator. Atmospheric pressure will hold casting ring and crucible former in place.

The spatulator shaft is attached to the rotating motor shaft and the investment is mixed under vacuum (15 to 20 seconds on the Whip-Mix equipment; 30 to 60 seconds with the Kerr). The vacuum inlets must be turned upright to minimize the contingency of having them filled with investment. The mixing bowl must be tipped rather warily from horizontal to vertical while vibrating the investment and causing it to flow from the mixing bowl into the ring. Vibration is transmitted through the rubber crucible former and casting ring to the mixing bowl. If the casting ring is carried to a vertical position too speedily, bubbles may be formed on the surface of the wax pattern adjacent to the sprue pin.

When the ring is filled with investment, the vacuum tube should be removed from the spatulator. When the Whip-Mix machine is used, vacuum may be terminated suddenly, but with the Kerr machine, it is prudent to remove the vacuum tube slowly and to continue mild vibration while doing so. Since the casting ring will drop away from the bowl upon removal of the vacuum, it must be held against the bowl during this operation.

The investment-filled casting ring should be set aside until the investment has hardened. Before the setting the bowl, spatulator, and vacuum line must be cleansed impeccably of any investment that they may have accumulated.

Vacuum investing equipment may be used also for vacuum mixing only, but the small-sized bowl will not prepare enough investment for two casting rings. If the bowl is overloaded, investment will be forced into the vacuum line and must be cleaned out promptly. The vacuum line and vacuum pressure must always be inspected before use.

Hygroscopic Technique

In the hygroscopic technique, after surrounding the wax pattern with a specially compounded investment, the casting ring is immediately immersed in a water bath at a temperature of approximately 100° F. The contact of the setting investment with the warm water brings about an added expansion, referred to as hygroscopic expansion, an expansion that probably is a prolongation of the normal setting expansion.

In most of the present hygroscopic expansion techniques, the degree of hygroscopic expansion sought is controlled by regulating the powder-water ratio. Generally the thicker the investment mix the greater will be the hygroscopic expansion. Also, the longer the delay in time before the investment is immersed in the water bath the less will be the hygroscopic expansion. With some investments the expansion may be increased by using warmer water.

After the investment has hardened, the ring is removed from the water bath and the burnout completed as for the thermal expansion technique.

Controlled Water-added Technique

In this technique a soft flexible rubber ring is employed instead of the conventional asbestos-lined metal ring. The pattern is invested normally. Straightaway a specific amount of water is added on the top of the investment and the investment is allowed to set, customarily at room temperature. It is contended that the degree of hygroscopic expansion caused by the added water may be controlled by the amount of water used.

It should be emphasized that several investing techniques can produce comparable results. The dentist or technician should familiarize himself with different methods to find the one that will work best in his hands.[18] In any technique, however, the fundamentals described here will be applicable.

REMOVAL OF THE SPRUE PIN. The sprue pin and base should not be removed for approximately 30 minutes. The edge and outside of the ring should be cleaned of all flakes of investment that might accidentally fall into

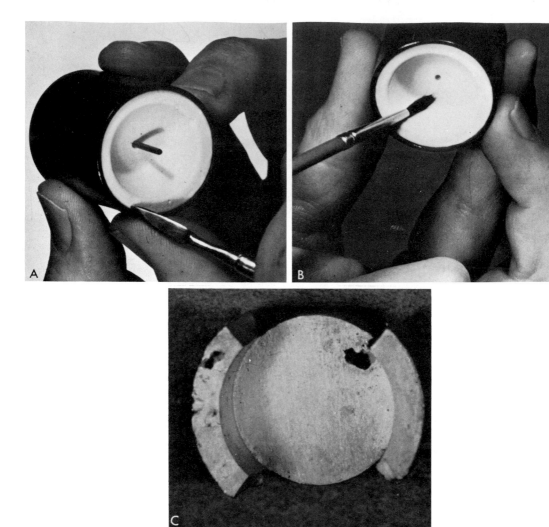

FIGURE 12-16.   *A*, Investment should be trimmed from edge of ring to prevent flakes from falling into sprue hole.

B, Dry brush may be used, holding ring inverted, to brush off investment chips after pulling sprue out.

C, Any bits of investment or charcoal from flux that get into mold will result in sharp, well-defined deficiencies as seen here.

the sprue hole. The pin is heated over a burner and carefully pulled from the investment. It is advisable, too, to check the edge of the investment at the sprue hole and to detach any small irregular edges that might inadvertently enter the mold during burnout or casting. (See Figure 12-16.)

Burnout

Elimination of the wax may be started as soon as the sprue pin has been removed (never before 30 minutes after investing), or it may be safely postponed indefinitely. While it is imperative to invest the pattern as soon as feasible to escape warpage, heating of the mold may be done at any suitable time. Once the burnout is started, the casting should be completed without the mold cooling, as reheating will cause a marked loss in strength in the investment, with the risk of frayed margins or an unacceptable casting.

The dental office or laboratory should contain an electric burnout furnace equipped with a pyrometer (Fig. 12-17). Calculated temperature control is essential in burning out the wax, and many failures may be traced to neglect of this precautionary measure. The pyrometer should be checked periodically, because it is not unusual to find these temperature-measuring devices to be inaccurate by as much as several hundred degrees. Dental gold manufacturers supply small cones of chemical compounds that melt at a specific temperature. These temperature indicators form an easy and precise way for checking the furnace temperature as registered on the pyrometer.

The temperature of the furnace should never be above 800° F. at the time the ring is inserted. Initial burnout temperatures above 800° F. cause too hasty heating, with danger of cracking the mold. The heating should be slow until the free water and the water of crystallization of the plaster have been evaporated. If the temperature is increased too quickly, steam may be formed and small pieces of investment literally will explode off the inside of the mold, giving a rough, defective casting. The furnace should be set on "low" during the first 20 minutes.

Slow heating is especially relevant with a cristobalite-type investment, since the inversion and thermal expansion occur rapidly over a narrow temperature range. The ultimate temperature should not exceed 1250° F. As a matter of fact, with a cristobalite-type investment, if the burnout is complete the casting may be made at a temperature as low as 1000° F. Thermal

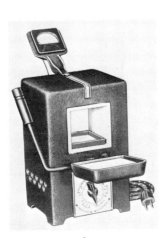
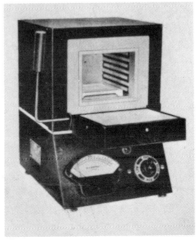

A   B

FIGURE 12-17. *Burnout furnaces.*

A, Jelenko.
B, Huppert.

expansion will have reached its crest at that temperature. If lower temperatures are used during burnout (900 to 1000° F.), the ring should be held at that temperature for time ample to assure complete wax elimination.

Prudence must be practiced to avoid heating the investment to a temperature that will decompose the gypsum that is present as a binder. If any traces of carbon still remain in the mold, the gypsum will break down at a temperature of only 1292° F. The sulfur that is liberated then will attack the gold alloy when it is forced into the mold. Gold that is contaminated by sulfur, or by chlorine in some investments, turns black, cleans up slowly on pickling, has low physical properties, and when cast is susceptible to corrosion and tarnish. If the temperature does not exceed 1250° F., there will be no probability of such contamination and the surface condition of the casting should be excellent. If the temperature of the mold is below 900° F., risk of subsurface porosity is increased.[19]

CASTING

Gold alloys may be cast repeatedly with no impairment of physical properties if the metal has not been abused. Nevertheless, as a safety precaution, it is expedient to use approximately one-half new gold for each casting. The old sprue or button should be cleaned on a charcoal block to remove any occluded gases or small pieces of adhering investment. This can be done conveniently just before the ring is to be removed from the furnace, and the mass of metal may be carried to the crucible or inlay ring while still hot, reducing the time required to make the casting. There is no reason for precipitancy except that if the investment contains the quartz form of silica, it will contract as the investment cools and perhaps result in an undersize casting; accordingly the casting must be made within 2 minutes after removal of the ring from the furnace. Metal should be used in a quantity that will fill the mold and still leave a dense sprue and modest-sized button.

Centrifugal, air pressure, or well-designed vacuum equipment may be used to make the casting (Figs. 12-18 and 12-19). As yet no difference has been demonstrated in the marginal sharpness or the physical properties of metal cast in any of these machines.

Cleaning Metal.   In cleaning an old button or sprue, the metal is placed on a charcoal block and melted (Fig. 12-20A). The molten metal should be sprinkled liberally with a reducing flux. A mistake frequently made at this point is to remove the flame from the metal and let it freeze. Exposed to air, the congealing metal will absorb gases and the primary purpose of cleaning the metal will be defeated. Instead, the air should be turned off and the gas flame played on the surface until the metal congeals (Fig. 12-20B). This flame is not so hot that it will keep the metal from solidifying, yet the alloy will be protected from occluded gases.

Fluxing.   Flux should be added just after the metal has liquefied, and another small amount should be added just before casting. This thin film of flux on the surface aids in guarding the metal against accidental oxidation

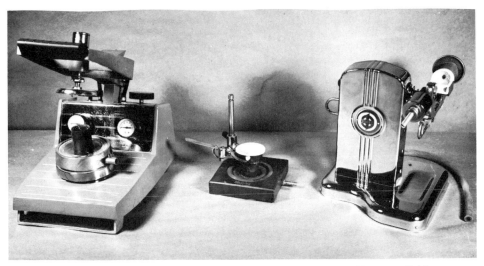

FIGURE 12–18. Various types of vacuum casting machines available.

during melting. The most popular fluxes are mixtures of borax and powdered charcoal. The charcoal acts as a strong reducing agent by combining with any oxygen to form carbon monoxide or carbon dioxide, neither of which contaminates the alloy. Such a reducing flux must be kept from falling or being blown into the sprue hole, because any charcoal particles entering the mold will be entrapped in the metal, quite possibly on a critical marginal area.

A good flux for casting may be made by grinding together equal portions of fused powdered borax and powdered boric acid. The black reducing

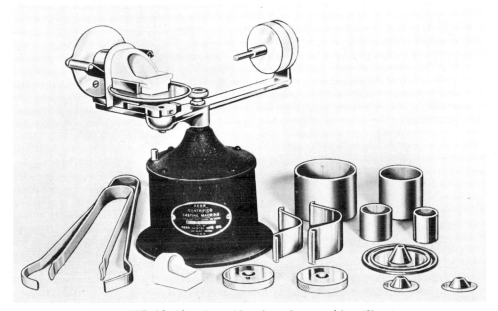

FIGURE 12–19. Centrifugal casting machine (Kerr).

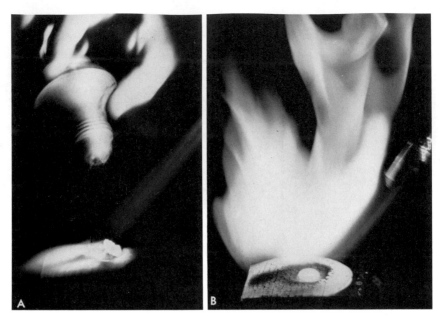

FIGURE 12-20.   *A*, Metal should be cleaned on charcoal block and liberally covered with a reducing flux.

B, After the metal is melted, the air is turned off and the metal freezes under protecting gas flame. When surface becomes frozen, torch may be removed.

flux, which contains charcoal, is handily applied with a salt shaker, but should be used only for cleaning old metal.

Melting Gold

Proper melting of the gold is of utmost consequence. Naturally the upper limit of the melting range must be exceeded so that the metal will flow into the mold. This temperature may be reached by various types of torches. Gas and air are adequate if the peak of the melting range is not over 1950° F. and if the gas has requisite B.T.U. The gas should be clean, as a high sulfur content may contaminate the alloy during melting. For higher melting ranges, oxygen and gas or acetylene must be used, but since they are exceedingly hot and a small mass of metal may be severely overheated, caution is mandatory.

The paramount factor to be considered during this melting procedure, beyond liquefying all the metal, is the hazard of oxidation. Dental gold alloys, particularly the harder types, contain metals that are easily oxidized during melting. As the metal solidifies the dissolved oxygen is expelled, leaving voids throughout the casting. This is called "occluded gas" porosity and ordinarily is manifested in a general pitting of the surface (Fig. 12-21). Such porosity offers a choice harbor for oral fluids or debris, with discoloration resulting.

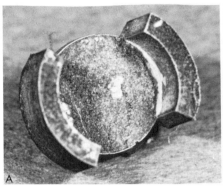
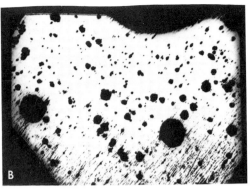

FIGURE 12–21. *A,* Mistreatment of gold results in black castings that do not clean up on pickling. Similar effects may result if investment is overheated, breaking down; the liberated sulfur attacks the gold.

B, Section through casting shown in *A* shows typical example of severe internal "occluded gas" porosity. Surface of casting is usually pitted.

Hardness, strength, and ductility are lost very soon in any porous area. If a gold alloy has been selected because of its applicable physical properties, it must be dense in order to retain these properties. Porosity resulting from occluded gas can be controlled by governed use of the torch and by protection of the metal by fluxing. The reducing zone of the flame should be used; this is the hottest area and the only portion that will avert oxidation of the metal (Fig. 12–22*A*). The appearance of the gold reflects the part of the flame that is being used. That is, whenever the gold has a scum or film on the surface, the metal is being oxidized (Fig. 12–22*B*); when the surface is shiny and mirrorlike (Fig. 12–22*C*), the metal is being reduced and the torch is in an appropriate position. A brush-type flame is desirable, since it is less hot and will cover a larger area of the gold. Its position should be adjusted until this shiny surface appears.

The color of the molten gold, when it has reached its specific state for casting, cannot be described succinctly; through repetition, recognition will come instinctively. It will be noted that as it is heated the alloy first becomes somewhat spongy and small globules of melted metal appear. This stage is followed by a gradual change of the bulk of alloy to spheroidal form. The reason for this adjustment from solid to liquid is that gold alloys have a melting *range*, rather than a melting *point*. In the earlier phases of heating, the lower fusing metals liquefy while the higher fusing metals remain solid. All the alloy soon melts and a spheroidal mass is formed; it has a dull red color at this point. Shortly thereafter the metal becomes almost transparent and begins to "spin." When the crucible of a centrifugal casting machine is shaken, the mass will roll around and will have assumed a light orange color. The gold is now ready to cast. Overheating the gold beyond this point does not burn out the base metal constituents, as was once believed, but it does heighten the danger of oxidation and will inevitably lead to frayed margins or a rough surface.

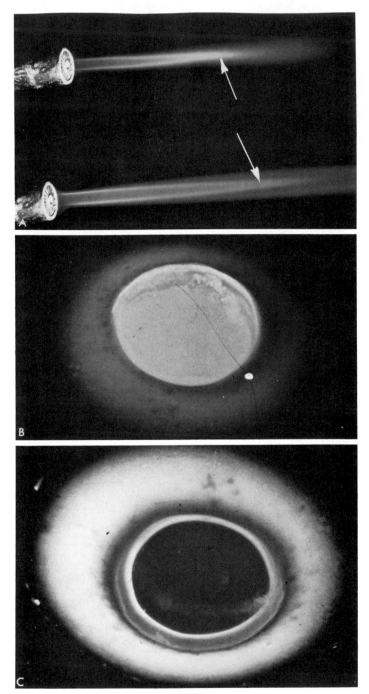

FIGURE 12-22.   *A*, Two different adjustments of torch. Flame at bottom is preferable as it is not so hot and covers wider area of gold. The reducing areas to be used for melting alloy are shown by arrows.

B, Scum on surface denotes oxidation.

C, Shiny, mirrored surface indicates that metal is being treated kindly and not oxidized.

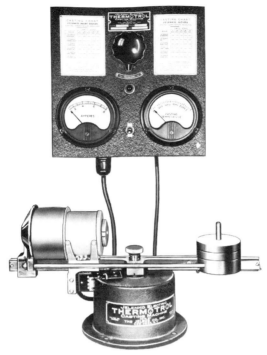

FIGURE 12-23.   Thermotrol (Jelenko).

There is an ingenious instrument for melting the metal electrically, and for casting at a definite, controlled temperature (Fig. 12-23).* Although it does not turn out castings that surpass in physical properties those that may be obtained using a well-handled torch, it does minimize the human variables.

CLEANING AND HARDENING THE CASTING

The casting may be a little dark, owing to surface oxidation from the investment, but it can be cleaned promptly by "pickling" in a 50 per cent solution of sulfuric acid or in solutions available from some dental gold manufacturers. If acid is used, the casting should be placed in a porcelain pickling dish or glass container, and the acid added and heated, but not boiled. After the acid has been poured off, the casting must be thoroughly washed in tap water. Acid may be re-used, but it should be changed regularly to mitigate any chance of contamination.

---

*Thermotrol, J. F. Jelenko & Co., Inc., New Rochelle, N. Y.

A casting should *never* be held with steel tongs, heated over a burner, and quenched in acid. Acid invariably contains traces of copper from previous pickling of gold castings, and placing the tongs in the acid will produce a galvanic current that will deposit a deep layer of copper on the casting, which will subsequently discolor in the mouth.

At this point the cavity surface of the casting should be examined with a magnifying glass. Any small nodules or irregularities that are present must be removed with a bur or very small knife-edge stone before trying the casting on the die or tooth.

The conventional medium-hard crown and bridge golds rarely are receptive to a hardening heat treatment, and since a later soldering operation will rid the casting of all effects from such treatment, the ring may be plunged into water as soon as the button loses its red color. It should *not* be quenched while still red, because the sudden drop in temperature may distort a fine margin or thin area.

In the area of casting it is the good fortune of the dental profession to have access to results of research in materials and their handling, including rules to be obeyed, directions to be taken seriously, and precautions to be heeded. Acceptance of these findings will leave small room for contamination and failure. Ignoring them is only indulging in the foolhardy practice of asking for trouble.

POLISHING THE CASTING

If the wax pattern was smoothed and polished before investing, if the investment was treated circumspectly during the burnout, and if the gold was not overheated, the casting will come from the pickling bath requiring minimal polishing.

The importance of a smooth, highly polished surface on a sound or dense casting cannot be overemphasized, since saliva can wash across it freely, tending to keep it clean and bright. A rough, poorly polished casting will hold saliva and debris and greatly accelerate the formation of deposits or a film that can become stained and unsightly. This discoloration may be mistaken for corrosion. Actually, chemical reaction of the metal is seldom involved and, as a rule, cleaning with a toothbrush and dentrifice will remove the deposit and restore the original color and luster, in the event that the surface has been polished and the alloy has not been contaminated.

The polishing routine to be described embraces the systematic use of progressively finer abrasive instruments and materials.[20] There are no short cuts. The final appearance will be disappointing if a step is omitted.

A separating disk,[a] * moved back and forth with very little pressure and kept as close as feasible to the casting, is used to cut off the sprue. It is followed by a heatless stone,[b] which blends the area of the cut-off sprue into

---

*See footnote on page 277.

the contour of the casting, but leaves a coarse surface. A mounted green stone,[c] of a finer grit, is then used over the area previously ground.

Because of the difficulty of polishing the sulci and maintaining the detail incorporated in the wax pattern, a dull No. 1/2 round bur[d] should be employed as a rotating burnisher, rather than a cutting instrument. A rubber point,[e] which can be kept sharp by rotating it against a heatless stone, will smooth the grooves of occlusal surfaces and other hard-to-reach areas that a round rubber wheel cannot touch.

A coarse 7/8-inch rubber wheel[f] is used with light pressure on larger surfaces. To preclude the formation of deep grooves, which might be made

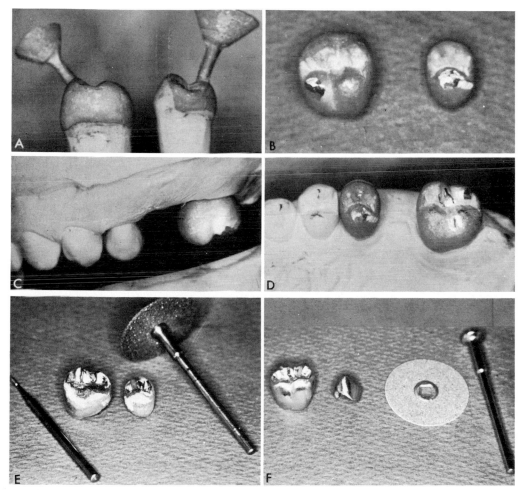

FIGURE 12–24. *Routine used to polish three-unit bridge. This varies slightly from that described in the text, but will produce excellent results.*

A, Castings pickled and seated on dies.
B, Sprues cut off and areas contoured.
C, Castings seated on working cast; occlusion being checked.
D, Premature contacts registered.
E, Occlusion adjusted and surfaces of castings stoned and burred.
F, Surfaces smoothed.

by rotating the rubber wheel in one direction only, the casting must be kept moving so that each successive cut is at right angles to the one previously made.

Next, a finer rubber wheel, the Green Burlew Disk,[g] will give a satin finish to all surfaces and prepare the casting for tripoli.

The occlusal and other finely carved surfaces may be polished with tripoli on a Robinson Bristle Disk, No. 11 Soft.[h] This brush is kept moving over the surfaces with enough pressure so that the bristles will spread out and reach all grooves and corners. It is followed by a 4-inch or larger lead center rag wheel,[i] well coated with tripoli. Medium pressure will effect the best surface.

The casting must be washed in a detergent[j] solution to remove all traces of tripoli before a reflecting surface is acquired from rouge applied with a rag wheel.[k] Every trace of rouge must be washed off. It is an antiflux and will hinder the flow of solder.

It is much less complicated to polish individual units satisfactorily rather than the assembled bridge.

After the bridge has been soldered, it must be pickled. If the retainers and pontics were polished separately before soldering, only light polishing

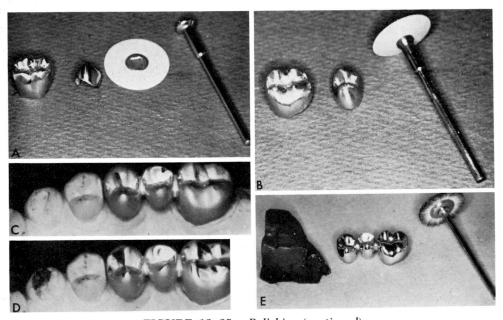

FIGURE 12–25. *Polishing (continued).*

A, Low polish produced by fine disk.
B, Smooth surface from rubber wheel.
C, Bridge soldered, pickled, and checked on cast for occlusion.
D, Occlusion corrected.
E, High polish produced by tripoli.

with tripoli, rouge, and No. 600 Carborundum powder† will be needed to prepare the bridge for cementation. After the bridge or crown is cemented, a higher luster can be achieved with a rubber cup and Amalgloss‡ or No. 600 Carborundum powder (Figs. 12–24 and 12–25).

CONTAMINATION AND FAILURE

A word should be said about the danger of contamination of the alloy. Certain contaminants, even if present in only minute amounts, have a profound effect on the physical properties. Usually the casting becomes brittle, the proportional limit is decreased, and the surface may be susceptible to corrosion. One of the possible contaminants, sulfur, was discussed earlier. A common hazard is mercury, and the effect of its absorption by gold is dramatic. Casting metal must not come in contact with amalgam scrap and dies, contouring pliers, or base metal of any type, since the action of metals, such as lead or antimony, is extremely detrimental. Different types of golds should never be mixed. The resulting metal may form a eutectiferous alloy, which is often quite brittle and has low resistance to corrosion.

Unquestionably casting failures should be infrequent, but they happen occasionally. Almost always the cause can be diagnosed readily. For example:

1. Rounded and shiny incomplete areas are indicative of incomplete burnout; the carbon left in the mold forms carbon monoxide, which acts as a strong reducing agent when the gold enters the mold.

2. Rounded margins that are dull instead of shiny may be attributed to inadequate casting pressure, to back pressure from improper orientation of the pattern in the ring, or to insufficient heating of the metal.

3. A sharp, well-defined deficiency, in a majority of times occurring at a margin, may be caused by the presence in the mold of some foreign object, such as a piece of investment or a bit of charcoal from the flux, or by the use of contaminated wax to form the pattern.

4. Frayed margins or a completely cracked mold are the result of burning out too rapidly, inaccurate powder-water ratio for the investment, or overheating the gold (Fig. 12–26).

5. Bubbles are associated with entrapment of air during investing or use of too much wetting agent.

*The materials indicated by superior letters are manufactured by the following:
a and d, The S. S. White Dental Mfg. Co., Philadelphia, Pa.
    b, Mizzy, Inc., Clifton Forge, Va.
    c, Chayes Dental Instrument Corp., Danbury, Conn.
c, e, and f, National Keystone Products Co., Philadelphia, Pa.
    d, The Ranson & Randolph Co., Toledo, Ohio.
    f, Dental Development & Mfg. Corp., Brooklyn, N.Y.
    g, J. F. Jelenko & Co., Inc., New Rochelle, N.Y.
    h, Buffalo Dental Mfg. Co., Inc., Brooklyn, N.Y.
i and k, William Dixon, Inc., Carlstadt, N.J.
    j, Lever Bros., New York, N.Y.
†Silicon Carbide Grain No. 600, The Carborundum Company, Niagara Falls, N.Y.
‡The L. D. Caulk Company, Milford, Del.

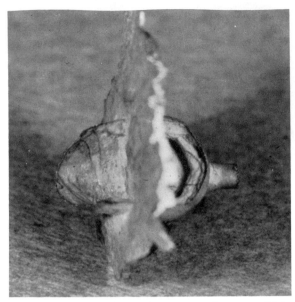

FIGURE 12–26.   Casting failure due to investment fracture. This may be caused from burning out too rapidly, overheating gold, or too thin a mix of investment.

CASTING ALLOYS

In few other facets of dentistry are there so many acceptable products as in that of the gold alloys used for castings. Many manufacturers supply a wide range of alloy compositions, each with physical properties that are tailor-made for the intended usage. On the basis of physical properties the dentist may well have a broader selection of alloys than does the engineer.

Choice of the gold alloy generally should be made on the basis of color, the facility with which the restoration can be polished, and the properties sought for the intended restoration rather than upon the advertising claims of the superiority of any one product.

There is no such thing as a universal alloy: that is, one that satisfies the requirements for all types of dental restorations. The rigorous demands to which a three-quarter crown retainer is subjected are entirely different from those made on a single inlay, and so are the characteristics desired in the alloy.

The American Dental Specification for Dental Casting Gold Alloys encompasses four types. They range from soft golds (Type I) for use in a simple restoration, such as a Class I inlay, to the very hard alloys (Type IV), which are used in the fabrication of partial dentures. The dental manufacturer may have four or five alloys within a given classification, each one varying slightly in its physical attributes.

A casting alloy for a given bridge unit, when other requirements permit, should be harmonious in hardness with the alloys that may have been used for restorations made previously for the patient. If this is not done, wear, burnishing, and masticatory shock could be uneven; also the rigidity vital to resist the transmitted forces, and flexing due to span length, must be inherent.

Rigidity is realized in part by using an alloy that is stiff after casting and soldering, and also by providing bulk in the casting. The thinner the occluding surface of a casting, the harder the alloy must be. Pinledges and many partial veneer crowns would be included in this group. Partial denture alloys must be used for many retainers, but first consideration should be given to conventional crown and bridge alloys.

Whenever a variation in hardness exists in the alloys placed throughout an arch, more frequent examination and equilibration should follow.

REFERENCES

1. Skinner, E. W., and Phillips, R. W.: The Science of Dental Materials. 6th ed. Philadelphia, W. B. Saunders Company, 1967.
2. Norman, R. D., Swartz, M. L., and Phillips, R. W.: Studies on the solubility of certain dental materials. J. D. Res., 36:977, Dec. 1957.
3. Sausen, R. E., Armstrong, W. D., and Simon, W. J.: Penetration of radiocalcium at margins of acrylic restorations made by compression and non-compression technics. J.A.D.A., 47:636, Dec. 1953.
4. Crawford, W. H., and Larson, J. H.: Dental restorative materials; amalgams, acrylics. J. D. Res., 33:414, June 1954.
5. Crawford, W. H.: Selection and use of investments, sprues, casting equipment and gold alloys in making small castings. J.A.D.A., 27:1459, Sept. 1940.
6. J. F. Jelenko & Co., Inc.: Dental Gold Structures. New York, The company, 1949.
7. The J. M. Ney Company: Ney Bridge and Inlay Book. Hartford, The company, 1958.
8. Phillips, R. W.: Studies on the density of castings as related to their position in the ring. J.A.D.A., 35:329, Sept. 1947.
9. Coleman, R. L.: Physical Properties of Dental Materials. (National Bureau of Standards Research Paper No. 32.) Washington, U. S. Government Printing Office, 1928.
10. Hollenback, G. M., and Skinner, E. W.: Shrinkage during casting of gold and gold alloys. J.A.D.A., 33:1391, Nov. 1946.
11. Hollenback, G. M.: Simple technic for accurate castings: new and original method of vacuum investing. J.A.D.A., 36:391, April-May 1948.
12. Asgars, K., Mahler, D. B., and Peyton, F. A.: Hygroscopic technique for inlay casting using controlled water additions. J. Pros. Den., 5:711, Sept. 1955.
13. Mumford, G., and Phillips, R. W.: Dimensional change in wax patterns during setting of gypsum investments. J. D. Res., 37:351, April 1958.
14. Phillips, D. W.: A scientifically correct inlay technique. D. Digest, 39:72, Feb. 1933. Controlled casting. J.A.D.A., 22:439, March 1935. Present-day precision inlay investing and casting technic. J.A.D.A., 24:1470, Sept. 1937.
15. Phillips, D. W.: Controlled casting. J.A.D.A., 22:439, March 1935.
16. Phillips, R. W.: Relative merits of vacuum investing of small castings as compared to conventional methods. J. D. Res., 26:343, Oct. 1947.
17. Lyon, H. W., Dickson, G., and Schoonover, I. C.: Effectiveness of vacuum investing in the elimination of surface defects in gold castings. J.A.D.A., 46:197, Feb. 1953.
18. Phillips, R. W., ed.: Symposium on dental materials—their use and recent developments. D. Clin. N. Amer., Nov. 1958.
19. Ryge, G., Kozak, S. F., and Fairhurst, C. W.: Porosities in dental gold castings. J.A.D.A., 54:746, June 1957.
20. Ficaro, J. P., Lemire, P. A., and Linton, C. C.: Personal communications.

chapter 13

THE PONTIC

SELECTING SHADES FOR PORCELAIN FACINGS OR VENEERS

For an indirect method of bridge construction, the shades of the facings should be selected before the abutment teeth are prepared. A paramount effort should be made to match approximating teeth, but corresponding teeth in the approximating quadrant and occluding teeth must be given some consideration too and should be checked. A compromise may be in order, since a marked contrast with any one of these areas might be noticeable.

In the direct technique, shades should be chosen with the retainers on the teeth. The color of the intact labial or buccal surface of a prepared tooth will be relatively unchanged if cement powder, mixed with a combination of 50 per cent water and 50 per cent glycerin, is placed inside the casting to mask the metal. Repetition with different trial mixes will assist in finding a shade, or a combination of shades, in the cement that will restore the natural appearance of the abutment. A notation of the powder combination should be placed in the patient's record so that the same mixture may be used when the prosthesis is cemented permanently.

At least two shade guides should be used, in case the first choice of facing is not obtainable at the depot. This will necessitate fewer staining modifications.

The patient should face a north, natural light, if possible. Lipstick, amount and color of rouge, earrings, spectacle frames, and clothing, as well as the color of the office walls, can influence shade selection. If one particular shade of lipstick is habitually worn by the patient, it may remain; but if excessive make-up is used, generally it is advisable that it be removed and that the patient's clothing be covered with a neutral drape.

Incisors, cuspids, and bicuspids should be matched, first on the incisal or occlusal, then on the cervical. If, owing to a high lipline, all the facing will be exposed during speaking or smiling, the shade of the facing must coincide in its entire length with that of the approximating teeth. If the cervical will not be exposed, no more than the incisal or occlusal one-half or two-thirds need be of major concern. Customarily only the occlusal half of molar facings must blend with the approximating and occluding teeth.

Shade and Form

Facings that will harmonize with the approximating teeth without some reshaping and subsequent reglazing can seldom be procured. They cannot be manufactured to fit individual cases and must be thought of as "blanks" to be worked into form, position, and alignment by the operator. Many facings are more translucent or more shiny than the teeth they will approximate, but this lack of harmony is largely overcome by the metal backing and luting material. Even a facing of correct shade will look out of place if overglazed. Harmonious form in the facing will lessen, to a degree, the requirement for exact shade matching; however, the closer the shade match, the happier the patient.

TYPES OF FACINGS

The porcelain facings regularly used are the pin, the flatback with a slot,* the Trupontic,* the Sanitarypontic,* the porcelain biting-edge,* and the reverse-pin. Overjet and vertical overlap, length of the space incisocervically or occlusocervically, width of the space, and frequently translucence, shade, and shade distribution will have a bearing on the type of facing used in constructing the pontic (Fig. 13-1).

Facings made of resin are on the market, but the authors use them rarely, and then only for *temporary replacement*.

Pin Facings

Two types of pin facings are recommended: the Dentsply† and the Harmony.‡ The Dentsply, or long-pin, facing has a porcelain component similar in contour and bulk to the flatback, or Steele's,* facing. The pins are at right angles to the metal-contacting surface. The porcelain is dense and of good quality.

The Harmony facing has a built-on bulk of porcelain to be adapted to the ridge so that only porcelain will have a static relationship to the tissue.[1, 2] The pins protrude from the bulkiest portion of the facing in a direction bisecting the angle formed by the two sections of the gold-contacting surface (Fig. 13-2).

When adapting a Harmony facing, on occasion there may be some

---

*The Columbus Dental Mfg. Co., Columbus, Ohio.
†The Dentists' Supply Company, York, Pa.
‡Harmony Dental Products Corp., Pasadena, Calif.

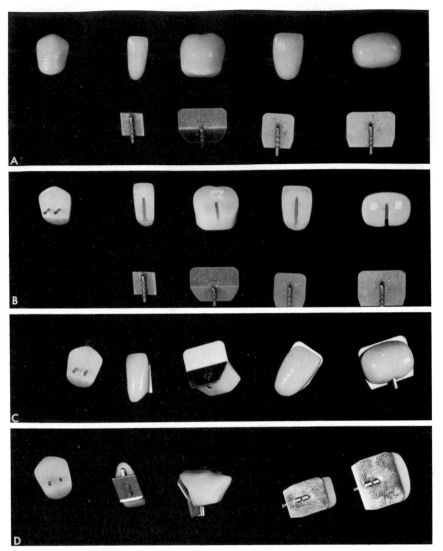

FIGURE 13-1. *Five of the facings discussed in this text.*

A, Left to right: Long-pin facing (The Dentists' Supply Co.); porcelain biting-edge; Trupontic; Steele's flatback; and Sanitarypontic. (The last four are supplied by the Columbus Dental Manufacturing Co.) An appropriate backing is seen under each facing.

B, Same facings, same order, and their backings as viewed from the lingual and the occlusal.

C, Backings in position.

D, Backings partly removed.

porosity in the bulky area. This can be filled in with low-fusing, add-on porcelain. The resulting glassy surface is salutary for contacting the ridge tissue.

The labial contour of the Harmony facing is not anatomic in an inciso-cervical direction. Two-thirds of the labial surface is natural; then the surface inclines somewhat toward the ridge. This is helpful in a high percentage of cases. For irregular alignment with a high lipline, and when there has

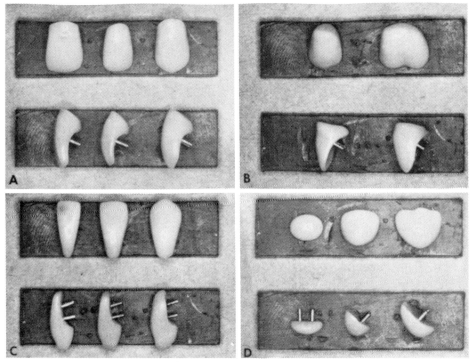

FIGURE 13-2. *Harmony facings.*

A, Maxillary anterior.
B, Maxillary posterior.
C, Mandibular anterior.
D, Mandibular posterior.

been more than average ridge resorption, the Harmony facing is superlative. It is adaptable in mandibular bridges when making bicuspid pontics with visible buccal surfaces and as a tip for contacting the ridge in molar areas.

Since the long-pin facing removes toward the labial or buccal, it can be adapted to almost all situations and types of occlusion. Excellent contour can be formed. Contact porcelain, which already exists on the Harmony facing, can be added to the Dentsply. The pin facing may be hollow-ground and tipped incisally or occlusally, for protection, or to permit insertion in very short spaces, or when the vertical overlap is long without a corresponding overjet.

Flatback Facings

The flatback facing can be used advantageously when the space is average or longer incisocervically or occlusocervically, provided the cusp or incisal edge contacts are normal or nearly so. In eccentric excursions there must be occlusal or incisal clearance to protect the porcelain. Almost always esthetic contours can be fashioned.

The Trupontic facing is hygienic, but in many cases it presents exasperating difficulties in adaptation and shaping. The labial convexities and angles and directions of cusp arms cannot always be made anatomically without displaying metal. The Trupontic facing, which also may be hollow-ground to shield the incisal or buccal margin, requires more length occlusally than the pin facing.[3]

Modifying a Pin Facing

A Dentsply pin facing can be altered so that when the pontic is built, the entire ridge-contacting surface will be porcelain. It must be ground to form and alignment, then shortened with a linguocervical bevel. A buccal plaster index is poured. The facing is grasped with a Graebner matrix* so that the pins are under the plate and the cervical half of the facing is exposed. Medium-fusing porcelain is built onto the lingual surface and over the cervical bevel of the facing with only minimal condensation (Fig. 13-3).

The facing is removed from the matrix and supported on a firing tray by a mound of silex. It is dried and fired to a low maturity. When placed on the working cast in the index, the contacting surface should have a plus contour. The facing is ground until contact with the ridge is continuous and the facing seats in the index. Embrasures must be formed and the cervical portion of the facing contoured to establish the correct contacting area. The facing is cleansed and fired to a suitable glaze (Fig. 13-4).

For this modified pin facing to be acceptable, the space for the pontic must have occlusocervical height only slightly less than that for the Trupontic facing; if the span is long, there must be room for a greater bulk of metal in the beam.

Mandibular Sanitary Facings

Two lower posterior sanitary facings are in common use: the Steele's Sanitarypontic and the Harmony pin-tip. They are used on all lower posterior bridges unless occluso-ridge crest dimension is too short for both gold and porcelain or unless the space is so far to the anterior to necessitate complete buccal tooth form. When esthetic considerations are a factor with the lower posterior pontic, either the regular Harmony facing (favored) or the Trupontic facing will be found superior.

Reverse-Pin Facing

The reverse-pin facing,[4] contrived from either a facing or a denture tooth, is very useful when pontics must be lapped or arranged irregularly, or

---

*The Cleveland Dental Mfg. Co., Cleveland, Ohio.

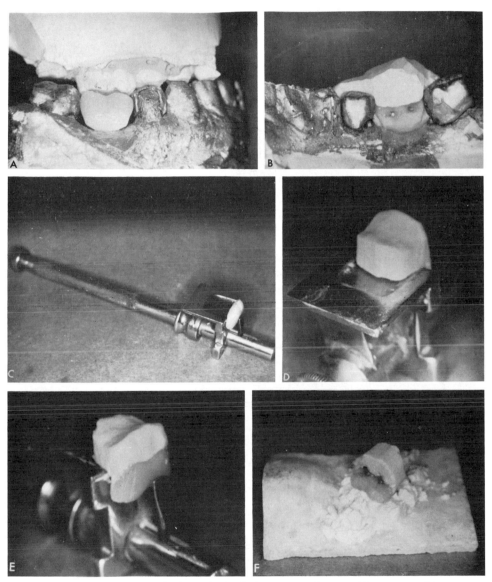

FIGURE 13-3. *A,* Buccal view of pin facing ground to position on working cast.
B, Lingual view.
C, Facing held by Graebner matrix.
D, Porcelain powder built onto facing.
E, Showing porcelain powder carried onto buccal surface.
F, Facing on firing tray.
(Courtesy of Mr. Russell J. Jones, Cleveland, Ohio.)

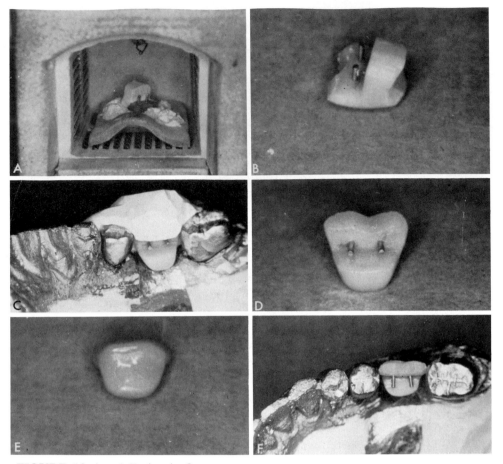

FIGURE 13-4. *A*, Facing in furnace.

B, Facing fired.

C, Facing contoured. Clearance between pins and added porcelain is sufficient to have bulk of metal in pontic for pinholes.

D, Facing glazed. Notice bevel along occlusal for protecting bulk of metal.

E, Highly glazed tissue-contacting surface.

F, Modified and glazed facing in position. (Courtesy of Mr. Russell J. Jones, Cleveland, Ohio.)

when space width or occlusion is not appropriate for standard types. It does not have a universal application, but it gives beautiful results in many situations.

SELECTION OF FACING

A mold guide should be used if available. The kind and mold of facing may be selected using diagnostic casts. However, this is done more often after the working cast has been articulated. If facings are selected and ground in on the diagnostic cast, they may be positioned in the space to determine the labial extensions of several types of retainer preparations.

Specific information concerning the facing should accompany the order. For example, it should read: "Steele's facing, upper right cuspid, mold 56G, New Hue shade 67." If the mold guide is not at hand, the order may read: "Steele's facing, upper right cuspid, 11.0 mm. long, 8.0 mm. wide at incisal, 6.0 mm. at cervical, New Hue shade 67." The facing chosen should be a little too wide and long so that there will be sufficient material for grinding to position and form.

GRINDING FACINGS TO PROPER POSITION AND FORM

Facings may be shaped and positioned on the working cast by (1) grinding to mesiodistal width; (2) adjusting to occlusocervical or incisocervical length, which includes adapting the facing to the ridge; (3) forming the mesiodistal convexities and occlusocervical contour; and (4) adjusting the long-axis inclination (see Chapter 14).

Width

The facing should be ground to the desired width with no attention being paid to mesiodistal contour (Fig. 13-5). The sides should be parallel incisocervically and labiolingually, although, in some instances, not parallel with the long axis of the facing because of the effect that must be produced in the space. Only in an occasional case, to create an irregularity by overlapping an abutment or another facing, should a mesial or distal cut converge lingually. If there is more than one pontic and the space is not ideal, it must be decided in advance which pontic should have normal measurements and which should be constricted or made wider. Usually the one nearer the median line is given true dimensions (Fig. 13-6).

Length

With the articulator closed, the facings should be placed against the ridge with the incisal or occlusal edges as nearly in alignment as possible and with only the excess of porcelain needed for contouring extending beyond the occlusal plane. The length should be studied from the lingual to see how much of the retentive slot will be left if the facing is a flatback, or how much of the cervical portion will remain if the facing is a Trupontic, or how close the retentive pins will be to the ridge if a long-pin facing is being used. The retentive pins should be at a point at least one-third of the distance from the ridge to the occlusal or incisal, but preferably in the cingulum region in anteriors. There must be a clearance between the pins and the ridge of not less than 1.0 mm. Approximately half of the slot or half of the cervical porcelain should remain. If these conditions cannot be met with the facings so positioned, they must be moved incisally or occlusally, and then be reduced in length on each end.

When adjusting the length incisocervically, the shade patterns of the approximating teeth will indicate whether to conserve the incisal or cervical

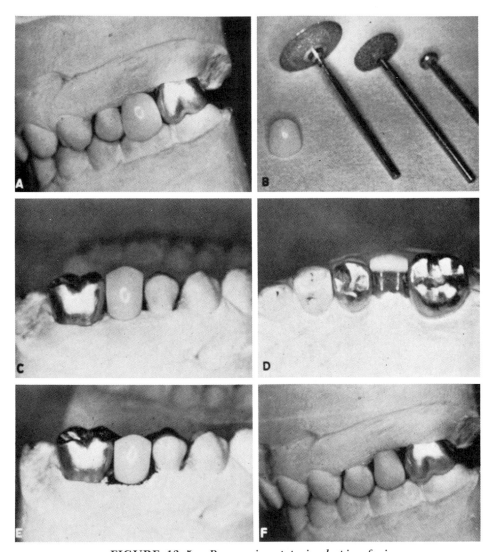

FIGURE 13-5.   *Progressive steps in shaping facings.*

    A, Facing selected is slightly wider and longer than the space.

    B, Facing and stones to be used in shaping and positioning facing.

    C and *D*, Cut to mesiodistal width, the facing is same width as distance between contact areas of retainers. Sides are parallel and do not cause facing to overlap abutments.

    E, Facing shortened occlusocervically. Ridge of working cast has been blackened with a pencil to aid in adapting facing.

    F, Facing contoured and in alignment. Note embrasure form, convexities at cervical and occlusal, and grooves.

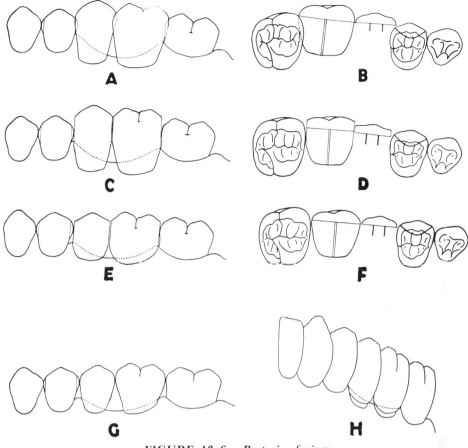

FIGURE 13-6. *Posterior facings.*

A and *B*, Facings chosen have excess width and length.
C and *D*, Cut to mesiodistal width.
E, Reduced in height.
F and *G*, Facings contoured.
H, Cementoenamel line and root form established.

of the facing. As a rule, the incisal or occlusal half will be ground less than the cervical.

The cervical is adapted to the ridge with the porcelain touching the ridge without interruption buccolingually or labiolingually. This fit may be realized by covering the ridge with black pencil markings, placing the facing in alignment against the ridge, and then grinding at the dark points of contact. (See Figure 13-10.) This and the incisal reduction are continued simultaneously until adaptation, length, and alignment of the facing meet specifications. If the ridgelap of the facing is altered with care, allowing the lingual surface to angle in toward the ridge, it can be aligned so that very little of the labial porcelain must be lost. The facing may be supported by modeling clay or soft wax during the marking process.

Contour

Convexities mesiodistally must conform to the anatomy of the tooth being replaced and also must be in harmony with the abutment teeth. Incisocervically the buccal or labial contour of the facing should follow the outline of the abutments and should be compatible with the arch form. Similar labial or buccal markings and incisal or occlusal edge form should be incorporated.

On the ridgelap of a flatback or a porcelain biting-edge facing, the lingual two-thirds should be reduced further with a 30-degree bevel, to enable an apron of gold to cover the slot in the porcelain (Fig. 13–7).

The contour of the facing from the simulated cementoenamel junction to the ridge cannot continue the normal tooth root form. If this were done, the facing frequently would extend so far apically beyond the gingival lines of the abutment teeth that the effect would be unsightly and artificial. Beginning at the cervical line, the facing must be curved lingually until it meets the ridge at an obtuse angle. The V-shaped space formed by the facing and the ridge must be greater than a 90-degree angle or it will form a food trap.

Grinding Harmony and Trupontic Facings to Form and Alignment

Harmony and Trupontic facings present problems in alignment dissimilar to those encountered with the flatback and long-pin facings. Adapting the porcelain-contacting area to the ridge so that the labial surface is in alignment with approximating teeth, with minimal grinding on the labial surface, is more time-consuming than adaptation of the ridgelap of other facings. It must be done with more caution to avoid scarring the cast. The

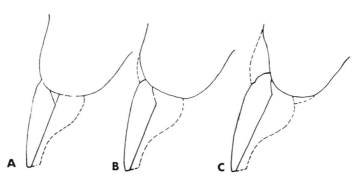

FIGURE 13–7. *Ridge adaptation of anterior facings.*

A, Ridge with minimal resorption. Cementoenamel junction ground into facing. Linguocervical beveled to make room for cast apron covering slot.

B and *C*, Progressive resorption. Facing is rounded into ridge. Incisal edge cannot be left exposed as shown here.

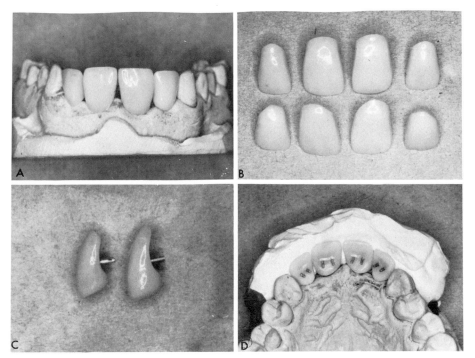

FIGURE 13-8. *Harmony facings.*

A, Four Harmony incisors aligned on diagnostic cast.

B, Facings removed and in position under unground facings.

C, Proximal view of one aligned and one untouched facing. Note incisal bevel on left.

D, Facings aligned with labial index before being attached to resin base.

tissue-contacting area must be outlined by the lingual and proximal embrasures of the facing itself. Labial or buccal alignment must be established prior to incisocervical length, or a gap may occur at the linguogingival margin of the facing (Fig. 13–8). Irregular ridge form magnifies the difficulties of securing adaptation and contact without pressure. The recontoured surfaces must be reglazed. (See Figures 13-9, 13-10, 13-11, and 13-12.)

Grinding Reverse-Pin Facings to Form and Alignment

To construct a reverse-pin facing, either a porcelain denture tooth or a pin facing of appropriate shade and slightly oversize must first be selected. Denture teeth are popular for this purpose, but it must be remembered that their shade distribution and translucence are less characteristic of human teeth than most bridge facings.

The tooth or facing is cut to width, length, and adaptation to the ridge, and is contoured following the designated sequence of operative procedures (Fig. 13-13). The pins, if present, are cut flush with the facing and partially removed by grinding with a round bur. The facing is placed in aqua regia

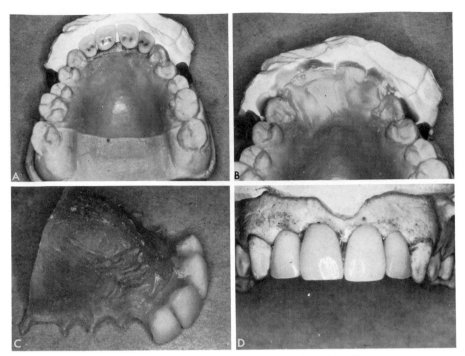

FIGURE 13-9.   *Harmony facings (continued).*

A, B, and *C,* Building and attaching base to facings.
D, Facings returned to cast.

and the remaining metal is dissolved. The incisal third is beveled, or angled, and the edge is hollow-ground. The facing is set, labial surface down, onto impression compound in a movable ring and taken to the drill press.

Drills, 0.025, 0.023, and 0.021 inch,* may be purchased, or they can be made from old carbide burs. The drill is lubricated with handpiece oil, and the holes, four or five in number and at least 1.2 plus mm. deep, are placed in the bulkiest part of the facing. They are distributed as widely as possible. For safety, the thickness of the porcelain should be measured before drilling, because a thickness of 1.0 mm. of porcelain should remain after the holes have been placed. If the facing is too thin, starting again with a new facing will save time (Fig. 13-14).

Protection

Facings must be protected on the incisal edge or bucco-occlusal margin. Pin, reverse-pin, and Trupontics, when recontoured here, can be beveled or hollow-ground to be covered and reinforced by the casting. This need in no way affect the shape of the labial or buccal silhouette (Fig. 13-15).

---

*Williams Gold Refining Co., Inc., Buffalo, N. Y.

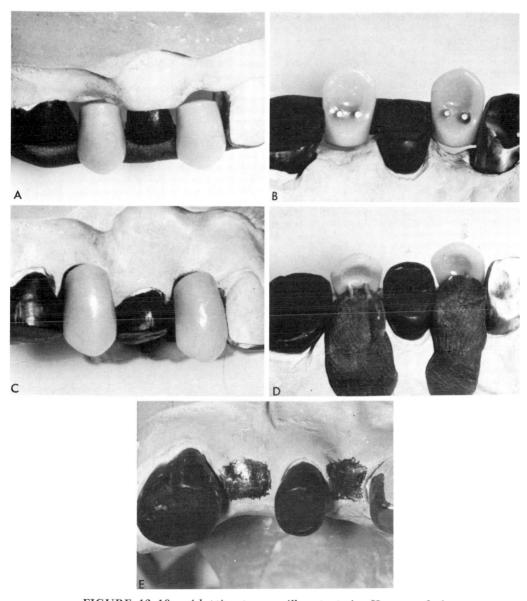

FIGURE 13-10. *Adapting two maxillary posterior Harmony facings.*

A and *B*, Checking facings for width. Bicuspid and molar are waxed to width, but without occluding surfaces.

C and *D*, Checking facings for length and for amount of contouring needed to adapt contacting surface to ridge.

E, Ridges on cast blackened with soft pencil to guide adaptation.

(Text continued page 298)

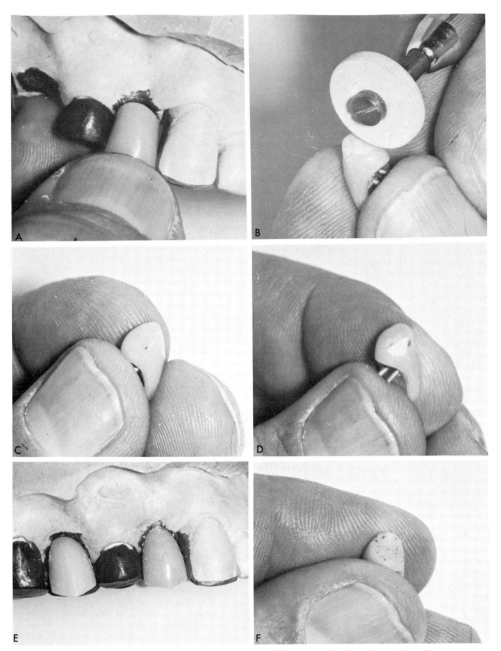

FIGURE 13–11. *Adapting two Harmony facings (continued).*

  A, After some shaping, facing is placed in contact with blackened ridge to mark area of contact.

  B, Further contouring with abrasive rubber wheel. Grinding on marked spot of contact.

  C, Marked spot will be reduced.

  D, Another mark after grinding spot shown in *C*.

  E, Process was continued until all of ridge area shows spots of contact.

  F, Two facings aligned. Occlusal edges have been shaped to clear opposing cast.

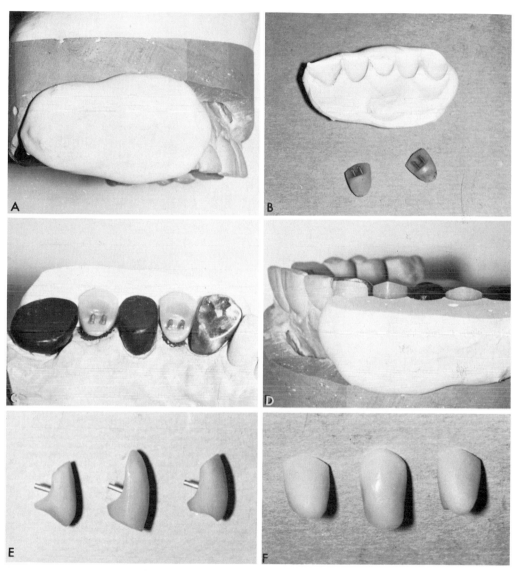

FIGURE 13–12. *Adapting two facings (continued).*

A, Plaster index on buccal of cast.

B, Index trimmed, and facings.

C and *D*, Index holding facings on cast.

E and *F*, Two shaped facings with one untouched. Ridge areas are concave buccolingually and a little convex mesiodistally. Occlusal is beveled to give space for metal.

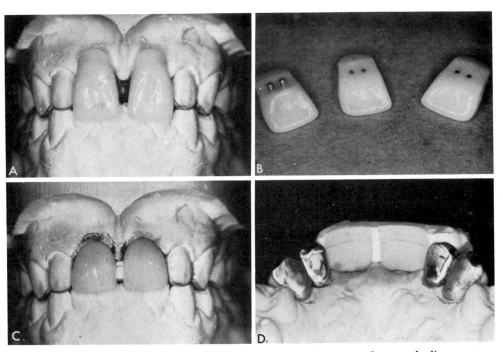

FIGURE 13-13. *Showing grinding reverse-pin facings to form and alignment.*

A, Denture teeth selected to be recontoured for facings.

B, With pins, and with pins cut off.

C, Ground to form and alignment.

D, Linguals showing adaptation to ridge and incisal areas that are hollow-ground for greater bulk of metal in casting.

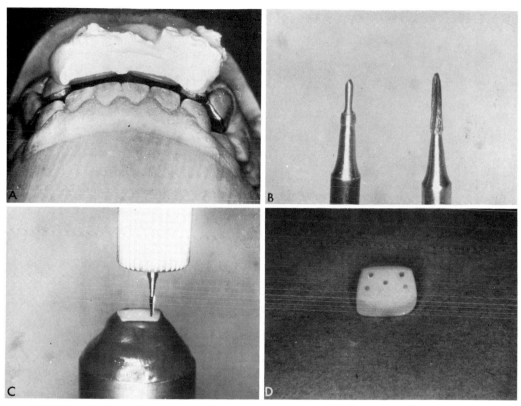

FIGURE 13–14. *Showing grinding reverse-pin facings to form and alignment (continued).*

A, Incisal clearance.

B, Drills made from carbide burs.

C, Facing mounted in compound. Holes are being drilled.

D, Facing prepared. Holes are widely distributed in bulky part of facing. Note concave incisal bevel.

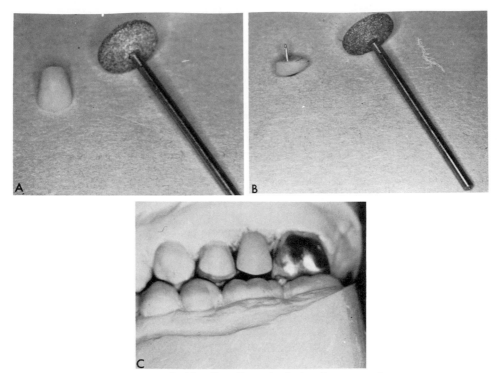

FIGURE 13–15. *Beveling pin facing for protection.*

A, Facing and stone.
B, Beveled facing.
C, Facing in position, showing clearance.

However, when the flatback facing is reduced on the incisal edge or bucco-occlusal margin, the shelf of porcelain cannot be covered with metal and the facial surface must be recontoured to eliminate the table, one possible cause for future fracture of the facing. This must be done before the facing is conformed to the ridge. Recontouring the surface will force a new alignment and a new angle of approach to the ridge. If the ridge adaptation were done first, realignment would nullify facing contact and subsequent efforts might not correct the situation.

MANDIBULAR SANITARYPONTICS

The selection of a Sanitarypontic or a Harmony porcelain tip is not critical when constructing a lower posterior bridge. These facings come in varying shades from light to dark. Since they are used for hygienic measures, rather than for esthetic reasons, matching the *exact* shade is not important.

If the facing is a little wider than the space, it can be reduced to size (Fig. 13-16). If it is a little narrower than would be specific for the case at hand, the mesial and distal edges can be beveled and the occlusal casting

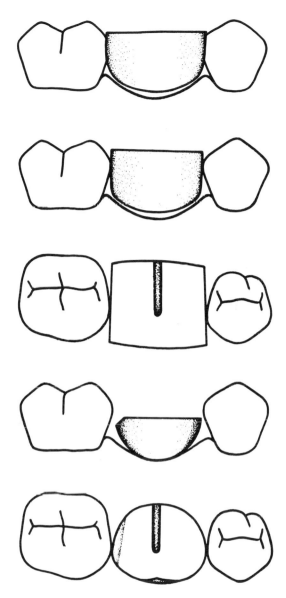

FIGURE 13-16. *Steps in shaping a Sanitarypontic.*

Top to bottom: Facing selected too wide and too high; facing reduced mesiodistally to permit placing between contact areas of retainers; facing contoured to give ample embrasure room and to approach ridge crest uniformly from all directions. Bevel will provide an adequate soldering surface; this may be done on each side. Buccal groove is indicated in porcelain.

contoured to accommodate to the space without resultant irregular form in the pontic.[5, 6, 7]

If the space is long occlusocervically, the facing should equal that length minus the thickness of the gold occlusal. If it is extra long and narrow mesiodistally, it may be better hygienically if the facing does not contact the mucous membrane, but stops about 3.0 or 4.0 mm. above the crest of the ridge. If the teeth and space are so short that the framework or facing, or both, would be weak, a facing may be contraindicated and a pontic fabricated of gold alone (Fig. 13-17) or one tipped with a Harmony pin-tip (Figs. 13-18 and 13-19) should be used. When the space is near the median line and is long occlusocervically, a Trupontic or a Harmony facing may have merit. (See Chapter 14, Pontic Form.)

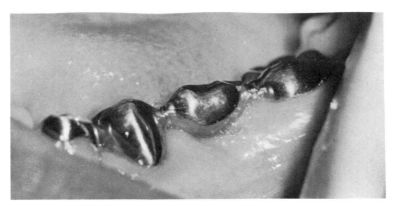

FIGURE 13–17.   All-gold pontic in short space.

Spaces of irregular ridge design compel irregular shapes in the under-portion of the pontic (Fig. 13–20). There are no rules to set forth; judgment must be used. If the space is malshaped because of tipped abutments, the apical section of the pontic should be no wider than the occlusal.

The height of the facing should allow for a minimal thickness of 1.0 mm. of gold in the thinnest sections of the occlusal casting, and it should touch the ridge with a rounded ridge-tip contact (Fig. 13–21*A*). The few exceptions almost always occur when replacing lower bicuspids. Sometimes here, be-cause it is visible, the pontic must be contoured so that it will be aligned buccally with the incisal and middle thirds of the cuspid or first bicuspid.

Except in the situation just noted, the convex underportion of the pontic should be centered over the ridge. The area in contact should never be more than one-third of the mesiodistal width of the space. The flat occlusal portion need not be parallel to the plane of occlusion. It can be tipped in any direction dictated by the positions of the opposing teeth. Viewed from the occlusal, the prepared facing should be widest mesiodistally in the areas that will be immediately below the connectors.

The mesial and distal surfaces of the facing should converge toward the

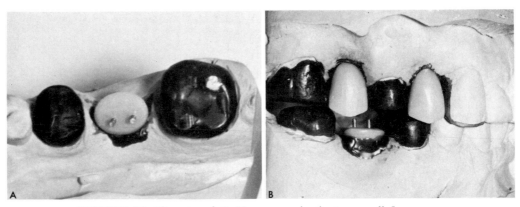

FIGURE 13–18.   *A* and *B*, Harmony pin-tip too small for space.

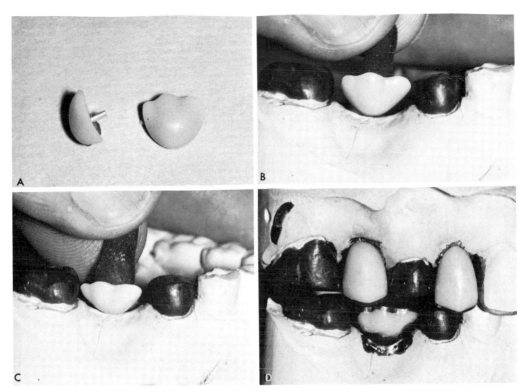

FIGURE 13-19.   *A*, Harmony mandibular posterior facing.
B, Facing has width and length desired.
C, Ridge-contacting surface rounded to lessen height. Ample space on occlusal.
D, Facing aligned and prepared for waxing simultaneously with retainers.

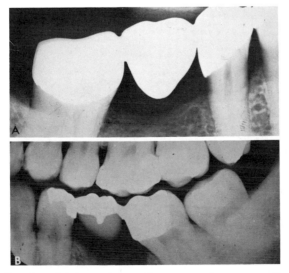

FIGURE 13-20.   Pontics with irregular outlines to conform to configurations of ridges.

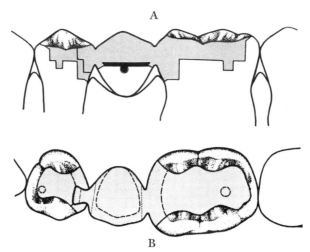

FIGURE 13-21. *A*, In the relationship between Sanitarypontic and ridge, contour should equalize mesial and distal embrasures; facing is beveled to increase soldering area on pontic casting and size of neck of occlusal rest shown here; backing is beveled toward facing to provide mechanical lock for wax and gold.

B, From occlusal, buccolingual width of the facing has been decreased with slight convergence toward mesial. Dotted line shows how backing is trimmed.

lingual to form adequate embrasure areas (Fig. 13–21*B*). Its buccolingual width should be reduced from one-fifth to one-third, this reduction being greater in the mesial half of the facing. When a larger soldering area must be provided on the proximal surfaces of the occlusal casting, the mesial and distal margins of the facing should be beveled. These bevels should be angled toward the ridge at a little more than 90 degrees and should converge lingually.

For hygienic reasons, resin is contraindicated as a veneer for lower posterior pontics. The all-gold pontic must be perfectly cast and polished when used in this area.

MANDIBULAR PORCELAIN-INCISAL FACINGS

The esthetic appearance of a lower anterior bridge may be enhanced by the use of the porcelain biting-edge facing. It is adapted in the same way as other flatback facings, except that all reduction in length must be made at the cervical to conserve the bulk and strength of the porcelain at the incisal edge. The angle formed by the incisal porcelain and the flat lingual surface should be increased slightly so that the casting can give more support along the incisal. This facing is indicated in the construction of mandibular anterior bridges only and should not be used except when the relationship is such that minimal lingual forces will be directed against the pontic.

STABILIZING THE FACING

When the facing has been aligned and contoured, and is being held in position on the working cast with modeling clay or soft wax, it should be secured in this position by a small quantity of sticky wax applied to the exposed linguoincisal edge and to the embrasures. The labial or buccal of the working cast should be coated with a separating medium or petrolatum, and a plaster index poured. This will be used to maintain the alignment of the facing during the waxing of the pontic. (See Figure 13–22.)

The index is made of impression plaster or quick-setting stone, mixed to a medium thick consistency and applied to the buccal surface of the facing, the abutment teeth, and the ridge, working the plaster into the proximal embrasures without extending it over the incisal or occlusal margin of the facing. When the plaster or stone has set, it should be removed and trimmed to workable size, retaining enough length and height so that the index will seat accurately and easily on the working cast and hold the facing and subsequent individual casting securely in position.

THE BACKING

After the facing has been cleaned, if it is a flatback or a Trupontic, a backing must be adjusted. The backing, which supports the pin for the retention of the facing, should be trimmed short of the margin on the mesial, distal, and incisal or bucco-occlusal, and it should be beveled toward the facing. Thus the waxed pontic will hold the backing in position, and there will be a mechanical lock between the backing and the cast metal.

The backing should be removed and the lingual and cervical portions of the facing, the ridge, and the index lubricated so that molten wax will not adhere to these surfaces.

The backing is then replaced on the facing and the facing is returned to the working cast, to be aligned and supported by the plaster index.

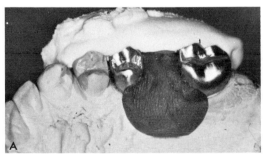 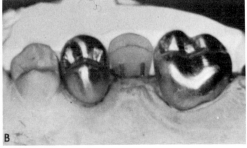

FIGURE 13–22. *A*, Facing stabilized with wax during making of buccal plaster index. *B*, Facing stabilized on working cast by plaster index. Index has been trimmed along occlusal to prevent interference with lateral excursions. Facing, pins, working cast, and index must be lubricated with Microfilm before wax is flowed into space.

If a broken-stress or nonrigid joint is to be used between the pontic and one abutment, it must be prepared at this time and be waxed with, or included in, the pattern for the pontic casting. Such connectors will be discussed at the end of this chapter.

WAXING AND CASTING

Against a Backing

Molten inlay wax should be flowed on the linguocervical of the facing, after which larger pieces may be softened, pressed to position, and attached. When the wax has been built to a sufficient height, the articulated casts should be closed and moved in eccentric excursions. The markings made in the wax will assist in carving the pontic to functional form (Fig. 13-23).

When more than one tooth is being replaced, pontics must be carved individually and to the exact dimensions required in the finished castings, with the wax surfaces free of flaws, and polished. Cast joints, to have resistance to deformation, sometimes must be so large[8] that embrasure form will be reduced and the underlying tissue overprotected. Acceptable size and form in the connector can be achieved more readily with solder or the subocclusal rest.

A large sprue pin must be used to avoid porosity in pontic castings. It must be attached to the pontic at such a point and at such an angle that the attachment will not destroy occlusal carving, and so that the gold will flow along the surface of the backing instead of meeting it at right angles.

When Using Pin or Reverse-Pin Facings

When a pin facing is used, the pins must be checked to see that they are parallel and at right angles to the facing, and the lingual and cervical, as well

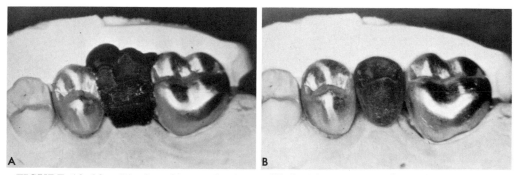

FIGURE 13-23. Waxing the pontic. Space filled with wax (*A*) and pontic carved (*B*).

as the pins, must be lubricated with one of several proprietary materials procurable.

The facing should be removed before the wax pattern is sprued, and carbon rods must be placed in the holes left by the metal pins. After casting, the carbon can be removed with a bur and the facing will then seat on the casting (Fig. 13-24).

Special alloy pins that do not fuse to the pontic casting may be used in the pinholes made by Harmony facings. They can be removed with little difficulty.

The reverse-pin facing must be lubricated and nylon bristles or plastic pins (0.002 or 0.003 inch smaller than drilled holes) placed in the pinholes (Figs. 13-25 and 13-26).[3] The pontic is then built, contoured, sprued, and cast, as described earlier. The facing cannot be seated on the casting until the pins and contacting surface have been "stripped." This is done with a special deplating machine or by a reverse connection in an electroplater. Usually less than 30 seconds at 1 ampere will effect the change in dimensions. The same result may be obtained by immersing the casting in aqua regia for tested periods of time. With either technique all margins, and surfaces not in contact with the facing, must be protected during the stripping process with a coating of lacquer.

It may be necessary also to countersink each hole to allow complete seating of the facing on the casting.

If the space is short occlusocervically and a facing cannot be ground to position and form without spoiling its strength or shade, it may be helpful to cast a pontic and veneer it with resin. For biologic reasons, all the pontic in contact with the ridge tissue should be metal. To secure uniform shading, this method of pontic construction is indicated many times when resin-veneered gold crowns are used as retainers.

The same alloy should be used in casting the pontic as was used in casting the retainers so that wear and contact shock during mastication will be equalized.

ASSEMBLY OF THE BRIDGE

After the casting has been cleaned and pickled, the sprue is cut off and that area polished to contour. The surface of the casting, against which the facing must fit, should be inspected closely for any bubbles or marginal burs that could interfere with seating the facing. These may be removed with a No. 700 bur. Any facing must be seated and removed from the casting without undue effort; otherwise there will be danger of cracking the porcelain.

When the facing has been seated, the pontic should be aligned on the working cast, using the plaster index. At this time the contacts, the adaptation to the ridge, the alignment, and the occlusion should be checked, and any needed corrections made (Fig. 13-27).

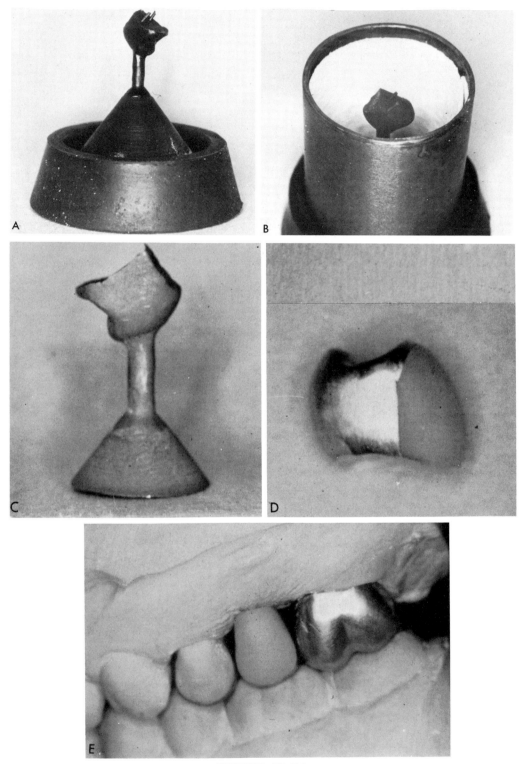

FIGURE 13–24.   Legend on facing page.

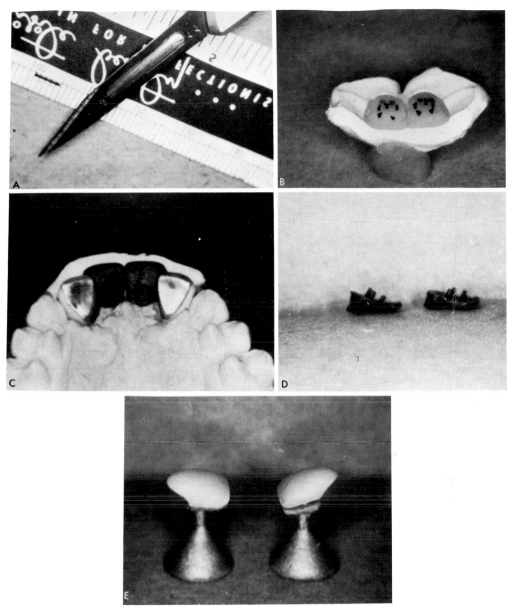

FIGURE 13-25. *A*, Bristle for cast pin cut to desired length.
B, Pins in place prior to waxing.
C, Pontics waxed.
D, Wax patterns.
E, Castings. Facings will not seat. No pressure permitted.

FIGURE 13-24. *Casting and fitting the pontic.*

A, Pontic pattern on sprue former. Sprue pin is attached to nonarticulating area at an angle that will cause the least turbulence in the molten gold. Carbon pins have been placed in pinholes. These will be drilled out after casting, and facing will seat.

B, Position of pattern in ring.

C, Pontic casting.

D, Pontic polished and facing seated. Margins should be polished and burnished around facing with a dull bur.

E, Pontic in position on working cast.

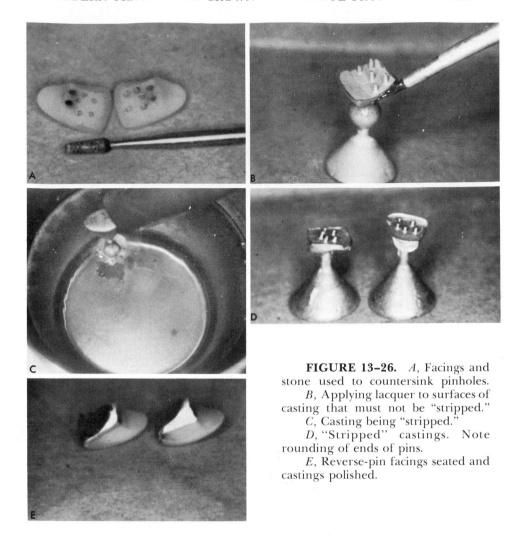

FIGURE 13–26. *A*, Facings and stone used to countersink pinholes.
B, Applying lacquer to surfaces of casting that must not be "stripped."
C, Casting being "stripped."
D, "Stripped" castings. Note rounding of ends of pins.
E, Reverse-pin facings seated and castings polished.

Although polishing may be postponed until after the bridge is assembled, better alignment and adaptation to the ridge will ensue if it is done before the bridge is rigidly assembled. The prevailing methods for polishing small gold castings can be employed if precautions are taken to prevent chipping the porcelain. Tripoli or rouge should not be used on the casting while the facing is in position, since these materials will stain the unglazed porcelain surface. Removal of the stain is practically impossible unless the facing is placed in an ultrasonic cleaner. After the pontic has been polished, the proximal surfaces may be cleaned with a dull bur.

THE NONRIGID CONNECTOR

The nonrigid connector, or broken-stress joint, should be used in bridge construction only where the span is short and the supporting alveolus is not extensively reduced or actively receding. When trouble might be encountered in preparing the abutments for a mutual path of insertion, when inlays are indicated as the retainers, or when an inlay or crown has been made previously and is in good condition, one nonrigid connector may be suitable in building the bridge. For this joint to be successful and nondestructive, the replacement must have the same type of occlusion along its entire length; that is, either natural teeth or a tissue-supported prosthesis.

The need for a broken-stress joint is limited, and whenever possible it should be bypassed in favor of the solder or rigid connector.

Two forms will be discussed. The first and the best, because in action it must be considered as semirigid, has been called the "subocclusal rest." The second, indicated only when used in connection with an abutment already

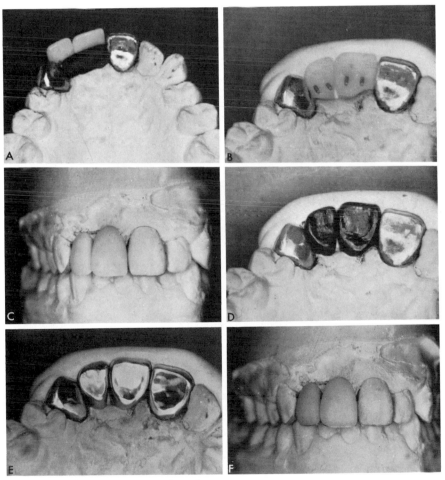

FIGURE 13-27. *A*, Facings selected.

B and *C*, Facings contoured and aligned.

D, Wax patterns for two anterior pontics. Note plaster index for keeping facings in alignment.

E, Pontics aligned on working cast with same labial plaster index.

F, Labial view of cast pontics.

restored, is known as the "dovetail occlusal rest." Lingual rests, used to support cantilever anterior pontics, may be placed in this classification.

The Subocclusal Rest

The subocclusal rest is frequently used when two inlays will act as retainers for the bridge. A solder joint will attach the pontic to the retainer in the stronger abutment (usually the posterior), and the subocclusal rest will be placed in the other inlay.

The subocclusal rest consists of a pin inserted into a prepared pinhole placed in the center of the contact area of the retainer. The pin should be 2.0 mm. long and may be made of 17-gauge high-fusing clasp wire. It must be square on the end, must closely fit the prepared hole, and should slant away from the occlusal at about 30 degrees (Fig. 13-28).

After the working casts have been articulated, or after the retainers have been cast in an indirect technique, the facing should be ground to position and form so that the center of the contact of the retainer on the weaker abutment will be on a level with the top of a Sanitarypontic, or behind a pin or flatback facing. The retainer is then removed from the cast, the pinhole is cut with a No. 35 inverted cone bur used as an end-cutting instrument, and the walls of the hole are smoothed with a No. 56 bur. Seventeen-gauge wire makes a serviceable pin, but 18-gauge or 16-gauge may be substituted in smaller or larger surfaces. It should be bent cervically just outside the orifice of the pinhole, to parallel or touch the backing over the facing. The pontic is waxed around the wire, and the gold is cast to it and the backing.

The subocclusal rest has several advantages over the dovetail occlusal rest. There can be no occlusal movement with it, and since it is placed in the center of the contact area, all embrasures are of normal size. It does not catch or retain food fibers, does not interfere in any way with the occlusion, and has maximal strength. There is one disadvantage: the retainers must be seated simultaneously and the preparations must approach parallelism.

The Dovetail Occlusal Rest

The dovetail occlusal rest is an extension of the pontic casting fitted into a dovetail-shaped rest seat prepared in the occlusal surface of the retainer (Fig. 13-29). The isthmus must be not less than 1.5 mm. wide and 2.0 mm. deep, and the rest at its extremity should measure 2.5 mm. at the widest point. A groove can be cut, 1.5 mm. wide, 1.0 mm. deep, and 2.5 mm. long, on the proximal surface of the retainer to receive a cast strut as a part of the rest. Theoretically this will prevent occlusal movement of the pontic. This type of rest partially fills the embrasure areas, and all too often must be placed to the lingual of the normal contact point.

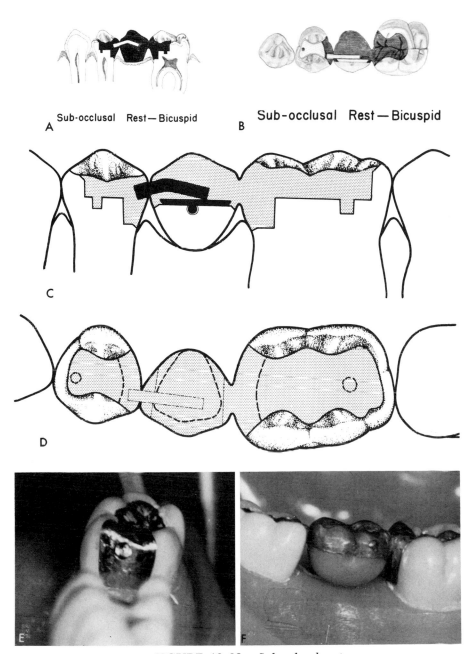

A, Sub-occlusal Rest — Bicuspid

B, Sub-occlusal Rest — Bicuspid

FIGURE 13–28. *Subocclusal rest.*

A and *B*, Cross sections, maxillary bicuspid. Pin, 2.0 mm. long, angles from occlusal at 30 degrees and fits into hole drilled to give semisnug fit.

C and *D*, Cross sections, mandibular bicuspid. Pin need not come into contact with backing on facing, but should be bent to clear occlusion.

E, Pinhole in mandibular molar is too high, since it includes beginning curve of marginal ridge.

F, Note desirable embrasure form at distal of pontic where subocclusal rest was used.

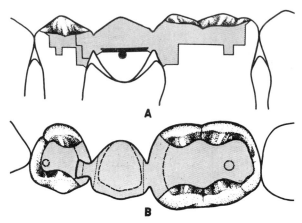

FIGURE 13–29.   Dovetail occlusal rest, cross sections in bicuspid.

The Lingual Rest

The lingual rest on an incisor should be positioned far enough incisally to support the pontic under biting force and to free the embrasure by not forming a shelf under which food may lodge. The rest seat should be angular, deep enough for the rest to complement the lingual tooth form, and fashioned so that lingual movement of the pontic will be impossible. This seat should be placed in metal (Fig. 13-30). A proximolingual inlay will suffice for support and will not be visible from the labial surface. The indiscriminate use of lingual rests is not recommended.

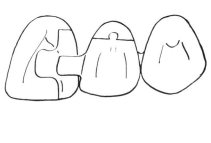

FIGURE 13–30.   Lingual rest, maxillary central incisor.

REFERENCES

1. Smith, D. E.: Improved porcelain facing design for fixed prostheses. J. South. California D. A., 23:34, April 1955.
2. Harmon, C. B.: Pontic design. J. Pros. Den., 8:496, May 1958.
3. Johnston, J. F.: Pontic form and bridge design. Part I. Illinois D. J., 25:272, May 1956.
4. Shooshan, E. D.: Reverse pin-porcelain pontic. J. Pros. Den., 9:284, March-April 1959.
5. Adams, J. D.: Planning posterior bridges. J.A.D.A., 53:647, Dec. 1956.
6. Boyd, H. R., Jr.: Pontics in fixed partial dentures. J. Pros. Den., 5:55, Jan. 1955.
7. Klaffenbach, A. O.: Biomechanical restoration and maintenance of the permanent first molar space. J.A.D.A., 45:633, Dec. 1952.
8. Dykema, R. W.: A Study of the Effects of Certain Variables on the Comparative Strengths of Soldered and Cast Bridge Joints. Master's thesis, Indiana Univ. School Den., June 1961.

Henderson, D., Blevins, W. R., Wesley, R. C., and Seward, T.: The cantilever type of posterior fixed partial dentures: A laboratory study. J. Pros. Den., 24:47, July 1970.

Lucia, V. O.: Modern Gnathological Concepts. St. Louis, The C. V. Mosby Company, 1961.

Miller, C. J.: Inlays, Crowns and Bridges. Philadelphia, W. B. Saunders Company, 1962.

Moulton, G. H.: Esthetics in anterior fixed bridge prosthodontics. J.A.D.A., 52:36, Jan. 1956.

Moulton, G. H.: Functional demands of a posterior crown or bridge. J.A.D.A., 66:534, April 1963.

Mount, J. F.: The importance of pontic design in the fixed prosthetic appliance. Georgetown Den. J., 33:8, Dec. 1966.

Schweitzer, J. M., et al.: Free-end pontics used on fixed partial dentures. J. Pros. Den., 20:120, Aug. 1968.

Selberg, A.: An exposition of pontics and their construction for fixed bridges. Illinois D. J., 9:440, Dec. 1940.

Tylman, S. D.: Relationship of the structural design of dental bridges to their supporting tissues. Internat. D. J., 13:303, June 1963.

Tylman, S. D.: Theory and Practice of Crown and Fixed Partial Prosthodontics (Bridge). 6th ed. St. Louis, The C. V. Mosby Company, 1970.

Wilson, W. H., and Lang, R. L.: Practical Crown and Bridge Prosthodontics. New York, McGraw-Hill Book Company, Inc., 1962.

chapter 14

PONTIC FORM

The whole of fixed partial denture construction can be embraced by three fundamentals: namely, fit, form, and function. The one of predominant importance, which does most to improve the two others, is form. The resultants of these basic requirements are cleanliness, comfort, and concealment. These also are enhanced by form.

In the construction of a crown, a retainer, or a pontic, form does not mean a slavish reproduction in all dimensions of the tooth to be restored or replaced. It should imply that, in the topographic anatomy of the given restoration, the customary convexities, concavities, cusp forms, and groove outlines of the tooth have been included or discernibly suggested, and that these have been so placed, and so modified if required, that

(1) the contact areas will guard the interproximal gingival tissue, but at the same time permit the formation of embrasures that allow food to massage that tissue;

(2) the buccal and lingual gingival tissues can be stimulated as well as protected;

(3) the supporting alveolar process will not be subjected to disintegrating forces;

(4) the escape of food will be facilitated;

(5) masticating efficiency will be kept at or restored to a proper level; and

(6) oral hygiene can be sustained with minimal endeavor.[1]

All these requisites can be met without undue difficulty when restoring one tooth. With thought and some extra effort a retainer can be made that performs according to these specifications.

The pontic may present greater problems. In it, form must be combined with shade to assure esthetically pleasing appearance. Anatomic form must be reproduced to maintain function, but concomitantly, modifications in form may be necessary to reduce the forces and torque on the abutments, and to promote tissue health and hygiene. Such modifications must be controlled so that the pontic will not seem like a foreign body in contact with the tongue and other mobile tissue.

Form is observed, reproduced, and modified in two ways. The peripheral quadrilateral or pentagonal plane form of the pontic may duplicate the

314

silhouette of the tooth being replaced, or it may be changed slightly to satisfy abnormalities in space width. The outline of the labial surface (Fig. 14-1), bounded by the incisal edge, the mesial and distal line angles, and the cementoenamel junction or the gingival line, is also a quadrilateral or a pentagon. It is smaller or narrower and inside the silhouette outline. The labial outline may copy the natural tooth or it may be altered in various subtle ways to suggest desired effects or harmonies with approximating and corresponding teeth. Plus or minus dimensions and long-axis directions may be simulated by minor contour changes at incisal angles or along proximal surfaces.

The majority of modifications proposed in this chapter concern primarily alterations in the labial surface outline. Beginning at the median line and moving around the arch to the molars, form will be considered for the sake of esthetics.

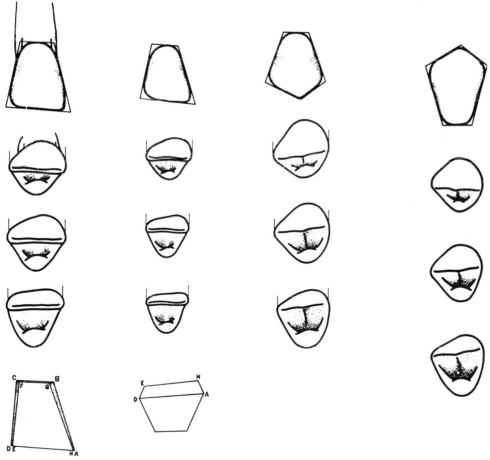

FIGURE 14-1. Geometric forms of silhouette (A-B-C-D) and labial surface outlines (E-F-G-H) of maxillary central and lateral incisors and maxillary and mandibular cuspids. Silhouettes of cuspids can be applied to bicuspids.

THE MAXILLARY CENTRAL INCISOR

When replacing the upper central incisor, one must be influenced not only by the silhouette and labial surface outline, the labial mesiodistal convexities and concavities, and the incisocervical curve of the tooth being replaced, if pre-extraction diagnostic casts are available, but also by these same anatomic features on the approximating central (Fig. 14–2). The long axis of the clinical crown of the central present in the mouth must be projected too, as a guide in positioning and aligning the facing (Fig. 14-3). Form and angulation developed in the pontic should be the same as on the natural tooth.

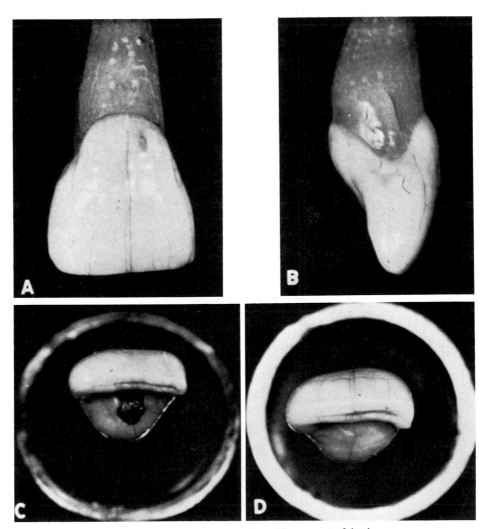

FIGURE 14-2. *Contour of maxillary central incisor.*

A, Labial. *B*, Proximal. *C* and *D*, Incisal.

A determined effort must be made to observe the convexities, concavities, and facets on associated teeth and to produce functional and harmonious form in crowns, pontics, and facings.

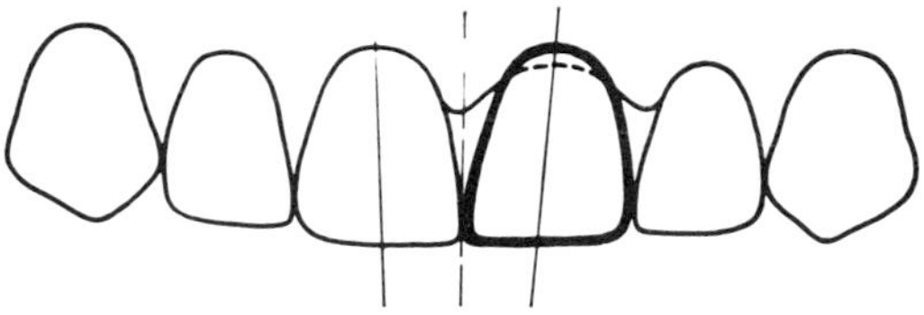

FIGURE 14-3. Form in the facing to harmonize long axes. The lines projected through the central incisors, which represent the visual long axes of the crowns, diverge cervically from the midline (broken line) to the same degree.

Unless changes are demanded for esthetics, the contour of the mesial surface of the central incisor abutment tooth should be reproduced in the retainer casting or in the veneer crown. The same outline, although not always the long axis or degree of rotation, must be transposed to the mesial of the pontic, studying the labial surface in sections before attempting to shape the facing for the expected effect. The facing *must* have sufficient bulk to make reshaping possible.

Incisal angles can be very expressive (Fig. 14-4). For instance, just a little too much rounding on the mesial can make an otherwise well-formed facing look out of place (Fig. 14-5). The illusion of decreased or increased width can be furthered to a degree by the form of the distoincisal angle (Fig. 14-6) and the distal outline of the silhouette. When the space is wider, the incisal or occlusal edge should remain the same from the mesial angle to the beginning of the curve of the distal angle. The distal angle and the distal fourth of the facing will tend to have characteristics similar to the distal of the abutment, but must be overcontoured to contact the approximating distal abutment or pontic. The major changes will be at the distoincisal and distocervical, where the angles become arcs of larger circles.

When the space is narrow, the change in contour is on the distal also, where the curve of the angle will be more confined and the surface flatter, but still suggesting the typal form of the natural tooth. (See Figures, 14-7, 14-8, and 14-9.)

The form in the same areas, and on the mesial too, affects the long-axis line. If the mesial and distal halves of a facing are the same, the long axis will be changed and the replacement will seem foreign to the environment (Fig. 14-10). However, if the mesiocervical and distoincisal segments of the facing have been given convex bevels, these will change the outline of the labial surface and increase the cervical divergence of the long axis (Fig. 14-11).

Other factors that help to fix the long-axis direction of the pontic facing are the angulation of the cervical half of the mesial surface outline and the mesiodistal convexities of the mesiocervical and the distoincisal fourths of the labial surface.

FIGURE 14-4. Areas of incisal angles that can add to or detract from esthetic appearance.

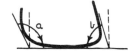

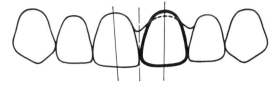

FIGURE 14–5. Excessive convexity at incisal angles changes the visual long axis of the pontic crown, destroying harmony.

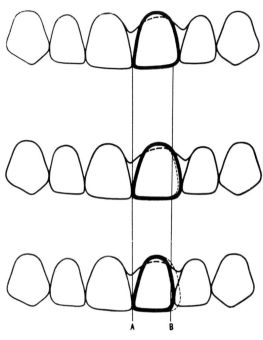

FIGURE 14–6. Treatment of silhouette in wide and narrow spaces when it is not feasible to alter abutment.

Lines A and B show the same mesiodistal length in the incisal edge of the replacement. Facings have been adapted to wider or narrower spaces by changing the convexity of the distoincisal angle and the bulge of the distal contact area.

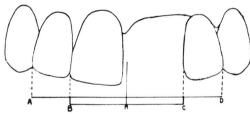

FIGURE 14–7. When single space is too wide, abutment and pontic can absorb equal amounts of excess.

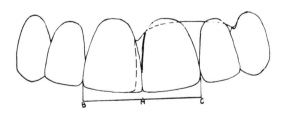

FIGURE 14–8. When single space is narrow, abutment and pontic may be reduced to absorb decrease.

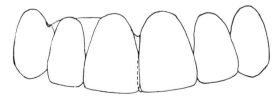

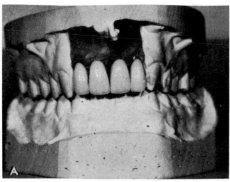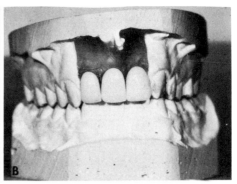

FIGURE 14-9. Four incisors missing. Four facings must be narrow individually (*A*); three facings may have too much width per unit (*B*). Usually wider facings will be more pleasing without it being obvious that (in number) one tooth has not been replaced.

Because of the usual resorption of the ridge tissue toward the lingual, pontic facings many times will be longer than the abutment teeth. To achieve the maximum in appearance, the correct cervical outline should be ground into the facing, even if there is an extension of porcelain beyond this reproduction of the cementoenamel junction (Figs. 14-12 and 14-13). In a majority of cases, establishing the form will suffice, but occasionally the root of the facing must be stained yellow, brown, or pink to accentuate the coronal portion of the pontic.

If the patient has a low lipline, exposing not more than the incisal one-half or two-thirds of the incisors, the interproximal embrasures can be widened discreetly in the gingival third (Fig. 14-14, heavy line) to allow easier access with the toothbrush and to permit a little more ridge coverage by the cingulum section of the pontic. If this is possible, the replacement will feel more natural to the tongue and perhaps will enable the patient to enunciate more clearly.

On many facings received from stock, the ridges running incisocervically the length of the labial surfaces must be removed. A facing with such ridges and grooves cannot be placed beside a tooth with a harmonious result (Fig. 14-15).

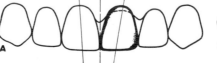

FIGURE 14-10.

FIGURE 14-11.

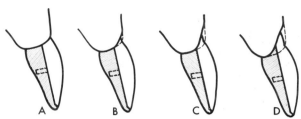

FIGURE 14–12.   Left to right: *A,* Full ridge, area of contact less concave. *B,* More ridge resorption; cementoenamel line ground into facing simulating a little gingival recession. *C,* Ridge resorption increased; facing longer; simulated cementoenamel line constant; contacting area more concave. *D,* Marked loss of ridge tissue toward lingual; facing shows much gingival recession. (See Figure 14–13.)

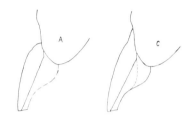

FIGURE 14–13.   *Cervical contour of labial surface.*

A — Correct. *C* — Incorrect.

FIGURE 14–14.

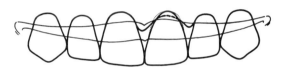

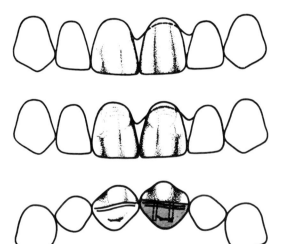

FIGURE 14–15.   Labial ridge reduced.

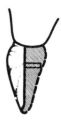

FIGURE 14-16. Grooves placed in cervical third.

After the facing has been ground to position, form, and alignment, and the surface has been smoothed, markings must be made similar to those found on the labial of the corresponding tooth (Fig. 14-16). Such grooves, indentations, peculiarities in formation, abrasions, or eroded areas can be intensified or softened, as the case requires, by staining, and by glazing to produce a surface texture typical of the given mouth.

THE MAXILLARY LATERAL INCISOR

The replacement of the upper lateral incisor will present somewhat different problems. Normally this tooth has a very constricted neck. If this is accurately transferred to the facing, the interproximal embrasures may be so large that the effect will be bad. To prevent this, it often becomes necessary to alter the silhouette slightly by widening the neck of the lateral facing (Fig. 14-17). This can be done without encroaching on the form of the labial surface enough to destroy harmony of relationship and without copying the central in form and angulation.

Many upper lateral incisor facings placed in the mouth fail to meet the requirements of form (Fig. 14-18) because (1) they are too flat mesiodistally; (2) they have almost square incisal angles, when the mesial angle should be less than 90 degrees and the distoincisal angle 90 degrees plus; or (3) because straight mesial and distal outlines, with almost square incisal angles,

FIGURE 14-17. Neck widened, changing silhouette, but outline of labial surface remains constant.

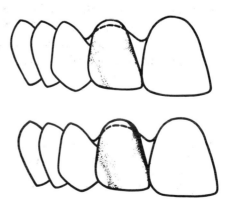

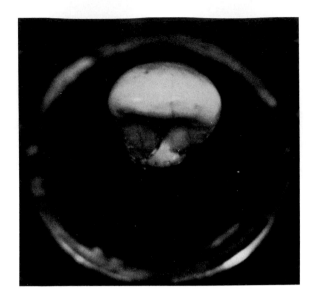

FIGURE 14-18. Incisal view of maxillary lateral incisor showing the normal mesiodistal convexity of the labial surface. Lateral incisors vary in this convexity, but usually it is more pronounced than on centrals.

are substituted for the ovoid type. This will bring the contact areas close to the incisal edge, whereas they should be well up toward the middle of the mesial and distal surfaces.

It is disconcerting to see a lateral incisor replaced by a pontic that appears to be a pyramid, with contacts at the incisal angles (Fig. 14-19), when actually the typal form of the teeth in that arch calls for the mesioincisal angle to be acute, with the contact at the angle, and the distal surface outline convex and contacting the cuspid much nearer the gingival line (Fig. 14-20).

It can be difficult to increase the cervical width of an upper lateral incisor facing and also retain the semblance of the mesial concavity so often found on this tooth, but it can be done in the outline of the mesial edge of the middle third of the labial surface (Fig. 14-21). A "hint" is all that will be needed.

Increasing the cervical width of the lateral incisor may be a further complication when the typical mesiodistal convexity of that area must be formed for the sake of harmony. At times the mesial embrasure must be closed as desired, but the distal may be opened in accordance with the design of the tooth being replaced. This illusion of convexity must be created in the mesial half of the labial surface of the facing without distorting the long axis.

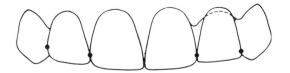

FIGURE 14-19. On left, contacts and form are normal; on right, facing is pyramidal and both contacts are close to incisal.

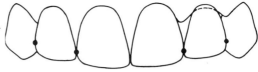

FIGURE 14–20. Contacts correctly positioned on each side.

THE MAXILLARY CUSPID

Upper cuspid facings, as received from the manufacturer, will be more acceptable than the incisor facings. The incisal edge, commonly abraded on the natural tooth, must be copied and protected (Fig. 14–22). It should be remembered that the contact areas of many upper cuspids are much closer to the gingival line than those on the central incisors or the mesial surfaces of the lateral incisors. Often they must be moved cervically or incisally, or adjusted for the anticipated long-axis angulation. If the mesial contact is shifted cervically, the distal contact will drop toward the incisal, the cusp will move mesially, and the crest of the cementoenamel junction will shift toward the distal. Many positions and forms can be suggested by the manipulation of these four points. (See Figure 14–23.) This angulation of the crown in pontic construction can be regulated by the mesial embrasure and the mesiolabial convexities. (See Figure 14–24.) The cuspid in the approximating quadrant should be the guide, with minor attention being given to the adjacent lateral and bicuspid.

The height of contour of the cuspid is not in the center of the tooth mesiodistally, but is to the mesial of the midline of the labial surface (Fig. 14–25). Frequently there will be a definite concavity or groove to the distal of the height of contour, which curves distally to fade out on the distal surface short of the cervical line. This may be obliterated by wear, but if observation of remaining teeth or diagnostic casts shows it to exist, it should be incorporated in the pontic. While the mesial half of this pontic must retain the contour of the cuspid, the interproximal embrasure on the distal may be enlarged for purposes of hygiene.

FACTORS CONSIDERED IN MAXILLARY
ANTERIOR PONTIC CONSTRUCTION

The contour of the lingual half of any upper anterior pontic will be governed not only by the length of span, quality and amount of the support-

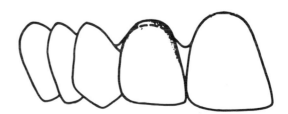

FIGURE 14–21. Mesiocervical concavity suggested by subtle grinding and change in labial surface outline.

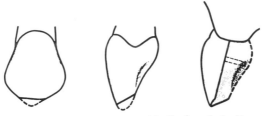

FIGURE 14–22.   Normal abrasion on cuspid. Facing is hollow-ground to make space for metal protection.

ing structure, and inciso-ridge measurement, but also by one other factor, the height of the lipline. The higher the lipline, the less the cervical half of the interproximal embrasures may be opened. (See Figure 14–26.) The use of less ridge coverage labiolingually and wider lingual embrasures will give access for brushing, flow of mouth fluids, and stimulation of the ridge tissue.[2, 3] (See Figure 14-27.)

The same type of construction is employed when the anterior pontic must be short incisocervically. The area of ridge covered is decreased at the expense of the normal cingulum contour. If the space is quite long from incisal edge to ridge crest, the ridgelap may become more ovoid if the lipline does not expose the contact. If that occurs, and all the incisors are missing, esthetic appearance might be improved with a removable bridge having a base to restore gingival contour.

MAXILLARY BICUSPIDS

When shaping an upper bicuspid pontic (Fig. 14-28), consideration must be given, first, to occlusocervical contour; next, to the relationship of the bucco-occlusal margin with the opposing teeth. It will not be enough to position or grind the facing so that it clears the opposing teeth in lateral or protrusive movements. This must be done, but the position and form of the facing must continue the symmetry of the arch.

When using the flatback or long-pin, it is axiomatic that the middle third of an upper bicuspid facing must be recontoured occlusocervically to remove excess convexity. However, with care in positioning the facing before adapting it to the ridge surface of the working cast, the amount of grinding on

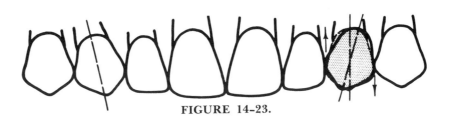

FIGURE 14–23.

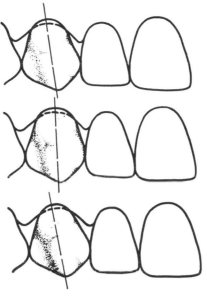

FIGURE 14-24.

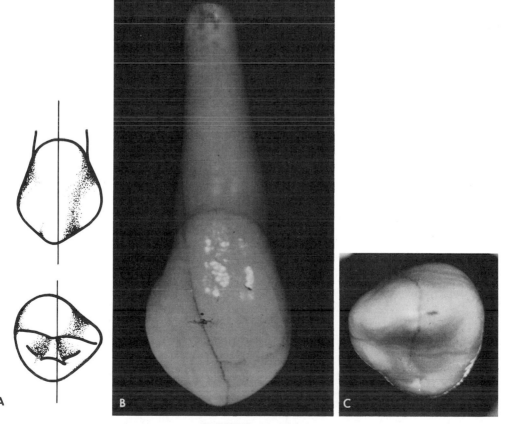

FIGURE 14-25

FIGURE 14-25. *A*, Height of contour is in mesial half of maxillary cuspid.
B and *C*, Labial and incisal views of maxillary cuspid.

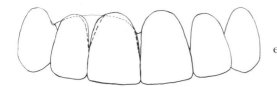

FIGURE 14–26. Dotted line shows how embrasures may be opened if lipline is low.

the buccal would be decreased, thus preserving the selected shade and reducing the amount of recontouring. (See Figure 14-29A.)

The mesial of a bicuspid pontic should be a near-replica of the missing tooth, with some increase in the size of the interproximal embrasure through exaggerated contour in the cervical third. (See Figure 14–29B.) On the distal margin, the contour may be changed to open the space and to reduce ridge coverage for better hygiene and tissue stimulation. Esthetic requirements in the upper bicuspid area rarely can be satisfied with a rounded pontic-tip, ridge-crest contact.

The mesial and distal developmental grooves on the buccal are two landmarks frequently ignored when shaping upper bicuspid facings. Designated by James Mark Prime[4] as the "ears" of the bicuspids, they are the boundary lines for small segments, buccal to and extending only a little way cervically beyond the contacts. The efficacy of such details must be stressed. (See Figure 14–29C and D.)

MAXILLARY MOLARS

The upper molar pontic need not be so exact in its reproduction of form and harmony on the buccal surface as do those nearer the median line. With the exception of the occlusal, all embrasures can be enlarged (Fig. 14-30A), even if the mesial outline must follow closely the pattern of the tooth being replaced. The surface next to the ridge can be reduced in all directions to make a narrower, almost rounded cone area. (See Figure 14-30B, C, and D.)

The buccal cusp relationship with the opposing teeth should be in harmony with the teeth remaining in the quadrant, and the occlusal one-half or two-thirds of the facing should conform to the normal buccal surface contour. Facings that permit hollow-grinding of the lingual portion of the buccal cusps are preferable. (See Figure 14-30D.) A flatback facing should never be used when it must be shortened unduly, or set out of alignment to accommodate either centric closure or lateral and protrusive excursions.

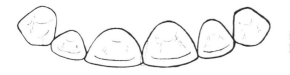

FIGURE 14–27. Cross section showing reduced ridge coverage of central and lateral pontics.

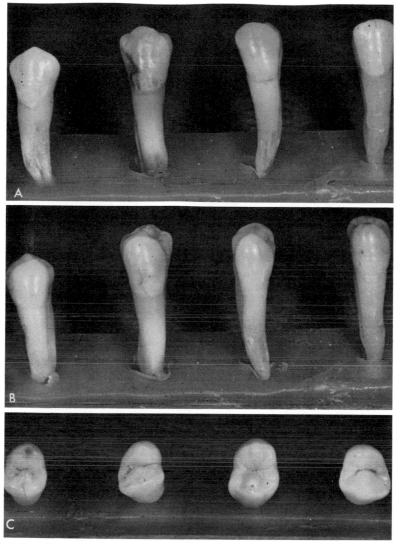

FIGURE 14-28. Buccal, lingual, and occlusal views of four maxillary bicupids. Lingual cusps are off center, narrower, and more pointed. "Ears" and spillways must be reproduced in pontic construction.

MANDIBULAR ANTERIORS

Lower central incisors can be made to look alike, but lower laterals must have a greater convexity in the mesial two-fifths. In many cases the embrasures around lower anterior pontics can be opened below the incisal half with an ovoid tip at the ridge, without any ridgelap (Fig. 14-31).

When shaping lower incisor facings, it will be advantageous to observe and copy (1) the angles of the incisal edge from the lingual to the labial surface and from mesial to distal, (2) the flat or very slightly concave area in the middle half of the incisal third of the labial surface of the central, and (3) the long axis.

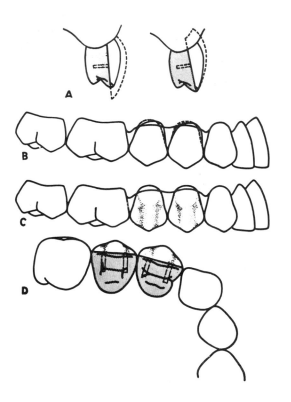

FIGURE 14-29.

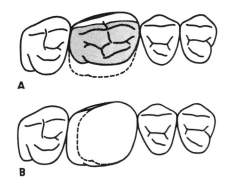

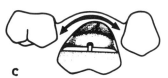

FIGURE 14-30.

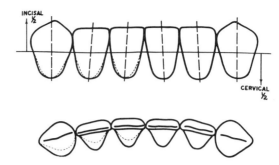

FIGURE 14-31. On left, dotted lines show outline of pontics with embrasures enlarged and ridge area reduced.

When a lower cuspid must be replaced, which fortunately is infrequent, it should duplicate its mate across the median line. Occlusion and space width sometimes will make reproduction impossible, but similar characteristics, such as angles and directions of the cusp arms, the contour of the mesiolabial line angle, the long axis, and the mesiodistal and incisocervical convexities of the incisal third, can be "implied," whatever the situation. Success in this effort comes from experience. This statement applies equally to all replacements.

MANDIBULAR BICUSPIDS

With much of the occlusal half of the buccal surface occluding with the opposing teeth, it is difficult to make lower bicuspid pontics using facings adaptable to the previously discussed situations. Such a method of replacement is not often essential, but when a facing other than the Sanitarypontic is indicated, the buccal anatomy, complex in its arrangement, should be duplicated.

The facing selected, usually a long-pin or Trupontic, must be cut down from the occlusal toward the cervical so that metal may absorb and dissipate the forces of occlusion (Fig. 14-32A).

This protective metal should take the outline of an inlay that provides a full occlusal restoration. Depending on the degree to which the cervical area of the pontic will be visible, the adaptation of the facing to the ridge will conform to the pattern developed for upper bicuspids, including a wider interproximal embrasure on the distal. (See Figure 14-32B.) When any display of metal is prohibited, the bridge must be fabricated using a porcelain

FIGURE 14-32. *A*, All-metal occluding surface on mandibular bicuspid. *B*, Increased distal embrasure.

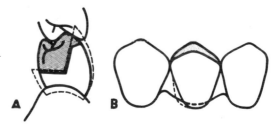

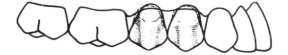

FIGURE 14-33.

veneer fused to the gold framework. A resin veneer would not be stable, and a base supporting tube teeth would not be tolerated by the tissue.

POSTERIOR PONTICS

When the form of a pontic has been modified (Figs. 14-33, 14-34, and 14-35) or exaggerated to promote self-cleansing, tissue stimulation, and comfort, and to reduce torque, leverage, and pressure on the abutments, it should not be expected that, as an individual unit, it will function with the same masticating efficiency as the lost tooth. However, it will replace much that was missing, it will add to the total of the working surfaces, and the reconstruction of the abutments may improve their relationship with the opposing teeth.

Solder joints should be placed in the area of normal contact in the buccal or labial halves (Figs. 14-36, 14-37, and 14-38); hence, it follows that the buccal half of the posterior pontic should fill the space. When viewed from the occlusal or incisal, the buccal or labial half or two-fifths of any pontic should have normal form, with the remaining lingual part decreasing rather sharply in width as it approaches the lingual line angles. This will result in a much narrower and much more convex lingual surface.

The distance from the tips of the buccal cusps to the tips of the lingual cusps should be shortened from one-fifth to one-third, with the lingual cusps becoming more pointed and having smaller surfaces contacting opposing cusps (Fig. 14-39). This will lessen leverages and other forces on the abutment teeth, especially if the spillways are deepened and repositioned a little to the lingual. To eliminate the flat or concave areas that are found proximally on natural teeth and that would be food traps, the lingual surface and those parts of the mesial and distal surfaces lingual to the contacts should be convex in form. (See Figure 14-40.)

When the alveolar process is questionable or receded, but the fixed partial denture remains the restoration of choice, buccolingual width of the pontics may be diminished as much as one-third, the units as a whole being set slightly to the lingual in the final assembly of the bridge. The lateral cusp plane thrusts can be equalized in this way.

In any case in which the abutment teeth and the edentulous areas are

FIGURE 14-34.

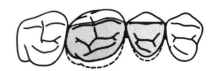

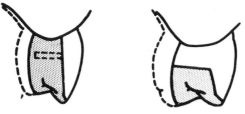

FIGURE 14–35.

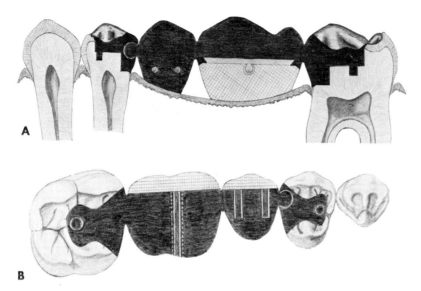

FIGURE 14–36. Buccal and occlusal cross sections of posterior pontics showing convex form, embrasures, and position of solder joints.

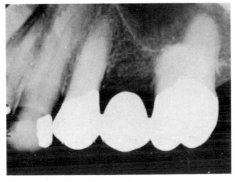

FIGURE 14–37. Cross sections of posterior solder joints. Placed at contact areas, they have a concave periphery.

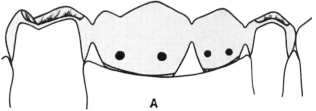

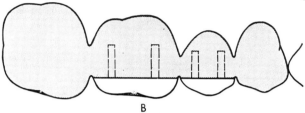

FIGURE 14-38. Cross section of solder joints.

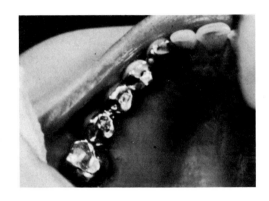

FIGURE 14-39. Reduced occlusal areas on the three pontics of a maxillary five-unit posterior bridge.

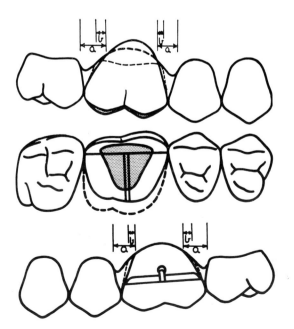

FIGURE 14-40. Reducing the area of contact between the pontic and ridge helps to establish convex surfaces on the proximals. Only the dark area in the center line will contact the ridge. This section becomes narrower as it approaches the lingual.

short occlusocervically, the amount of tissue covered by the pontic, and the resultant stagnation, will become a problem. Again at the expense of the lingual half, the occlusal surface of the pontic must be altered. Reduction of the buccolingual width, and much wider embrasures, will partially rectify the situation, but its solution will depend largely on patient instruction and compliance with such instruction.

Governed Reduction

The amount of reduction of the lingual half of any posterior pontic will be governed by the length of the span, the quality and amount of the supporting structure, and the occluso-ridge measurement.

When the span is long, lingual modification of the individual posterior pontic will be mandatory to lessen the load carried by the abutment teeth during the closing of the jaws on a food bolus. This decrease in the length of the cusp plane will not bring about a lack of balance. Sufficient cusp plane surface will remain on the lingual portion of the pontic to continue the contact with the opposing teeth, because in lateral excursions cusp tips in such areas seldom, if ever, will move into contact with the cusp tips of the opposite jaw. Even then, balance would be continued by the occluding surfaces of the abutments.

RIDGE CONTACT

The contact of any pontic with the ridge tissue deserves special attention. If biologic acceptance and hygienic measures are to be possible, it must touch the ridge, but without pressure. In its over-all contour the pontic must conform to the shape of the ridge, yet it must never be concave in two directions (Fig. 14-41A and B). Buccolingual or labiolingual ridge form demands that the area approximating the ridge be concave, but mesiodistally it should be barely convex.

There may be an occasional exception when the facing adapts to the tissue. The ridge contact should be in the form of an irregular "T" (Fig. 14-41C), with the crossarm under the facing, or it may be only a narrow strip running at right angles to the crest of the ridge. The amount of convexity on either side of this contact area is minor (Fig. 14-41A and B), but this will be enough to prevent a saucerlike food trap. Such form can be developed in far more than half of the pontics, making it easy to keep the tissue-contacting area clean by passing floss mesiodistally under the pontic. The area of contact of the pontic will be smaller than the ridgelap, which in turn is much smaller in circumference than the outline of the pontic. Mesiolingual and distolingual segments of the ridgelap should be convex in form and peripherally should clear the tissue about 0.2 mm. for convenient cleansing. If the pontic extends just over the crest of the ridge lingually (Figs. 14-41A and 14-42D), the tongue will be more comfortable.

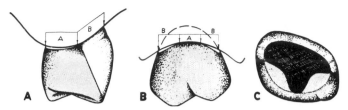

FIGURE 14-41. *A*, Shows slight space between pontic and ridge in area marked "A," but the facing is in contact.

B, Clearance is lateral to area "A."

C, Shows area covering ridge. Dark "T" will be in contact.

A mandibular posterior Sanitarypontic facing or pin-tip should be contoured to have the height of convexity over the ridge crest. The occlusal half or one-third of the pontic, narrower buccolingually and with wider lingual embrasures, should stimulate normal tooth contours, then should curve symmetrically to the contacting line. The embrasures should permit the passage of small or medium bits of food. The line of contact should be no more than half the mesiodistal dimension of the pontic (Fig. 14-43).

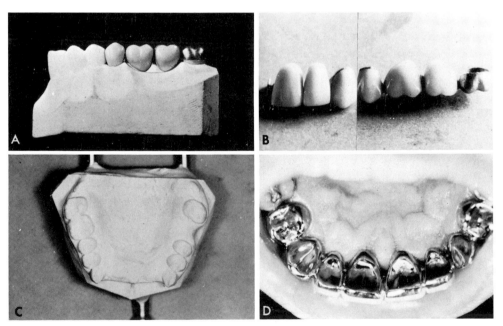

FIGURE 14-42. *Ridge contact, area of coverage, and embrasure form of posterior and anterior pontics.*

A, With less resorption, facings should lap ridge.

B, Embrasure form, anterior and posterior pontics.

C, Diagnostic cast for anterior bridge.

D, Anterior bridge, incisal view; excessive ridge coverage by central incisor pontics will make it more difficult to maintain hygiene and tissue tone.

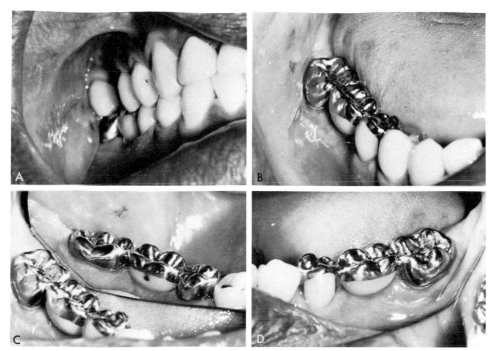

FIGURE 14–43. *A*, Buccal contour of mandibular posterior pontic. Occlusal one third has same inclination as molar and bicuspid retainers.

B, Occlusal of pontic is narrower than molar retainer.

C, Buccal and lingual views. Ridge-crest contact is approximately one-half length of pontic.

D, Embrasures permit passage of food particles.

REFERENCES

1. Johnston, J. F.: Pontic form and bridge design. Part II. Illinois D. J., *25*:339, June 1956.
2. Klaffenbach, A. O.: Anterior fixed bridge prosthesis including acrylic resins. J.A.D.A., *34*:670, May 1947.
3. Moulton, G. H.: Esthetics in anterior fixed bridge prosthodontics. J.A.D.A., *52*:36, Jan. 1956.
4. Prime, J. M.: Lecture before Indianapolis Study Clubs, 1925.

Adams, J. D.: Planning posterior bridges. J.A.D.A., *53*:647, Dec. 1956.

Boyd, H. R., Jr.: Pontics in fixed partial dentures. J. Pros. Den., *5*:55, Jan. 1955.

Cunningham, D. M., and Dykema, R. W.: A case report (fixed bridge). Alum. Bull. Indiana Univ. School Den., Jan. 1956.

Davis, M. C., and Klein, G.: Combination gold and acrylic restorations. J. Pros. Den., *4*:510, July 1954.

Gill, J. R.: Treatment planning for mouth rehabilitation. J. Pros. Den., *2*:230, March 1952.

Hagerman, D. A., and Arnim, S. S.: The relation of new knowledge of the gingiva to crown and bridge procedures. J. Pros. Den., *5*:538, July 1955.

Henry, P. J., et al.: Tissue changes beneath fixed partial dentures. J. Pros. Den., *16*:937, Sept.-Oct. 1966.

Shelby, D. S.: Esthetics and fixed restorations. D. Clin. N. Amer., March 1967, pp. 57–70.

Yock, D. H.: Indications for the use of plastic resins in crown and bridge prosthesis. J.A.D.A., *46*:505, May 1953.

chapter 15

SOLDERING

Solder is an alloy used to unite metal surfaces. Gold solder is similar in composition to a casting alloy, with the difference that tin is added to lower the melting range.[1] The requirements of a dental solder are numerous and rigid. It must flow readily at a temperature at least 100 to 150° F. below the fusing point of the parts to be joined, and must have strength to combat deformation or fracture. It should have a color, a polished luster, and a resistance to tarnish and corrosion comparable to that of the cast alloys. These characteristics can be maintained by a knowledge of the fundamental factors that control the accuracy, properties, and clinical behavior of the solder joint.

The gold content of a solder is usually signified in reference to its fineness, i.e., 1000 fine is pure gold, and 700 fine is 700 parts gold and 300 parts other metals. Often, however, the manufacturer may designate solder in terms of carat, the carat referring to the carat of the gold to be soldered, rather than to the solder itself. For example, an 18K solder does not contain 18 parts in 24 of pure gold, but is to be used with an 18K gold alloy (Table 15-1).

The safest and most sensible way to select a solder is from its melting range, even though traditionally the carat designations have been used. The upper limit of this range should be *at least* 100° F. below the lower limit of the melting range of the casting gold or plate on which the solder is to be

Table 15-1. APPROXIMATE COMPOSITIONS OF DENTAL GOLD SOLDERS

	FOR 16K (.560 fine)	FOR 18K (.650 fine)	FOR 20K (.729 fine)	FOR 22K (.809 fine)
Gold	56.0	65.0	72.9	80.9
Silver	21.4	16.3	12.2	8.1
Copper	16.3	13.1	9.9	6.8
Zinc	4.8	3.9	3.0	2.1
Tin	1.5	1.7	2.0	2.1
Melting Range	1355– 1435° F.	1420– 1490° F.	1465– 1515° F.	1535– 1590° F.

used. Many people refuse to believe that sometimes 16K solder may require a higher temperature for fusing than 18K. Nevertheless this is true, because so much depends on the composition other than the gold content.

A soldering assembly is a mass of set soldering investment, trimmed and cleaned and holding the parts to be joined in the exact relationship that should ensue following the operation. It should be poured to a minimal thickness of ½ inch, should extend not less than ⅛ inch beyond the terminal castings, and should be from ⅛ to ¼ inch wider than the widest casting contained in the assembly.

The requirements for successful and rapid soldering include stability and contact of the pieces to be joined, access, cleanliness, and controlled heating. Theoretically there should be a clearance of 0.005 inch between the pieces to be soldered, which amounts to contact for all practical purposes. A good solder will flow into such minute openings by capillary action. The wider the space to be filled with solder, the weaker the joint, but even more important is the greater shrinkage during solidification of the metal, and the resultant distortion.

SOLDERING INVESTMENT

The composition of a soldering investment is much like that of conventional casting investments, with quartz preferred to cristobalite as the refractory agent.[1] Quartz reduces the thermal expansion and thus the dimensional change during soldering. Just as the contraction of gold during casting must be compensated for, so the contraction of the solder must be balanced in part by the setting and thermal expansion of the investment. The compositions of soldering investments are adjusted accordingly.

ASSEMBLY OF THE BRIDGE

When the pontic has been polished, cleaned, and aligned, the plaster index should be luted to the working cast and the linguocervical of the pontic waxed to the ridge (Fig. 15-1). If all units of the bridge are posterior to the cuspid, the cervical half of the lingual of all units should be blocked out with modeling clay so that the occlusolingual plaster index will not extend into undercuts. The individual parts of the bridge must be cleaned and assembled in the index and luted to position with the relationship that existed on the cast. The interproximal areas between all units must be filled with wax (Fig. 15-2). The exposed surfaces of the plaster of Paris should be painted with a separating medium, soaked in water to fill air pockets, and the soldering assembly should be poured, using an accepted soldering investment.

If the bridge is short, with no more than three joints to be soldered, this operation may be completed at one time (Figs. 15-3, 15-4, and 15-5). If the

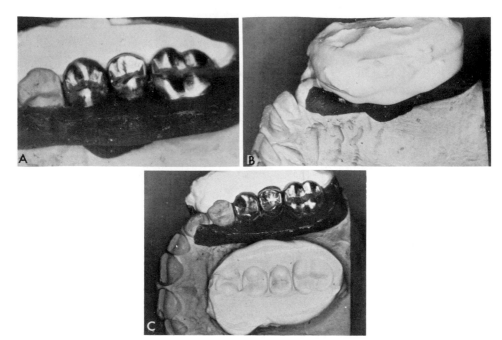

FIGURE 15–1. *A*, Buccal index in position to stabilize pontic during making of occlusal index; modeling clay is used to outline area of occlusal index.

B, Occlusal index poured.

C, Index separated.

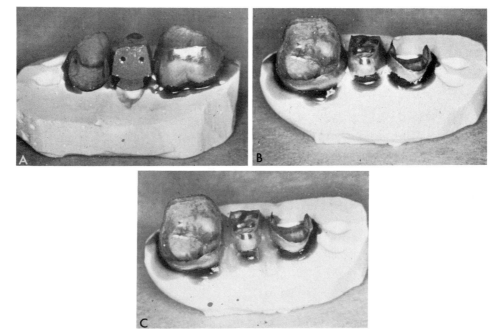

FIGURE 15–2. *A*, Bridge units assembled in occlusal index and secured with wax; index trimmed under pontic to enable poured investment to hold pontic securely.

B, Units luted on lingual.

C, Embrasures filled with wax to prevent soldering investment entering.

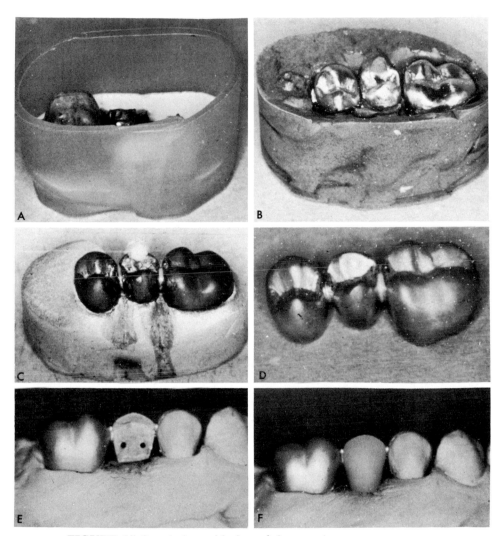

FIGURE 15-3. *A,* Assembly boxed for pouring.
B, Soldering assembly before trimming.
C and *D,* Soldered bridge; note size, form, and position of joints.
E, Bridge seated on working cast; metal contacts unscarred ridge.
F, Facing in position; it is barely narrower than space.

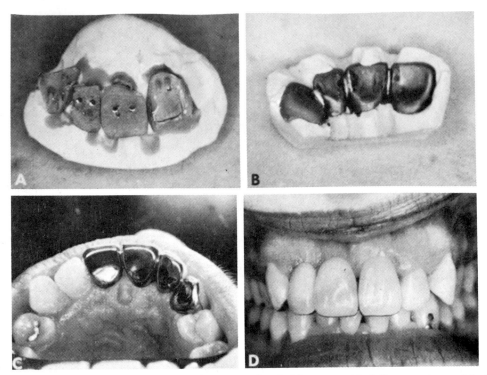

FIGURE 15-4. *A*, Four units of an anterior bridge assembled for pouring soldering assembly. Joint areas are not yet waxed. Parts presumably are separated by correct distances. Spaces for retentive fingers of investment have been cut under incisal edges of pontics.

B, Soldered bridge. Joints are long and relatively thin. Observe investment holding incisals of pontics.

C and *D*, Lingual and labial views of cemented bridge. Joints do not encroach on embrasure form. Tissue is clear for massage by food. Solder is not visible from labial.

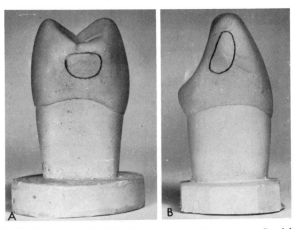

FIGURE 15-5. *A* and *B*, Ideal location and contour of solder joints.

bridge is longer, with more than three solder joints, it is safer if one middle joint is left unsoldered in the first assembly. Then the two parts of the bridge can be realigned, either in the mouth or on the working cast, another index made, and the soldering operation completed in the second assembly.

PREPARATION OF THE ASSEMBLY

Access for soldering may be secured by trimming the assembly to size, beveling the edges, and cutting spear-shaped grooves in the investment that

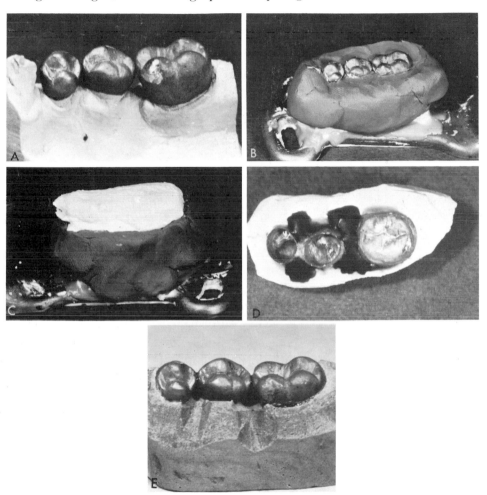

FIGURE 15-6. *Preparation of soldering assembly.*

A, Castings for splint on working cast.

B, All areas blocked out with modeling clay except those to be included in the plaster index.

C, Plaster index poured.

D, Castings assembled and secured to plaster. Areas to be soldered are protected from investment by wax.

E, Soldering assembly washed, trimmed, and fluxed. Since no facings are involved, surfaces to be soldered may be approached from either side. Joints can be smaller because no support will be required. Approximate contact, access, and cleanliness are demonstrated here. Correct application of heat completes the four requisites for soldering.

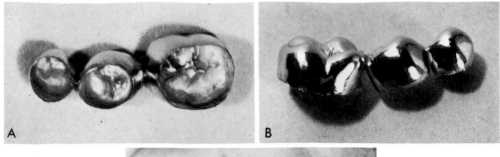

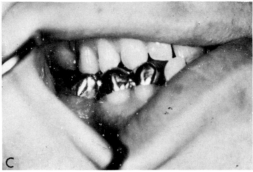

FIGURE 15–7.   *Soldering splint.*

A and *B*, Solder joints are about one-half the size required for a bridge; embrasures are not filled and hygiene should be easy.

C, Splint seated.

lead to and expose the surfaces to be soldered (Figs. 15-3*C*, 15-4*B*, and 15-6). These areas must be wide enough and deep enough for the flame to approach the surfaces from all directions. The wax, originally placed in the embrasures to help to provide access and to prevent particles of soldering investment from falling between the surfaces during trimming, can be flushed away by a stream of boiling water. Any loose pieces of investment will be removed at the same time. Following the elimination of the wax and debris and while the assembly is still hot, a minimal amount of flux should be applied to the contact areas. The heat from the metal will melt the flux base and allow it to enter the embrasure. Excessive flux can be a nuisance. (See Figure 15-7.)

FLUX AND ANTIFLUX

Flux, a borax-containing material, is a substance that maintains the cleanliness of the metals to be united and facilitates the flow and attachment of solder. It burns out during the soldering process, leaving negligible residue. Flux may be procured in either powder or paste form. The paste is easier to control. One of the best available is a paste manufactured according to Dr. Cook's formula.* Any soldering flux with a petrolatum base should be

*The S. S. White Dental Mfg. Co., Philadelphia, Pa.

stirred occasionally, especially if the jar is stored in a warm area, as heat will cause the suspended borax to settle and reduce the fluxing potential of the material at the top of the container.

An antiflux is any substance that precludes the attachment of solder. One of the best examples is gold rouge. It can be mixed with chloroform and painted on critical areas very near the joint and will hinder the union of solder with these parts. It must be kept away from the point at which the solder will be applied and from the crevice into which the solder must flow to create the joint. The need for it is limited.

HEATING THE ASSEMBLY

The soldering assembly should be heated to a temperature of 900 to 1000° F. in a furnace, or over a Bunsen burner flame, the block being supported by a wire screen. It should be placed to one side of the screen until it has dried, *not* directly over the flame. It is the belief of many operators that the assembly will be sufficiently hot when it has been dried, and that the torch is then needed only to heat the areas to be joined. However, experience proves that the assembly should be heated to a higher point, so that on application of the torch flame the castings held in the investment will become a dull red almost instantly.

WARNING: Overheating the investment may cause warpage and a breakdown of the ingredients, releasing elements such as sulfur and chlorine that can attack the metal. Chemical attack of the alloy will lead to brittleness and susceptibility to corrosion in the oral environment.

SOLDERING TECHNIQUE

Solder may be placed at the desired area in strips, but the size and form of the joint can be better controlled if the solder is cut into pieces and applied with tweezers.

Solder will accumulate at the hottest area of the metal. When a small pointed flame from the torch has brought the joint area to a dull red, a piece of solder should be placed in the embrasure and the flame should be directed around the crevice into which the solder must flow. Only the reducing point of the flame should contact the metal. If the cardinal principles have been observed, the solder will flow at once into the contact area. Molten solder acts somewhat as a solvent for the surface of the casting and penetrates beyond the surface, but a strong junction can be obtained without marked diffusion.

When lack of flux or contamination inhibits the flow of the solder, causing it to "ball" or "hang" on the surface of the metal, the torch flame should be removed and the unattached solder taken off, if possible. The castings are refluxed, a new piece of solder is applied, and the flame is again directed as described previously.

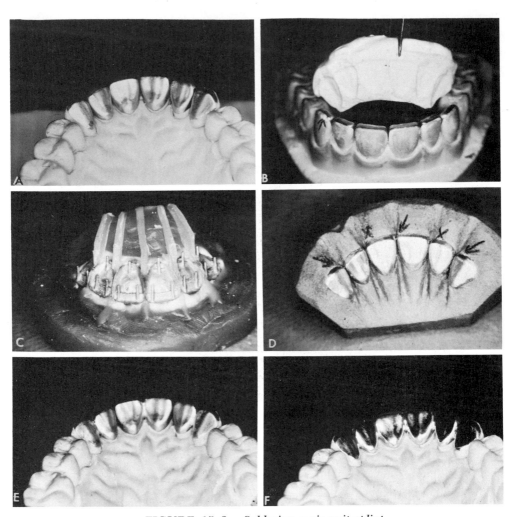

FIGURE 15-8. *Soldering a six-unit splint.*

A, Six pinledges on cast.

B, Lingual plaster index.

C, Castings assembled in index; embrasures waxed.

D, Soldering assembly trimmed; arrows point to the three joints that will be soldered in first assembly.

E, Three double units returned to cast; a new index was made and a new assembly poured; two remaining joints were then soldered.

F, Six-unit splint with five solder joints.

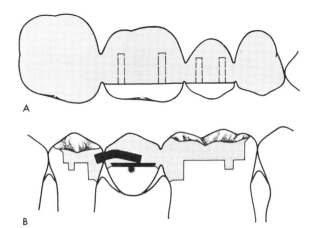

FIGURE 15-9. Cross sections of solder joints.

When the solder does not react quickly, it can become oxidized; the base metal constituents are then burned out and the melting range is raised. Much of the clinical success of a soldered bridge is dependent on maintaining the physical properties of the gold alloy in the abutment castings. These alloys are never inert. At elevated temperatures, induced by overheating in an attempt to cause solder to flow, the grain structure increases with an accompanying loss of ductility. The resultant brittleness can lead to fracture under masticating forces. Therefore care in soldering is important to assure maximal physical properties in the assembled bridge.

If the soldering assembly has been carefully heated and the torch flame correctly adjusted and applied, the time required for the soldering operation will be short. When molten metal solidifies, there is some shrinkage, which can be controlled suitably by having the units in contact, by properly heating the soldering assembly, and by producing no more than three joints in any assembly (Fig. 15-8).

When the soldering has been finished, the assembly should cool until the metal is black before being placed in water; the investment is then removed and the metal is cleaned. Rapid quenching from a high temperature will induce distortion.[2, 3, 4]

A good solder joint must have a complete and concave peripheral attachment, circular or elliptical in form (Fig. 15-9). No joint is acceptable if it has pits, irregularities, or open sections resulting from inadequate fluxing, debris, or insufficient heat. It should be centered at the contact areas of the castings, extending into the embrasures only far enough for strength. Solder must not extend to the margin of the retainer, because this can cause warping or rounding of the margin and will interfere with finishing the cemented casting. There are no laws governing the size of solder joints other than those set up through the judgment of the operator. The greatest measurement of the joint ideally should never be at right angles to the line of force directed against the prosthesis. Since this rule must be violated many times in the construction of anterior bridges, joints in these areas must approach perfection.

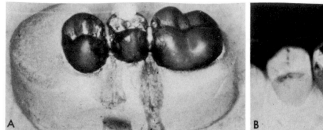
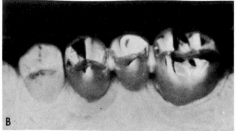

FIGURE 15–10.   Soldered bridge is black (*A*), but color and luster can be returned (*B*), by pickling and by using rubber wheels, pumice, tripoli, and No. 600 Carborundum powder.

PICKLING

The bridge should be placed in a porcelain pickling dish and a solution of 50 per cent hydrochloric acid* should be poured over it. The acid is heated until the surface of the gold is free of oxide; then the acid is poured off and the prosthesis is removed. Any greenish tint in the acid is evidence of copper or silver salts. If dirty acid is used for pickling, an electrolytic deposit of copper is suddenly formed. This will lead to corrosion. Copper pans and iron tongs should not be used in connection with acid because they contaminate the gold alloy. The soldered bridge should never be pickled by holding it over a flame and then plunging it into acid, because of the possibility of a joint breaking during heating, or distortion occurring from the sudden change in temperature.[3] (See Figure 15–10.)

If necessary, the solder joints may be contoured, using knife-edge stones or disks, and should be polished, using rubber wheels, pumice, tripoli, and No. 600 Carborundum powder (Fig. 15–11).

The prosthesis is now ready for trial in the mouth.

---

*Fifty per cent sulfuric acid may be used and it gives off less fumes. Hydrofluoric acid is excellent, but it is too dangerous for general use.

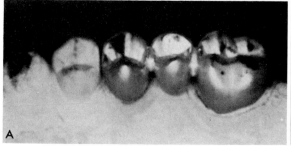
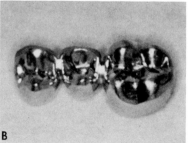

FIGURE 15–11.   *A*, Equilibration of soldered, unpolished bridge on working cast. Note markings from articulating paper.
B, Bridge polished, washed, and ready for try-in.

REFERENCES

1. Taylor, N. O., and Teamer, C. K.: Gold solders for dental use. J. D. Res., *28*:219, June 1949.
2. Steinman, R. R.: Warpage produced by soldering with dental solders and gold alloys. J. Pros. Den., *4*:384, May 1954.
3. Ryge, G.: Dental soldering procedures. D. Clin. N. Amer., Nov. 1958, p. 747.
4. Perdigon, G. J., and Van Eepoel, E. F.: Minimizing solder joint warpage in fixed partial denture construction. J. Pros. Den., 7:244, March 1957.

Dykema, R. W.: A Study of the Effects of Certain Variables on the Comparative Strengths of Soldered and Cast Bridge Joints. Master's thesis, Indiana Univ. School Den., June 1961.

J. F. Jelenko & Co., Inc.: Crown and Bridge Construction. A Handbook of Dental Laboratory Procedures. The company, 1964.

Simpson, R. L.: Failures in crown and bridge prosthodontics. J.A.D.A., *47*:154, Aug. 1953.

Winslow, M. B.: Fixed splint and bridge assembly. J.A.D.A., *51*:47, July 1955.

chapter 16

GLAZING AND STAINING FACINGS

A ground, unglazed porcelain facing is rough, porous, and irritating, stains readily, and is an inviting area for plaque and bacterial growth. It should never be placed in contact with mucous membrane, either static or mobile. Although some vacuum-fired facings can be given a semipolish after contouring, even these surfaces cannot be considered acceptable. "Any number of excuses may be made for using an unglazed surface, but the tissue will not accept any of them."[1]

Reglazing pontic facings can be done by rubbing dry porcelain powder into the pores and firing the facing to fuse the exposed ground surface, or by applying a coating of an overglaze and firing it at the temperature suggested by the manufacturer. The first method mentioned generally overfuses the facing, thereby changing form and fit and reducing the physical properties.

Overglazes for restoring the surface texture and finish to ground porcelain facings have reacted favorably in accelerated solubility tests using synthetic saliva. When applied in a thin layer, never over 0.006 inch thick, they are transparent and do not alter the shade of the surface to which they are applied. Whether the overglaze is one that fuses at 1945,* 1762,* or 1600° F.,† if directions are scrupulously followed and if the glaze is adequately fired, it does not seem to dissolve, lose its luster, or change its surface texture in the oral environment. When the overglaze is fused at less than 1825° F., the holding period should be at least 1 minute. If the piece is overfired, the surface texture, although substantial, will be glassy and artificial looking. Usually, however, this appearance can be improved satisfactorily by lightly rubbing the surface with a very fine sandpaper disk.[2]

---

*Steele's Super Glaze, The Columbus Dental Mfg. Co., Columbus, Ohio.
†The S. S. White Dental Mfg. Co., Philadelphia Pa.

APPLYING THE GLAZE

After the facing has been ground to form and alignment, it must be boiled in water to remove wax and grit, scrubbed with a detergent, washed, and dried with a clean towel (Fig. 16-1).

With the facing mounted on a facing holder, or prepared toothpick, and steadied with the finger, dry glazing powder, picked up on a clean napkin, should be rubbed into all ground surfaces that will not be in contact with metal later on (Fig. 16-2). If inadvertently any powder is pushed into the slot and lingual surface or gathers around the pins of a facing, it must be brushed off with a semistiff bristle brush.

Glazing powder should be mixed to a creamy consistency, using the liquid medium found in the Glazing Kit.* A liquid made by placing equal quantities of glycerin and water in a bottle and heating the combination in a double boiler is suitable also. This mixture is complete in about 10 minutes.

The mixture of powder and liquid, mobile but not runny, is applied in a thin, even coat to all ground surfaces, again being careful to keep it away

---

*Steele's Super Glaze, The Columbus Dental Mfg. Co., Columbus, Ohio.

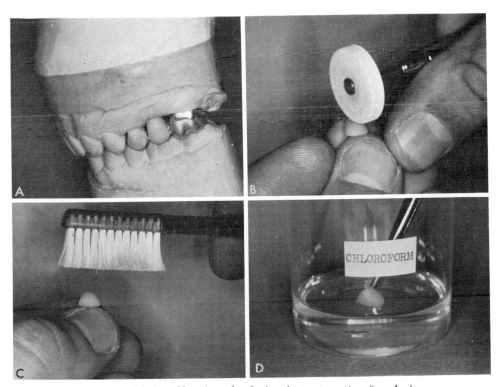

FIGURE 16-1. *Cleaning the facing in preparation for glazing.*

A, The recontoured facing on the soldered and equilibrated bridge.
B, Smoothing the facing with a rubber wheel.
C, Scrubbing facing with a detergent.
D, Dipping facing in chloroform to remove any remaining wax particles.

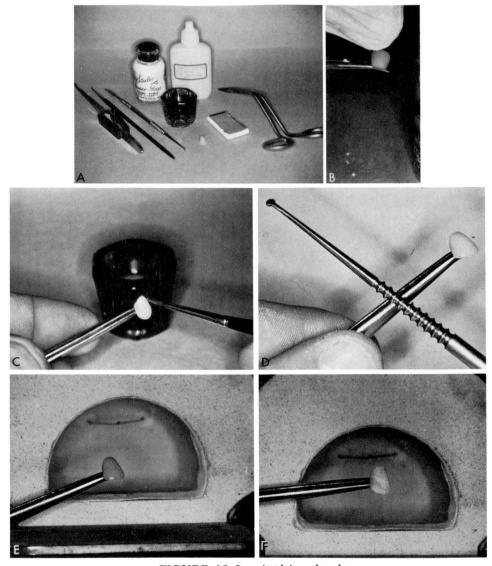

FIGURE 16–2. *Applying the glaze.*

A, Armamentarium needed for glazing facings: tongs, brush, vibrator-spatula, glaze (one that fuses at 1945° F. or 1762° F.), Dappen dish, liquid, tray covered with platinum, and furnace tongs.

B, Rubbing powder onto facing.

C, Applying glaze with brush.

D, Vibrating facing to spread glaze evenly.

E and *F*, Drying glaze before furnace door so that evenness of application, and quantity, may be verified.

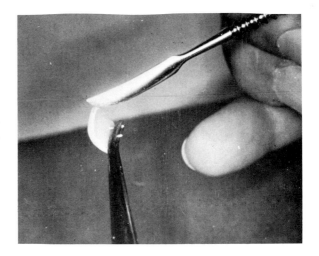

FIGURE 16-3. Removing misplaced glaze powder with instrument.

from, or to remove it from, the slot or any portion of the facing that will be in contact with the casting. The facing should be held before the furnace door to dry, or rotated above a clear-burning Bunsen burner flame, and should then be examined for evenness and thickness of the glaze. If any area has been missed or has a coating that is too thin, no attempt should be made to patch the spot. All glaze must be rubbed off and reapplied. To repeat: any powder on any surface that will come into contact with a casting surface must be removed with an instrument blade or fine brush (Fig. 16-3).

FIRING THE GLAZE

There are inexpensive furnaces having restricted upper-temperature ranges* (Fig. 16-4), which can be used for glazing and for firing low-fusing porcelain. A burnout furnace should not be used, since the muffle will be contaminated by the gas from the wax.

The facing should be placed on a small firing tray, or sagger, which has been covered with a sheet of 0.001 platinum foil, or which contains a mound of flint or fine silex powder. Platinum foil is preferable to ground silex because if the platinum touches the glaze, it can be peeled away, whereas silex must be broken off, sometimes spoiling the contour or glaze of the facing (Fig. 16-5).

After being preheated in front of the open muffle, the facing is placed in a furnace no hotter than 900° F., and the temperature is increased by 100° every minute. The current is turned off when the fusing point of the glaze has been reached. The furnace temperature is dropped to 900° F.; then the door is opened and the furnace is cooled to 500° F. The sagger is removed to the bench and covered with a glass beaker.

The first application of glazing material is expected to serve only as a

*K. H. Huppert Co., Chicago, Ill.; Barkmeyer (The J. M. Ney Company), Yucaipa, Calif.

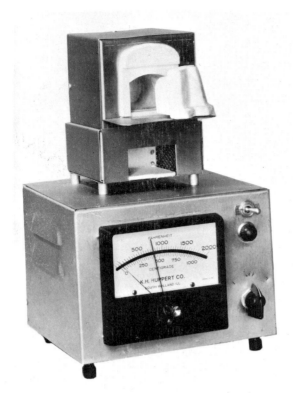

FIGURE 16-4.   Glazing furnace (Huppert).

filler for the pores of the porcelain; a second layer probably will be needed to provide a smooth, semiglossy surface. However, if characterization of the facing is required, the stains should be applied following the fusing of the initial coat. After the stains have been dried and examined, they should be fired at the designated fusing point, raising and lowering the temperature in the usual manner. Glaze is again applied, matured, and cooled, as previously described, although the fusing temperature must be lowered and the time increased in order to preserve the shade of the stains.

Facings should be resurfaced to have a luster harmonizing with approximating and corresponding teeth, except that the highest possible glaze should always be placed on Sanitarypontics and on porcelain surfaces to be clasped.

STAINING

Two kits of stains are widely accepted. One fuses at 1762° F.,* the other at 1600° F.† The 1762° F. group must be used with the glaze that is fired at 1945° F. or 1762° F. The second type, which is fired at 1600° F., is coupled with the glaze that fuses at the same temperature; no holding time is used with this combination.[1]

*Steele's, The Columbus Dental Mfg. Co., Columbus, Ohio.
†The S. S. White Dental Mfg. Co., Philadelphia, Pa

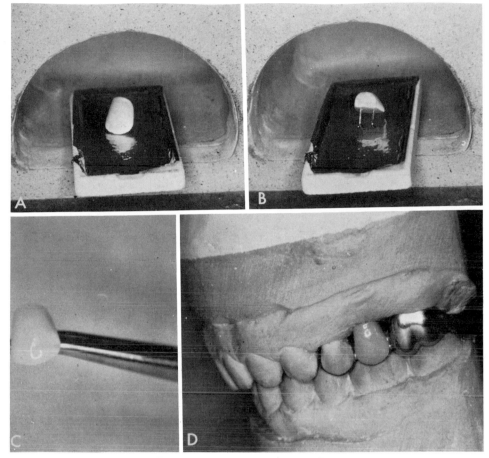

FIGURE 16-5. *Firing the glaze.*

A and *B*, Facing on firing tray in door of furnace.
C, Facing glazed.
D, Glazed facing returned to bridge.

Hairline Check

Stains must be applied to facings in a very subtle form, producing only a hint of the simulated object. A hairline check is made by using brown stain plus a very little black, with one part of the diluting agent added to four parts of stain. It should be neither thin nor ropy when mixed. It is applied with a very small brush in a rather wide strip; then, drawing the brush from cervical to incisal, alternately on each side of the stain, a narrow, hairlike, sometimes intermittent line is formed. It may be in the center of the tooth, and if so will follow the long axis; but if the check is nearer the margin, it probably will angle slightly toward the proximo-cervical.

Decalcified Areas

Decalcified spots are made from white stain with no diluting agent added. These are often in the cervical third and lateral to the center of the tooth, irregular in form, and frequently crescent-shaped, surrounding a pin point of caries that will show up as a brown dot. The white stain should be feathered around the edges.

Restorations

Silicate or resin fillings may be outlined with a fine brown line and shaded with white. Such a characterization is seldom desired by the patient, since it could denote a lack of pride in the upkeep or repair of the teeth.

Enamel Cracks

Cracks in enamel may be copied, and in an anterior bridge replacing one or two teeth can be of great help in establishing esthetic harmony. Gray stain is placed on the facing, with one edge a straight line and the remainder spread, thinned, and feathered toward the distal for a distance of 1.0 mm. plus at the incisal, narrowing as it reaches the end of the line, which may be from 3.0 to 5.0 mm. long. To the mesial, the surface is shaded with white, not too heavily, thinning out quickly in about 0.6 mm.

After stains have been fused, they are covered with a layer of glaze, which is fired at the same temperature with a holding time of 1 minute (Fig. 16-6).

A reverse-pin facing and a pin facing in a light shade may be effectively stained along the incisal edge or proximal margins of the metal-contacting surface before the pontic is waxed. These stains do not require an overlay of glaze.

When staining bonded Ceramco* porcelain veneers to simulate the

_____

*Ceramco, Inc., Woodside, N.Y.

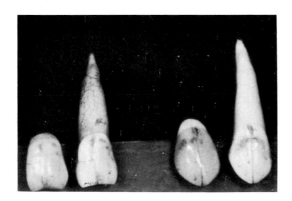

FIGURE 16-6.   Stained facings.

appearance of separation between the individual units, a fine line of Steele's Superstain, made up of half brown stain and half diluent, will be painted at the junction of the units. A groove, made by a flexible diamond disk, should be provided. Since there appears to be some fluxing action at higher temperatures, inducing flow between the porcelain and the stain, this firing temperature should not exceed 1720° F.

SEATING THE FACING

When the facing has cooled and is tried on the pontic, the increased width caused by the overglaze may make it necessary to use a sandpaper disk on proximal edges to allow the facing to seat on the casting without interference.

Facings may check and have a tendency to be more friable if preliminary heating, or cooling, is not done with care.

REFERENCES

1. Pettrow, J. N.: Personal communication.
2. Kipp, R. P.: Personal communication.

chapter 17

CHECKING AND CEMENTING CROWNS AND BRIDGES

The occluding surfaces of the polished bridge should be dulled with a Burlew disk, after which the bridge must be washed before being placed in the mouth. Doubtless it will have been cleansed thoroughly beforehand, but repeating the process after the patient is in the chair will allay any suspicion of carelessness. In order that the patient may be more acutely aware of premature contacts, and more helpful in detecting them when the bridge is first placed in the mouth, it is an accepted practice not to anesthetize the abutment teeth at this time. Placing the metal in warm water before seating will do much to minimize discomfort.

SEATING AND CHECKING A FULL VENEER GOLD CROWN CASTING

The casting should be seated on the tooth with a mallet and orangewood stick. If it does not seat, the inside must be scrutinized again for irregularities, which now will have a shiny, burnished appearance. If a plus-contact obstructs seating, it must be polished further, this process being repeated until the casting can be seated. When the contact is deficient, it must be rebuilt by adding solder.

With dental floss secured to the forefinger of each hand and with about a 2-inch length between the fingers, the floss is held taut and at a 30-degree angle to the occlusal plane. One finger, either inside or outside the arch, is kept stationary after the floss reaches the occlusobuccal embrasure, and the floss is forced through the contact area by downward pressure from the other hand. A buccolingual movement of the floss will hasten the entry into the cervical embrasure. A snapping-through should be avoided because of the probable injury of the gingival papilla.

356

Testing the Contact

The strength of the contact will be demonstrated by the resistance to the passage of the floss unless one (or both) of the approximating surfaces is rough or carious. If the interproximal soft tissue at the site chosen for testing is healthy, and if the alveolus is normal radiographically, the contact form and pressure may be considered correct for that mouth and the opposition to the passage of the floss can be viewed as a standard by which the contact strength of a restoration may be judged. An instrument was built for making such a test,[1] but since it is not available commercially, experience and judgment must suffice.

If the restoration seats, another check of the control or tested area should precede an appraisal of the newly established contact, adding or subtracting pressure until, after final shaping and polishing, resistance to the floss is the same at the two contacts.

Checking for Overextension and Underextension

When the casting has been seated, an explorer point may be used for locating overextensions. After the occlusion has been registered with articulating paper, the casting is removed and occlusal and cervical alterations are made outside the mouth to escape overheating of the tooth and trauma to soft tissue. Marking, removal, and adjustment are continued until optimal occlusion has been reached, after which the contact areas and cervical margin must be re-evaluated for strength and position. If the casting is short and fails to cover the preparation, the crown must be remade, as repair is impossible. The exposed tooth surface and its concomitant roughness will set up tissue irritation, which cannot be excluded or controlled, and sensitivity and caries may develop.

Smith[2] writes:

"The fourth basic step in achieving a satisfactory crown is the fitting in the mouth. This amounts to a checking of the gingival fit and correction of the contact and occlusion. If the marginal fit is inaccurate, the crown should be discarded and the preparation re-evaluated, corrected if necessary, and a new impression made. Before the marginal fit can be checked, the crown must be completely seated. Excessive contour on the proximal contact areas will prevent the complete seating of the crown. This excess must be reduced, and normal contact must be developed. Final seating may be done by tapping the crown with a steel instrument and mallet. Positive seating may be sensed through the feel and ring of the instrument. The margin of the crown may be examined then by using an explorer. An easily accessible point on the crown margin where the preparation margin is readily discernible by tactile examination is selected. With the point directed toward the gingival margin, the explorer is passed over the crown down onto the root surface. If the marginal fit is good, the passage of the point will be smooth. If the passage is interrupted by bumping over a prominence, it means that the preparation is not completely covered, and that the crown is not in place or that it is short. If the passage is interrupted by the point dropping off of the crown to the tooth, the crown is either too long or not in close apposition with the tooth. A further check of the marginal fit may be made by reversing direction of the point so that it is directed toward the occlusal surface, and is passed from the tooth surface below the crown margin up and over the casting. If the passage is smooth, the marginal fit is good. If the point catches under the margin of the casting, it is an indication that the margin is either too long, or is not in apposition with the tooth. If, in the passage, the point drops over an irregularity of the tooth, and then contacts the crown, it is an indication that the preparation is not completely covered.

"This procedure is repeated at a number of points around the gingival margin, and if any of the above irregularities are evidenced, correction is attempted. The seating of the crown is double checked, overextensions are reduced, and the margins are rechecked. The contour of the crown is checked, and the axial surfaces from the margin occlusally are shaped to be in harmony with the surrounding tissues. If the tactile examination is satisfactory, a bite-wing roentgenogram is taken as a check of the interproximal fit, and if this proves satisfactory, the marginal fit of the crown is accepted.

"*Summary.* The construction of cast crowns that possess accurate marginal fit requires: first, understanding; second, ability; and third, conscientious execution. . . . Crowns with accurate marginal fits should contribute to the preservation of teeth and the health of surrounding tissues."

INITIAL SEATING AND CHECKING FIT OF A BRIDGE

After the temporary coverings have been removed from the preparations and the abutments cleaned, the bridge should seat with minimal frictional retardation. If a long period of time has elapsed between taking the impression for the working cast and the completion of the bridge, a constant application of pressure to the seated bridge may be advisable for several minutes so that the abutments will reposition themselves to conform to the path of insertion. There should be no permanent or marked change in the position of the abutment teeth or of the opposing teeth during this period of construction, although a minor temporary shift should have no adverse effect. A major discrepancy or excessive difficulty in seating will oblige the breaking of one or more of the solder joints and reassembly and resoldering of the segments.

After seating the bridge, the cervical adaptation of the retainers should be checked with explorers and bite-wing radiographs. Also, occlusion, strength of contact, alignment, pressure of the pontics against the ridge, and color matching must be examined.

Equilibration

Articulating paper or tape of one color will show the location and extent of any high spots in centric; another color should be used for eccentric movements. It will color all surfaces that touch, but the point of premature contact will be burnished and is the area to be altered. This routine must be continued until there can be comfortable closure in centric and in all excursions. If the working casts were accurately related on the articulator, and if carving and assembly were done with care, only minor adjustment should be necessary.

Considerable adjustment may be expected when a bridge has been constructed using casts related by a wax centric occlusion registration. Wax is notoriously inaccurate when the teeth are brought into contact and should not be used if the Kerr Bite Frame or some other equally satisfactory means of mounting is at hand.

A bridge constructed by the indirect technique should be returned to the working cast after soldering, and before polishing, for occlusal equilibration. If the opposing cast has been poured in stone, closure against the soldered bridge must be done with delicacy so that the cast will not be abraded. If the cast is worn or distorted, the bridge could be completed and polished with gross occlusal imperfections remaining.

After discrepancies in occlusion have been eliminated and the bridge has been polished, the facing may be glazed before the patient appears. This is psychologically advantageous; also it is easier at this time to check the shade of the recontoured facing.

Contacts, Alignment, and Ridge Adaptation

The strength of contact must be checked with floss. If one of the retainers was unintentionally polished to a point at which it no longer has the desired form or enough pressure against the approximating tooth, the bridge must be invested and the area recontoured by the addition of solder. A cemented bridge with a weak contact will be constantly annoying, owing to the packing of fibrous foods. Not only is the patient unhappy, but, worse than that, a resorption of the supporting structure around the abutment tooth may result. To maintain alignment, the bridge must be reinvested.

In checking alignment, the relationship of the buccal cusps of the prosthesis with the buccal cusps of the opposing teeth must be observed, to ascertain whether the patient might bite the cheek or lip (Fig. 17-1). This can happen in the posterior area wherever cusp tips or buccal margins approximate an end-to-end closure. The maxillary buccal cusps should have an overjet, with the mandibular cusps curving slightly toward the center of the opposing tooth. Although errors in this relationship can be remedied after the bridge has been cemented, to do so at this late stage may necessitate grinding a porcelain facing that cannot be reglazed. The facing can be

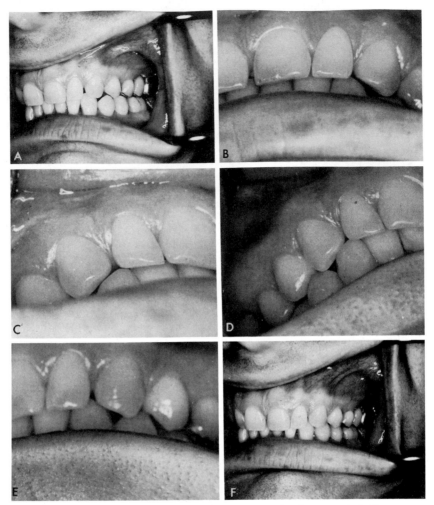

FIGURE 17–1. Checking occlusion and alignment in the mouth before cementation. *A*, *B*, and *C*, Bridge in position; alignment correct, but contact premature. *D*, *E*, and *F*, Occlusion corrected; teeth occluding.

smoothed, but the pores cannot be filled and the patient will be continually conscious of a rough spot. Therefore this matter demands attention at the time the occlusion is being adjusted and before any cementation.

If the ridgelap of the metallic portion of the pontic contacts the tissue too forcibly, this must be recontoured and the ridge surface of the pontic repolished. Floss should be passed under the bridge, from front to back, to disclose the contact relationship with the tissue. A little clearance is tolerable, although contact without pressure is to be sought.

When all changes have been made in occlusion, alignment, and contact, the metal parts that have been ground should be repolished. If stains are needed to add character or to enhance shading, or if adjustments in occlusion, ridge relationship, or alignment have included work on the facing, final glazing can be done during the time the patient is in the chair. Glazing is discussed in Chapter 16.

The facings should be fixed to the pontics, preferably with zinc phosphate cement. The bridge is now ready for cementation.

CAVITY VARNISHES

Zinc phosphate cement, because of its clinical behavior manifested throughout the years and its excellent handling characteristics, still remains the permanent luting agent usually recommended for the fixed gold alloy restoration.

There is, however, increasing evidence that the acidity of zinc phosphate cement may be somewhat greater, and that this type of cement may remain acidic longer, than previously believed.[3] Every precaution should be taken to shield the underlying dentin and the pulp from the aggravating effects of phosphoric acid; hence, the role of the cavity varnish deserves thoughtful consideration.

There are a number of commercial cavity varnishes and little difference generally exists in their composition.[4] They are natural rosins or synthetic resins that have been dissolved in a solvent such as chloroform. The solvent rapidly evaporates to leave a thin, shellaclike film on the tooth surface. Other buffering salts, such as zinc oxide or calcium hydroxide, have been added in a few products, but these compositions have not proved to be superior to the usual inert rosin or resin-type varnish. Selection of a given brand should be based on handling characteristics. The brand of varnish that will flow most evenly over the tooth surface and that is the most readily discernible is the material of choice.

A continuous, thin film of varnish, placed over the cut tooth surface, guards the dentin and pulp in two ways. First, the varnish tends to minimize any seepage of deleterious fluids that may occur around the cemented restoration. Secondly, and of more moment, the varnish will minimize the penetration of any acid that may be present in the zinc phosphate cement. Thus, the possibility of irritation to the pulp from leakage or acid is greatly diminished.[1]

From the foregoing discussion, it is apparent that the varnish is particularly indicated in a deep cavity preparation, where little dentin may remain to protect the tooth against thermal or mechanical shock or from irritants. In such a situation, the varnish may be salutary in maintaining both pulpal health and patient comfort. In a cavity preparation in which a minimum of at least 1.0 mm. of dentin remains, the dentin acts as an insulator, and the use of varnish is of less consequence.

The varnish is painted onto the surface of the prepared cavity immediately before the restoration is to be seated. The tooth surface is dried and the varnish applied. It may be painted on with a small camel's-hair brush, or a pledget of cotton may be employed to carry the varnish into the deeper areas of the cavity preparation. A small wire loop is supplied for application of one commercial product. Because of the difficulty in attaining an intact layer of varnish and the propensity for small holes to form as it dries, two or three coats should be applied. The aim of the multiple applications is not to build up the thickness of the layer, but rather to fill in many of the voids that normally form as the first layer dries and to make possible a more complete coating and better protection for the underlying tooth structure.

Regardless of the method favored, the varnish should be thin. If the varnish becomes thick or viscous upon storage, it should be thinned by the addition of the solvent customarily supplied with it. Chloroform or ether are, in the main, acceptable as thinners. Naturally there is no precise way to determine the appropriate "thinness" except through use and observation. The danger lies in having the varnish too thick, not too thin. A thick consistency will not flow out over the tooth surface, thus will not wet it and will prevent a good marginal seal. The film thickness of the varnish is extremely low and retention of the restoration is not reduced.

CEMENTATION

Cementation will involve the following factors:
(1) a clean, dry crown or bridge;
(2) isolation of the area of operation;
(3) clean, dry tooth or abutment teeth;
(4) a saliva ejector in position;
(5) a cool, clean mixing slab and spatula;
(6) sufficient quantities of cement powder and cement liquid;
(7) an instrument for applying the cement to the inner surfaces of the castings and to the teeth;
(8) an orangewood stick and mallet;
(9) a cotton roll to cushion the biting pressure against the seated crown or bridge;
(10) cavity varnish; and
(11) brush or instrument for applying varnish.

Although discomfort from cementation is not prolonged,[5] many patients are grateful for anesthesia during this procedure, and some insist on it. The anesthetic is prone to decrease the flow of saliva, making it less of a problem to keep the bridge and cement dry during the setting period.

After the abutment teeth have been isolated and dried, older operators may prefer to clean the prepared tooth surfaces with phenol, then to remove the phenol with a pellet of cotton soaked in alcohol and dry the abutments with warm air. Recent research indicates that such so-called sterilizing agents serve no useful purpose and increase the likelihood of further pulpal irritation. It will suffice to scour the cavity preparation with pumice to remove any remaining fragments of the temporary restorative material, wash, and then dry with warm air.

Dental cements do not actually adhere in a chemical sense to the tooth surface or the metal. There is no attraction of unlike molecules. They must not be relied on to hold the casting in place. Such a concept can lead only to failure. The cement serves merely as a luting material to occupy the small space that exists between the restoration and the tooth. Even with a casting that visually fits perfectly, a minute crevice is present that must be occupied by the cement. It is also theorized that the cement, provided it will extrude into a sufficiently thin film, will work its way into the irregularities in the tooth structure and in the cavity side of the casting. Upon hardening, the cement furnishes a certain amount of mechanical retention for the restoration. To keep this intimate adaptation and to avoid leakage, it is imperative that solubility be minimized and adequate strength be retained to avert fracture of these small projections of the cement.

Zinc Phosphate Cement

There are many acceptable brands of cement, and selection should be based upon objective handling characteristics rather than inherent properties. Zinc phosphate cement, which is also used as a cement base, is made from a mixture of a powder and a liquid, the powder being essentially zinc oxide and magnesium oxide, while the liquid is phosphoric acid and water, with metallic salts used as buffers.[6] The water in the liquid is added in a definite concentration to control the setting time. This water balance is critical, and every precaution should be taken to preserve it. Even minor deviations will markedly influence the setting time, and the consistency of the mix will vary accordingly. An increase in the water content accelerates the set, whereas a decrease retards it. If the liquid is exposed, it will either absorb or lose moisture from the air, depending on the humidity of the room. For this reason the bottle should always be kept tightly stoppered and the liquid should *not* be placed on the slab until the operator is ready for mixing.

The neck of the bottle must be kept clean. Agitation of the liquid is not necessary and results only in a smeared cap. If a precipitate appears, the liquid should be thrown away. Precipitation or cloudiness in liquid may result from evaporation and from any crystallized liquid that is allowed to gather inside the cap or around the neck of the bottle. The last portion should be discarded also, because repeated opening of the bottle over a long period of time alters the water content of the liquid through evaporation.

The importance, clinically, of careful manipulation cannot be overemphasized, since the present cements are the weakest link in the otherwise strong chain of dental castings. At best they have a relatively low strength and are in a measure soluble in mouth fluids, particularly the weak organic acids commonly present in the oral environment (Fig. 17–2).[7] When handled correctly, in conjunction with a well-fitting casting, they do their job, but improper manipulation of even fine commercial brands, of which there are many, produces inferior chemical and physical properties and precludes success.

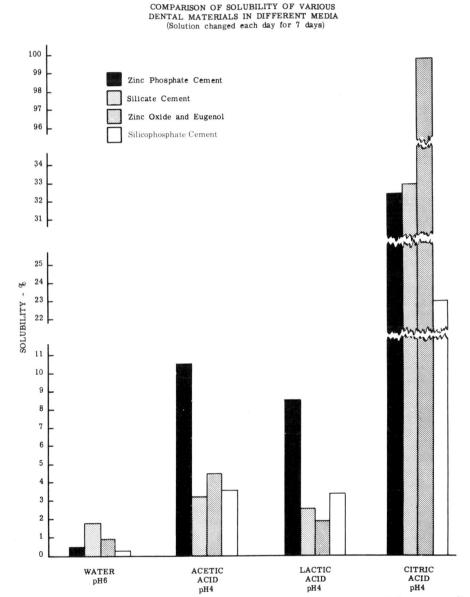

FIGURE 17-2. Solubility of various types of dental cement in different media. Although all show low solubility in distilled water, they are quite easily eroded in other acids that may be present in the oral cavity.

Mixing Technique. The technique for mixing cement is easily learned; nevertheless it does call for watchfulness as to detail in the working of the materials. The principal factor controlling the solubility, as well as the strength, is the powder-liquid ratio. Solubility is directly related to the amount of powder that can be incorporated into the liquid. The really soluble portion of the cement is the crystalline matrix that forms around the original particles of powder. With a greater amount of powder present in the mix, less of this matrix will be formed and the cement will be stronger and less soluble. For any consistency, as much powder as practicable must be incorporated. Obviously, to seat a well-fitting casting, a thin mix and film of cement will be mandatory; still, this consistency must contain a maximal amount of powder. The only way that this can be accomplished is by the use of a cool slab, approximately 60 to 75° F., yet it must not be below the dew point. A warm slab will speed the chemical reaction and the cement will set before enough powder can be incorporated.

The mixing slab should be of heavy glass, clean, and free of scratches. When the powder is placed on the slab, it should be divided into five or six equal parts (Fig. 17-3). The liquid should then be measured and the first portion of powder thoroughly mixed into it. Before the second bit is added, the mass should be spatulated, using a rotary motion, until it is completely homogeneous. A good rule is to mix each increment for approximately 20 seconds, with a total mixing time of $1\frac{1}{2}$ to 2 minutes. The mix should be smooth and free of lumps or clots. The determination of consistency that offers optimal properties becomes a matter of judgment acquired only through experience.

Cementing Procedure. A coating of cement is applied to the inner surfaces of the crown or retainers. After using maximal finger pressure, seating is completed using an orangewood stick or metal instrument and mallet (Fig. 17-4).

After the saliva ejector has been removed, a cotton roll should be folded and placed on the occlusal surface of the prosthesis and the patient should be asked to close in centric. This position is held without lateral or protrusive movement until the cement has set, which will be approximately 3 to 5 minutes. If the luting material is resin cement, any excess must be removed from the embrasures *before* setting takes place and *before* the patient is asked to close and apply pressure.

After the cement has set,* the cotton rolls are removed and the patient is permitted to rinse. Excess cement around the margins of the retainers should now be removed, using scalers or chisels, and explorers. It must be stressed that no cement should be allowed to remain in the gingival crevices or the interproximal areas (Fig. 17-5). Occasionally the cement will be very hard to remove from the area just cervical to the contact. When this cannot be done with dental floss, vigorous lateral excursions by the patient will break the adhesion or locking of such cement fragments. After the oral

---

*Zinc phosphate cement may be considered as "set" when it is unyielding to an instrument, fractures under pressure, and has lost its surface luster.

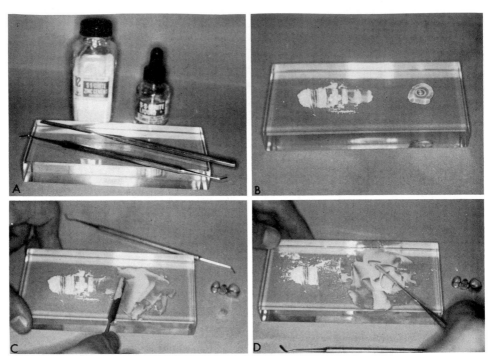

FIGURE 17-3. *Cementing bridge with zinc phosphate cement.*

A, Cement powder, liquid, slab, spatula, and instrument for applying cement.
B, Powder in separate piles, and liquid.
C and *D*, Mixing technique.

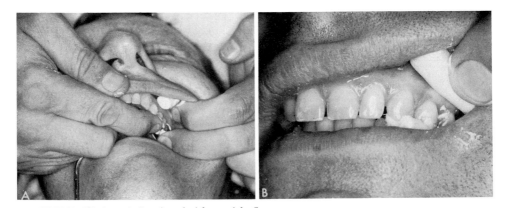

FIGURE 17-4. *A*, Seating bridge with finger pressure.
B, After bridge is tapped to place with a mallet and stick, patient is asked to close on cotton roll.

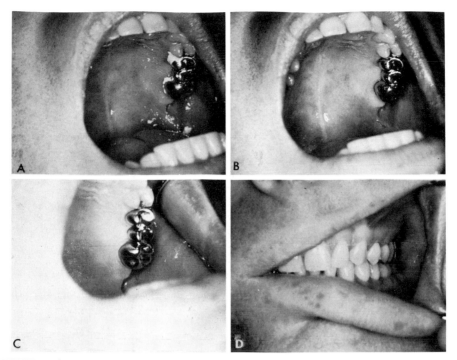

FIGURE 17-5. *A*, Cemented bridge before removing excess.
B, Cemented bridge—cement removed.
C and *D*, Two views of maxillary posterior bridge made six months after cementation. Occlusion and tissue tone are good.

cavity has been freed of debris, the occlusion should be rechecked and any roughened areas repolished.

If the abutment preparations are long and have parallel walls, it may be advantageous to drill a hole, with a No. ½ round bur, through the centers of the occlusal surfaces of the retainers to afford the cement an escape occlusally as well as cervically. After the cement has set and the bridge has been polished, a very small cavity can be prepared at the site of the occlusal perforation and the void can be filled with gold foil.

After cementation, any unfinished margins must be polished lightly with a finishing bur and flour of pumice and No. 600 Carborundum powder, applied with a revolving rubber cup.

It is detrimental for the zinc phosphate cement, exposed at the margins of a cemented restoration, to have immediate or early contact with saliva. For example, the 5-day solubility of a zinc phosphate cement immersed in water 10 minutes after the start of the mix is approximately 10 times greater than solubility of cement that is kept free from moisture for 24 hours prior to contact with water. With this in mind the dentist may wish to coat the margins of the cemented gold restoration with a cavity varnish before dismissing the patient.

ERRORS. The most common causes of trouble in use of zinc phosphate cement can be attributed to the use of liquid that has changed either through exposure to the atmosphere or by contamination or faulty mixing technique.

The probable causes of cement *setting too slowly* are (1) a mix that is too thin (that is, not enough powder has been incorporated); (2) a mix that has been spatulated too long (increased spatulation time increases setting time); or (3) a mix using liquid that has lost water because of inappropriate care.

Mixing on a warm slab, insufficient spatulation time, or adding powder too rapidly will cause cement to *set too fast.*

If more powder than is needed for the mix has been placed on the mixing slab, the surplus must *never* be returned to the bottle, as it may have come into contact with the liquid, and if so it can influence the properties and action of subsequent mixes.

REMEMBER: Liquid is *never* added *to* a mix. Another mix must be made if the ratio of powder to liquid has resulted in a mix too thick for the intended use.

As previously discussed, it is recognized that zinc phosphate cement has inherent shortcomings of solubility and disintegration in oral fluids, and low strength. Furthermore, it is an acidic material that can engender pulp reaction unless ample protection is given to the underlying tooth structure.

Silicophosphate Cement

Silicophosphate cement is a combination of zinc phosphate and silicate cements. Although this type of cement now and then is employed for the cementation of cast restorations, its major use is as a luting agent for the cementation of jacket crowns or porcelain inlays. This preference is based upon esthetics, inasmuch as zinc phosphate cement is opaque whereas silicophosphate cement is somewhat translucent.

In many respects, a silicophosphate cement surpasses zinc phosphate cement.[8] It is a little less soluble in the dilute organic acids present in the oral cavity. The fluoride in the powder increases the resistance of the adjoining enamel to caries if microleakage should occur at the margins. The compressive strength is also at a higher level than that of zinc phosphate cement. Thus, the retentive properties imparted to the restoration by the cement are similar to or an improvement on those of zinc phosphate cement.

Unfortunately the manipulative characteristics are not so good. This type of cement may set faster and does not extrude into quite so thin a film. If a technique can be developed for mixing the cement and placing the restoration so that there will be commensurate working time and a minimal film thickness, the silicophosphate cements are completely satisfactory. To do this, a thinner consistency may be required than would normally be the case when the cement is utilized as a posterior restorative material. It may be mixed in a manner about the same as used for zinc phosphate cement, rather than as used for a silicate cement. The addition of the powder in small increments and a longer period of mixing extend the working time, facilitate manipulation, and provide a more desirable consistency.

Zinc Oxide-Eugenol Cement

Zinc oxide-eugenol cements are being advocated for use in the permanent cementation of fixed restorations.[9] Certainly this type of cement has many qualities that would recommend it for such usage. It is kind to the cut dentin, adapts better to the walls of the prepared cavity than any other cement, and is slightly less soluble in the fluids in the oral cavity.[10] Regrettably it is not strong, having a compressive strength approximately one-fifth that of zinc phosphate cement. Likewise, it has poor resistance to abrasion and attrition. Contrary to popular opinion, the strength cannot be increased significantly by the addition of polystyrene. Only compounds such as ortho-ethoxybenzoic acid will appreciably increase the strength, but solubility increases upon the addition of that chemical.

STRENGTH. The low strength of the cement is of special concern when it is used as a permanent cementing medium. The theory of mechanical retention and the role of the cement in this regard have been discussed. If this theory is correct, then the restoration can loosen only if these small projections fracture. If these small projections do fracture under stress, the mechanical retention of the cement is lost. Logically, the stronger the cement, the more resistant to fracture these tiny projections will be and the greater is the mechanical retention stemming from the cement. Strength is one of the principal properties that must be taken into consideration in selecting a luting agent. The newer zinc oxide-eugenol permanent cements have been formulated with a view to increasing their relatively low strength, which may be done by incorporating various additives.

Several cements have a polymer added to the zinc oxide powder to serve as a reinforcing agent. A more habitual technique is to substitute o-ethoxy benzoic acid (usually referred to as EBA) for a portion of the eugenol. In those products, quartz or alumina also generally are added to increase the strength even more.[11]

The compressive strength of these products approaches that of zinc phosphate cement, and the retentive characteristics are inclined to parallel their strengths, i.e., the higher the strength of the cement, the greater the retention.

The relative ability of certain of these cements to retain the casting, as contrasted to zinc phosphate cement, is illustrated in Figure 17-6. Inlays were cemented into standard one-surface cavity preparations, and the tensile force essential to removal of the castings was measured. With two of the zinc oxide-eugenol cements, the stress exerted to unseat the castings was comparable to that required when the same restorations were cemented with zinc phosphate cement. Other zinc oxide-eugenol cements exhibited less retentive capabilities. It is difficult to predict whether the reduced retention in those cases would result in a loosening of the clinical casting or bridge when subjected to stress. Since this type of cement does comprise an entirely different class of material than zinc phosphate cement, and thereby different criteria for evaluation, there must be long-term clinical observations before they can be adopted unequivocally for all types of cemented restorations.

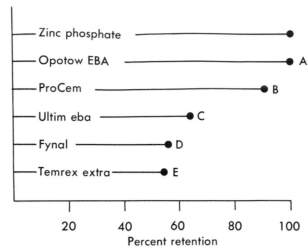

FIGURE 17–6. The tensile strength required to remove one-surface inlays cemented by means of five commercial permanent zinc oxide-eugenol cements is compared to the force required to remove the same inlays cemented with zinc phosphate cement. The mechanical retention provided by two of the products, A and B, is essentially equal to zinc phosphate cement, but considerably less in the case of the other three formulations.

In most instances, the insertion of a cement base when it is indicated and the routine use of a cavity varnish in a deep cavity preparation give sufficient pulp protection from the irritating effects of the zinc phosphate cement. If, by the proper use of bases and varnishes, postoperative sensitivity is not considered questionable, then there is no point in using a zinc oxide-eugenol cement. On the other hand, sensitivity does sometimes occur despite these precautions. Such situations can often be foreseen on the basis of the depth of the cavity, condition and history of the pulp, and past experience. A zinc oxide-eugenol cement is the material of choice in such cases.

Eugenol attacks most dental resins, causing them to soften and craze. Therefore these cements should never be used for the cementation of resin jacket crowns. Any resin facing should be kept from contact with the eugenol by a coating of silicone grease. As some of these formulations are very tenacious, petrolatum or silicone grease should be applied to the adjacent teeth to make easier the removal of excess cement from those surfaces.

The mixing procedure for zinc oxide-eugenol is not so exacting as it is for other types of cement. The mix may be made either on a paper mixing pad or a glass slab. Temperature affects the rate of setting to a degree; cooling the slab will help to retard it.

The EBA type cements have a rather peculiar fluidity. They flow under pressure for a longer period of time than do the zinc phosphate cements and some of them are apt to have a somewhat higher film thickness. The casting should be seated with adequate pressure as soon as possible after mixing the cement and the pressure *maintained* until the cement hardens. Only in this way can a minimal film thickness be obtained and the casting completely seated.

Resin Cement

Resin cements are at present used infrequently. Their composition is very much like the direct acrylic filling resins. Fillers such as quartz may be added to reduce the coefficient of thermal expansion.

The one characteristic in which a resin is superior to other types of cements is its insolubility in oral fluids. Acrylic resins do not adhere to tooth structure; they rely upon mechanical retention, just as other cements. Notwithstanding the minimal solubility, a resin cement should not be relied upon to compensate for the inadequacies of an ill-fitting casting. They do pose some handling problems. Removal of excess cement is more trying, and the time at which the flash is removed is critical.

Another resin cement system has now been introduced in the United States. Such cements, e.g., Durelon,* are referred to as carboxylates.[12] A polyacrylic acid liquid is mixed with a zinc oxide powder. It is claimed that during setting a chemical bond occurs between the cement and the inorganic part of tooth structure. This type of cement will be widely used, but more data on its adhesive properties and further histologic evidence as to its biologic characteristics are needed before it can be suggested for daily use in the cementation of crown and bridge prostheses.

---

*Premier Dental Products Company, Philadelphia, Pa.

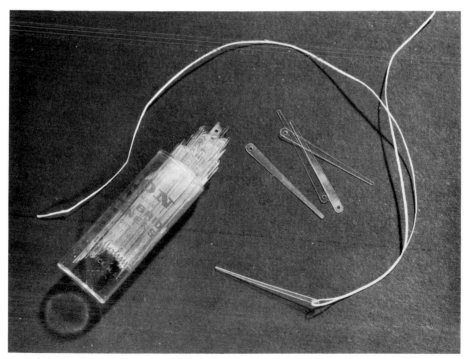

FIGURE 17-7. ZON Dental Bridge Cleaners. Very helpful for pulling dental floss or tape through embrasures of a bridge so floss may be moved from back to front, and also the reverse, between pontics and tissue. This is imperative in keeping surface clean and tissue healthy. (Johnson & Johnson, New Brunswick, N. J.)

POSTOPERATIVE TREATMENT

Whether the cemented unit be a crown or a bridge, an appointment should be scheduled within the 24 to 72 hours following, at which time the occlusion, gingival crevices, tone of the gingival tissue, and mouth hygiene should be checked (Fig. 17-7). The occluding surfaces should be examined closely for premature contacts that may develop on marginal ridges, cusp planes, or in sulci. After using articulating paper, only the shiny portion that does *not* retain a stain should be reduced with a round bur or stone. This reduction then should be feathered into the surrounding surface. The occlusion must be checked again, and the process repeated if indicated.

If within a few days there is complaint of soreness, sensitivity to cold or sweets, or slight sensitivity to heat, the occlusion should be checked again, because as a rule these symptoms show a premature contact or interference. It may be found that the occluding area must be constricted to reduce leverage, torque, or rotation, or that a cusp, marginal ridge, or sulcus must be reduced to prevent trauma in the direction of the long axis.

A few minutes should suffice to make an equilibration. However, the patient should be contacted within 48 hours to ascertain the effectiveness of the treatment. If the symptoms persist, the prosthesis and the abutment teeth should be re-examined.

At future visits crowns and bridges should be viewed with concern at the cervical margins for caries, using sharp explorers or scalers. Radiographs may not disclose marginal lesions.

It appears that the profession now has three types of luting materials, one of which, if used carefully, has established a record for satisfactory performance. With any one, emphasis is still on a dry field for seating, high standards of cavity preparation, and a meticulous fit of the casting.

REFERENCES

1. Lindquist, J. T.: A study of the intra-arch relationships in normal human dentures. Master's thesis, Indiana University School of Dentistry, 1951.
2. Smith, G. P.: The marginal fit of the full cast shoulderless crown. J. Pros. Den., 7:231, March 1957.
3. Norman, R. D., Swartz, M. L., and Phillips, R. W.: Direct pH determinations of setting cements. I. A test method and the effects of storage time and media. J. D. Res., 45:136, 1966.
4. Phillips, R. W.: Cavity varnishes and bases. D. Clin. N. Amer., March 1965, p. 159.
5. Lynn, L. M., and Ludwick, R. W., Jr.: Method to reduce pain during cementation of restorations. J.A.D.A., 53:563, Nov. 1956.
6. Skinner, E. W., and Phillips, R. W.: The Science of Dental Materials. 6th ed. Philadelphia, W. B. Saunders Company, 1967.
7. Norman, R. D., Swartz, M. L., and Phillips, R. W.: Studies on the solubility of certain dental materials. J. D. Res., 36:977, Dec. 1957.
8. Swartz, M. L., Phillips, R. W., Norman, R. D., and Oldham, D. F.: Strength, hardness and abrasion characteristics of dental cements. J.A.D.A., 67:367, 1963.
9. Horn, H. R.: The cementation of crowns and fixed partial dentures. D. Clin. N. Amer., March 1965, pp. 65–81.

10. Phillips, R. W., Swartz, M. L., Norman, R. D., Schnell, R. J., and Niblack, B. F.: Zinc oxide and eugenol cements for permanent cementation. J. Pros. Den., *19*:144, 1968.
11. Civjan, S., and Brauer, G. M.: Physical properties of cements based on zinc oxide, hydrogenated rosin, o-ethoxybenzoic acid, and eugenol. J. D. Res., *43*:281, 1964.
12. Smith, D. C.: A new dental cement. British D. J., *124*:381, Nov. 1968.

Baraban, D. J.: Cementation of fixed bridge prosthesis with zinc oxide-rosin-eugenol cements. J. Pros. Den., *8*:988, Nov.-Dec. 1958.

Ewing, J. E.: Temporary cementation in fixed partial prosthesis. J. Pros. Den., *5*:388, May 1955.

Gerson, I.: Cementation of fixed restorations. J. Pros. Den., *7*:123, Jan. 1957.

Hedges, P. G.: Occlusion as it relates to fixed restorations. J. Pros. Den., *13*:499, May 1963.

Schorr, L., and Clayman, L. H.: Cementing a large fixed bridge. J.A.D.A., *55*:415, Sept. 1957.

Selberg, A.: A full cast crown technique. J. Pros. Den., *7*:102, Jan. 1957.

Simpson, R. L.: Failures in crown and bridge prosthodontics. J.A.D.A., *47*:154, Aug. 1953.

Sullivan, E. J.: Cementation and esthetic problems in crown and bridge procedures. J.A.D.A., *51*:34, July 1955.

chapter 18

PORCELAINS AND PORCELAIN FURNACES

For many years fused porcelain has been recognized as a restorative material that is compatible with oral soft tissues and that has superior esthetic qualities. Even though it is extremely friable and does not produce a mechanically sound restoration under an adverse occlusion, it has enjoyed continuing and growing popularity in the construction of jacket and veneered crowns and bridge pontics. With the advent and use of the aluminous porcelains, strength has been increased, and with the observation of all measures to prevent breakage, the incidence of fracture has been reduced dramatically. However, crowns constructed with aluminous porcelain cores or occluding surfaces are not capable of replacing veneered crowns in severe situations.

THE COMPOSITION OF PORCELAIN

Dental porcelain is formed by mixing and firing minerals, principally feldspar, kaolin, and quartz, plus fluxing substances and pigments.

Feldspar is a double silicate of aluminum and potassium, and at the normal firing temperatures for dental porcelains fuses and acts as a matrix, binding the small, irregularly shaped refractory crystals of kaolin and quartz together. It makes the porcelain vitreous and translucent when fired. Feldspar functions as a flux and surface glaze as well as a matrix.

Kaolin is a hydrated aluminum silicate resulting from the decomposition of feldspathic minerals. The name often is given to any porcelain clay that does not discolor when fired. The greater the quantity of kaolin, the more the opacity of the porcelain is increased.

Quartz imparts stiffness and hardness to the mass during and after firing. It acts as a refractory skeleton for the contracting kaolin and feldspar.

Aluminum oxide (Al_2O_3) may replace silica as a component of dental porcelain. McLean[1] has developed a method for bonding this material chemically as a reinforcing agent with dental porcelain or pigmented glasses. While it has a strong opacifying effect, it measurably strengthens the porcelain.

374

Fluxes are added to increase fluidity of the mixture and to absorb or remove certain objectionable impurities. Sodium and potassium carbonates, borax, glass, and occasionally lead oxide, are used. The fusing point of a porcelain may be varied by the quantity of flux incorporated.

The *pigments* used to color porcelain may be oxides of tin, nickel, cobalt, titanium, chromium, iron, or gold, or metallic gold and platinum. Fluorescence, as well as shade, may be a product of the pigmenting materials.

PORCELAIN REACTIONS TO FIRING

It is usual for dental porcelains to have been fired once or more during their manufacture. This is known as "fritting," and by this process chemical reactions can be controlled, maturing temperatures can be lowered, and shrinkage will be lessened.

During the firing cycle in the construction of a crown all porcelains must go through several phases of physical changes. First is the biscuit stage, in which very little shrinkage has occurred; the mass is an opaque white with no color sheen, and it is easily contaminated by oil from the fingers or by other debris that may penetrate the excessively porous surface. As a rule, this stage is ignored in the laboratory. The porcelain is brought to a low maturity, erroneously referred to as a "high biscuit." Next is maturity, or vitrification, which may be divided into low, medium, and high phases. Third is a state of glaze. Fourth is coalescence, or the formation of an overglazed and rounded form.

Maturity will be evident when true color and translucence can be seen, when shrinkage has occurred, and when there is a slight sheen on the surface of the porcelain. The degree of sheen and translucence will depend on the extent of maturity.

The state of glaze brings a light-reflecting luster to the surface. This stage may also be divided into low, medium, and high. Low is just over the border from maturity and might be esthetically desirable in some mouths. Occasionally a low-glaze porcelain can be vulnerable to water sorption, which from a hygienic standpoint would be undesirable.[2] A medium glaze will be suitable in the majority of mouths. A high glaze is to be avoided, because it is very close to coalescence and results in an abnormal sheen, rounded corners, and loss of detail.

Porcelains may be divided into low-fusing and high-fusing. Low-fusing porcelain is one that fuses under 1945°F., or the melting point of pure gold; high-fusing porcelain is one that fuses above 1945° F. The available commercial subdivisions are low (1600 to 2000° F.), medium (2000 to 2300° F.), and high (above 2300° F.). A high-fusing porcelain surpasses one in the low-fusing range in that the fusing temperature is not so critical, and staining, glazing, and repairing are less complicated, especially if done after the form, contact, and occlusion have been established. However, the many merits of some low-fusing porcelains should not be ignored.

Low-fusing, medium-fusing, and high-fusing dental porcelains are made for both air and vacuum firing. The more recent categories include those manufactured for the purpose of being bonded to metal structures and the aluminous porcelains. The bonding porcelains also come in low-firing and medium-firing ranges and for both atmosphere and vacuum firing, while the aluminous porcelains have a firing range below 2050° F.

Air-fired Porcelain

Air-fired porcelain has excellent physical properties, which are clinically comparable to those of vacuum-fired porcelain. Porcelain fired in atmosphere does have many air spaces between the particles to interfere with, or "scatter," light transmission.[3] Entrapped air or gas within a jacket or veneer creates or increases opacity.

Vacuum-fired Porcelain

Vacuum-fired porcelain has some characteristics that differ from those of air-fired porcelain. It has certain claimed superiorities, some justified and some academic. There is a general increase in the strength of the porcelain, which probably is more significant in jacket crowns than bonded veneers.

The porcelain will have greater translucence. Almost without exception, vacuum-fired porcelains have an opaque shade to match each body shade, and this close match in color reduces variation in shade when the thickness of the veneer varies from area to area.[4]

When building a vacuum-fired jacket crown, it is necessary to cover the platinum matrix with an opaque. This is an integral part of the crown, and, as with the veneer, should duplicate or harmonize with the plotted shade pattern.

It is easier to obtain a smooth, nonpitted surface on the glazed porcelain. There will be more uniformity in color when several operators are using the same porcelain. Porcelain for vacuum firing can have a finer and graded particle size, thereby increasing the wet strength of the material and making it less difficult to carve a built-up mass.

Shade is markedly affected by vacuum firing, and formulas must be worked out by each practitioner through experimentation. The lessened number of air spaces decreases the internal reflective surfaces. Thus, with opacity reduced and density increased, it becomes impossible to reproduce precisely the shades made with air firing.

THE FURNACE

The furnace has three important parts: the control system, the indicating system, and the heat chamber. The control system, or transformer, regulates the amount of electrical energy passing through the heating element, which in turn determines the amount of heat generated in the muffle. There can be fluctuations due to the amount of current usage on the lines. These are often seasonal, or they may vary, depending on the time of day, which reduces the effectiveness and accuracy of automatic furnaces.

The pyrometer is a warning system in that it indicates the temperature within the muffle. It does *not* decide when the work is completed. The degree or extent of firing must be judged visually by reflected light, not by the temperature indicated by the pyrometer. Owing to its normal location close to or on top of the muffle, fluctuation in the temperature of the pyrometer itself leads to erratic readings. Pyrometers can be adjusted easily, and all should be checked routinely. If adjustment cannot be made to within 50 degrees of accuracy at 2300° F., then the instrument should be returned to the factory for examination.

In the muffle, heating is by convection and radiation. In vacuum firing, heating is predominantly by radiation. Heating elements may be exposed or surrounded by refractory substances. Each furnace muffle develops its own spot or area of highest heat, and that spot can be at any place in the interior of the muffle. The major factors for premature burnout of muffles are (1) too-rapid heating for the first 1000° F. (heating should be 50° F. per minute); (2) too-rapid or forced cooling of the muffle; or (3) firing over 2500° F. (just one such instance can reduce by one-half the potential life of the muffle). A new muffle, or one that has been repaired, should be degassed at 2450° F. from 2 to 4 minutes before the insertion of any porcelain ware.

Inside the muffle will be seen a protruding thermocouple, the end of which must be welded. A thermocouple is a combination of two dissimilar

FIGURE 18-1. Jelenko vacuum furnace with vertical muffle. Maximal temperature 2500° F.

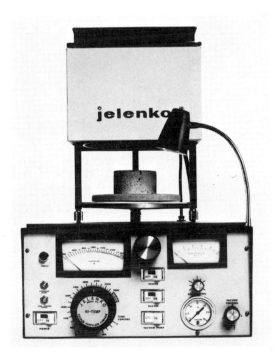

wires that generates a current as the welded end is heated. This current is then translated into temperature on the pyrometer. Various combinations of metals are used, depending on the temperature to which they are to be subjected. For high-fusing porcelain work, the wires are pure platinum and alloys of platinum; for low-temperature furnaces, the wires are base metal alloys. For the thermocouple to register the heat within the muffle precisely, it must be parallel to the roof. When checking temperature for accuracy, gold foil or a Tempil* pellet should be placed directly under the tip of the

*Tempil Corp., New York, N. Y.

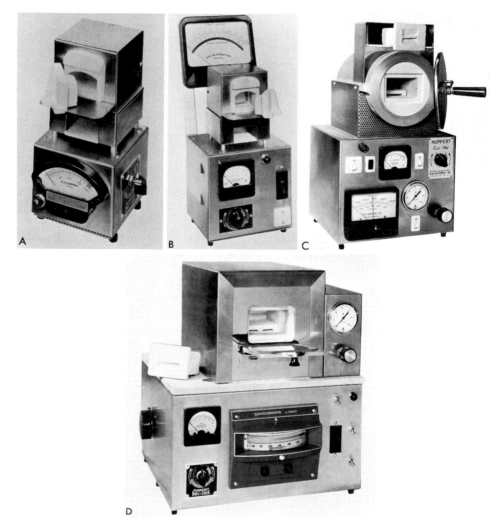

FIGURE 18–2.   *Huppert furnaces.*

A, Glazing furnace, maximal temperature 2000° F.
B, Air-firing furnace, maximal temperature 2500° F.
C, Vacuum furnace, bench model, maximal temperature 2560° F.
D, Vacuum furnace, maximal temperature 2500° F. Floor model is almost identical.

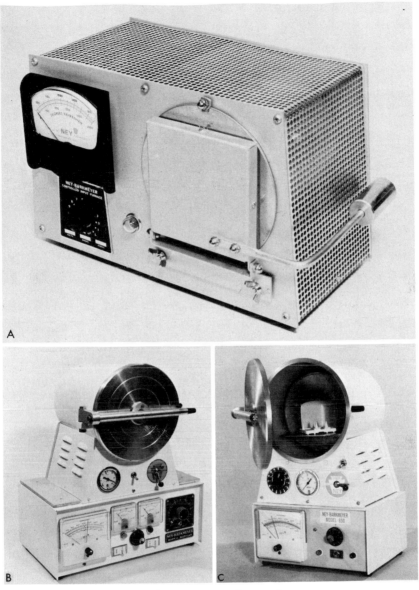

FIGURE 18-3. *Ney-Barkmeyer furnaces.*

A, Glazing, staining, and burnout unit. Maximal temperature 2000° F. Separate muffle should be used for burning out casting rings, because gas will impregnate muffle walls and may discolor porcelain as it fuses.

B and *C*, Vacuum furnaces. Maximal temperature 2500° F.

thermocouple. The pyrometer reading should always be correct for the highest temperature at which the furnacc will be used.

Furnaces for vacuum firing are considerably more complex in design than those for air firing. The furnaces available vary in the degree of automation and also in the orientation of the muffle. Furnaces that have vertical muffles, such as the one manufactured by Jelenko (Fig. 18-1),

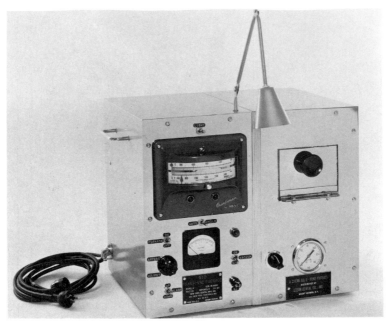

Figure 18–4. Stern Transi-Vac automatic porcelain furnace. Maximal temperature 2500° F.

require lower firing temperatures than those with horizontal muffles, irrespective of whether they are being used for air or vacuum firing.

There are porcelain furnaces (Figs. 18-2, 18-3, and 18-4) manufactured by other firms, all achieving similar results. There are differences in details. The ease with which muffles can be changed and pyrometers regulated, and the way the instrument will fit into or onto the available space should be considered when purchasing a furnace. The authors have found that a small, inexpensive furnace for glazing and staining facings is indispensable to any office, and well worth having, even if a larger vacuum furnace with a maximal temperature range is at hand.

REFERENCES

1. McLean, J. W., and Hughes, T. H.: The reinforcement of dental porcelain with ceramic oxides. British D. J., *119*:251, Sept. 21, 1965.
2. Pettrow, J. N.: Practical factors in building and firing characteristics of dental porcelain. J. Pros. Den., *11*:334, March-April 1961.
3. Vines, R. F., and Semmelman, J. O.: Densification of dental porcelain. J. D. Res., *36*:950, Dec. 1957.
4. Mumford, G.: Personal communication.

Hodson, J. T.: Preliminary study of dental porcelains. J. South. California D. A. *26*:334, Sept. 1958.
Hodson, J. T.: Some physical properties of three dental porcelains. J. Pros. Den., *9*:325, March-April 1959.

chapter 19

ESTHETIC CRITERIA IN A PORCELAIN RESTORATION

Three components of any porcelain restoration – form, surface characteristics, and color – are complementary to one another in achieving an admirable esthetic result. Their importance to the success and acceptance of a crown or veneer lies approximately in the order stated.[1]

PERIPHERAL FORM

A faithful duplication of the form of the patient's natural dentition generally leads to the most pleasing end result. Although occasionally an increase or diminution in over-all size of the tooth is mandatory, the basic curves and angles present in the outline form should remain the same. The restoration should be viewed from one angle and the silhouette made to conform. The direction is then changed and the process repeated. This is done from the right side, front, left side, lingual, and incisal; if each stage is performed capably, the ultimate contour will be correct. It is almost impossible to arrive at this ideal form if the crown is shaped in a haphazard manner.

The working cast must record in detail the surfaces of the adjacent teeth, particularly in the embrasures, with as little as possible of the cast representing the gingival tissue being trimmed away for access. Areas that must receive concentrated consideration are the mesial and distal incisal angles, the concavities and convexities at the labial line angles in the gingival third of the crown, and the thickness of the incisal edge labiolingually.

CAUSES AND EFFECTS OF GROSS DIMENSIONS

Development of satisfying form in a veneered crown is dependent absolutely on sufficient reduction of tooth structure and the formation of a metal framework without excessive bulk in either the cervical collar or the incisal third. A great many veneered units have inordinate mesiodistal width in the cervical half because of shoulders that are too narrow, or that were not extended far enough into the proximal embrasures, or because a chamfer was substituted for the shoulder. The same situation may ensue, even though the tooth was correctly prepared, if the metal framework was made or left too thick in the labial half.

Crowns often have an exaggerated labial or buccal convexity incisocervically in the cervical half because of too little reduction of the tooth and too much metal. Incisal edges will be too thick labiolingually for the same reasons. Heavy incisal edges are especially noticeable in mandibular incisors, and from some angles in the uppers too, and they should be avoided for esthetic reasons, even if function is not disturbed. All these abnormalities detract seriously from appearance.[2]

It may be out of the question to make a shoulder of desirable width on a small tooth. To compensate, the metal framework for a veneered crown can be made quite thin on the labial half, dispensing with the labial collar, the porcelain veneer to be built against the tooth itself in the manner of a porcelain jacket crown. This technique is also a good one to employ when the gingival crevice is shallow or when recession makes it impracticable to extend the preparation apically to meet the gingival tissue.

It should be remembered and emphasized that almost all teeth have flat or concave triangular areas at the cementoenamel junction on the proximal surfaces, with the apex of the triangle pointing toward and just under the contact. When a restoration is built that adds to the tooth contour in these proximal portions, the gingival tissue is displaced, probably both buccally and lingually, is abnormally stimulated during incising and mastication, and frequently reacts adversely.

The visual effect of overcontoured crowns is one of crowding, of a mass of material, and an accentuation of the darkness sometimes associated with embrasures. Overcontouring crowns on the labial surfaces in the cervical half or third makes the teeth appear too prominent, overprotects gingival tissue, and gives an appearance of grossness. This oddity in form does not change the contour of the lip while it is in repose, but it creates a situation that is very noticeable when the patient is laughing or speaking.

SURFACE CHARACTERISTICS

A tooth smoother than normal will give an impression of larger size, and the converse is also true. A glassy porcelain surface is always incompatible with enamel. Overprominent, exaggerated, and unnatural ridges and grooves on the labial surface of a veneered crown, doubtless associated with the forms of denture teeth and facings, add nothing to the beauty of a restoration and are seldom found on a human tooth.

Copying the heights of contour and existing irregularities on the surfaces of adjacent or corresponding teeth is recommended, although some latitude exists. Heights of contour are those areas from which a maximal amount of light is reflected. Vertical highlights suggest greater length, horizontal highlights give an illusion of width. Changes in contour and the resulting highlights can be used to alter the apparent long-axis inclination of a tooth. For example, a vertical highlight running from near the mesioincisal angle of an incisor toward the distogingival angle will suggest that the tooth has a mesial tilt.[3]

Many times it is obligatory to contour wax, resin, or the biscuited restoration in the patient's mouth, examining the moistened surface and comparing it with the adjacent teeth. This procedure is most significant when a single crown is to be placed among natural teeth. When a pair of central incisors or six anterior teeth in one arch are being restored, the dentist's knowledge of natural tooth morphology becomes of paramount importance.[4]

COLOR AND LIGHT

To make a veneer simulate the appearance characteristics, texture, and color of a tooth can be difficult, and matching natural teeth may be an impossibility. This stems from the fact that teeth are composed of a layer of enamel, usually translucent, which overlies a core of dentin, relatively opaque. A certain amount of light is reflected from the enamel surface, and the remainder either passes completely through, as in the area of the incisal edge of some teeth, or passes through to the dentinoenamel junction, where it is reflected back through the enamel. The light reflected from the outer tooth surface undergoes no change, but that passing into the tooth emerges, having acquired the color attributes of the enamel and dentin.

Before these effects can be described and fully understood, the components of the visual sensation from a colored object must be explained. These are:

hue, that quality of sensation through which an observer is aware that one color is green and another red;

brightness, represented at its extremes by white and black, with gray as an intermediate, and indicative of the amount of light reflected from a matte-colored surface; and

saturation, that property that makes one sample of a pair of the same hue appear more intense or pure.

Since enamel is generally translucent, much of the light passes through it and is lost in the darkness of the oral cavity. Thus the incisal edges of many teeth lack brightness and will be gray in color. Toward the gingival one-third, the enamel becomes thinner and light is reflected from the basically yellow dentin core. Here the hue changes to yellow and becomes progressively more saturated. Directly at the gingival marginal area, some light is transmitted to the tooth through the red and translucent gingival tissues. This area then has a reddish hue superimposed on the yellow.

Psychological Primary Colors

The eye resolves all colors into a set of psychological primary colors: red, yellow, green, blue, black, and white. The basic color of the tooth being yellow, it can deviate in only one of three ways:

(a) in hue, by being a reddish yellow (orange) or a greenish yellow; (b) in brightness, either reflecting more or less light than a median gray; (c) in saturation, either by being a stronger or weaker yellow.

One other factor or effect is known as contrast enhancement. When a light and a dark color are juxtaposed (i.e., gingiva and tooth), each appears respectively lighter and darker than it would separately. When yellow and gray are approximated, the gray tends to take on the complementary hue to yellow (i.e., blue), so that in a strongly yellow tooth the incisal edge frequently appears blue gray. Red next to yellow often seems to make the red appear bluish red and the yellow a greenish yellow.

The fact that color has three basic attributes is of consequence in blending porcelain powders. For instance, if a yellow shade is correct in hue but is too saturated and needs dilution, then it must be diluted with a gray of similar brilliance rather than with a bright white modifying color.

Using a rating scale of 0 to 100 (0 being black and 100 white), the body colors of the New Hue shade guide vary in brightness from a maximum of 72 for shade 61 down to a minimum of 56.5 for a shade 87. The white modifier for Ceramco air-fired porcelain rates at 71 and would be suitable to modify the saturation of shade 61. However, for the other shades a mixture of the Ceramco white modifier with gray modifier, which has a brightness of 39, would be required.

If the nearest shade of porcelain powder to match a natural tooth is too orange (because it contains too much red), then the hue can be changed by the addition of a yellow-green porcelain of slightly greater brightness, since the green, in canceling out the effect of the red, forms a gray color. To change the saturation of a given specimen of porcelain, a modifier of the same hue and brightness but more intense or saturated in hue should be added.

These examples of the modification of hue, brightness, and saturation are indicative of the ways in which the color of a porcelain can be effected.

Additive and Subtractive Primary Colors

Two other sets of primary colors affect color matching. The first, or additive group, consists of red, green, and blue. If lights of these hues are mixed and the brightness and saturation are right, a white light will be reproduced, the combinations of red and green giving yellow, and so on.

The second group, or subtractive primaries, are those that affect the admixture of pigments. In this case the pigment absorbs all the component colors in white light except one, which is reflected. These colors are yellow, magenta, and cyan (bluish green). When all these colors are mixed, all light is absorbed and black results.

As light falls on a natural tooth, yellow is transmitted to the middle third of the tooth from the gingival and gray is transmitted from the incisal. The two colors mix by the additive system and form the gradation found in this area. When this tooth is reproduced in porcelain by placing a tapered layer of gray over a yellow core of porcelain, the light reflected from the middle third area will be formed by the system of subtraction. As a rule, gray porcelain contains slight amounts of other colors, such as yellow or blue, and these will tend to give a color lacking clarity. The addition of red hues, such as are found in cervical blend stains, will counteract this.

Matching Natural Tooth Shades

Since the optical properties of dentin, enamel, and fused porcelain are dissimilar, it is in the main only by chance that an exact shade match is made. The aim is to select and reproduce a shade that *blends* with the natural teeth.

Blending must be by eye and by instinct. No preblended shades match manufactured shade guides exactly, and it is difficult to match a natural tooth with the manufactured shade guides. The use of a denture tooth shade guide for veneered crowns predicates two errors in the color selection. It is recommended, therefore, that for veneered crowns a personal shade guide be made by using small castings of the metal and applying the appropriate porcelain to build a tooth-shaped unit (Fig. 19-1). For a jacket crown shade guide, tooth-shaped buttons of each powder and of some combinations should be fired.

The superior results attainable make this extra effort well worth while.

Adjuncts to Shade Selection

When the shade is to be selected, the patient should be seated with the head erect and at the operator's eye level. The operator should be able to

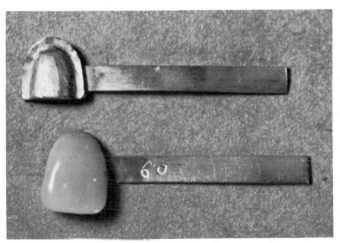

FIGURE 19-1. Suggested shade guide specimen for bonded porcelain veneer crowns.

stand between the patient and the light source, which preferably is a window with a northern exposure. A slightly overcast sky is best. A bright sky has light with a larger blue component, and early morning and late afternoon sunlight has a larger yellow component. The former would tend to enhance green color in the tooth, the latter yellow.

The room should have neutral gray walls or at least not be painted with brilliant colors.

Color Selection

The shade pattern for any crown should be worked out and recorded before the preparation is started. Tonal fatigue will start approximately 6 minutes after the operation begins on the tooth; after looking at an object closely for only a few minutes, it is no longer possible to differentiate color areas and variations accurately. Lipstick must be removed. When choosing the gingival color, the lips of the patient should be raised and the incisal covered. In selecting the incisal shade, the patient's lips should be in speaking position to give a more specific concept of the incisal shade and to eliminate any influence from the gingival third of the tooth. Then the selections must be verified with the entire tooth exposed.

The tooth and shade guide specimens must be positioned so that the minimum of light is reflected from the contours of the surfaces, and then observed quickly for match. If reflectance is a problem or if there are a number of different hues in the tooth, it is helpful to half-close the eyes and move away from the patient to gain an impression of the general qualities of the match.

Color Distribution Chart

Color selections and distribution should be charted after scrutinizing the tooth from frontal, profile, and standing positions, and with different sources or angles of light and environment. This will establish a reliable picture of the existing conditions.[5] To select the number from the series in a shade guide that is the closest match to the tooth will not give sufficient information. It is essential that the distribution of the incisal and gingival shades and their overlapping combinations be designated on the color chart or prescription as they are seen on the tooth and the approximating and corresponding teeth.

The color distribution chart of the labial surface of the tooth, drawn to exact anatomic form should be divided into thirds, incisocervically and mesiodistally (Fig. 19-2). This will assist in appraising and locating the irregular outline where the gingival color overlaps the mesial and distal surfaces and blends with the incisal shade, areas of incisal translucence, and also such characteristics as calcified areas, check lines, or stains. The chart should list

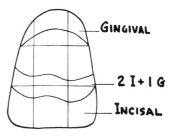

FIGURE 19–2.   Color distribution chart.

or indicate everything seen on the tooth that must be included in the restoration to have an esthetic and harmonious result.

It is desirable to have duplicate shade guides, and if a laboratory is being employed to construct the jacket, to send with the order a copy of the color distribution chart and the specimens used in matching the tooth.[6, 7, 8]

Control of Shade

In the construction of a porcelain veneered crown, several factors combine to control the ultimate shade. The first is the color of the metal; the second, the opaque color; and the third, the color and translucence of the body and incisal porcelain.

If the tooth preparation and the metal frame have been correctly contoured, there will be enough room for an opaque layer that will obliterate the metal color. If space is at a premium, then some sacrifice in thickness of body porcelain and intensity of body color, rather than opaque, is necessary. Otherwise, in any combination the resulting crown would be gray in appearance.

To some extent the opaque color shows through the body color and influences the shade. When a crown is made with a variable thickness of body porcelain, the opaque shade must match the body shade exactly or there will be a variation in shade from area to area. The limited number of opaque colors in Ceramco air-fired porcelain causes some difficulties in this regard, and these colors frequently must be modified. It is somewhat easier to obtain consistent results with the vacuum-fired porcelains, which have a separate opaque shade matched to each body shade.

Of course, the fact that the opaque does affect the color of the veneer can be used to advantage when grayness of the incisal (or apparent translucence) must be increased or when yellowness in the cervical one-third must be enhanced. Modifiers can be added to the opaque to achieve these effects.

Staining

When single crowns or a number of anterior crowns on one side of the arch are being made, staining may be mandatory to attain a degree of blending with the natural teeth. With a knowledge of available modifiers and stains, an accurate prescription for the color can be made and recorded on a diagram of the tooth. The authors often have been forced, especially in veneer construction, to modify body and incisal porcelain colors and to resort to surface staining in order to realize the maximal esthetic result.

Steele's stains, when fused to Ceramco porcelain, have a low-fusing temperature of approximately 1720 to 1740° F.

REFERENCES

1. Johnston, J. F., Mumford, G., and Dykema, R. W.: Porcelain Veneers Bonded to Metal Castings. Practical Dental Monographs. Chicago, Year Book Medical Publishers, Inc., March 1963.
2. Johnston, J. F.: Porcelain veneers bonded to precious metal castings. J. Canad. D. A., 26:657, 1960.
3. Mumford, G.: Recent Studies in Porcelain and Porcelain Jacket Crown Construction. Paper read before the Partial Prosthodontics Section, American Dental Association meeting, Philadelphia, Oct. 1961.
4. Shelby, D. S.: Practical considerations and design of porcelain fused to metal. J. Pros. Den., 12:542, May-June 1962.
5. Theofilis, B. G.: The porcelain jacket crown. Senior thesis, Indiana University School of Dentistry, June 1955.
6. Jones, R. J.: Personal communication.
7. Dunton, H.: Personal communication.
8. Moskey, M. S.: Personal communication.

Clark, E. B.: The color problem in dentistry. D. Digest, 37:499; 571; 646; 732; 815; 1931.
Committee on Colorimetry, Optical Society of America: The Science of Color. New York, Thomas Y. Crowell Company, 1953.
House, M. M., and Loop, J. L.: Form and Color Harmony in the Dental Art. Copyright 1939 by M. M. House.

chapter 20

THE VENEERED GOLD CROWN: INDICATIONS, CONTRAINDICATIONS, AND PREPARATION OF TEETH

A veneered gold crown is a full cast crown having the labial or buccal surface, and portions of the proximal surfaces, faced with fused porcelain or resin (Fig. 20-1). Many times a part, and sometimes all, of the occlusal surface will be veneered when porcelain (not resin) is a component. The resistance of a veneered crown to the forces of occlusion compares favorably with the full veneer gold crown. It may be used as a single-unit restoration, as a bridge retainer, or on abutments supporting or retaining removable partial dentures. In its capacity to blend satisfactorily with or duplicate consistently the shade variations of natural teeth, a veneered gold crown is inferior only in a minor degree to the jacket crown.

To achieve this harmony and to maintain a healthy gingiva, it must be kept within the confines of the form, contour, and dimensions of the original tooth. There are exceptions when the malposition of a tooth, or the excessive width or narrowing of an edentulous space, cannot be improved by orthodontic intervention. However, the effect of altered contour on the health of the gingival tissues and the possibility of damage to the supporting structures by increased forces, due to changes in occlusal form or by an increase in incisal width or thickness, must be carefully appraised.[1]

The major items of concern associated with the construction of veneered crowns and bridges are

(1) selection of shade pattern before preparation is started;
(2) tooth preparation;
(3) making castings that have fit, smoothness, minimal porosity, and resistance to deformation, and that reproduce or continue the narrow bands of natural contour in the cervical area;

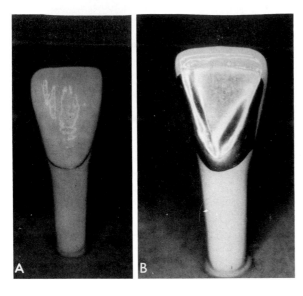

FIGURE 20-1. *A*, Labial view of porcelain veneered gold crown. *B*, Lingual view.

(4) building crowns to normal or agreeable tooth form;
(5) matching human tooth shades;
(6) assembly of units;
(7) durability; and
(8) maintenance or repair.

The extension of the veneer will be governed by

(1) the esthetic standards set for the individual case;
(2) whether porcelain or resin is to be used for the veneer;
(3) the relationship of the tooth to be restored with the adjacent teeth;
(4) occlusion; and
(5) the amount that the tooth can be reduced.

INDICATIONS

The objective of any operative procedure on a tooth is, essentially, the conservation of tooth structure.[2] If this concept is accepted, the veneered gold crown cannot be considered a conservative restoration, since with it occur[3, 4] maximal tooth reduction and extensive contact with gingival tissue. Nevertheless, it is indicated on any tooth when a full crown is justified from a restorative or preventive standpoint, when it can be made to correspond to its environment or its application will enhance esthetic properties, when there must be maximal retention and it can be contrived, and when function will be assured.[5, 6]

The veneered gold crown may be used on any vital tooth if, after the cervical shoulder has been prepared, there is sufficient coronal dentin to resist fracture, or if the remaining tooth structure can be buttressed and rebuilt to prepared form with a cast pin-retained core or with a pin-retained and supported amalgam. It also can be used on a pulpless tooth[7] if a post can be placed in the root canal to support a cast core, or if the tooth can be rebuilt otherwise to prepared form. It may be the restoration of choice when a jacket crown might be broken or abraded in a short time owing to the occlusion, or when the length or shape of the tooth to be restored is such that only a well-fitting metal restoration will have prolonged retention.

CONTRAINDICATIONS

The veneered gold crown is contraindicated on a tooth with a pulp of a size that makes it impossible to prepare the tooth correctly, and on a tooth with a very short clinical crown that will have insufficient retention and stability after it has been reduced to allow space for metal and porcelain or resin.[8]

PREPARATION OF THE TOOTH

Preparation of a tooth can be facilitated and problems can be diminished by

(1) close study of the radiographs and casts and an evaluation of potentialities;
(2) remembering that exposed labial and proximal contours may decrease very rapidly in diameter just inside the gingival crevice;
(3) realizing that insulted gingival and periodontal tissues do not always repair perfectly; and
(4) recognition of the form and depth of the reduction called for in the prepared tooth crown to secure retention and permit reproduction of normal tooth contour and bulk of material for shading.

A certain bulk, as much or more than is wanted for a jacket crown, is necessary to produce the requisite color and translucence in a porcelain veneer or the desired shade in a resin veneer. The preparation will be a combination of the jacket crown and the full veneer gold crown preparations if compatible form and color and a minimal display of gold are to ensue.[9, 10, 11]

To ascertain the receptivity of a given tooth to a preparation for a veneered crown, the following factors must be assessed:

(1) length of clinical crown;
(2) labiolingual bulk in the incisal one-third of an anterior tooth;
(3) presence or lack of a well-defined cingulum on an anterior tooth;
(4) convexity of the cervical enamel fold;
(5) width of the pulp horns in relation to mesiodistal width of the neck of the tooth;

   (6) relation of the pulp to the incisal edge or occlusal surface of the tooth;
   (7) assumed relation of the pulp to the labial or buccal surface;
   (8) position of contact areas (labially or lingually to normal position);
   (9) depth of gingival crevice;
  (10) height of curves of gingival crevice on mesial and distal surfaces; and
  (11) direction of dictated path of insertion.

Factors 1, 2, 3, and 11 must be considered together if the tooth is to be used for a bridge abutment because the preparation must resist torque and leverage. Incisocervically or occlusocervically the finished preparation should be more than half the length of the seated restoration and also should have metal encircling the cingulum or linguocervical without a shoulder encircling the tooth. On a tooth that is thin in the incisal half, or short, unless there is contrived augmented retention, the stump generally will be incapable of resisting dislodging forces because of the reduction needed for the framework and porcelain on the incisal or on the buccal cusp.

Criteria to Guide Reduction of Tooth

The mesiodistal measurement of the pulp horns may make the tooth impractical for a veneered crown preparation, or impossible if the neck is constricted. The tooth must be reduced enough for the crown to have shade and bulk without altering embrasure form, which may not be feasible if there has been no pulp recession. If such reduction is out of the question, a veneered crown should not be used.

In order for a veneered crown to be well constructed and to meet the best esthetic standards, there must be a clearance of 2.0 mm. along the incisal edge of an anterior tooth or the buccal half of the occlusal surface of a posterior. This requirement eliminates some teeth that have pulp chambers irregular in contour and pulp horns extending quite far incisally or occlusally.

The proximity of the pulp to the labial or buccal surface cannot be demonstrated radiographically, but must be estimated. The probability that the pulp is too close to that surface for proper depth in the preparation of this area (usually 1.4 mm.) should be weighed, because exposures of the pulp in these areas are not uncommon. While endodontics is a valuable adjunct to restorative dentistry, every effort should be made to avoid it. The greatest possibilities for maximal service are still to be found with the use of vital teeth.

The more shallow the gingival crevice and the higher, larger, and more convex incisally or occlusally the proximal curves of the cervical line, the more difficult it is to make the shoulder and cervical margin conform to the curves and to prepare a tooth for a veneered crown with the expectation for satisfactory long-range appearance. There is an alarming tendency, when using an ultra-speed handpiece, to make a flat labiolingual seat on a veneer preparation at the immediate expense of the entire cervical enamel fold and of the proximal gingival and supporting tissue, with a heightened prospect of gingival tissue irritation and recession.

Protracted observation of patients for whom preparations have been extended cervically to meet or to go beyond the periodontal attachment has convinced the authors that this is bad practice, whether it be done labially, lingually, or proximally. Regardless of the depth of the crevice or the area, 1.0 mm. under the gingival crest is ample for any preparation, and 0.5 mm. will suffice for most. The extension of the preparation apically should not exceed one-half the depth of the crevice, especially if it is shallow.

Casts should be analyzed with a surveying instrument to determine a path of insertion most acceptable by all abutments and closest to meeting the criteria just set forth.

Increasing Retention.   When there is no exposed convex cingulum, or when it is not expedient to expose it, a finishing line must be formed in the sulcus, and stability and retention obtained by two pinholes in the lingual (or cervical) third of the surface, parallel to the path of insertion and 1.5 mm. deep. If the stump is very short because of form or original measurement, these two pinholes, plus two others much closer to the incisal edge, will retain the casting following cementation. A No. 701 bur can be used for the holes whenever tooth and pulp size permit. If the dentin lateral to the pulp is narrow, smaller holes may be made with a drill.

Retention on a short posterior tooth can be increased by proximal and lingual grooves or by proximal boxes with posts going into the cervical seats. Occlusal posts may be extended into cusp areas, preferably the lingual because of less reduction there.

Using Accelerated Speeds

There are numerous combinations of instruments, used in variable sequences, with which a diligent operator can use accelerated speeds to prepare teeth to receive veneered gold crowns. When using ultra-high speeds it is good judgment for the novice or the operator who makes such preparations infrequently to reduce contacting surfaces with a disk. In this way there is less chance of scarring an approximating tooth. The opening made with a disk should be wide enough so that in cutting the tooth circumferentially with a carbide bur it can pass freely through the opening.

The shade should be selected and a shading pattern made before preparation is begun.

Sequence of Steps in Preparation of Maxillary Central Incisor.   Very often the authors will use the set of instruments shown in Figure 20-2, and will follow this routine:

(1) Incisal reduction is made with a 169L carbide bur. A labiolingual groove is cut across the incisal edge to the depth wanted. Cutting is continued mesially and distally, and the tooth is shortened one-half at a time.

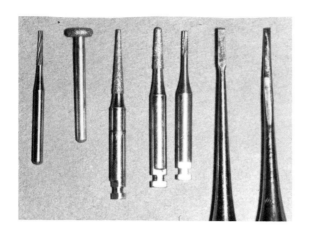

FIGURE 20-2.   Left to right: 169L-FG carbide bur (Densco); 110P-FG wheel diamond (Starlite); ¼D-L latch tapered diamond stone (Densco); 1D-T latch tapered diamond stone (Densco); 556 latch carbide bur (S.S.W.); #10 straight Tarno chisel (S.S.W.); #22-23 Wedelstaedt chisel.

(2) Proximal reduction is done with a 169L bur, with no attempt to form a shoulder at this time.

(3) Labial reduction is accomplished with a 169L bur. A groove is made in the labial surface to the depth desired (to be done in two planes, incisal half and cervical half), and first the mesial, then the distal is prepared. (See Figure 20-6 *B, C, D,* and *E.*)

(4) An outline of the shoulder is made on the labial and proximals at the gingival crest with a 169L bur. The mesial terminus of the outline must go farther lingually so that the finished shoulder will let the line of junction between frame and veneer be covered by the approximating tooth or pontic.

Linguoproximal terminations of the shoulder will be controlled by the width of the embrasures, presence or absence of an interdental papilla, and the position of the tooth (i.e., labioversion, torsoversion, and so forth). To conceal the metal framework effectively, the terminal point should be beneath or to the lingual of the center of the contact area. (See Figure 20-3.)

(5) Using a 169L bur or tapered diamond stone, the axial wall of the lingual surface (cingulum) is reduced, forming a knife-edge margin. The depth of this cut should be 0.5 to 0.7 mm.

(6) The concave lingual surface is prepared with a 110P Starlite diamond wheel stone to a minimal depth of 0.5 to 0.7 mm. Occluding areas, either centric or excursion, should be 0.2 mm. deeper. Slow speed is used.

(7) With slow speed the axial walls are finished with a ¼ D-L Densco tapered diamond stone.

(8) A chamfered finishing line is established on the proximal and lingual surfaces with a 1D-T Densco tapered diamond stone and these surfaces are finished with the same stone at slow speed.

(9) The labial and proximal shoulder is extended apically into the gingival sulcus, using a No. 556 or 557 S.S.W. carbide bur with slow speed. Another size may be substituted. The shoulder should be 0.7 mm. wide and 0.5 mm. into the crevice, or no more than one-half the depth of the crevice if it is very shallow.

The added cutting on the labial and proximal surfaces should end

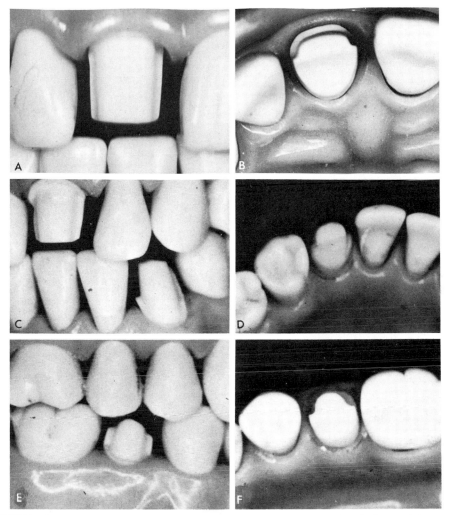

FIGURE 20–3. *Preparations suitable for cast gold crowns with bonded porcelain veneers.*

A, Maxillary central incisor, labial view.

B, Maxillary central incisor, incisal view.

C, Maxillary central and mandibular cuspid; note extension of shoulders into inter-proximals on central and mesial of cuspid.

D, Mandibular cuspid, incisal view.

E, Mandibular bicuspid, buccal view.

F, Mandibular bicuspid, occlusal view.

abruptly on each side in a half groove made parallel to the cervical half of the labial or buccal contour of the prepared tooth, even if one, or both, grooves open lingually to the incisal edge on an anterior tooth. It is important that the groove be just as wide proximally as on the labial or buccal so that the veneer may have the right shade and contour interproximally. On small teeth or on those with constricted necks, the shoulder may of necessity have to be less than 0.7 mm. wide. If so, there can be a question about shade and contour.

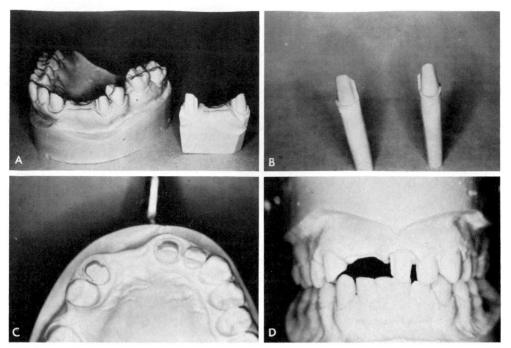

FIGURE 20–4. *Cast and dies showing a maxillary central incisor and a maxillary cuspid prepared for veneered gold crowns.*

A, Working cast and cast to be sectioned for dies.

B, Dies trimmed.

C, Note that shoulders on mesial of cuspid and on both mesial and distal of central incisor are far enough toward lingual so that boundaries of veneers will not be seen.

D, Lingual surface of cuspid preparation clears occluding teeth by 0.5 mm. or more in all positions.

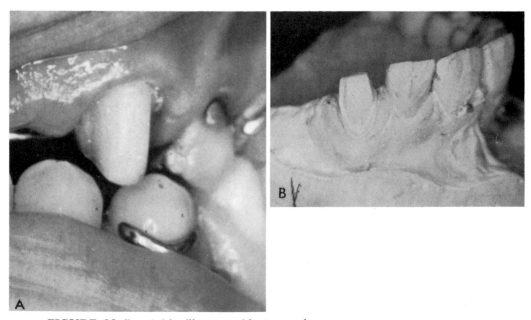

FIGURE 20–5. *A*, Maxillary cuspid prepared.

B, Cast of prepared mandibular cuspid. Shoulder on mesial extended lingually.

(10) Using slow speed, corrections are carefully made in the cervical finishing line with ¼D-L and 1D-T diamond stones.

(11) The shoulder, which should be part enamel and part dentin, is smoothed with a chisel.

Examples of finished preparations are shown in Figures 20-3, 20-4, and 20-5.

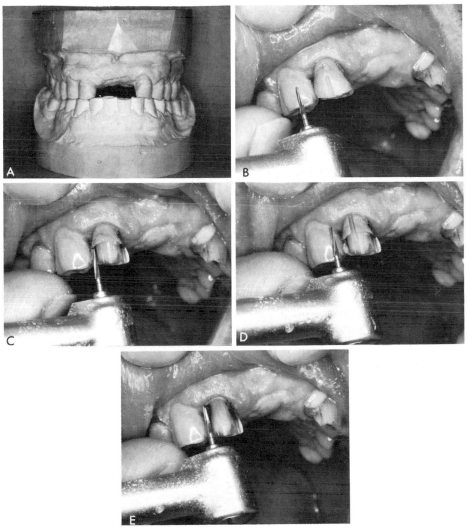

FIGURE 20-6. *A*, Occluded diagnostic casts. Maxillary lateral incisors and cuspids will be prepared for veneered gold crown retainers.

B, Groove cut in incisal half of labial surface.

C, Surface reduced to right and left of groove. Groove guided depth of proximal extensions of cutting.

D, Groove cut in cervical half of labial surface. This groove is in another plane diverging less or not at all from the long axis of the tooth. Groove in incisal half ends at height of contour; this groove begins there and ends at gingival line, or, with gingival recession, at cementoenamel line.

E, Labial surface reduced. Cuts stop at contact areas.

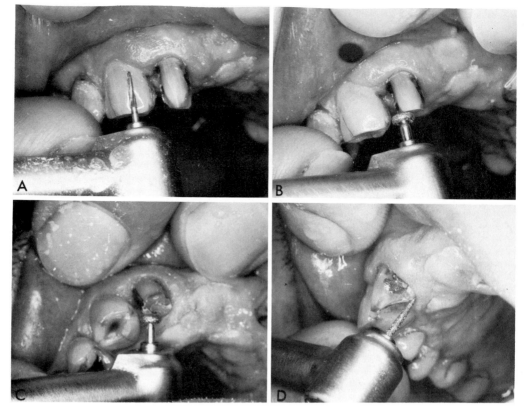

FIGURE 20–7. *A,* Proximal surfaces have been made parallel.
B, Incisal is shortened.
C, Lingual surface is contoured.
D, Lingual wall of cingulum is reduced.

There are many variations in sequence. This is a personal matter and may vary from tooth to tooth. Figures 20-6, 20-7, and 20-8 illustrate another concept.

PREPARATION OF OTHER TEETH

The basic steps are the same for other anterior and for posterior teeth. The buccal half of the occlusal surface should be cut to a depth of almost 2.0 mm. for bulk of metal and a veneer over the outer one-third of the buccal occlusal border. The lingual half of the occlusal surface and the occluding portion of the lingual surface must have a clearance of 1.0 mm. or more. The linguoproximal finishing line is chamfered. The set of instruments, which may be augmented by wheels or larger tapered stones, is shown in Figure 20-9.

Five other programs of instrumentation for this preparation are delineated in Tables 20-1, 20-2, 20-3, 20-4, and 20-5.

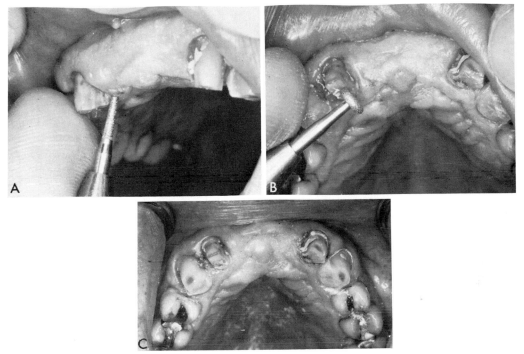

FIGURE 20–8.   *A*, Labial and proximal shoulder has been cut. Proximal and lingual chamfer is made with round-end diamond stone.

B, Lingual surface is reduced to give desired clearance in all relations.

C, Incisal view of four preparations.

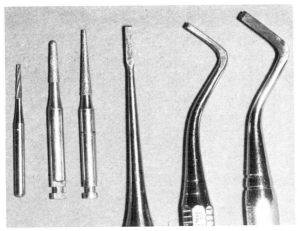

FIGURE 20–9.   Left to right: 169L-FG carbide bur (Densco); 1D-T latch tapered diamond stone (Densco); ¼D-L latch tapered diamond stone (Densco); #10 straight Tarno chisel (S.S.W.); #8-9 double-ended enamel hatchet (Am. Den.)*; #10-11 double-ended enamel hatchet (S.S.W.).

*American Dental Manufacturing Co., Missoula, Mont.

Table 20–1.

INSTRUMENT	TO BE ACCOMPLISHED	R.P.M.
71L Premier "Ela" carbide	Peripheral reduction except lingual of anteriors. Occlusal or incisal reduction. Buccal or labial shoulder grossly outlined.	150,000
3½ J Densco diamond	Lingual surface reduction of anteriors.	8,000 to 10,000
1D Densco diamond	Irregularities smoothed and angles rounded.	8,000 to 10,000
701 or 702 Premier "Ela" carbide	Shoulder positioned cervically and made square.	5,000

Table 20–2.

INSTRUMENT	TO BE ACCOMPLISHED	R.P.M.
700 or 701 R & R carbide	Complete peripheral and incisal or occlusal reduction.	150,000
123 SSW diamond	Convex lingual surface reduction.	150,000
557 SSW steel bur	Shoulder extended into gingival crevice.	6,000
1D-T Densco diamond	Lingual chamfer extended into gingival crevice.	150,000
Sandpaper disks (any brand)	Irregularities smoothed and angles rounded.	6,000

Table 20–3.

INSTRUMENT	TO BE ACCOMPLISHED	R.P.M.
1D or 2D Densco diamond	Peripheral reduction of posteriors. Labial, proximal, and incisal reduction of anteriors.	150,000 to 200,000
123 SSW diamond	Occlusal reduction of posteriors. Lingual reduction of anteriors.	150,000 to 200,000
701 SSW carbide	Buccal or labial shoulder.	150,000 to 200,000
1D-T Densco diamond (worn) or 44 SSW carborundum stone	Irregularities smoothed.	4,000

Table 20-4.

INSTRUMENT	TO BE ACCOMPLISHED	R.P.M.
701 R & R carbide	Buccal, lingual, and occlusal reduction.	150,000 to 200,000
700 or 699 R & R carbide	Mesial and distal reduction.	150,000 to 200,000
1D-T or 1D-C Densco diamond	Location and contour of cervical margin.	150,000 to 200,000
170L SSW carbide	Finish labial or buccal surface and shoulder.	150,000 to 200,000

Using Conventional Speeds

For beginning students, conventional speeds may be advantageous. If so, the steps in the preparation of either an anterior or posterior tooth are as follows:

(1) reduction of the mesial and distal surfaces,

(2) reduction of the buccal and lingual surfaces, and

(3) reduction of the incisal edge or occlusal surface;
    (NOTE: The order of 1 through 3 is not important.)

(4) effacing of angles so that the cervical finishing line at this time has continuity and lies at or just under the gingiva;

(5) preparation of a cervical shoulder on the labial or buccal half;

(6) extension of shoulder lingually into anterior interproximal so that contact line of frame and veneer will be hidden by tooth or pontic to the mesial; and

(7) modification of angles and smoothing irregularities. (See Figure 20-10.)

Table 20-5.

INSTRUMENT	TO BE ACCOMPLISHED	R.P.M.
701 or 701-L Densco carbide	Occlusal or incisal reduction. Peripheral reduction of posteriors. Labial and proximal reduction of anteriors. Gross outline of shoulder.	150,000
1½J Densco diamond	Lingual reduction of anteriors.	150,000
¾D or 1D Densco diamond	Irregularities smoothed. Location and contour of cervical margin. Shoulder finished.	150,000
Sandpaper disks (any brand)	Preparation smoothed.	600

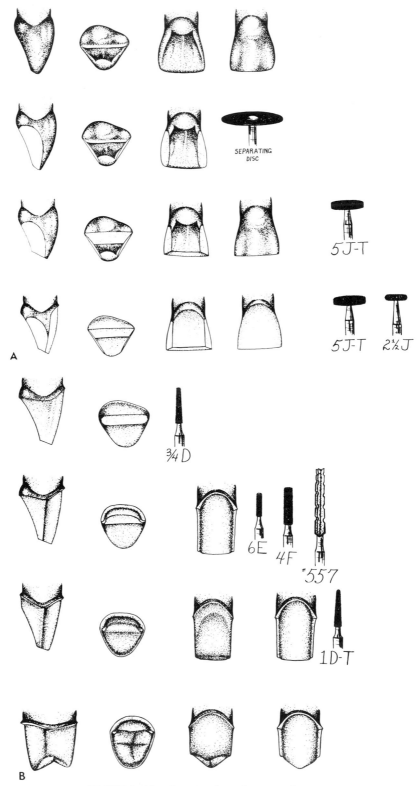

FIGURE 20–10.   *See legend on opposite page.*

MESIAL AND DISTAL SURFACES.   The mesial and distal surfaces should be reduced with a disk, using the straight handpiece for better control. Started on or just inside the marginal ridges, these cuts must be carried cervically to the gingival line, or if the gingival line has receded, just beyond the cementoenamel junction, following the planes of the surfaces buccolingually. One proximal cut should be parallel to the path of insertion or converge only a few degrees toward the incisal edge or the occlusal surface. The other must be compatible and should supply as much mechanical retention as is possible from the inclination of the tooth.

LABIAL OR BUCCAL AND LINGUAL SURFACES.   The labial or buccal and lingual surfaces are reduced in the same way as for a full veneer crown, except that the outer surface must be cut deeper and be more convex in the occlusal half. Extension should be to the gingival line.

INCISAL EDGE OR OCCLUSAL SURFACE, AND AXIAL ANGLES.   A wheel stone is used for the reduction of the incisal edge, and wheel, inverted cone, and knife-edge stones and fissure burs for the occlusal surface. The preparation on the occlusal should duplicate roughly the contours of the original surface, except that the buccal cusp or the labioincisal dimension should be shortened not less than 2.0 mm. The lingual cusp and marginal ridge areas should have clearance of at least 1.0 mm. in all excursions. The four walls are then connected at the axial angles to form a line at and following the height of the gingival crest, using a long tapered diamond, sandpaper disks, or flat surface or concave diamonds. For a crown that is to be veneered with resin, incisal or occlusal clearance need be no more than 1.2 mm.

At this point a copper band should be trimmed, marked for position, and laid aside if such an impression is to be taken.

THE SHOULDER.   To make shading and normal contour practicable on the exposed surface, there must be a cervical shoulder (a chamfer is not sufficient) on the labial or buccal half or four-sevenths of the tooth (Fig. 20-5).

The shoulder should be approximately 0.7 mm. in width, but if the tooth is large or if the pulp has receded, it can be as wide as 1.0 mm. This will entail further cutting pulpally in the cervical one-half or one-third, which may be done with a No. 557 or 556 bur, followed by an end-cutting bur or a cylindrical or tapered stone. Conversely, on small teeth or on those with constricted necks the shoulder may have to be less than 0.7 mm. The shoulder should end abruptly on each side in a half-groove made parallel to the cervical half of the labial or buccal contour of the prepared tooth. It is of consequence that it be just as wide at its proximal termination as it is on the

---

FIGURE 20–10. *Preparation.*

A, Top to bottom: Uncut tooth; mesial and distal surfaces; incisal edge (this can precede or follow reduction of labial and lingual surfaces); labial and lingual reduction.

B, Top to bottom: Corners rounded (if band impression will be used, band should be fitted at this point); shoulder prepared; all angles rounded and finishing line established. Preparation on a maxillary bicuspid.

labial surface so that the veneering material may have abundant thickness for shade without abnormal overcontour in that area.

The shoulder and the remaining proximal and lingual margins should be extended uniformly 0.5 or 0.6 mm. under the gingiva. The chamfered cervical finishing line on the lingual should connect the mesial and distal of the shoulder, at the same time rounding the lingual angles. It should be made with a tapered, round-point stone.

On mandibular cuspids and first bicuspids, the mesial shoulder can be extended lingually onto the cingulum or lingual surface so that the metal frame will be hidden by the approximating tooth. The curvatures of the reduced labial or buccal surface should approximate the contour of the uncut surface until the preparation approaches the incisal or occlusal third, where it must curve more sharply toward the lingual surface. This must be rechecked after the shoulder is completed.

PREPARATION OF TOOTH USING A POST AND CAST CORE

Many times teeth requiring veneered gold crowns will have had endodontic therapy and will present to the restorative dentist with much of the internal crown structure lost. At one time such teeth would have been cut off at the gingival crest and restored with Davis or Richmond crowns. The practice today is to salvage the remaining coronal dentin, supplement that with a cemented post and core, and then shape the tooth structure and casting to prepared form.

There are advantages to be derived from the application of this concept:
(1) long-term retention is better with a crown secured over a cemented core (since it appears that restorations, cemented to some tooth structure, are less apt to become loose); and
(2) the incidence of root fracture is practically nil because of controlled leverages.

The technique to be discussed here for a post and cast core is most suitable for anterior teeth. Bicuspids and molars can be rebuilt to prepared form either by castings or by pin-retained alloy restorations. (See Full Veneer Crown Preparation.)

REDUCTION OF RESIDUAL TOOTH STRUCTURE.   The coronal structure that remains is prepared to near dimensional form (Fig. 20–11 A, B, and C) with the preferred burs and stones. Any undercuts in and on the lingual surface that could interfere with removal of the post and wax pattern for the core are obliterated (Fig. 20–11 D) and the root canal is enlarged to accept the post. (Twelve-gauge or 14-gauge high-fusing clasp wire is most often used unless the tooth is very small.) The authors believe that enlarging the canal can be done with greater safety with a series of round burs (Fig. 20–11 E) than with reamers. Then the coronal third of the canal should be smoothed with a tapered stone.

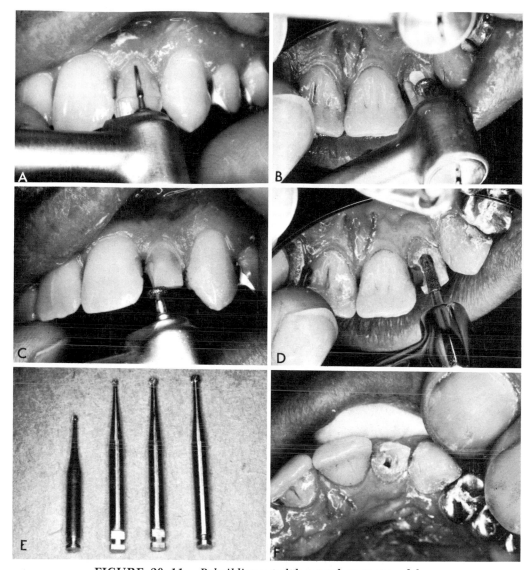

FIGURE 20–11. *Rebuilding a pulpless tooth to prepared form.*

A, Reducing remaining coronal dentin.
B, Removing lingual undercuts.
C, Establishing incisocervical length.
D, Enlarging pulp chamber and obliterating remaining lingual undercuts.
E, Graduated sizes of round burs for opening canal.
F, Canal opened.

FITTING THE POST.   The post should extend into the root a distance equal to the length of the proposed restoration. The wire is cut so that it will reach the end of the enlarged canal and extend 4.0 or 5.0 mm. beyond the incisal edge of the carved pattern. That part to be covered with wax must be notched irregularly so that the wax will withdraw with the post, and be secure and not turn on the wire (Fig. 20-12 *A* and *B*).

WAXING THE CORE.   The post is removed and softened inlay wax is

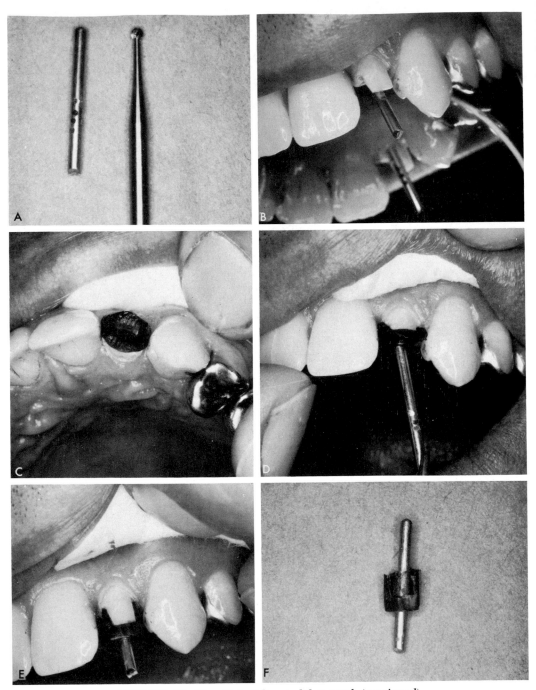

FIGURE 20–12. *Rebuilding pulpless tooth (continued).*

A, Post, and bur for final enlarging of canal.

B, Post in canal showing extra length beyond incisal. Notches will hold wax firmly.

C, Wax forced into pulp chamber and filling lingual concavity.

D, Forcing warmed pin through wax until it seats in canal.

E and *F,* Carved pattern for cast core, on and off tooth.

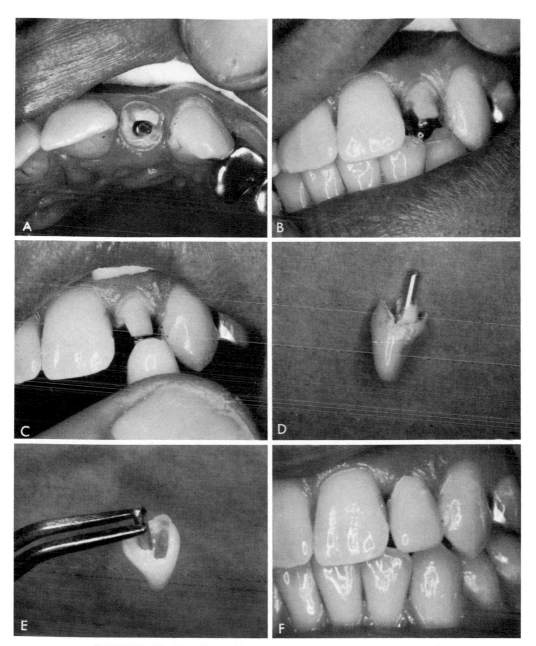

FIGURE 20–13. *Temporary crown for prepared pulpless tooth.*

A, Short post in canal.
B, Crown form fitted to cervical of tooth. Teeth are occluded.
C, Crown form containing filling resin.
D, Temporary crown removed.
E, Temporary crown trimmed and ready for seating.
F, Crown seated.

forced into the lingual depression (Fig. 20-12 *C*). The post is warmed and forced through the wax and seated in the canal (Fig. 20-12 *D*). The pattern is carved to form (Fig. 20-12 *E* and *F*).

Temporary Crown. A shorter wire is fitted into the canal and a resin crown form is adapted to the tooth (Fig. 20-13 *A* and *B*). The crown form is filled with resin and forced on the lubricated tooth stump (Fig. 20-13 *C*). When the resin has hardened it is removed (Fig. 20-13 *D*) and trimmed (Fig. 20-13 *E*). It is fixed to the moist tooth with a fragile mix of temporary cement (Fig. 20-13 *F*).

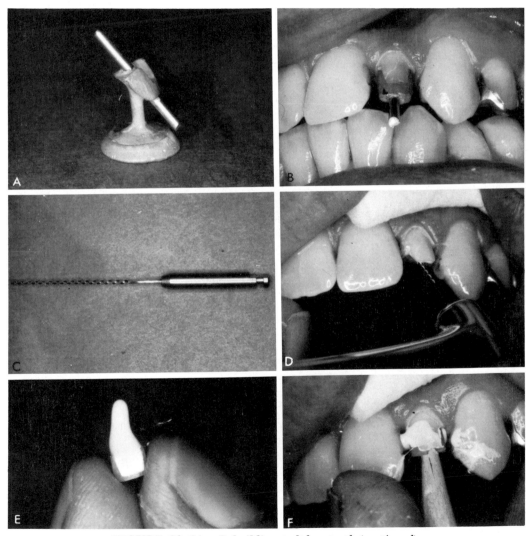

FIGURE 20–14. *Rebuilding pulpless tooth (continued).*

A, Casting (see Fig. 20–12 for pattern).
B, Cast core seated for check on fit.
C and *D*, Spirec drill for carrying cement into canal.
E, Post and core covered with cement.
F, Post and core cemented.

FINISHING THE PREPARATION.   The casting is made (Fig. 20-14 *A*) and fitted (Fig. 20-14 *B*). Zinc phosphate cement is carried into the canal (Fig. 20-14 *C* and *D*) and painted over the contacting surface of the casting (Fig. 20-14 *E*). The casting is rotated into place and seated with light mallet pressure (Fig. 20-14 *F*).

When the cement is set the preparation is completed, and after the impressions are made the tooth is covered.

*   *   *   *   *   *

The shade should have been selected before preparation of the tooth was begun.

REFERENCES

1. Wheeler, R. C.: Complete crown form and the periodontium. J. Pros. Den., *11*:722, July-Aug. 1961.
2. Nuttall, E. B.: Personal communication.
3. Johnston, J. F., Mumford, G., and Dykema, R. W.: Porcelain Veneers Bonded to Metal Castings. Practical Dental Monographs. Chicago, Year Book Medical Publishers, Inc., March 1963.
4. Kahn, A. E.: Partial versus full coverage. J. Pros. Den., *10*:167, Jan.-Feb. 1960.
5. Wilson, W. H., and Lang, R. L.: Practical Crown and Bridge Prosthodontics. New York, McGraw-Hill Book Company, Inc., 1962.
6. Miller, C. J.: Inlays, Crowns and Bridges. Philadelphia, W. B. Saunders Company, 1962.
7. Abramson, I.: Role of endodontics in crown and bridge prosthesis. J. Maryland D. A., (No. 1) *1*:28, 1958.
8. Hagerman, D. A., and Arnim, S. S.: Relation of new knowledge of the gingiva to crown and bridge procedures. J. Pros. Den., *5*:538, July 1955.
9. Dykema, R. W., Johnston, J. F., and Cunningham, D. M.: The veneered gold crown. D. Clin. N. Amer., Nov. 1958, p. 653.
10. Brecker, S. C.: Crowns. Philadelphia, W. B. Saunders Company, 1961.
11. Pincus, C. L.: Esthetic variations in jacket crowns and bridge restorations involving periodontal and other deformities. Its application to oral rehabilitation. New York J. Den., *24*:132, March 1954 (Abstract).

Meadows, T. R.: Clinical comparison of cast gold crowns with acrylic and with fused porcelain veneer facings. J.A.D.A., *66*:772, June 1963.
Youdelis, R., et al.: Full coverage restoration of pulpless anterior and bicuspid teeth. S. Afr. J. D. A., *22*:112, April 15, 1967.

chapter 21

THE CONSTRUCTION OF BONDED PORCELAIN VENEER CROWNS

As early as 1887 dental restorations utilizing bonded porcelain veneers were constructed by Dr. Charles Land after his observation that the platinum matrix has an affinity for porcelain. For a number of years following 1907 frameworks for crowns and bridges were made of an iridioplatinum alloy over which a high-fusing porcelain was fired.[1] Later came swaged, brazed, and cast platinum cores and ferrules.[2]

The resulting veneered restorations and prostheses were failures because of inadequate fit, brittleness, and poor bonding of the porcelain.[3] Platinum lacked the requisite physical and working properties for good dental restorations; it was frangible and easily contaminated when alloyed with iridium, rhodium, and palladium.[4, 5] Adding to these difficulties were casting investments that could neither compensate for the increased metal shrinkage nor withstand the high burnout temperatures necessary to assure complete castings.

Since 1950 investigation and clinical testing of restorations veneered with porcelain have been intensified and expanded by manufacturers, teaching institutions,[5, 6] and independent practitioners. Coleman, Klaus, Shell, Taylor, Vining, Wain, and many others from the research laboratories of several manufacturers of dental alloys and porcelains have contributed notably to the progress made in porcelain veneered restorations. Brecker, Cunningham, Dunton, Hobo, Jones, Kramer, Lew, Lyon, Moskey, Mumford, Ridge, Teteruck, and Vu thi Thin are among those who have assisted in the evaluation of the materials used and in the stabilization and rationalization of means of application.

With the techniques now developed, building and bonding or fracture of the porcelain veneer should not be listed as problems. It may be said that bonded porcelain veneer crowns are now acceptable in almost every respect to a great majority of dentists and patients, but they are frustrating, ineptly used, and badly constructed by the less perceptive and persevering members of the dental profession and the technicians' craft.

410

The authors use Ceramco porcelain, both air and vacuum fired,* and Ceramco Microfine alloy;† techniques for their use will be described. These products are manufactured to be in balance.‡ In practice there are some other gold alloys and one or more cobalt chromium or nonprecious metal alloys that seem to have a satisfactory balance with Ceramco porcelain.

Other combinations of porcelain and alloy are obtainable in both high-fusing and low-fusing ranges and for either air or vacuum firing. Among them are Stern's MF-Y gold alloy and Gold-Bond porcelain§ and Micro-Bond Hi-Life gold alloy and porcelain.**

WORKING DIES AND CASTS

Polysulfide rubber impressions are excellent for making dies and working casts.[7, 8] (See Chapter 9, The Working Cast.) Gingival displacement can be achieved efficiently with Westwood alum yarn, Gingi-Pak cord, Hemodent cord, or Pascord, and Hemodent Hemostatic solution. Only one full mouth impression need be made. The areas of the prepared teeth are poured with Vel-Mix[9, 10] or a similar improved stone; the set stone is removed after 1 hour and a complete arch working cast is poured into the same impression. The first cast is sectioned to make the dies; the intact working cast is used to contour and align an individual crown or to assemble a splint or fixed partial denture (Fig. 21-1). (See also Figure 21-5 C and D.)

The opposing casts must be related with care and mounted on an adjustable articulator. When the dentist is demanding of himself in this matter, he will have suitable "tools" and can fashion crowns or bridges requiring minimal corrections.

CASTINGS

The next step in bonded porcelain veneer crown construction is producing the casting. To be worthy of cementation, a cast restoration must fit, must have surface smoothness and density, and either through bulk or inherent physical properties must be capable of resisting deformation.

"Fit" in a casting for a porcelain veneered crown may have manifold definitions. To the authors it means a snug adaptation (without binding) of the metal to the entire cut surfaces of the tooth, covering all the prepared

---

*Ceramco, Inc., Woodside, N.Y.

†J. F. Jelenko & Co., Inc., New Rochelle, N.Y., and Julius Aderer, Inc., Long Island City, N.Y.

‡Veneering porcelain and alloy are said to be in balance when the contraction of the two materials has been synchronized so that the alloy, after the veneer has been fired, contracts just enough more than the porcelain to place the porcelain under compression. This reduces checking and increases strength.

§Stern Dental Co., Inc., Mount Vernon, N.Y.

**Howmedica, Inc., Chicago, Ill.

NOTE: All companies have well written and explicit pamphlets that describe the techniques for using their materials. Some details of frame design and cervical extension differ from those delineated in this text.

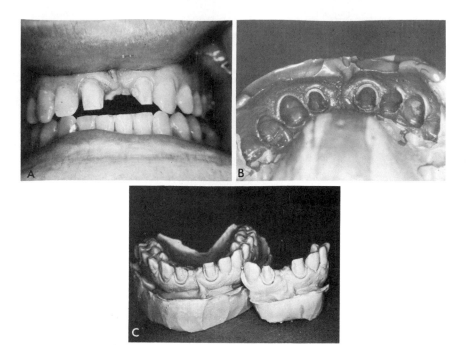

FIGURE 21-1.   *Construction of a veneered bridge.*

A, Central and lateral incisor abutments prepared.
B, Rubber base impression.
C, Two casts that were poured in one impression. The smaller will be sectioned for dies.

tooth surfaces after polishing, but with *no extension of the casting cervically beyond the margins of the preparation,* and natural contour and adequate bulk in the cervical fifth. To others it may mean close adaptation of the casting to the tooth structure only in the cervical fourth or fifth, with the remaining area etched to provide more freedom for seating and flow of cement. However, a cast framework for a bonded porcelain veneer crown cannot have the same degree of frictional retention as a well-fitting partial veneer crown. It must seat without pressure. When the pattern is lined with soft wax, removal and seating will abrade the inner surface and help to establish the desired type of fit. (See Figure 21-2*A*.)

Forming the Wax Pattern.   A casting that fits must duplicate the form and dimensions of a wax pattern that also fits. The metal frame must support the porcelain bonded to it, and since any flexure of the metal will cause checking or outright fracture of the veneer, it is essential that the wax pattern have no internal creases. If this is attained, it matters little how the pattern is formed. The authors use stone dies, lubricated and dipped in a dish of molten Kerr's blue sprue wax, which gives a smooth, well-adapted inner surface to the pattern. Also, because of the softness of this inner layer, the investment can more effectively expand the pattern during setting. The contour is built up with a wax that meets the specifications for indirect inlay waxes.

The wax pattern for a casting to be veneered should be carved first to full dimensions in order to place exactly contact areas and form embrasures;

then the surface to which the veneer will be bonded is cut back to the contour most suitable for veneering (Fig. 21–2). (See also Figure 21–5 *E* and *F*.) This cutback should be at least 1.0 mm. deep toward the center of the tooth at every point on the labial or buccal surface, but as the incisal edge is approached, the depth must be increased for a minimal clearance of 1.5 mm. between the wax pattern and the opposing teeth. Clearance over the buccal cusp and occlusal surface of any posterior unit should be approximately 1.5 mm. On a maxillary bicuspid or molar crown, the surface to be veneered preferably will terminate halfway down the lingual slope of the buccal cusp or cusps, but not at a point in contact in centric closure.[10, 11]

There should be no sharp angles within the area to be veneered; still there should be an invisible right angle where the surface of the veneer meets the flat face of the casting. To assure complete casting the buccocervical collar in the wax pattern should be left approximately twice as thick as it will be after the casting is prepared for veneering. When the pattern is finished, all surfaces that will be exposed should be as smooth as possible.

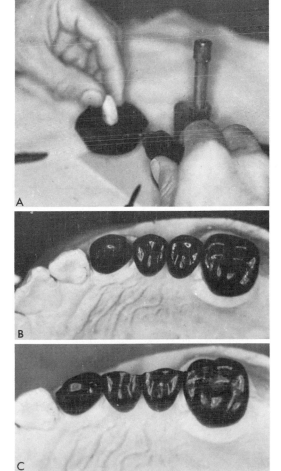

FIGURE 21–2. *A*, Dipping lubricated die into molten sprue wax to give inner surface of pattern a smooth, unblemished surface.

B, Wax patterns for a crown and two pontics carved to full contour. Each of these three units will be veneered with bonded porcelain.

C, Wax patterns cut back to best form for veneering.

A porcelain veneered gold crown is built with the incisal edge "unsupported" by overlying metal. This is an esthetic virtue and a mechanical necessity. The only incisal edge fractures seen by the authors have occurred when an attempt was made to protect the incisal edge with a lingual metal veneer, which is always too thin to resist deformation under incising forces.

Although the incisal edge should be reproduced in porcelain, it is advisable that the areas on the lingual surface, making contacts in centric occlusion and the beginnings of the eccentric movements, should be metal. This subsequently permits some occlusal adjustment without leaving a rough, unglazed porcelain surface. For the same reason (equilibration) the occlusal surfaces of posterior crowns or pontics are left unveneered unless the absolute in esthetic results is requested by the patient. (For selecting shade and shade pattern, see Chapter 13, The Pontic.)

Spruing. It was once thought that patterns must be sprued in an unorthodox manner in order to make castings without voids. (See Figure 21–3 *A* and *B*.) While a considerable number still attach sprues so that the gold enters the mold and circulates, standard spruing is now generally accepted (Fig. 21–3 *C*). Sprue sizes from 10-gauge to 12-gauge (never less than 14-gauge) are indispensable. Venting can do no harm, but is no longer thought to be imperative unless the pattern is large and the veneering area

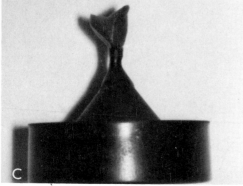

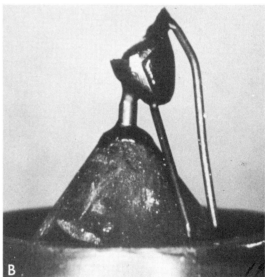

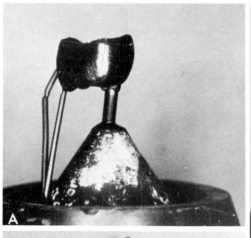

FIGURE 21-3. Three wax patterns sprued for casting Ceramco alloy.

is thin and extensive. If a vent is used, an 18-gauge wax rod is extended from a point near the periphery of the thin section of the pattern to the face of the crucible former, about 2.0 mm. from the casting ring (Fig. 21–3 *A* and *B*). When investing a posterior pattern, spruing should be the same as for a full veneer gold crown. Some continue to place a 10-gauge or 12-gauge sprue on the tip of a cusp perpendicular to the plane of the occlusal surface (Fig. 21–3 *A*). When sprued in this manner, an 18-gauge vent is used. With the second method the gold will enter the mold and circulate in a manner that ordinarily might cause turbulence. In any case the air will be forced ahead of the gold and out into the vent, making certain a complete casting.

Investing. Ceramigold* investment has been used by the authors for some time. The prescribed liquid-powder ratio is 6.5 cc. of Ceramigold liquid and 2 cc. of water per 60 grams of powder; but for most clinical cases 12 cc. of Ceramigold liquid, and *no* water, mixed with 60 grams of powder gives very satisfying results. Ceramigold investment seems to accept these variables in the liquid-powder ratio with no significant differences in the end product.

MIXING TECHNIQUE.   The liquid is placed in a clean mixing bowl, the powder is added, and the mix is stirred by hand until the powder is wetted. It will be quite stiff, but its fluidity will increase if it is mechanically spatulated for 20 seconds in vacuum. The pattern is then hand invested. The mixture is applied to the pattern with a brush and the remainder is poured into the ring. The pattern and sprue former are oscillated into place in and on the ring. The investment must bench-set for not less than 1 hour.[12]

The ring is placed in a cold furnace and over a period of 1 hour is heated to 1300° F. It is heat-soaked at this temperature for an additional 30 to 45 minutes, when it is ready for casting.

Casting. A special Wesgo† Type A high-heat crucible is used in a centrifugal casting machine, which is wound to give a slightly higher casting pressure than is usual. A gas-oxygen torch‡ is employed for melting the alloy. The crucible is preheated, but neither an asbestos liner nor flux is used in it. Asbestos might contaminate the metal, and flux could remove some of its vital trace elements. The metal in the crucible is heated in that part of the flame just beyond the end of the light blue zones.

As the alloy melts, a scum appears to form on its surface. With continued heating this scum disappears, the button becomes shiny, and the metal is in condition for casting. After the casting ring has bench-cooled until the button becomes dark, it is quenched in water and the investment is removed.

This investment is very compact and is difficult to remove from the casting. By grooving the sides of the investment block, it can be split, which helps to expose the metal. When the bulk is taken off, the remaining mass is

*Whip-Mix Corporation, Louisville, Ky.

†Western Gold and Platinum Co., Belmont, Calif.

‡Linde Oxweld torch #W17 with a 125 M4 multiflame tip, Linde Co., Div. of Union Carbide Corp., Speedway, Ind.

Torit #77 with A and B tips (for soldering) and C tip (for casting), Torit Mfg. Co., St. Paul, Minn.

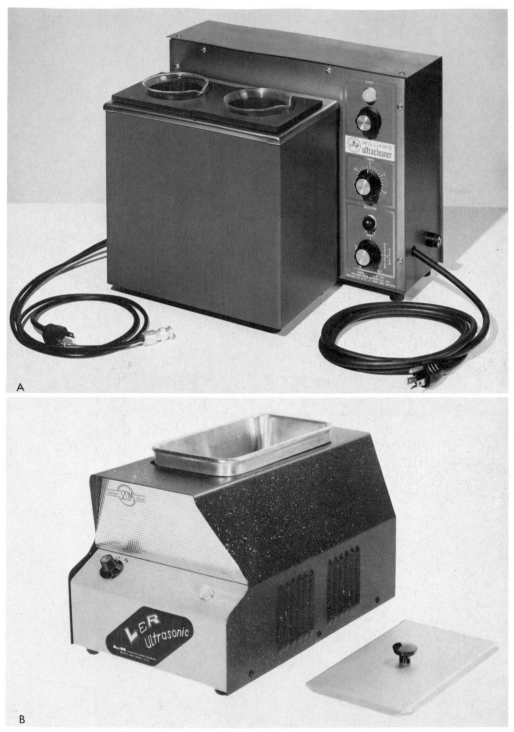

FIGURE 21–4. *A*, Williams Ultracleaner. *B*, L&R Ultrasonic Cleaner.

soaked in hydrofluoric or hydrochloric acid to soften that which remains so that the greater part can be washed away with a brush under running water. The casting and attached fragments should be placed in a polyethylene receptable containing one of the acids and then into an ultrasonic cleaner.* (See Figure 21–4.) The casting must be washed with care. Hydrofluoric acid must be handled circumspectly, and milk of magnesia, the best antidote, must be at hand.

---

*Williams Gold Refining Co., Inc., Buffalo, N.Y.
L & R Mfg., Co., Des Plaines, Ill.

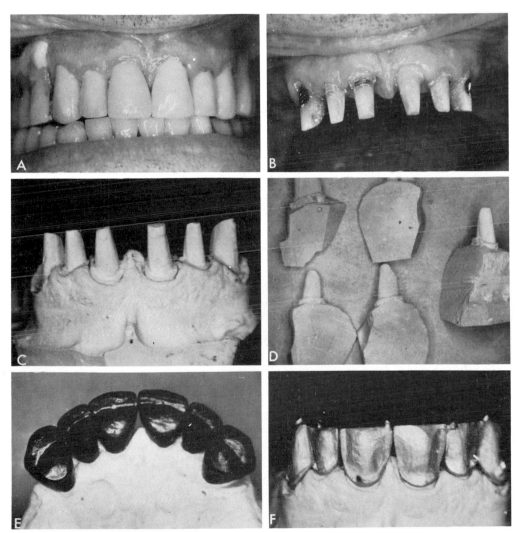

FIGURE 21–5. *A,* Six maxillary anterior teeth with abraded resin veneered gold crowns.
B, Crowns removed, showing excessively prepared teeth. No further cutting was done.
C and *D,* Stone cast and sections for dies.
E, Wax patterns on working cast. Cast and dies were poured in the same polysulfide rubber impression.
F, Castings seated on working cast. Heavy sprue pins were attached to lingual surfaces; vents to other surfaces. Labiocervical collar is heavy.

The sprue is removed by a carborundum or a Kro-Go† disk (Fig. 21–5 F).

Finishing the Casting.   Those surfaces of the casting that are not to receive porcelain are finished with stones and rubber wheels. The contacts and occlusion should be checked and rectified on the articulated working casts, and also in the mouth if practicable. This is important because only minimal alterations should be made in the contour of the frame after the veneer has been glazed.

The area to be veneered must be enlarged or extended. The cervical

---

‡Precision Dental Mfg. Co., Chicago, Ill.

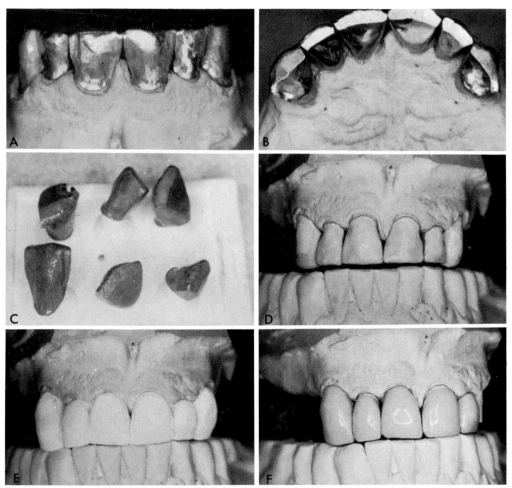

FIGURE 21–6.   *A*, Castings contoured for veneering. Incisal angles are rounded. Cervical collar is thinned. Surfaces to be veneered have been stoned.
   B, Incisal view of castings. Labial margins round; lingual margins precise.
   C, Castings degassed and metal conditioner (Ceramcote) fired.
   D, Opaque fired.
   E, Body porcelain applied ready for first firing.
   F, First application of body porcelain fired.

collar will be excessively thick and must be thinned and given chamfered form (Fig. 21–6 A). When finished and seated the collar must be hidden by the gingiva. All internal angles on the veneering surface must be rounded. Porcelain should not be built into or over a sharp angle. In the first situation it can pull away or warp the casting; in the second it cleaves along the crest of the angle upon shrinking. The proximal and linguoincisal margins must be right angles so that the porcelain and gold can form approximately a 90-degree butt joint (Fig. 21–6 B).

PREPARING THE FRAME FOR VENEERING

After all exposed surfaces of the casting have been smoothed with rubber abrasive wheels, the area to be veneered with porcelain is roughened with a coarse wheel stone without organic binder. The casting must be pickled for 30 minutes in hydrofluoric acid in a polyethylene container placed in an ultrasonic cleaner. Up to 8 hours in the acid may be necessary without use of the ultrasonic cleaner. Gold manufacturers recommend other procedures that may be substituted, but hydrofluoric acid works best for the authors.

When veneering a crown with Ceramco vacuum-fired porcelain the casting is washed and degassed. (See Table 21–1.) This procedure will remove any gas contamination resulting from the casting process and will obviate one potential cause of porosity in the porcelain veneer. If Ceramcote is applied (Fig. 21–6 C), it is dried and fired in a vaccum of 1825° F., the vacuum is released, and the firing is continued in air up to 1925° F.

Britecote,* a conditioner that gives a bright gold color and a lumpy surface, can be applied. It has the same firing schedule as Ceramcote, or it can be set on the casting with a torch.[13] The value of Britecote or other conditioning agents, developed to eliminate the need to use hydrofluoric acid for cleaning, seems to be limited. When used under some of the very light enamel porcelains, with a thin layer of opaque, Britecote occasionally can aid in securing subtle esthetic values.

VACUUM-FIRED VENEERS

Regardless of the combination of materials used, certain factors remain constant for all vacuum-fired porcelains fused to metal. The metal should be degassed in the vacuum. Each addition of opaque and porcelain, either body or incisal, should be vacuum fired *except* the glaze firing, which is *always* done in air. Vacuum firing increases considerably the intensity of the color and the translucence of the porcelain; therefore, a shade guide of vacuum-fired

---

*Ceramco, Inc., Woodside, N.Y.

TABLE 21–1. FIRING SCHEDULE FOR PORCELAIN-FUSED-TO-GOLD PORCELAIN (CERAMCO)

BIOFORM VACUUM-FIRED PORCELAIN	TEMPERATURE	TEMPERATURE INCREASE	VACUUM OR AIR
Degassing Casting			
Fired	1200 to 1860° F.	75° per minute	28 inches vacuum
HOLD	1860° F. — 10 min.		28 inches vacuum
*Paint-O-Pake			
Fired	1200 to 1720° F.	75° per minute	28 inches vacuum
	1720 to 1860° F.	75° per minute	air
Remove immediately and cool under cover.			
Regular Opaque			
Fired	1200 to 1720° F.	75° per minute	28 inches vacuum
	1720 to 1820° F.	75° per minute	air
Remove immediately and cool under cover.			
Body and Incisal Porcelain			
Fired	1200 to 1700° F.	75° per minute	28 inches vacuum
	1700 to 1800° F.	75° per minute	air
Remove immediately and cool under cover.			
Glaze and Stain			
Fired	1200 to 1800° F.	75° per minute	air
Remove immediately and cool under cover.			
New Hue Vacuum-fired Porcelain	(Firing the same as Bioform vacuum-fired Porcelain).		

*Paint-O-Pake not available in New Hue shades.

porcelain is mandatory.[14] Porcelain powders designed for air firing cannot be used for vacuum firing unless they are modified by the addition of opacifiers and pigments.

The degree of vacuum used and the time of application vary from one brand of porcelain to another. Water will boil at room temperature under reduced pressure, and so will some of the veneering porcelains near their fusion temperature. Because this would increase the porosity of the porcelain rather than decrease it, the last part of each firing of these porcelains must be completed in air.

Glazing must be carried out at normal atmospheric pressure.

Table 21-1 shows a schedule of times and temperatures for firing Ceramco porcelain.

Building a Vacuum-fired Ceramco Veneer

The Opaque.   The opaque is mixed with distilled water to a consistency of thick cream and applied to the surface of the casting. By alternately vibrating and drying the surface with gauze, a layer 0.35 to 0.4 mm. thick is built up. The surface is brushed smooth and the opaque is dried. (For firing schedule, see Table 21-1.)

The opaque material will have shrunk during the firing so that it is now 0.3 mm., or less, in thickness (see Fig. 21-6 D).

AIR FIRING. For air firing, the casting is placed in the furnace at 1200° F. The temperature is increased 100 degrees per minute until 1800° F. is reached. This same firing schedule is used for all ensuing bakes. Immediately on reaching 1800° F. the casting is withdrawn from the furnace and placed under a cover to cool.

The Body Porcelain. The crown is now ready for the application of the veneering porcelains. The body porcelain is mixed to a consistency of very thick cream and applied to the casting with a spatula. By alternate vibrating and blotting with gauze, the crown is built to a slight overcontour in all dimensions to compensate for the anticipated shrinkage. Sufficient excess must be added near the margins to prevent the porcelain from pulling away from the metal (Fig. 21-6 E and F). The incisal and labial surfaces of the crown are trimmed with a sharp blade to create space for the incisal or the enamel-colored porcelain. The amount removed will depend on the shade distribution of the natural tooth to be matched. Margins must be feathered to avoid a distinct line of demarcation between the two porcelains.

The Incisal Porcelain. The incisal porcelain, because of its coarser particle size, is mixed to a thin consistency and flowed onto the surface with a brush. It is built up in layers to correct contour, moisture is removed with gauze, and the surface is smoothed with a large soft brush. The crown is dried in front of the open muffle. After the firing cycle has been repeated, the surface of the porcelain should have a semiglazed appearance. If more porcelain must be added in spots to complement form, the glaze should be removed from the crown before this is done (Figs. 21-7 and 21-8). Wet porcelain powder can be applied with more facility to a ground surface and, when fired, the surface texture will be more uniform.

Again it is dried and fired as described for other vacuum or air firing. Final alterations in contour and topographic anatomy are made at this stage, using small, mounted Carborundum stones. The stones should be wet. The surface is smoothed with wet white abrasive disks or a wet Dedeco* white rubber porcelain polishing wheel; otherwise, the porcelain must be subjected to the glazing temperature for such a length of time that contours and anatomic detail will be obscured or rounded.

GLAZING. Before the crown is glazed, all debris must be removed from its surface. This may be effected by (1) placing it in an ultrasonic cleaner (see Figure 21-4), (2) boiling it in chloroform, or (3) brushing it under running water. It is dried and preheated in front of the furnace for 2 to 3 minutes, then placed in the furnace at 1200° F. and carried to 1800° F., raising the temperature 75 to 100 degrees per minute, according to furnace characteris-

---

*Dental Development Mfg. Corp., Brooklyn, N.Y.

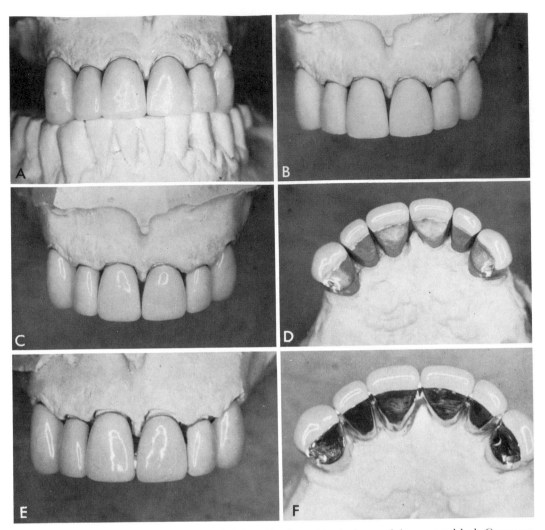

FIGURE 21–7.   *A*, After second firing. Body and incisal porcelain were added. Contour incorrect.

    B, Contoured for third firing.

    C, After third firing, labial view.

    D, Incisal view.

    E, Six-unit splint soldered.

    F, Lingual view after being polished.

tics. The degree of glaze desired will not be the same for all patients, and there will be dissimilar effects if the glazing temperature is varied between 1780° F. and 1810° F. The higher the temperature, the more glossy the surface becomes. If the surface is too glossy when the crown is tried in the mouth, the labial surface should be rubbed lightly with a fine sandpaper or cuttlefish disk held in the fingers. When the application of surface stains will assist in blending and harmonizing the color or shade pattern with the adjacent teeth, it is done at this stage, using normal staining procedures. (See Chapter 16, Glazing and Staining Facings.)

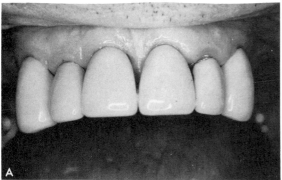
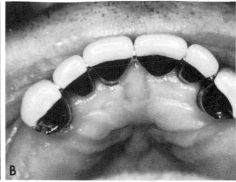
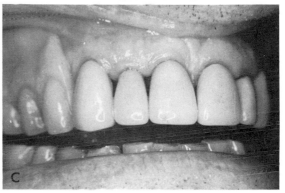

FIGURE 21-8. *A* and *B*, Six-crown splint cemented.
C, Supporting a Class I precision attachment partial denture.

After the porcelain has been fused, the casting is pickled in 50 per cent hydro*chloric* acid (not hydro*fluoric*). Any small pieces of porcelain adhering to the exposed metal surface are removed with stones, and the scratched surface is finished with a fine rubber wheel, followed by tripoli applied with a brush until the surface is completely free of any blemishes.

After adding and glazing the porcelain veneer, final polishing of the metal is accomplished with tripoli, or Motloid Polishing Agent,* followed by Amalgloss or No. 600 Carborundum powder mixed with water, or Buehler's AB Alpha polishing Alumina, No. 2,† mixed with a few drops of a liquid detergent.[10]

Ceramco alloy, as well as all other alloys used to support bonded porcelain veneers, can be finished to an exceptionally high luster (see Figure 21-7 *F*); all resist tarnish in the oral environment as well as standard crown and bridge alloys. Each will remain clean if the patient maintains a satisfactory level of oral hygiene.

CROWN WITH PORCELAIN SHOULDER

When the crown is to be made without a labiocervical collar of gold, another technique is employed for the wax pattern. A piece of 0.001 plati-

*Motloid Co., Inc., Chicago, Ill.
†Buehler, Ltd., Evanston, Ill.

num foil is burnished to overlap the shoulder cervically and incisally about 2.5 mm., or a complete platinum matrix may be made. Adaptation to the shoulder should be close. The pattern is waxed and carved to form but is not extended labially over the platinum foil (Fig. 21-9). Spruing is the same as described before, except that, to ensure casting over the platinum foil, an auxiliary sprue or vent must be attached very close to the cervical of the labial wax wall. The casting is cleaned, polished, and conditioned for veneering.

The opaque is applied to the surface of the casting, but not to the foil collar, and fired. The veneering porcelains are built to oversize form and then a V-shaped ditch is cut at the cervical, exposing the platinum. After firing, the crown is contoured, the platinum is reburnished against the die, and porcelain is added to complete the form of the crown. The ditch is overfilled and the crown is fired for the second time. If more porcelain is needed, it is added and the crown is again contoured and glazed. Before cementing, the platinum is peeled off the porcelain (Fig. 21-10).

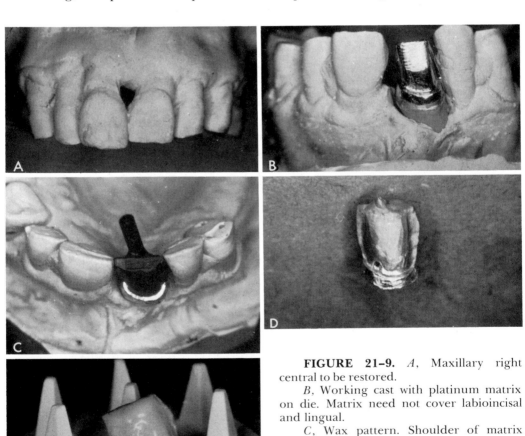

FIGURE 21-9. *A*, Maxillary right central to be restored.

B, Working cast with platinum matrix on die. Matrix need not cover labioincisal and lingual.

C, Wax pattern. Shoulder of matrix not covered.

D, Casting. Cervical discrepancy not important.

E, Opaque applied and fired. Cervical shoulder not covered.

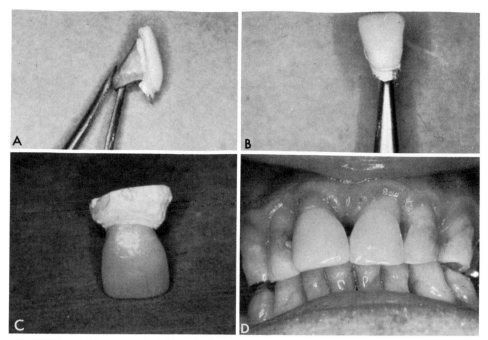

FIGURE 21–10. *A* and *B*, Cervical ditch and marginal shrinkage.
C, Crown supported by ceramic investment for glaze firing.
  D, Porcelain veneered crown without labiocervical collar of gold on maxillary right central incisor. Crown fits against prepared tooth as a jacket crown.

This method of construction is indicated when recession has gone beyond the cementoenamel junction, when recession is foreseen, or in any situation in which esthetic considerations are paramount. Strength and retention are not sacrificed in a single-unit restoration. However, if the crown were a retainer for a bridge, subject to leverage or torque, the frame might not withstand deformation and the veneer could be checked.

This technique demands more care in handling during construction, especially if the crown is used as a retainer. It is an excellent restoration esthetically and possibly is less irritating to the gingiva. Certainly, if recession did occur, it would be longer before dissatisfaction with appearance would require the tooth to be reprepared and another crown constructed.

VENEERS WITH INTRACORONAL ATTACHMENTS

A porcelain veneer can be built around the female section of a precision attachment or semiprecision rests (Sherer, McKay*) that have been positioned and soldered to the casting (Figs. 21-11, 21-12, 21-13, and 21-14).

---

*The female portion of a Sherer rest is formed in the wax pattern and made by casting.
  The female section of the McKay mortice rest (The J. M. Ney Company) is prefabricated and incorporated in the wax pattern, and metal is cast around it.

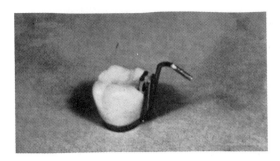

FIGURE 21–11.   Molar gold crown with complete porcelain veneer built around precision attachment. In the construction of a small percentage of clinical cases, a discernible warping of this attachment was noted. Adjustment was done quickly.

Two rules MUST be followed. The receptacle (female) portion of a precision attachment must be totally surrounded by metal so that no porcelain will be in contact with it. (See Figures 21–12 and 21–13 C.) Warping will then be minimal and can be remedied with a sizing tool. Seating of the male part will not cause internal stress and check the veneer.

The female component must be made of a platinum alloy so that it will not be affected by the high soldering and firing temperatures. The solder used to attach the component to the casting MUST be a *high-fusing solder*.[10, 13]

VENEERS UNDER CLASPS

When a porcelain veneer crown is being built to support a clasp,[15] the designed rest seats or ledges and any lingual retentive undercuts and proximal guiding planes are surveyed and carved into the wax pattern for the frame. Heights of contour and retentive undercuts are surveyed and ground into the porcelain just prior to glazing. When a crown is to be clasped, the

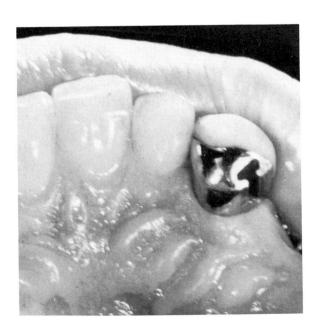

FIGURE 21–12.   Cuspid crown with veneer and precision attachment.

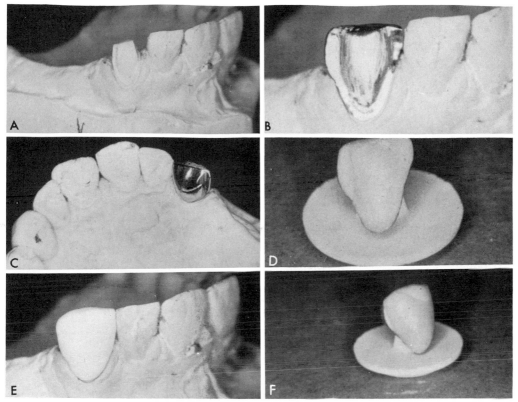

FIGURE 21–13.   *A*, Working cast.
B, Cast framework ready for veneering.
C, Casting, lingual view. Sherer rest seat. Cingulum contoured for cast retentive arm of clasp.
D, Opaque fired.
E, Body and incisal built.
F, First firing; shrinkage along margins.

glaze should be higher than is wanted on many other restorations, because the smoother surface has less abrasive action on the inner surface of a clasp. With a lesser glaze, now and then a wrought wire retentive arm will leave a faint gray metallic mark on the crown surface. The porcelain veneer crown is quite helpful in the preparation of mouths for clasp-retained partial dentures (Fig. 21–15).

CEMENTATION

The dentist may use the cementing technique of his choice, but it should be noted that he should resort to temporary measures for only short periods of time. When an abutment tooth must be slightly repositioned because of movement from its original alignment, a petroleum jelly and cement powder luting material may be used, but for just a few hours only. Removing a

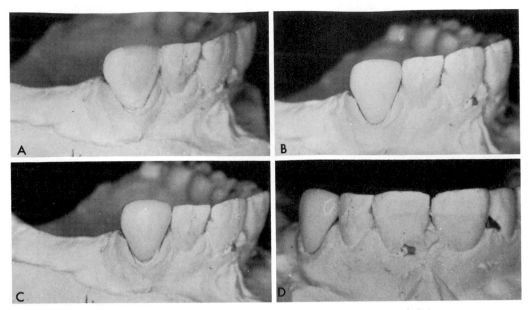

FIGURE 21–14. *A*, Porcelain added to plus contour before second firing.
B, Veneer contoured after second firing.
C and *D*, Veneer glazed.

cemented prosthesis or having it loose on a tooth may result in an internal pressure that will check the veneer. The authors strongly recommend immediate permanent cementation.[10] Teeth are seldom sensitive if they have been prepared watchfully and covered so that they were not subjected to premature contacts, lateral movement, or torque. A cavity varnish such as Copalite should be used, since it has no adverse effect on cementation and does

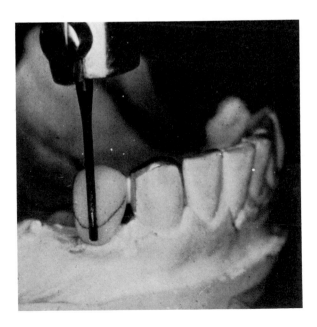

FIGURE 21–15. Bonded porcelain veneer contoured to provide correct survey line for clasping.

afford some protection to the pulp against the acid in the cement mix. (See Figure 21-8.)

* * * * * *

All phases of building a veneered crown or bridge can be done in the office laboratory. The extra equipment needed is not excessively expensive, but some CLEAN working space is very important. If all ceramic work is sent to a laboratory, impressions, dies, shade selections, and shade patterns must be flawless and instructions must be clearly stated. The ideas of the dentist must be well founded and must prevail.[16, 17]

REFERENCES

1. Brecker, S. C.: Porcelain fused to gold. J. California D. A. and Nevada D. Soc., 36:425, Dec. 1960.
2. Tylman, S. D.: Theory and Practice of Crown and Fixed Partial Prosthodontics (Bridge). 6th ed. St. Louis, The C. V. Mosby Company, 1970.
3. Perlman, T. H.: The use of platinum and porcelain in dental restorations. Aust. D. J., 26:118, June 1954.
4. Perlman, T. H.: Further observations on cast platinum and baked porcelain restorations. D. Digest, 56:298, 1950.
5. Brecker, S. C.: Porcelain baked to gold—a new medium in prosthodontics. J. Pros. Den., 6:801, Nov. 1956.
6. Johnston, J. F., Dykema, R. W., and Cunningham, D. M.: The use and construction of gold crowns with fused porcelain veneers—a progress report. J. Pros. Den., 6:811, Nov. 1956.
7. Phillips, R. W., and Schnell, R. J.: The Use of Rubber Impression Materials. Practical Dental Monographs. Chicago, Year Book Medical Publishers, Inc., May 1962.
8. Johnston, J. F., Dykema, R. W., Mumford, G., and Phillips, R. W.: Construction and assembly of porcelain veneer gold crowns and pontics. J. Pros. Den., 12:1125, Nov.-Dec. 1962.
9. Dykema, R. W., Johnston, J. F., and Cunningham, D. M.: The veneered gold crown. Dent. Clin. N. Amer., Nov. 1958, p. 653.
10. Johnston, J. F., Mumford, G., and Dykema, R. W.: Modern Practice in Dental Ceramics. Philadelphia, W. B. Saunders Company, 1967.
11. Johnston, J. F., Mumford, G., and Dykema, R. W.: Porcelain Veneers Bonded to Metal Castings. Practical Dental Monographs. Chicago, Year Book Medical Publishers, Inc., March 1963.
12. Schnell, R. J., Mumford, G., and Phillips, R. W.: An evaluation of phosphate bonded investments used with a high fusing gold alloy. J. Pros. Den., 13:324, 1963.
13. Jones, R. J.: Personal communication.
14. Bazola, F. N., et al.: A customized shade guide for vacuum-fired porcelain-gold combination crowns. J.A.D.A., 74:114 8, Jan. 1967.
15. Dykema, R. W., Cunningham, D. M., and Johnston, J. F.: Modern Practice in Removable Partial Prosthodontics. Philadelphia, W. B. Saunders Company, 1969.
16. Johnston, J. F., et al.: The dentist and the ceramic technician. J. Tennessee D. A., 48:83-91, April 1968.
17. Katz, S. R.: Aesthetics in ceramics. J. Canad. D. A., 32:224, April 1966.

Hagen, W. H. B.: Combination gold and porcelain crown. J. Pros. Den., 10:325, March-April 1960.
Lund, M. R., and Bonlie, D. R.: Baked porcelain restorations without the use of the platinum matrix. J. D. Res., 40:94, 1962 (Abstract).

Lyon, D. M., Cowger, G. T., Woycheshin, F. F., and Miller C. B.: Porcelain fused to gold—evaluation and esthetics. J. Pros. Den., *10*:319, March-April 1960.

Morrison, K. N., and Warnick, M. E.: Investment compounded specifically for ceramic procedures. J. D. Res., *38*:762, July-Aug. 1959 (Abstract).

Morse, F. F. E.: Porcelain fused to metal. Comparisons of the air-fired and vacuum-fired porcelain jacket crowns and porcelain fused to precious metal. Den. Pract. & Den. Rec., *13*:99, Nov. 1962.

Mumford, G.: The porcelain fused to metal restoration. Dent. Clin. N. Amer., March 1965, p. 241

Mylin, W. K.: Present status of porcelain fused to metal restorations. J. Kentucky D. A., *14*:152, July 1962.

Pruden, K. C.: Abutments and attachments in fixed partial dentures. J. Pros. Den., 7:502, July 1957.

Pruden, W. H., II: Porcelain veneer crown. J. Pros. Den., *10*:955, Sept.-Oct. 1960.

Shell, J. S., and Nielsen, J. P.: Study of the bond between gold alloys and porcelain. J. D. Res., *41*:1424, Nov.-Dec. 1962.

Teteruck, W. R., et al.: The fit of certain dental casting alloys using different invest ng materials and techniques. J. Pros. Den., *16*:910-27, Sept.-Oct. 1966.

Thin, Vu thi: A Study of the Brinell Hardness of Metals Used in Conjunction with the Porcelain Fused to Metal Technic. Master's thesis, Indiana University School of Dentistry, June 1962.

Warnick, M. E., and Morrison, K. N.: Porcelain-faced crown technique. D. Digest, *68*:60, Feb. 1962.

Wheeler, R. C.: The implications of full coverage restorative procedures. J. Pros. Den., 5:848, Nov.-Dec. 1955.

chapter 22

THE CONSTRUCTION OF BRIDGES WITH BONDED PORCELAIN VENEERS

Bridges that include units with bonded porcelain veneers may be fabricated either before or after the veneers are fired. If this is done *prior* to the application of porcelain, the solder must have a melting point very close to that of the casting alloy so that the bridge will not warp or come apart during the firing of the veneer. If bridges are soldered *after* veneering, standard gold solders may be used.

Air-fired veneers seem to tolerate the soldering operation with no ill effects. With vacuum-fired Ceramco units, a great number of fine bubbles may appear on the surface, and while their tops can be removed by polishing with a rubber wheel, the natural glazed surface of the porcelain is thus destroyed, and pits remain that may collect debris.

When veneered units are to be joined (either for bridge construction or splinting), the proximal surfaces that will be soldered must be contoured to provide enough area for the joint — larger for bridges, smaller for splinting. The longer the span, the larger the joints must be. Also, joints formed with the special solders must be a little larger if the frame for a bridge is assembled before veneering, as clinical experience and critical observation show that such joints may be less perfectly formed and therefore perhaps more liable to break.

PONTIC DESIGN

Pontics may be designed to have alloy, porcelain, or both, in contact with the ridge tissue. The authors prefer a pontic frame similar to that used with a long-pin facing, in which half or more of the ridge-contacting surface will be highly polished and correctly contoured metal, with a labiocervical or

431

buccocervical rim of porcelain. An all-porcelain ridgelap entails a more complicated technique.

The incisal edge of an anterior pontic should be reproduced in porcelain, but the lingual section, which will occlude in centric and in the beginnings of eccentric movements, should be metal in order to make future equilibration and repolishing easier. The occlusal surface of a posterior pontic is usually veneered only on a portion of the lingual inclines of the buccal cusps. The outline and area of the veneer on any pontic should simulate that of a veneer crown without a labial collar of metal on the tooth

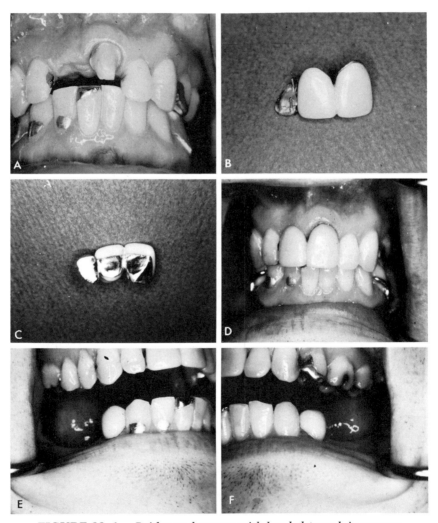

FIGURE 22–1. *Bridge and crowns with bonded porcelain veneers.*

A, Maxillary central incisor missing. Central incisor abutment prepared for veneered gold crown; lateral incisor prepared for pinledge.

B, Fused porcelain veneers on central incisor retainer and central pontic.

C, Lingual showing unsupported incisal edges of porcelain.

D, Bridge cemented. Gingival tissue covered cervical gold collar in eight days. Clasped mandibular bicuspids are restored with gold crowns with fused porcelain veneers.

E and *F*, Crowns with clasps removed.

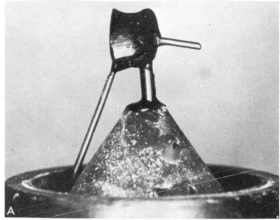

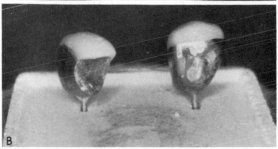

FIGURE 22-2. *A,* Pontic pattern sprued. Handle extends from lingual surface.

B, Handle supports pontic in firing tray.

being replaced. In thickness, the pontic veneer should approximate that of the veneers on adjacent retainers so that the shades will match or blend (Fig. 22-1).

Before investing the pattern for a pontic, a section of 18-gauge wax rod, 2.5 or 3.0 mm. long, is extended to form a handle at right angles from near the center of the lingual surface, although at a point that will not interfere with occlusion (Fig. 22-2). Pontics are hard to control, and this handle will expedite not only the application and firing of the porcelain, but also the grouping of the components of the fixed partial denture for soldering.

FABRICATION OF BRIDGE PRIOR TO BAKING VENEERS

Soldering Assembly

The castings are finished with stones and burs and polished with a rubber wheel. The units to be soldered are assembled on the working cast, and an occlusal or linguoincisal plaster index is formed. The units are seated in the index, and to facilitate its ready removal after the soldering assembly has hardened, any plaster past the heights of contour should be cut away, because difficulty in removal may fracture the soldering investment. The units are luted to the plaster, and the embrasures are filled with wax (Figs. 22-3 and 22-4).

Whip-Mix high-heat soldering investment, which will stand the shock of rapid heating without cracking, is mixed to a stiff putty and vibrated into the retainers and around the projections on the lingual surfaces of the pontics until a base of investment ¼ inch thick is formed. After setting for at least 30 minutes, the assembly is boiled in carbon tetrachloride or chloroform to melt and dissolve the wax. The index is removed and the investment block is trimmed. (Hot water may be used to remove the index, but cautiously, inasmuch as water will further soften an already weak investment.)

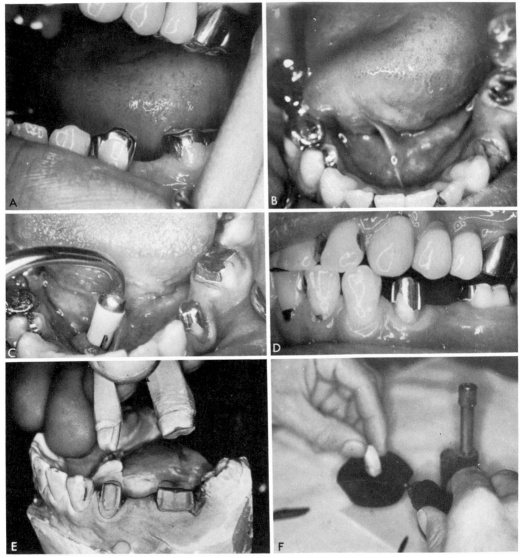

FIGURE 22–3. *Assembly of fixed prosthesis.*

A, Mandibular posterior space.
B, Restorations removed from abutments.
C and *D*, Abutments rebuilt to prepared form with castings.
E, Working cast and dies. One rubber base impression.
F, Dipping lubricated die prior to waxing pattern for retainer.

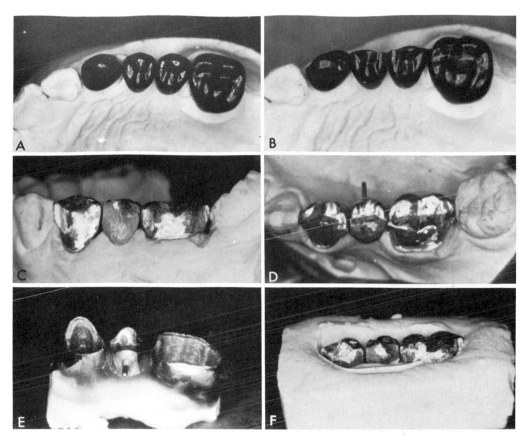

FIGURE 22-4 *A* and *B*, Wax patterns for opposing bridge. First waxed to full contour, then cut back to form for veneering.

C, Cast retainers and pontic for mandibular bridge.

D, Occlusal view of castings showing handle on pontic. This will secure it in soldering assembly.

E, Ready to pour soldering assembly. Contacts and embrasures protected by wax.

F, Soldering assembly.

Soldering

There is no call to enlarge the embrasure areas of the soldering block, as the intense, small flame of the soldering torch (Torit #77 with an A tip) will heat the area readily (Fig. 22-5).

A small amount of Ceramco flux is mixed with water to a paste, and the joint areas are fluxed. The assembly is placed in a cold furnace, speedily heated to 1300° F., and removed. A gas-oxygen torch is adjusted so that the flame measures about 3 inches, with a blue inner cone ³/₈ inch long. The castings are heated to a bright red, and pieces of Ceramco high-fusing gold solder are applied. The solder is heated until it slumps into place, at which stage the castings will have taken on a glossy appearance. A greater quantity of solder seemingly is needed to form a joint of specific size than is required to form a joint of like size with a standard gold solder.

The assembly is bench-cooled before being placed in water to aid in the

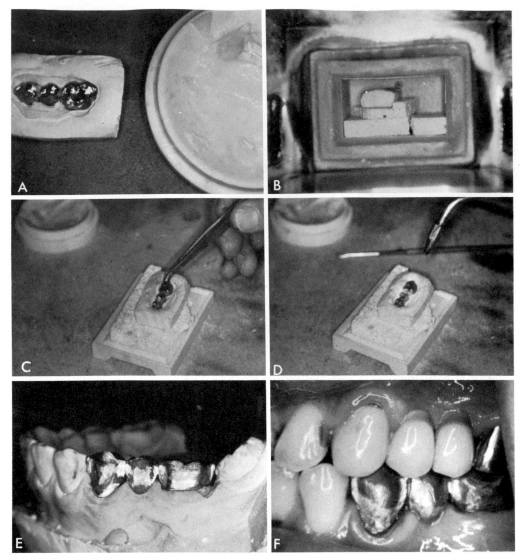

FIGURE 22–5.   *A*, Soldering assembly fluxed.

B, Drying.

C, Placing small pieces of solder.

D, Soldering.

E, Soldered and prepared frame on working cast. Cervical collar has been reduced and surfaces stoned.

F, Occlusion adjusted in mouth.

removal of the investment. It is pickled in 50 per cent hydrochloric acid to remove the flux. The cast handles are cut off and the castings are repolished to the rubber wheel stage. The veneering areas are ground with a coarse stone. The frame is equilibrated on the working cast, but it may be tried in the mouth also to determine fit and to recheck the occlusion. Prior to the application of the veneering porcelain, the bridge is placed in hydrofluoric acid and then degassed.

Veneering

Assembled units are veneered in the same way as a single unit, except that the pontics must be built to fit the ridge. Following the opaque bake, a piece of cigarette paper is cut to fit over the ridge area, moistened, and adapted to the cast (Fig. 22-6 *B*). The framework is then placed on the working cast over the cigarette paper, which will act as a separating medium between the stone and the porcelain to be built to contour against the cast (Fig. 22-6 *D*).

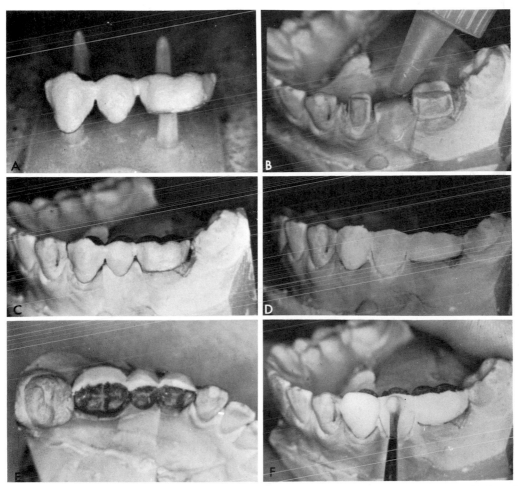

FIGURE 22-6. *A*, Prepared and degassed assembled frame with opaque applied and fired.

B, Cigarette paper adapted to ridge of working cast.

C, Frame seated over paper separating medium.

D, Body porcelain applied.

E, Occlusal view. Body porcelain tapered toward occlusal to make space for incisal porcelain.

F, Adding incisal porcelain.

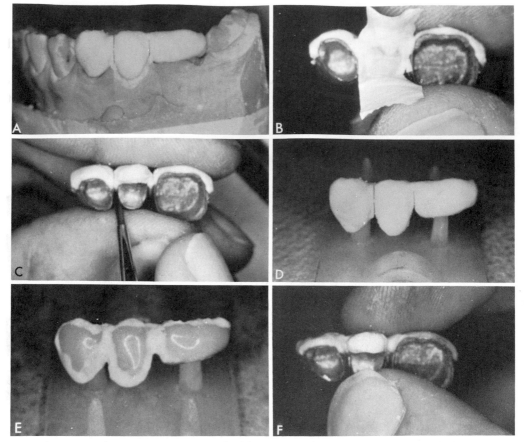

FIGURE 22-7.   *A*, Units separated with razor blade.

B, Cigarette paper attaches to pontic and must be removed.

C, Cleaning embrasures and casting surfaces not to be veneered.

D, Bridge on firing tray. Being divided, porcelain will shrink toward three centers.

E, On firing tray for second baking. Porcelain added to lines of separation, to contacting surface of pontic, and to other areas lacking contour.

F, Excess porcelain on pontic.

The veneers are built to full contour with body porcelain, with some excess to compensate for shrinkage. The area for the incisal (or occlusal) color is cut away, and the incisal porcelain is applied (see Fig. 22–6 *E* and *F*). After being carved to form, the unit veneers are separated by a razor blade. The cut must be made in the embrasure down to the previously bonded opaque layer to allow shrinkage of the porcelain toward several centers, thereby avoiding warpage of the framework (Fig. 22-7 *A*, *C*, and *D*).

The bridge is removed, and the cigarette paper, which invariably remains attached to the porcelain, is peeled away. Porcelain that has flowed into the proximal embrasures is removed with carvers and a moist brush (Fig. 22–7 *B* and *C*). The bridge is placed on a firing tray with the supports fitting up inside the abutment castings. A wide selection of trays should be at hand from which to choose one with suitable spacing between the points. At times muffle repair clay must be used, or a heavy piece of nichrome wire must be bent to form a custom-made support.

After firing, shrinkage will be found where the razor blade was used for separation and at the gingival area (Fig. 22–7 *E* and *F*). Another layer of porcelain must be added to the lines of separation, and the cervical must be overcontoured to assure that a small surplus of porcelain will remain after the second firing.

The ridge area of the working cast is blackened with a lead pencil so that, with the graphite acting as a marking agent, the bridge can be ground to fit the ridge intimately (Fig. 22-8 *A* and *B*). The general contours of the

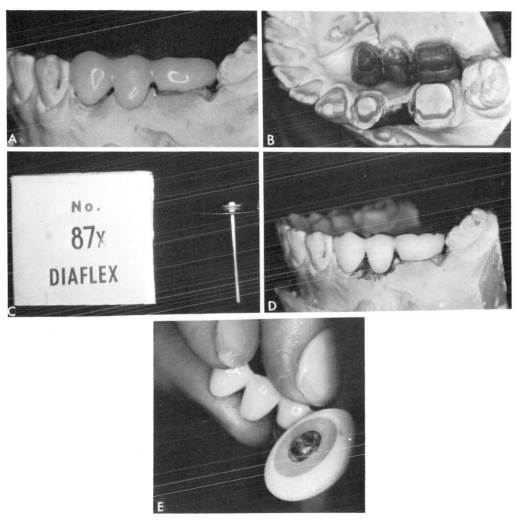

FIGURE 22–8.   *A*, Excess on pontic prevents seating of bridge.
B, Recontouring contact surface of pontic.
C, Flexible diamond disk.
D, Contoured veneers.
E, Smoothing veneers before glazing.

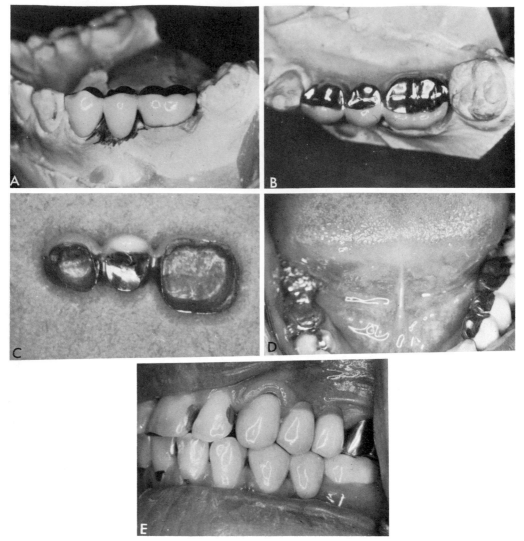

FIGURE 22–9.   *A*, *B*, and *C*, Polished and glazed bridge.
D and *E*, Bridge cemented. Bonded veneers on maxillary prosthesis.

buccal or labial surfaces are produced, using a Busch Silent stone.* The
interproximal surfaces and the contact areas are shaped with a Horico No.
87X diamond disk. This disk, being flexible and very thin, makes it possible
satisfactorily to form fine grooves between the units, which may be stained to
heighten the effect of separation. (See Chapter 16.) After contouring and
smoothing, the porcelain is glazed and the finished bridge is polished as has
been described (Figs. 22-8 *C*, *D*, and *E* and 22-9).

*Pfingst & Company, Inc., New York, N.Y.

FABRICATION OF BRIDGE AFTER
BAKING VENEERS

Soldering Veneered Units

Veneered units can be assembled and soldered without damage to the porcelain or to its surface texture, provided neither the soldering investment nor the flux contacts the veneer (Fig. 22-10). The fixed partial denture units or those to be splinted are assembled in a plaster of Paris index, and baseplate wax is flowed over the porcelain surfaces to prevent contact with investment. The soldering assembly is poured with Whip-Mix high-heat soldering investment, which must set for a minimum of ½ hour. This high-heat investment has little strength; therefore it must be reinforced to preclude fracture of the assembly, particularly when long spans are to be soldered. U-shaped stainless steel wire rods, with the tips placed inside the crowns and extending from one side of the assembly to the other, are used for reinforcements.

The soldering assembly is placed in warm water, and the index is removed. Any investment covering the wax on the porcelain surfaces is carefully cut away, and any minute particles of wax must be removed by boiling the assembly in chloroform. To avert any overflow onto the porcelain when the assembly is heated, only minimal amounts of Ceramco flux are used. It should be dried in front of the open furnace muffle for 20 minutes or more, after which, during a 10-minute interval, it is slowly introduced into the furnace (Figs. 22-11 and 22-12).

A .560 fine (or 14 carat) solder, which will fuse at about 1435° F., is the most practical for this operation. Regular crown and bridge solders are preferred to the higher fusing solders used to unite the parts prior to the application of porcelain veneers, because they fuse at lower temperatures, will fuse much more rapidly, will flow more quickly, and according to clinical observation the joints are superior, especially as to form and the absence of blemishes. By comparison, the solders designed solely for use with the

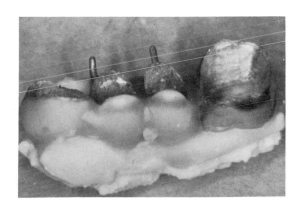

FIGURE 22-10. Glazed veneers covered with wax to protect surface from soldering investment.

veneering alloys are sluggish and have a very high fusing range. Many of these joints have discernible defects.

When a .560 fine solder is to be used, the furnace should be heated, and when a temperature of approximately 1550° F. is reached, the assembly is removed and the solder is applied to the joint areas in small pieces and in such quantity as judgment dictates. It is placed again in the furnace and left until the solder flows and the parts are well joined. The bridge or splint is cooled under a cover to room temperature before being placed in water to free it from the investment.

It is then pickled in 50 per cent hydrochloric acid to remove the flux and is polished, using the polishing Alumina (mixed with a detergent liquid),

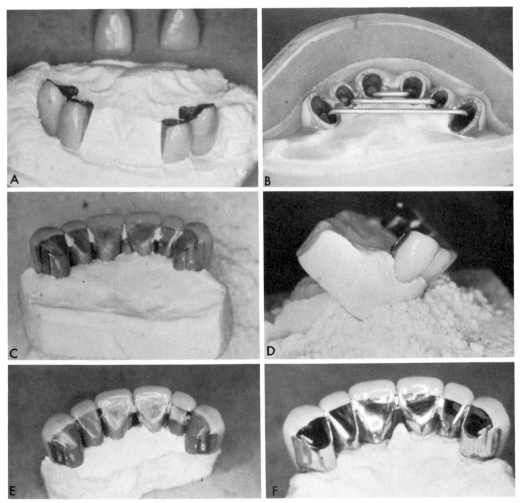

FIGURE 22–11.   *A*, Units of a splint being assembled in plaster index.
B, U-shaped stainless steel supporting rods in place, ready for pouring soldering assembly.
C, Units fluxed.
D, On firing tray to be placed in furnace for heating.
E and *F*, Six units soldered and polished.

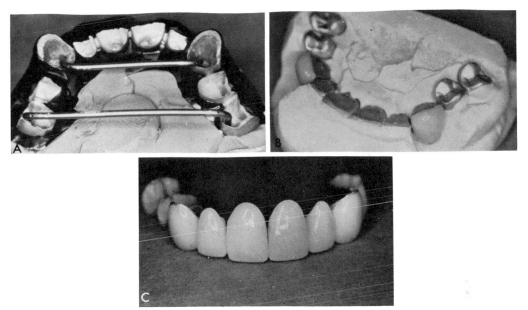

FIGURE 22–12.   *A,* Ten-unit bridge. Cuspid retainers are veneered crowns with porcelain bonded prior to assembly of prosthesis. All other units cast from standard crown and bridge alloys. Solder joints to be made from standard gold solder.

B, Soldering assembly trimmed so that no investment will touch porcelain veneers. Bicuspid units and incisor pontics soldered before this assembly. Four joints to be soldered.

C, Assembled bridge.

Amalgloss, or No. 600 Carborundum powder. Each will give a very high gloss to the surface of the metal.

See Chapter 16 for a discussion of cervical and incisal staining.

CONSTRUCTING A TEMPORARY RESIN BRIDGE

A temporary bridge, or splint, can be made before the abutments are prepared. Wax pontics can be made on a duplicate diagnostic cast and an alginate impression then taken. Shallow preparations are made on the abutments and, with the wax removed and the bridge area loaded with filling resin, the impression is seated on the prepared and lubricated cast. The resin bridge is removed, trimmed, and polished (Figs. 22-13, 22-14, and 22-15).

It may be necessary to ream the retainers before it will seat in the mouth. The prepared teeth and the surrounding tissue are coated with petroleum jelly, the retainers are coated internally with more resin, and the temporary covering is seated (Fig. 22-16).

When the resin has polymerized, the bridge is removed and the margins are trimmed. Luting is done with a weak mix of temporary cement over moist teeth.

The occlusion can be adjusted before and after cementing.

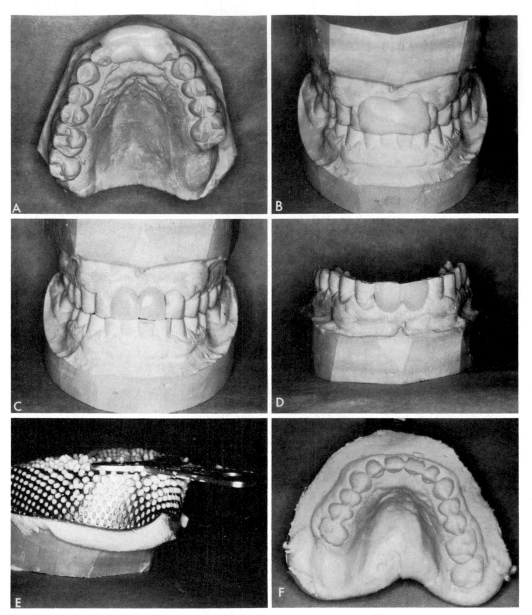

FIGURE 22–13.   *Construction of a temporary six-unit maxillary anterior bridge before preparation of abutments.*

A and *B*, Wax placed in edentulous central incisor area.
C and *D*, Central incisor pontics carved to form.
E and *F*, Alginate impression of cast with pontics.

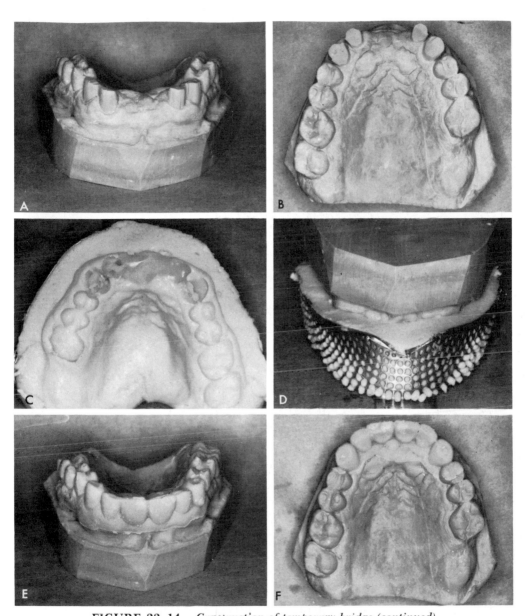

FIGURE 22–14. *Construction of temporary bridge (continued).*

A and B, Shallow preparations on abutment teeth on cast.

C, Bridge area filled with resin.

D, Loaded impression seated on cast.

E and F, Impression removed. Untrimmed bridge still in place.

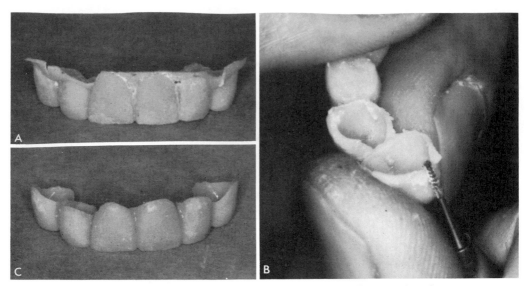

FIGURE 22-15.   *Construction of temporary bridge (continued).*

A, Resin bridge removed from cast.
B, Trimming margins.
C, Trimmed and polished bridge.

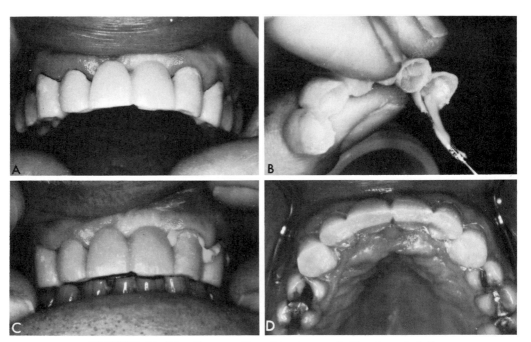

FIGURE 22-16.   *Construction of temporary bridge (concluded).*

A, Bridge does not seat fully on abutments.
B, Retainers have been reamed. Resin is placed inside.
C, Bridge seated. Excess resin forced outside.
D, Finished temporary splint fills space, covers and holds teeth in exact relationship.

REFERENCES

Johnston, J. F., Dykema, R. W., Mumford, G., and Phillips, R. W : Construction and assembly
  of porcelain veneer gold crowns and pontics. J. Pros. Den., *12*:1125, Nov.-Dec. 1962.
Johnson, J. F., Mumford, G., and Dykema, R. W.: Porcelain Veneers Bonded to Metal Castings. Practical Dental Monographs. Chicago, Year Book Medical Publishers, Inc., March
  1963.
Johnston, J. F., Mumford, G., and Dykema, R. W.: Modern Practice in Dental Ceramics.
  Philadelphia, W. B. Saunders Company, 1967.

chapter 23

THE PORCELAIN JACKET CROWN, PART I

INDICATIONS, CONTRAINDICATIONS, PREPARATION OF TEETH, AND BUILDING CROWNS USING VACUUM-FIRED AND AIR-FIRED PORCELAINS

A single-unit restoration held in much esteem today by the profession and the discriminating public is the jacket crown.[1] The word *jacket*, while not eminently technical, has been used by the profession at large to denote a porcelain or resin restoration that covers the clinical crown and terminates at or under the gingiva. It can preserve the vitality and health of the individual tooth and associated structures and maintain or satisfactorily re-establish esthetic appearance. It is used on fractured, carious, discolored, malaligned, or abraded teeth, and when the occlusion is favorable and it is constructed over a balanced preparation, it has a long life in most mouths (Fig. 23-1).

The jacket crown is contraindicated on very short teeth that would have minimal retention when prepared, many times on maxillary anteriors when the opposing teeth occlude with the cervical fifth or incisally beyond the end of the prepared tooth, or when the lingual surface is very concave and there is no cingulum on the tooth to be restored. On short teeth a veneered gold casting must be considered, but when the occlusion or tooth form is less than ideal, a jacket crown with the contacting area made of *aluminous* porcelain may be the preferred restoration.[2]

Jacket crowns are suspect also in mouths in which the teeth are grossly abraded and there is evidence of a heavy, strong, and active musculature, and when the patient is addicted to the use of a pipe or holder. *Veneered crowns* are mandatory in these instances.

If a porcelain jacket crown, which has fit, occlusion, contour, and harmonious shading, is to be constructed, there must be a broad concept, and skills that can be developed only through long hours of practice. Ceramic technique is highly personalized, and experience or a desire for perfection and an intimate knowledge of the working properties of the materials involved are expected. To grasp all the significant details of this subject, the

448

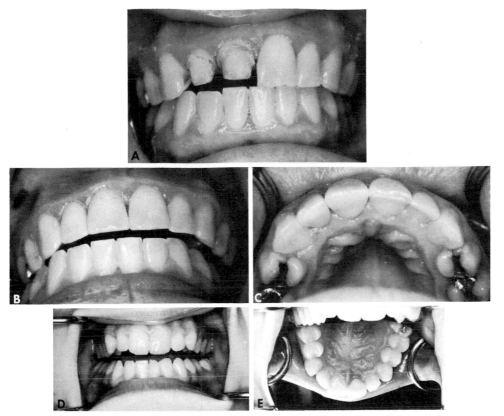

FIGURE 23–1. *A,* Maxillary central and lateral incisors partly prepared for jacket crowns. Because of fractured incisal edges, teeth had been restored with resin crowns when patient was an adolescent. Following normal gingival recession, margins were exposed.

B and *C,* Teeth rebuilt with porcelain jacket crowns. Teeth were reprepared; shoulders were placed in gingival crevices.

D and *E,* Labial and incisal views of jacket crown on left maxillary central incisor.

student (dentist or technician) must discipline himself in considerable arduous albeit fascinating preparatory study. Otherwise the result can be disappointing failure.[3]

Some of the finest examples of dental art are seen in porcelain jacket crowns, and the greatest professional gratification to be derived from clinical restorative dentistry can come from the construction and seating of such restorations. If the operator is proficient in preparing a tooth for a porcelain jacket crown and is capable of its fabrication, or has access to the services of a dependable technician, then *porcelain is the material of choice* for both anterior and posterior teeth.[4, 5]

PREPARATION

A balanced preparation is one that is made on the tooth so that the space between the mesial and distal walls and the approximating teeth will be as nearly as possible equal.[1, 2, 6, 7, 8] The length of the prepared tooth stump must be at least two-thirds of the longest incisocervical measurement of the restoration. To give general support during incising and at the mesial and distal incisal angles, the incisal edge of the preparation should be parallel with the incisal edge of the finished crown. Balance will distribute forces, reduce torque, and minimize breakage and unseating. (See Figure 23-8.)

Preparation of a Maxillary Central Incisor
Using Ultra-High Speed

A preparation can be cut in minimal time using ultra-high speed, although not more precisely than with slower techniques. With high speeds a totally indirect impression technique is best, but with the long established step-by-step method and slower cutting, copper band impressions can be made for the dies.[2]

One set of instruments used when making this preparation is shown in Figure 23-2. A hoe can be substituted for one or both chisels.

Proximal Surfaces.   The preparation is started on the proximal surfaces with a long tapered fissure carbide bur (Fig. 23-3). The bur is placed on either the labial or the lingual and the cut is made to produce a cervical shoulder at the gingival crest as wide as the smallest diameter of the bur. Cutting should be within the tooth to forestall mutilating the adjacent surface. Proximal cuts should approach parallelism and converge lingually about the same degree as the planes of the uncut surfaces.

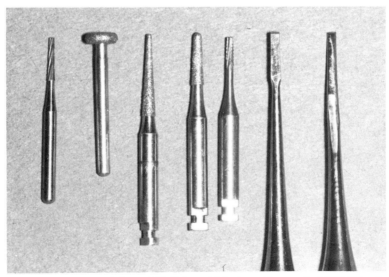

FIGURE 23-2.   Left to right: 169L-FG carbide bur (Densco); 110P-FG wheel diamond stone (Starlite); ¼D-L latch tapered diamond stone (Densco); 1D-T latch tapered diamond stone (Densco); 556 latch carbide bur (S.S.W.); #10 straight Tarno chisel (S.S.W.); #22-23 Wedelstaedt chisel.

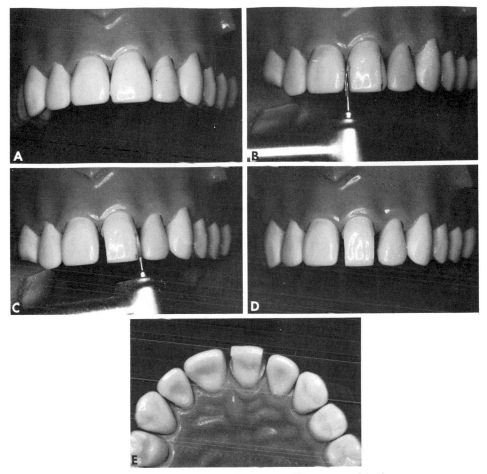

FIGURE 23–3. *Preparation on maxillary central incisor.*

A, Labial view of field.
B, Cuts outlined. Bur in position.
C, First proximal reduction. Bur in place for second cut.
D and *E*, Labial and incisal views of proximal cuts.

Incisal Edge and Lingual Surface. The incisal edge (Fig. 23-4) and the lingual surface are reduced with a round-edge wheel diamond stone. Preparation of the incisal edge may follow the routine described for the porcelain veneered crown. Incisal clearance should be 1.5 mm., with the flat surface at right angles to the line of thrust from the occluding teeth. The lingual reduction should be approximately 1.0 mm. in depth.

Labial Surface. Preparation of the labial surface (Fig. 23-5) is also the same as for the veneered crown. The section to the incisal of the height of contour is grooved to a depth of 1.0 mm. and reduced uniformly mesially and distally. Then the cervical area is grooved (in another plane) and reduced (Fig. 23-6).

The Shoulder. With slow speed the shoulder is extended 0.5 mm. into the gingival crevice (Fig. 23-7), using a cylindrical or tapered diamond stone

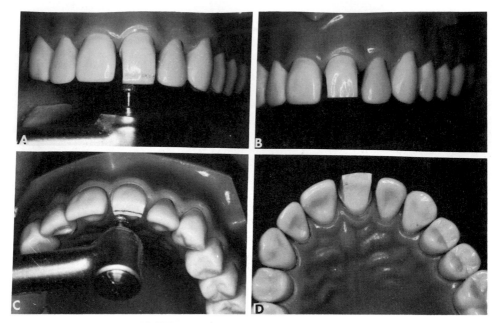

FIGURE 23-4. *Preparation (continued).*

A, Incisal reduction outlined.
B, Incisal shortened.
C, Depth of lingual reduction marked on incisal.
D, Lingual reduced to height of contour on cingulum.

or a fissure or end-cutting bur. Some operators favor a small, narrow wheel stone (Fig. 23-6 *E*) that must be supplemented interproximally by other stones or burs. The shoulder is finished with a hoe or chisel. The shoulder should angle apically 5 degrees from the long axis of the tooth.

The vertical surfaces, angles, and corners are smoothed with sandpaper disks (Fig. 23-7 *C*). When the gingival crevice is deeper than usual, the preparation may go farther into it. When recession has bared the cementoenamel line, the preparation should stop there (Fig. 23-8).

Preparation of a Maxillary Anterior Tooth Using Slow Speeds

The step-by-step preparation of an anterior tooth using slow speeds can be accomplished by

(1) reduction of the mesial and distal surfaces without forming a shoulder;

(2) reduction of the incisal edge (steps 1 and 2 may be reversed);

(3) reduction of the lingual surface, one-half at a time (the first cut to be used as a guide for the remaining half);

(4) reduction of the labial surface, one-half at a time (steps 3 and 4 may be reversed);

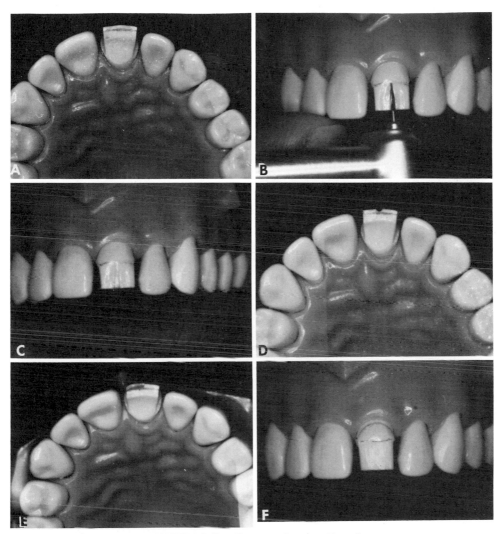

FIGURE 23–5. *Preparation (continued).*

A, Depth of labial reduction marked on incisal.
B, *C*, and *D*, Cutting groove, incisal three-fifths of labial surface.
E and *F*, Reduction of labial surface incisally from height of contour.

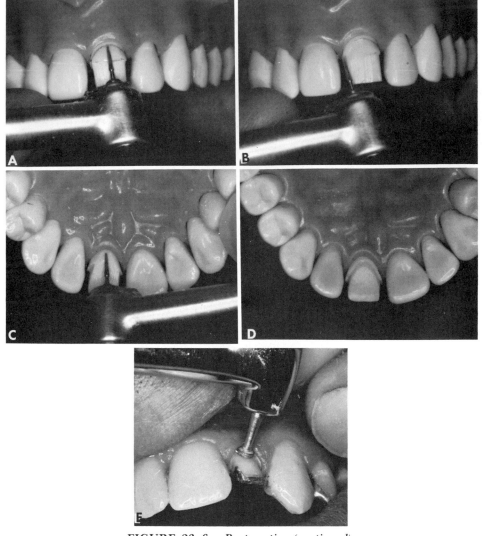

FIGURE 23–6. *Preparation (continued).*

A, Grooving cervical segment of labial surface.

B, Reducing cervical segment.

C, D, and *E,* Reducing lingual of cingulum; shoulder partially formed, but not extended into gingival crevice.

    (5) rounding the angles to fashion a continuous cervical finishing line at the gingival crest;

    (6) fitting the copper band;

    (7) further reduction of the tooth and preparation of the shoulder; and

    (8) rounding all angles except at the shoulder (Figs. 23–9 and 23–10).

Axial Preparation Before Shoulder.   The mesial and distal slices are made using a disk in a straight handpiece, with the impregnated surface of the disk toward the pulp. The cut should be made through the tooth structure to the gingival line, and without forming a cervical shoulder it should converge a few degrees both incisally and lingually.

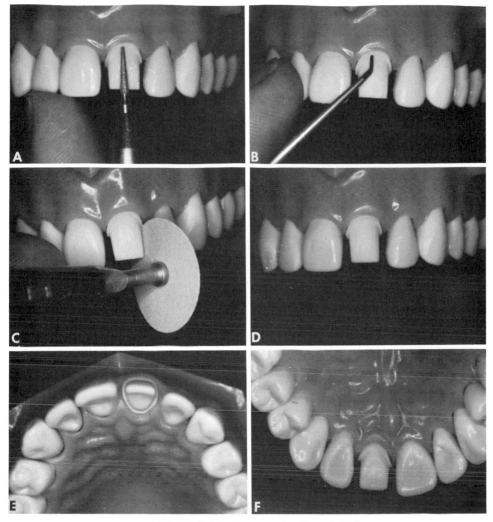

FIGURE 23–7. *Preparation (concluded).*

A, Extending shoulder into gingival crevice.
B, Toilet of shoulder.
C, Smoothing vertical surfaces.
D, *E*, and *F*, Finished preparation.

The incisal edge can be reduced with a wheel stone of appropriate size, and ordinarily this same stone may be used to reduce the labial surface. The clearance at the incisal edge should be 1.5 mm. plus, at right angles to the line of force from the opposing teeth, and evenly from mesial to distal. It is not important that the incisal reduction be at right angles to the long axis of the tooth.

The lingual surface should be prepared with a round-edge wheel stone. The natural contour must be approximated, with 1.0 mm. clearance at all points or paths of contact. The labial reduction, conforming to or slightly increasing the convex tooth contour in the incisal half, must be deep enough

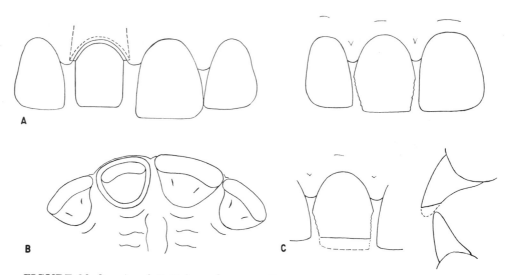

FIGURE 23-8. *A* and *B*, Balanced preparation.
C, Incisal reduced for thickness of material and for resistance to thrusts from opposing teeth.

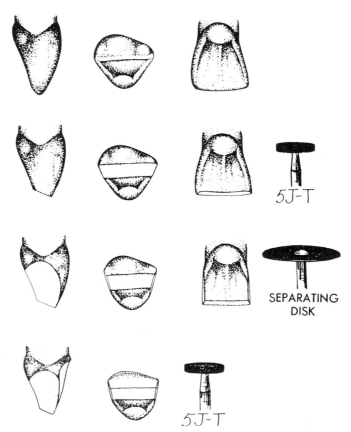

FIGURE 23-9. *Preparation of a maxillary central incisor.*

Top to bottom: Uncut tooth; reduction of incisal edge (this can precede or follow proximal slices); proximal slices made; labial surface cut.

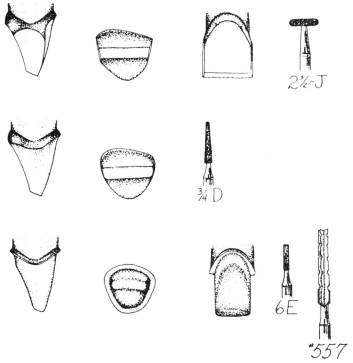

FIGURE 23–10. *Preparation (continued).*

Top to bottom: Lingual surface reduced; corners rounded, band fitted at this time; shoulder cut.

so that the outline of the underlying tooth structure cannot be seen or so that cement will not adversely alter the shade of the crown. The incisal edge and angles must be observed for assurance that this has been done.

The four angles are rounded so that the temporary cervical margin is at and copies the contour of the gingival crest. Thus far the same rotating cutting instruments and instrumentation have been used as were specified for the veneered crown preparation.

It is to be noted that the reduction of teeth for jacket crowns should be done only partially with accelerated speeds. The preparation can be made as far as a chamfered cervical, using the same stones or burs and the accelerated speeds designated for the veneered crown. However, the shoulder should be completed and positioned more deliberately and can be done very successfully by the methods to be discussed in this chapter. If a copper band is to be used, it should be adapted prior to cutting the shoulder.

Copper Band Fitted (If Needed). A copper band can be fitted and contoured with the least difficulty before the tooth is further reduced and the shoulder cut (Fig. 23–11). *For rubber impression materials,* the band must clear the tooth by 0.3 mm. at all points. *For impression compound,* it should be of such size that, when slipped over the preparation, the cervical portion will be flared a very little and extend a little less than 1.0 mm. into the gingival crevice. *For either kind of impression,* it should be cut to conform to the outline of the gingival margin.

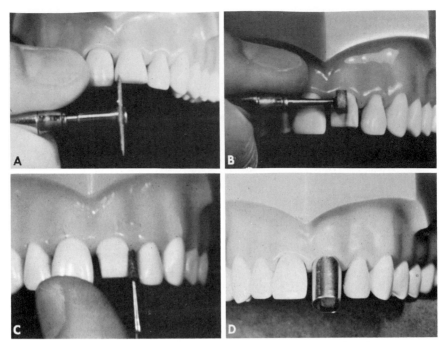

FIGURE 23-11. *Preparing tooth for fitting band.*

A, Proximal cut without shoulder.

B, Labial surface reduced one-half at a time with wheel stone flat surface parallel to long axis.

C, Corners rounded with long tapered stone and reduced labial surfaces smoothed.

D, Copper band fitted to cervical contour.

Forming the Shoulder.   With the use of a cylindrical or tapered stone, the tooth structure around the cervical half of the tooth should now be reduced more to outline the shoulder and to make the walls converge 5 to 7 degrees toward the incisal (Fig. 23-12). The shoulder, 0.7 mm. wide, can be cut with a No. 557 or an end-cutting bur or with a cylindrical diamond, and finished with hand instruments to smooth the enamel and dentin. It should simulate the curves of the gingival line and extend into the crevice 0.5 mm., or one-half the depth of the crevice. The shoulder should incline (Fig. 23-13) into the crevice from 5 to 10 degrees, forming an angle of approximately 85 to 80 degrees apically toward the long axis of the tooth (Fig. 23-12).

All axioproximal line angles and mesioincisal and distoincisal point angles must be rounded so that they will not act as cleavage points to induce fracture of the crown (Fig. 23-13), yet the taper should not be increased. If the surface of the preparation is smooth, it will be easier to secure an unblemished impression.

Nuttall's Method.   Nuttall[9] uses a somewhat different but logical technique in the preparation for a jacket crown, reducing the labial, mesial, distal, and incisal, and forming the shoulder on these segments of the cervical. He says:

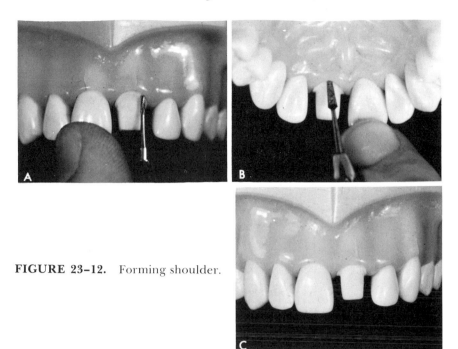

FIGURE 23–12.   Forming shoulder.

"The steps in a routine preparation for the complete porcelain veneer crown may be satisfactorily executed by the average willing operator. However, producing the lingual shoulder often presents difficulties in its clinical management which may be overcome by employing the following approach to the problem [Fig. 23–14].

"The enamel should be reduced mesio-distally at the lingual gingival area with a 4 mm. diameter mounted wheel (#34 Starlite) with abrasive on all surfaces. The initial reduction must establish a shoulder the same thickness of the instrument and extending into the gingival crevice. [See Fig. 23–14 *A*.]

"A 9 mm. diameter 'safe-on-inside' wheel (#39 S I Starlite) can be used to round the lingual proximal angles and to extend the shoulder in an interproximal direction. [See Fig. 23–14 *B*.]

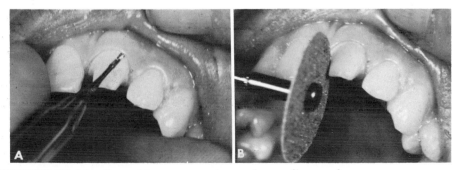

FIGURE 23–13.   Smoothing preparation and rounding angles.

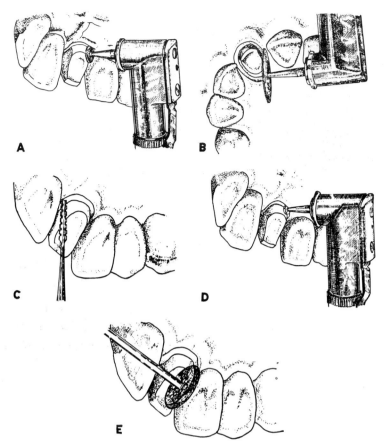

FIGURE 23–14. Preparation of the lingual shoulder on a maxillary central incisor. (Courtesy of Dr. E. B. Nuttall.)

"The lingual and proximal shoulders can be connected with a #700 tapering crosscut fissure bur. [See Fig. 23–14 *C*.]

"The shoulder finishing instrument (#45 Starlite) should have abrasive only on the periphery and be used to finish the lingual shoulder. [See Fig. 23–14 *D*.]

"The lingual enamel must be removed now with a round edge mounted wheel of suitable diameter (#32 R Starlite). [See Fig. 23–14 *E*.]

"RATIONALE. The procedure of lingual preparation is frequently approached incorrectly, the enamel being completely removed before the shoulder is prepared, and since dentine does not resist the axial penetration of rotary instruments, this usually results in a lingual shoulder which is too wide.

"In the procedure suggested and illustrated, the enamel in the cingulum area prevents the extension of the preparation in an axial direction. Thus a shoulder of uniform width may be completed to the desired depth."

The technique devised by Nuttall is simple, rapid, and safe. It can be used readily by the novice if he will have the instruments available in the order of use.

Modifications. On an upper lateral or a lower incisor, because of the constricted neck in relation to the width of the pulp, a No. 556 or 56 bur should be used to make a narrower shoulder. Ideally the shoulder should be the same width on both the mesial and distal surfaces, but it may be necessary to make one side wider and one narrower in order that the prepared tooth stump will more closely approximate the center of the space to give balanced support to the crown.

Some clinicians favor a preparation without a shoulder on lower incisors and other small teeth, a heavy chamfer being substituted for the shoulder. Labially it is placed in the gingival crevice, while on the lingual the margin generally is found at the height of contour on the cingulum. The incisal edge of the prepared tooth must be wide both mesiodistally and labiolingually, and it is theorized that a thin layer of enamel should be left covering the dentin so that there will be no elasticity in the tooth stump. This preparation and the crowns constructed for it are effective only in the hands of the truly expert clinician.

Preparation on Pulpless Tooth

When an anterior tooth has been fractured or mutilated by caries, or is pulpless, it must be restored to prepared form with a cast core supported by a post in the root canal (Figs. 23-15 and 23-16) or by pins extending into the dentin, or it may be rebuilt with resin, which is considered by some to have advantages esthetically. When a metal core is used,[2] the depth of reduction on the labial surface should be greater, so that the extra thickness of the crown will completely hide the prepared tooth stump. If additional tooth reduction and crown bulk are not possible, an opaque liner that will mask the prepared tooth can be used in constructing the crown (Figs. 23-17 and 23-18).

THE DIE AND WORKING CAST

The gingival tissue must be displaced laterally or prepared surgically before a polysulfide rubber impression is taken. The preparation segment of the impression is poured with stone and is set aside for 1 hour. It is removed and sectioned and the replica of the prepared tooth is trimmed to die form (Figs. 23-19 and 23-20).

An elastic impression exactly duplicates the prepared area and the tooth contour beyond it. In jacket crown construction, the undercut that extends cervically beyond the shoulder causes considerable inconvenience in the removal of a platinum matrix. A technique planned to overcome this has the undercut waxed out approximately 3.0 mm. apically from the margin of the shoulder, the wax diverging from 3 to 5 degrees. A suitable copper band (that is, one that will have 0.3 to 0.5 mm. clearance at all points) is closed on one end with impression compound, the interior is coated with rubber ce-

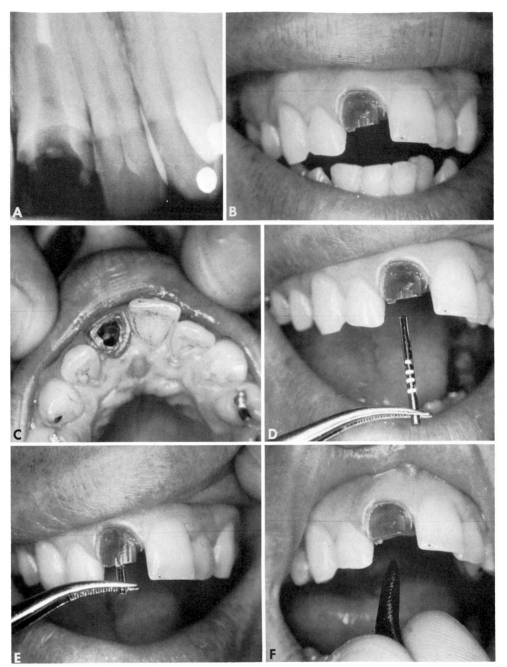

FIGURE 23–15. *A*, Radiograph of maxillary central incisor. Canal has been enlarged to receive post.

B and *C*, Darkened tooth has been semiprepared. Shoulder not extended into crevice.

D and *E*, Post cut to length, serrated, and tried in canal. Extends beyond incisal edge to give area for pliers to grasp it when pattern is removed.

F, Placing cone of wax into canal.

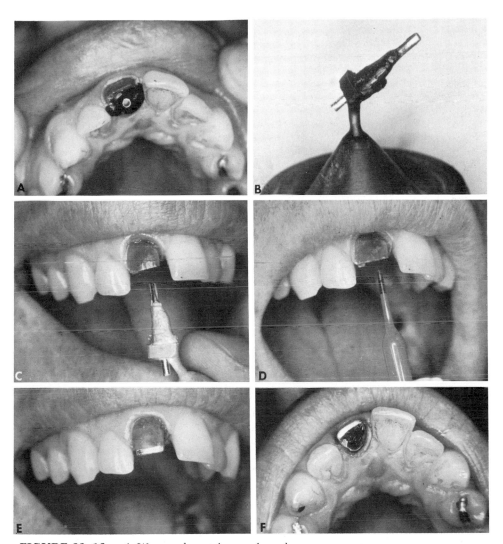

FIGURE 23–16.   *A*, Wax and post in canal ready to carve pattern.
B, Pattern sprued.
C, Casting being fitted.
D, Placing cement in canal. Casting must be seated with light mallet pressure.
E and *F*, Casting cemented. Preparation completed.

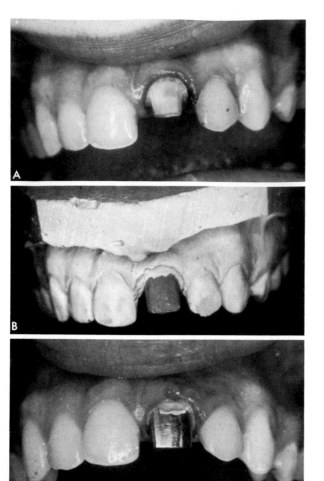

FIGURE 23–17. *A*, Tooth stump too short and too conical to support jacket crown. Two porcelain crowns built for this tooth had fractured; one resin crown came off.

B, Cast ferrule designed to restore tooth to correct prepared form.

C, Completed preparation.

ment, and a polysulfide rubber impression is taken of the stone die, which no longer has a cervical undercut. The impression is silver-plated (see Chapter 10) and a stone core is poured and trimmed (Fig. 23-21).

The silver-plated die is seated in the original rubber base impression and luted to it with baseplate wax, and an intact full arch working cast is poured in stone and allowed to set for 1 hour. The gingival area around the die is cut away to a depth of 3.0 to 4.0 mm. on all sides. If the root of the silver-plated die was lubricated with petrolatum, it can be removed from the cast.

The working and opposing casts should be mounted on an articulator capable of being guided in protrusive or lateral excursions by the approximating and posterior teeth. If only a single anterior crown is being built, and if the matured porcelain form can be taken to the tooth to adjust occlusion, it is permissible to dispense with the articulator.

The original dies, *with* the cervical undercuts, should be preserved, so

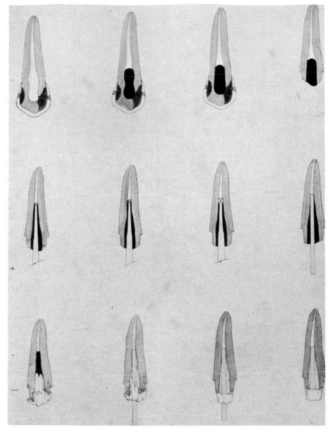

FIGURE 23–18. *Rebuilding maxillary cuspid to prepared form.*

Top row: Filling canal and preparing remaining coronal structure.
Middle row: Enlarging canal and fitting post.
Bottom row: Forming pattern, fitting casting, finished preparation.

that the curves of the uncut tooth beyond the shoulder can be observed and extended onto the cervical of the crown.

TEMPORARY PROTECTION

Careful protection of the tooth can contribute much to jacket crown success.[10] If the gingival tissue is pushed aside from the shoulder only enough so that later the field may be dry during cementation, normalcy will recur almost immediately and the probability of gingival recession will be minimized. Temporary crowns should have the strength to withstand ordinary chewing and dislodging motions, and should be adjusted to the occlusion to forestall any change in tooth position. All rough edges and sharp points must be removed after fitting.

Self-curing resin should be used for the temporary crown (Fig. 23-22). It can be fabricated on a cast over a simulated preparation, rather than on

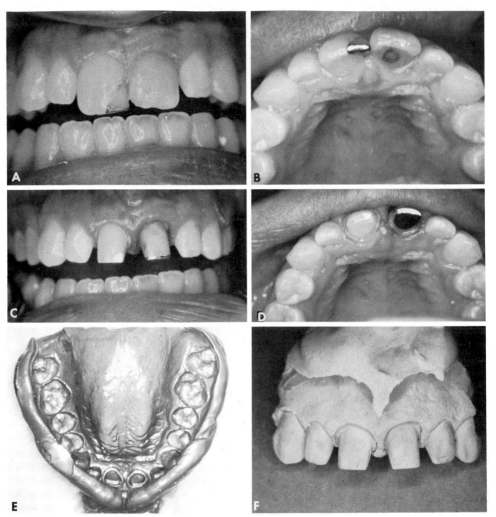

FIGURE 23–19.   *A* and *B*, Adolescent patient. Left maxillary central pulpless. Right central has receded pulp, due to blow, fracture, and restoration.

C and *D*, Teeth prepared. Pulpless tooth restored to prepared form with cemented cast core. Incisal angle of right central recontoured with cement.

E, Complete arch polysulfide rubber impression.

F, Cast of prepared area.

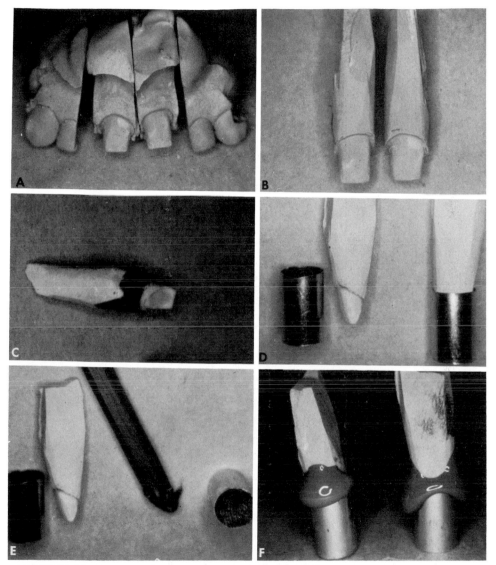

FIGURE 23–20.   *A* and *B*, Cast sectioned for stone dies.
C, One stone die showing cervical contour undercut waxed out.
D and *E*, Fitting and preparing copper bands for impressions of stone dies.
F, Elastic impressions of stone dies.

the tooth. While the effect of the heat generated during curing of the resin will not be experienced, there are the disadvantages of poor fit and time used in adjustment. The preparation on the cast may be lubricated or covered with tin foil and the crown form trimmed to fit the shoulder. Incisal and cervical shades should be selected, mixed, and distributed inside a crown form or an alginate impression, which must be seated in alignment, and the resin given time to polymerize. The contacts of a crown form should be perforated with a No. 6 bur so that the temporary cover will have the width to maintain the space. Before it is cemented with zinc oxide and eugenol

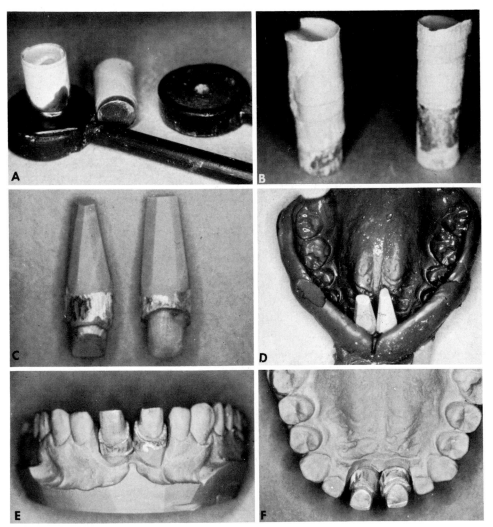

FIGURE 23–21.   *A,* Impression attached for plating with silver.
B, Roots poured.
C, Dies.
D, Placed in same impression from which stone dies were poured.
E and *F,* Working cast was not articulated because matured crowns were fitted in mouth.

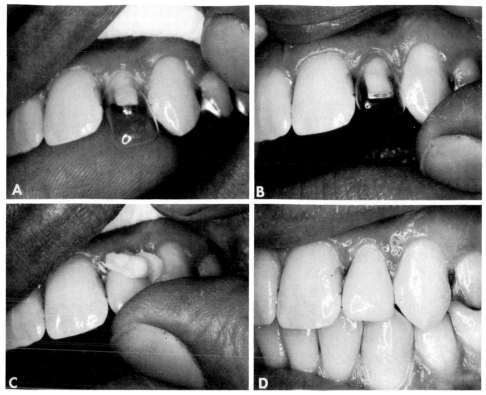

FIGURE 23–22.   *Temporary covering for prepared tooth.*

A and *B*, Fitting celluloid crown form.
C, Crown form filled with resin and seated.
D, Luted temporary crown. Crown form remains in this instance.

over a lubricated stump, it should be machined internally to seat, trimmed at the cervical, and adjusted to the occlusion.

Many operators fabricate the temporary crown on the prepared tooth. If the tooth to be restored is mutilated, it is recontoured with wax on the diagnostic cast and an alginate impression is made. Then, with resin in the tooth being rebuilt, the impression is seated in the mouth over a lubricated stump. Soft tissue is protected by petroleum jelly. When the resin has begun to stiffen, the impression is removed; while it is still slightly flexible, the temporary crown is taken off, given time to harden, and trimmed. It is seated with a zinc oxide and eugenol luting material on the stump, and the crown is polished.

Although shading will probably not satisfy the patients, they are disposed to accept this situation for short periods. Better shade distribution is possible when the temporary crown is built on a prepared cast. Resiliency of the resin will allow removal, whenever expedient, without destroying the crown.

For shade selection and distribution, see Chapter 19, Esthetic Criteria in a Porcelain Restoration.

THE MATRIX

The matrix, which should be made of 0.001 inch dead-soft platinum foil, is the foundation for the construction of the crown. Platinum seems to have an affinity for porcelain and will not discolor it. It can be adapted to many shapes without destroying its continuity of surface. The one drawback is that it has an annoying attraction for most contaminating elements or substances. It should be kept in an envelope or clean box, away from all metal grindings. Porcelain has an equal affinity for contaminants, particularly those harbored on the platinum foil. Green discoloration around the gingival of a fired jacket crown usually is caused by the die, but internal porosity is the result of a number of contaminating influences on the platinum.[11]

A platinum matrix should be softened or cleaned by heating in the area of combustion, *not* in the cone of a Bunsen burner flame. It may be annealed or heated in the furnace to a temperature 25 to 50 degrees higher than the fusing point of the porcelain to be used. This is especially important before vacuum firing, when the matrix must be degassed at 2450° F. if high-fusing porcelain is being used.

The instruments needed for forming a matrix are scissors, cotton pliers of stainless steel or some noncorrosive metal, an orangewood stick pointed on one end and flattened on the other, a burnisher shaped like a nailhead on one end and with near-parallel sides on the other, soldering tweezers, a mallet, a swage, and a small, fine-grit wheel stone. Usually a marked cardboard guide is included by the manufacturer in the envelope with the platinum (Fig. 23-23).

The proximal joint concept is a product of evolution, and it appears that the reasons for placement here were founded on Pettrow's[11] research on functional breakage. When the tinner's joint is placed on the lingual surface of a maxillary anterior die, there will be a line of cleavage in the lingual surface of the porcelain crown. Since this surface receives the thrust from the opposing teeth, the possibility of fracture is increased. One of the fundamentals of jacket crown construction is that bulk adds strength. Generally one of the proximal quadrants of a jacket has the greatest thickness; therefore, if the folded joint of the matrix is moved to that surface, the crown will be stronger.

Technique—Proximal Joint. Before the matrix is formed, the die must be scrubbed with chloroform to remove the oils or other contaminants from the impression. A rectangular piece of platinum is used (Fig. 23-24 *A*), approximately 5.0 mm. wider than the longest incisocervical measurement of the preparation. It is applied to whichever proximal surface will be thinner in the finished crown. It is held in position and pushed around the die with the thumb and first finger (Fig. 23-24 *B*), then held tight with the thumb and finger of the other hand (Fig. 23-24 *C*). The platinum is molded to the shoulder with a wedge-shaped orangewood stick or a plastic burnisher (Fig. 23-24 *D*). The protruding ends of the platinum are grasped with cotton

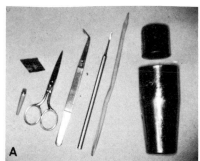

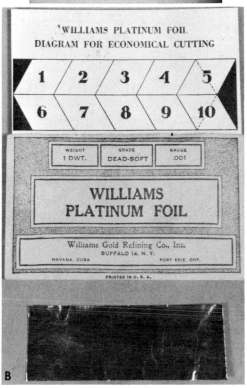

FIGURE 23–23. *A*, Instruments used in forming a platinum matrix: die and platinum, scissors, pliers, burnisher, orangewood stick, swage.

B, Platinum foil and diagram for cutting.

pliers (Fig. 23-24 *E*) and pulled close against the proximal surface of the die. While the platinum is being held in position with the fingers, the flaps are trimmed to 1.5 mm. in width (Fig. 23-24 *F*). On this same side, the platinum at the incisal edge is cut away at a 45-degree angle; on the opposite proximal surface, it is slit or cut from the top to the edge of the die (Fig. 23-24 *G*). The two incisal tabs are shortened in length to approximately 1.0 mm. (Fig. 23-24 *H*).

A tinner's joint is formed with the bend placed at the midline of the platinum extension (Fig. 23-25 *A*). The added 0.001 inch of platinum on this surface will not materially lessen the strength of the porcelain crown. After the tinner's joint has been made, the labioincisal flap is folded over the lingual (Fig. 23-25 *B*), then the lingual flap is folded over the incisal edge toward the labial surface (Fig. 23-25 *C*).

The platinum is burnished from incisal to cervical and all wrinkles are eliminated (Fig. 23–25 D). The burnishing is continued over the shoulder and down onto the apron, which should be about 3.0 mm. in width. Before swaging, the matrix is removed and the collar is trimmed to approximately 2.5 mm. in its shortest dimension and made square with the long axis of the matrix so that it can be seated and will stand without toppling. The die and the matrix are placed in the swage, and the matrix is adapted to the surface of the die. After swaging it is removed with sticky wax, and the sticky wax is melted off with a torch flame because the oxidizing areas can be controlled more thoroughly than with a Bunsen burner flame. The matrix is heated to a cherry red to render it less brittle and to remove any impurities.

The matrix is replaced on the die and burnished while being wrapped with and held in position by twisted gauze (Fig. 23–25 E). It is examined for wrinkles (Fig. 23–25 F); if any are found, they must be obliterated by burnishing, as they function as cleavage lines and thereby weaken the crown.

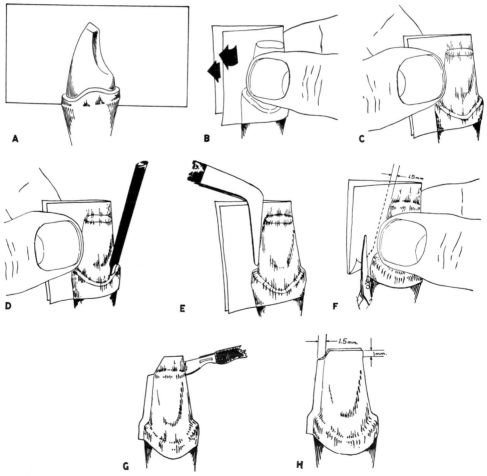

FIGURE 23–24.   Matrix construction.

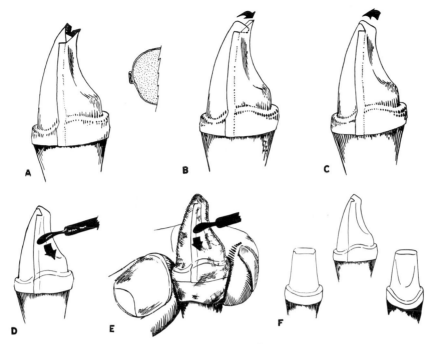

FIGURE 23-25. Matrix construction (continued).

The excess platinum of the tinner's joint over the shoulder can be stoned away. This indentation will not serve as a line of cleavage.

Before reseating of the die and matrix, all areas of the working cast that may contact the porcelain during building the crown are painted with a solution of chloroform and clear acrylic powder. This seals the surface of the stone so that water from the porcelain mixture will not be drawn off into the cast.

Technique — Lingual Joint. The foil must be placed on the labial of the die so that it covers both the shoulder and the incisal edge; it should be held in position by the first finger while the die is grasped by the thumb and second and third fingers. The ends are pulled together around and at the center of the lingual surface. With the matrix held in this position and using the flattened end of the orangewood stick, the platinum is burnished to conform to the labial and proximal surfaces and shoulder of the die. The platinum is grasped with the cotton pliers and closed tight against the lingual surface so that the excess and the two ends project from and at right angles to the lingual surface. The platinum is cut at the corners from the topmost labial edge to the incisal of the die. The lingual is opened and a triangular piece is removed on each side, making the second cuts continuous with the incisal edge and at right angles to the first. The labioincisal extension is cut off, leaving about 3.0 mm. to be folded lingually over the incisal and onto the lingual surface. The lingual flaps are closed again and the folds drawn tight with the cotton pliers. The flaps are trimmed so that the lingual extension of each is 1.5 mm. Either the right or the left flap is narrowed by one-half and

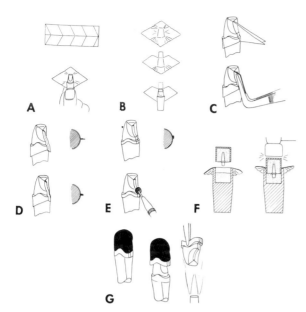

FIGURE 23–26.   *Construction of platinum matrix.*

A, Diamond of platinum pushed against die.

B, Flap cut and burnished over linguoincisal.

C, Ends pulled tight on lingual surface.

D, Flaps trimmed and folded to start tinner's joint.

E, Fold continued to left, completing tinner's joint; excess platinum taken off shoulder.

F, Matrix swaged on die for closest possible adaptation.

G, Matrix covered with sticky wax, removed, and wax melted off.

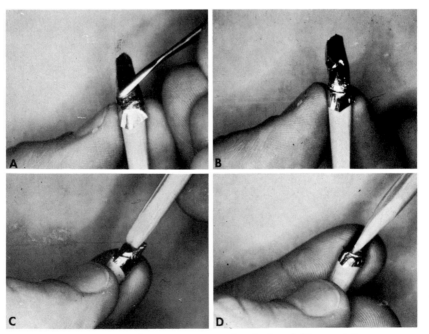

FIGURE 23–27.   *Instrumentation in burnishing matrix.*

A, Platinum being burnished to labial surface and shoulder.

B, Labial burnished, ready to cut incisal flap.

C, Burnishing tinner's joint.

D, Burnishing shoulder.

both are readapted to the lingual surface. The longer flap is folded over the shorter, the bend being made at the margin of the shorter flap (Fig. 23-26).

Folding is continued in the same direction, to form a tinner's joint. The folded lingual surface and shoulder must be burnished with the orangewood stick (Fig. 23-27). The matrix is covered with sticky wax and removed. The irregular apron is trimmed evenly so that 2.0 mm. of platinum foil will extend cervically at all points beyond the shoulder to stiffen the matrix during manipulation and waxing. The wax is melted off and the platinum is annealed at the same time. The matrix is replaced on the die, burnished with the stick and, with the use of a swage, is given the closest possible adaptation to the die. This is essential in the construction of any jacket crown. Again the matrix should be covered with sticky wax and removed. After the wax has been melted off, the matrix is placed on the die, wrapped in gauze, and burnished incisocervically to remove or smooth any minute wrinkles. It is returned to the working cast after the stone around the shoulder of the die is trimmed away, so that the platinum will not be distorted.

A small, fine-grit wheel stone can be used on the shoulder area of the matrix to remove three of the four layers of platinum in the tinner's joint.

BUILDING AND FIRING THE CROWN

It should be stated again that dental ceramics must be an expression of the individual. There are no substitutes for enforced experience, a penchant for perfection, and an encompassing knowledge of the equipment and materials to be used, but the technique and art can be learned by anyone who is willing to expend the effort.

Before constructing a jacket crown of fused porcelain, the dentist or technician should remember these three points:
1. "There are no short cuts in ceramics except not to do it."[12]
2. The firing of porcelain is accumulative; it is a combination of temperature plus time that equals maturity.
3. Equally pleasing crowns can be built from either vacuum-fired or air-fired porcelain.

Assuming that the die, or reproduction of the prepared tooth, is exact, there are three factors that must be combined in their application and use to create a porcelain jacket crown: the platinum matrix, the furnace, and the porcelain.

The platinum must be adapted to the die intimately, *without wrinkles,* and with minimal thickness in the area of the tinner's joint. The eccentricities of the furnace must be recognized, the firing chamber must be clean, uncontaminated, and capable of being closed to contain the heat, and the pyrometer must be adjusted within the range of acceptable accuracy. Distilled water must be used with the porcelain powder to form the paste from which the jacket will be built to oversize form for firing.

Mixing the Powder.   The proportions of gingival and incisal powders should be placed on separate glass slabs. The powders (for example, two parts No. 6, one part No. 4, and six parts No. 8) must be incorporated thoroughly before the addition of distilled water. Heavy spatulation with a metal instrument must be avoided, else the porcelain will be contaminated by metallic particles. Porcelain is an abrasive, and minute bits of the metal will be transferred to the powder if pressure from the spatula is accompanied by movement (Fig. 23-28). When a heavy cream consistency has been reached, the mix, while remaining on the slab, should be vibrated to remove air bubbles. The porcelain can be mixed and kept in a mound with the spatula. It must remain moist during the working period and be covered between firings. Dry porcelain powder cannot be worked, so water should be added and the mix vibrated before each build-up. This will help to eliminate entrapped air and will aid condensation. Moist porcelain powder will build with more ease and will be freer of bubbles if applied to the matrix with a spatula or bladed instrument rather than a brush. Excess beyond the angle of the shoulder can be trimmed away.

Cervical Contact Technique

The First Firing or Foundation.   During firing, porcelain will shrink toward its bulkiest area and toward the surface to which it is attached. The first bake in making a jacket crown can establish the cervical fit if the porcelain is contoured to place the bulk in the cervical fourth and to appose the marginal area. The first application of porcelain should be very thin over the incisal half or two-thirds of the matrix and overbuilt in the cervical fifth or fourth. Porcelain of the gingival shade should be used (Fig. 23–29).

Condensation is gained through light vibration from a serrated instrument and by absorbing the surface moisture with clean gauze. Vibration should be restrained so that the porcelain will not roll or flow out of position, and blotting should take place immediately upon evidence of any moisture on the surface. When moisture no longer comes to the surface, it can be

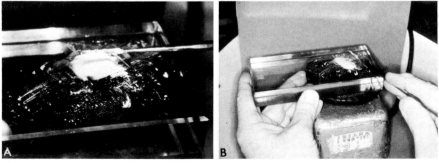

FIGURE 23–28.   *A,* Mixing measured portions of porcelain powder and water. *B,* Vibrating mix.

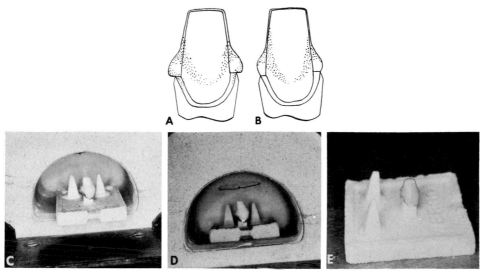

FIGURE 23–29. *First bake.*

A, Cross section of first application of porcelain.
B, Cross section of first application after firing.
C, First application drying in muffle opening.
D, In muffle; note relation to thermocouple.
E, After firing.

taken for granted that condensation is sufficient, although it cannot be complete because of the shape of the particles.[13, 14]

Air-Fired 2400° Porcelain. The "green" porcelain crown should be placed on top of the furnace, or in the preheating chamber, for a minimal time of 10 minutes, and dried completely and slowly so that no cracking will occur. The temperature at which the porcelain is inserted into the furnace is not critical, but in order that there will be no possibility that steam formation will cause an explosion within the crown, it should be placed in front of the open muffle at approximately 1200° F., or lower, and moved into position, ½ inch each move, over a 3 to 5 minute period.

The accepted firing rate of all dental porcelain is sustained by increasing the temperature 50, 75, or 100 degrees per minute. Practice with the available furnace will determine how the transformer should be manipulated. The initial firing of high-fusing porcelain should be carried to the maturation temperature shown in Table 23–1. When the directions are met, the firing tray should be removed and covered with a beaker or glass until the crown is cool enough to handle. It is returned to the die, again wrapped in gauze, and the platinum apron is burnished from the shoulder toward the apex of the root. It is removed and replaced a number of times to be certain that there is no binding. A crack in the porcelain caused by undersize of the crown due to shrinkage poses no problem.

The Second Firing. The die is placed in the working cast and held so that the lingual of the crown may be supported by one finger covered by a clean gauze, and the crown is built to the incisal height with gingival porce-

Table 23–1.   FIRING SCHEDULE

PORCELAIN	DEGASSING	OPAQUE	BODY	GLAZE
1130° C.* VITA	2100° F. for 6 minutes	Dry for 5 minutes before open muffle	Dry for 15 minutes before open muffle	Insert in muffle at 1950° F.
		Then 1600–1950° F. HOLD 1 minute	Then 1600–1950° F. HOLD 1 minute	HOLD 2–4 minutes
	TOTAL Vacuum	TOTAL Vacuum	TOTAL Vacuum	WITHOUT Vacuum (Hobo)
2100° F. BIOFORM	2150° F. for 6 minutes	Dry for 5 minutes before open muffle	Dry for 15 minutes before open muffle	1850–2100° F.
		Then 1600–2100° F. in 5 minutes	Then 1600–2100° F. in 5 minutes	HOLD 2–4 minutes
	TOTAL Vacuum	TOTAL Vacuum	TOTAL Vacuum	WITHOUT Vacuum
1875° F. APCO Air-fired ADD-ON			Dry for 6 minutes before open muffle	
			Then 1200–1875° F. Temperature rise 50° per minute	
2400° F. STEELE's TRUBYTE Air-fired	2450° F. for 6 minutes	Dry for 10 minutes before open muffle OR in preheating chamber	1st bake: 1200–2350° F. Remove and cool	1200–2400° F.
				HOLD 2–6 minutes
			2nd bake: 1200–2400° F. Remove and cool	EXAMINE for sur- face texture and luster. REMOVE when texture and luster are as desired
				Cool under glass

NOTE: FURNACE TEMPERATURE SHOULD INCREASE AT RATE OF 50 to 100° F. per MINUTE.

*FIRING SCHEDULE, Vita 2070° F. Porcelain. (Johnston, J. F., Mumford, G., and Dykema, R. W.: Modern Practice in Dental Ceramics. Philadelphia, W. B. Saunders Company, 1967.)

DEGASSING	OPAQUE	BODY	GLAZE
2050° F.	1850–2000° F.	Same as Opaque	2000° F.
	30° per minute	1st Bake	
HOLD 10 minutes	HOLD 2 minutes	2nd Bake (if needed)	HOLD 3–5 minutes
Vacuum 28 inches	Vacuum 28 inches	Vacuum 28 inches	NO Vacuum
ADD-ON (Vita Korrektur)	1500–1720° F.		Can be done with matrix removed.
	Temperature rise 45° per minute		
	NO Vacuum		
STAINS	900–1700° F.		Can be done with matrix removed.
Steele's Super-Stains	Temperature rise 50° per minute		
	NO Vacuum		

lain. Porcelain is added to the labial surface, and the cast is vibrated with a serrated spatula that is moved in one direction only. (Flow of the porcelain can thus be better controlled.) Moisture appearing on the surface is blotted with the gauze. Anatomic contour at this time is not consequential.

The lingual of the crown is built in the same way, the porcelain being applied with a sliding motion of the spatula and by vibrating and blotting.

With guidance from the color distribution chart, gingival porcelain is trimmed off the labioincisal and proximal surfaces at an angle. This is replaced and the contour of the crown restored with the incisal shade. Incisal porcelain is more difficult to handle because of the coarser particle size needed to produce translucence. It should be flowed on with a brush and built up from 1.0 to 1.5 mm. longer than the finished crown (Fig. 23-30).

The crown should receive final condensation by burnishing or "whipping" with a large sable's-hair brush. Then the proximal surfaces should be dampened with the die in the cast, and the die and crown removed. The cervical portions must be trimmed to approximate contour, but slightly beyond the margin of the shoulder. From 0.5 to 1.0 mm. of porcelain (either gingival or incisal, or both, depending on the color pattern) should be added to each proximal surface.

With the same technique described previously, the crown is dried on top of the furnace or in the preheating chamber and placed in the furnace. It

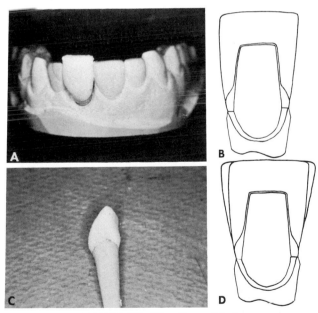

FIGURE 23-30. *Second bake.*

A, Die and crown in working cast; incisal has been built longer than approximating teeth to compensate for shrinkage.

B, Cross section of first and second applications of porcelain.

C, Die removed, ready to increase bulk at contacts.

D, Cross section before second firing, showing added porcelain at contact areas.

need not be directly under the thermocouple; neither should it be close to the furnace door. The firing schedule listed in the Table 23-1 should be followed.

Contouring.   A Busch Silent stone is used to remove the excess at the incisal and to contour the crown. However, at the gingival margin a concave carborundum or a flexible diamond disk may be used. The crown should be placed on the die and the excess on the proximal surfaces observed (Fig. 23-31), so that when these surfaces are contoured there will be equal pressure mesially and distally on the approximating teeth. This will add to the safety and comfort of the cemented crown. Contacts must have strength comparable to that in other sections of the mouth (Fig. 23-32).

The occlusion must be adjusted at this time. If articulated casts have been used, this can be done in the laboratory, or the crown may be taken to the mouth. When a crown is to be adjusted in the mouth, the apron of the platinum matrix must be trimmed to a width of 0.4 mm. or less.

The Third Firing.   The crown is brushed with detergent and water, and washed. Any elusive black specks at the surface can be effectively removed by boiling in nitric acid, but those that are embedded must be ground out. The crown is dried and the surface rubbed with dry porcelain powder; if a small bubble or irregularity developed in the surface of the crown during the second firing, or if it becomes necessary to add to the contour, the mix of porcelain should be 75 per cent of high-fusing porcelain and 25 per cent of low-fusing, or 1875°,* porcelain. It is then returned to the furnace and carried to maximal fusing temperature and held at this temperature. During the holding period, the crown should be examined for luster and surface texture. When texture and luster are as desired, it is removed from the furnace and covered to cool slowly.

Fitting.   The finished crown should be tried on the tooth before the matrix is removed so that contacts and occlusion may be checked (Fig. 23-32). If any adjustment is made, the ground surface should be covered with an overglaze. If a contact area is lacking to a minor degree in convexity or strength of pressure, this too may be corrected by use of an overglaze, which should be mixed thicker and added in greater bulk.

---

*Steele's Apco, The Columbus Dental Mfg. Co., Columbus, Ohio.

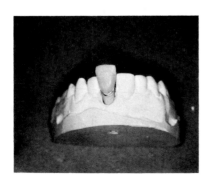

FIGURE 23–31. Contouring. Crown after second firing. Contacts, length, occlusion, and contour must be checked and corrected.

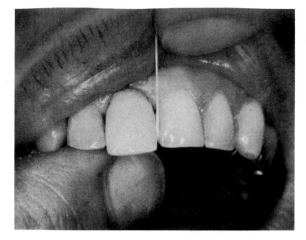

FIGURE 23-32. Testing contact strength when fitting and contouring crown.

The matrix can be removed with a pair of straight-beak tweezers by grasping the platinum apron and rolling it toward the center of the crown. Removal of the platinum can be facilitated by the presence of water. The action here has never been explained, but the clinical phenomenon exists. If the matrix was made quite smooth before the crown was built, it should be removed with little effort.

If the shoulder of the preparation has been made 0.5 to 0.8 mm. in width on the labial surface and if the incisocervical contour of the tooth has been followed in the preparation, the porcelain should have plentiful thickness to disguise or hide the prepared tooth stump and the underlying cement completely.

If for some reason the preparation could not be made sufficiently deep, or if the tooth is pulpless and has become quite dark, prior to building up the crown, a layer of opaque porcelain should have been applied by brush to the matrix and fired to a low maturity (Figs. 23-33 and 23-34).

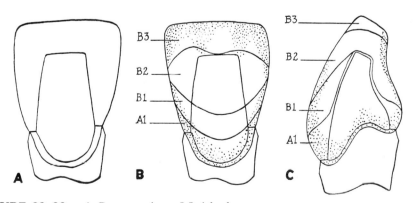

FIGURE 23-33. *A*, Cross section of finished crown.
B and *C*, Cross sections showing layers of porcelain: A1, initial application, gingival; B1, second application, gingival; B2, first application, incisal; B3, second application, incisal or incisal mixed with a translucent porcelain.

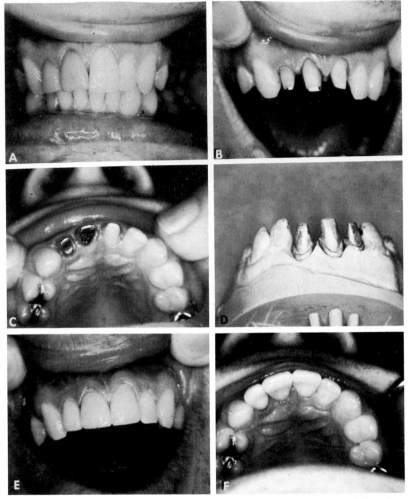

FIGURE 23–34. *Construction of three porcelain jacket crowns on a pulpless lateral and central and a vital central.*

A, Discolored maxillary right central and lateral incisors.

B and *C*, Three teeth prepared. Pulpless teeth built up to prepared form by cast cores, with posts extending into root canals.

D, Working cast. Dies are silver-plated with stone roots. Roots were coated with petrolatum before cast was poured.

E and *F*, Crowns after cementation.

Cervical Ditching Technique

A clinical case will be used to illustrate this technique for jacket crown construction. The teeth were prepared, extending the shoulders into the gingival crevices approximately 0.4 mm. A working cast with removable silver-plated dies was made and a platinum matrix was formed on each die. (See Figures 23-19, 23-20, and 23-21.) The technique to be described is for any porcelain, has an unlimited application, and is probably used more than any other.

Application of the Opaque. The opaque is mixed to a thin, creamy consistency by spatulating and vibrating to help to eliminate any air bubbles. It is applied to the matrix with a spatula and, by alternate vibration and drying, is built up evenly over the matrix surface, except on the shoulder, to a thickness of approximately 0.4 mm. (Fig. 23–35). The opaque is dried in front of the open muffle or in the drying chamber of the furnace. The firing schedule designated for the porcelain being used (Table 23-1) is followed for the opaque and all subsequent firings.*

---

*The firing schedule suggested by the manufacturer should be the basis for trial firings.

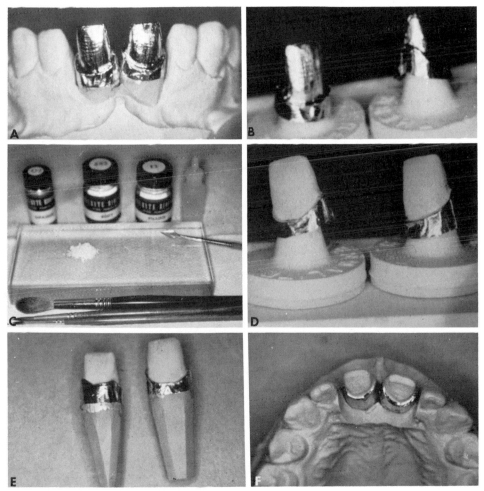

FIGURE 23–35. *A,* Platinum matrices formed. They were made with proximal joints, were burnished, swaged, and reburnished, then removed with a covering of chilled sticky wax.

B, Matrices on firing trays. To be placed in furnace for degassing and burning off of other impurities.

C, Armamentarium for applying opaque.

D, Opaque applied.

E and *F,* Opaque fired. Opaque was necessary because of darkened pulpless teeth.

The tray is removed and placed under a cover to cool. The matrix with the fired opaque is placed on the die and the shoulder is readapted.

Building the Crown

FIRST FIRING.   Body and incisal porcelain are mixed to a thick, creamy consistency on separate slabs (Fig. 23-36). The crown is built up to contour with the body porcelain applied with a spatula. The die is vibrated with a serrated instrument, and the moisture that comes to the surface is absorbed with a clean gauze pad (Fig. 23-37). Porcelain is added, vibrated, and dehydrated until the crown is overcontoured. This is all done with the die in the working cast. The proximal and incisal excess is trimmed, leaving some porcelain overlapping the approximating teeth, and the surface is burnished and smoothed with a large brush, using a whipping motion. The incisal edge and the labial surface are carved away to provide space for the incisal color.

This is added and condensed by vibrating, dehydrating, burnishing, and brushing. It is built about 1.0 mm. overlength. The crown is removed, and the grooves formed by the overlapping proximal porcelain are filled with body and incisal so that the crown has extra contour in all dimensions. The lingual is roughly carved to form, but with excess thickness. The die is removed from the working cast, and the cervical porcelain is carved away to form a V-shaped ditch exposing the platinum shoulder of the matrix (Fig. 23–38). It is dried and placed in the furnace. After firing it is removed and covered while cooling.[9, 15, 16, 17]

SECOND FIRING.   The adaptation of the matrix to the shoulder is checked on the die and improved if distorted. When placed in the working cast, the mesiodistal measurement of the crown is sometimes too wide. If so, the contacts must be reduced by grinding with a Busch Silent stone or a Dedeco rubber porcelain wheel so that the die, with the crown in place, will seat in the working cast with equal pressure mesially and distally (Fig. 23–39).

The ditch at the cervical is filled with body-colored porcelain and considerably overcontoured. Porcelain is added wherever shrinkage from the first firing has minimized the contour. The firing cycle is repeated, and after

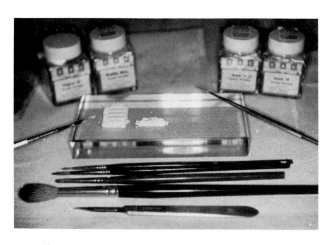

FIGURE 23–36.   Equipment for building porcelain crown.

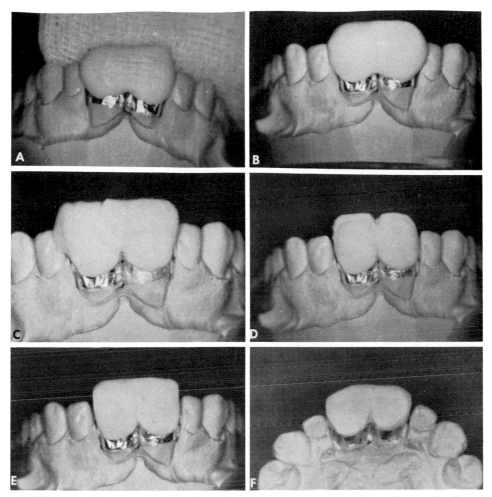

FIGURE 23–37. *A,* Gauze is held against the lingual surface of the dies, and body porcelain is built on the labial surface in a solid mass. Approximating teeth have been coated with lacquer to prevent absorption of moisture from porcelain. Cast was vibrated with serrated instrument and moisture absorbed by gauze as soon as it came to surface.

B, Mass of porcelain condensed by vibrating, absorbing moisture, and brushing.

C, Lingual porcelain added.

D, Body porcelain trimmed and incisal porcelain added.

E and *F,* All porcelain condensed and matrices cleaned.

cooling the crown is roughly shaped, using stones and rubber porcelain grinding wheels. If the cervical ditch is undercontoured, porcelain is added and the firing cycle is repeated. The crown may receive its final shaping on the working cast. Preferably it will be taken to the mouth in the low maturity stage so that occlusion and contacts may be re-established and contour and minute anatomic irregularities checked. Contacts must be very carefully tested and, at the mouth-checking stage, should seem to be tight. Occlusion must be meticulously developed. Staining should be done at this stage.

FINAL FIRING.   Final firing or glazing is done in atmosphere because, if

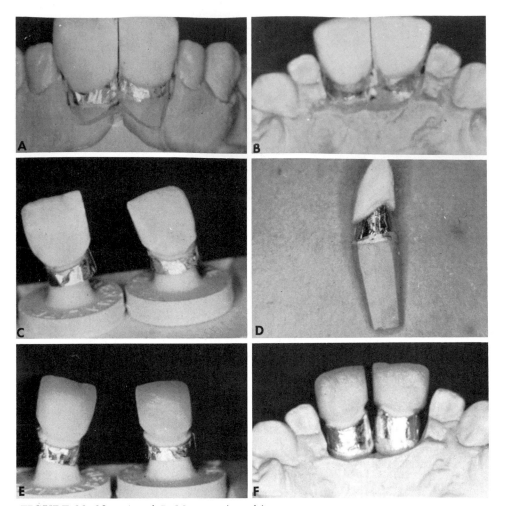

FIGURE 23–38.   *A* and *B*, Mass sectioned into two crowns.
    C and *D*, Cervical porcelain carved away to form ditch. Shrinkage will be toward incisal and will not disturb fit of matrix.
    E and *F*, Crowns after first firing.

done in vacuum, a pitted surface will generally result. Pitting or bubble formation caused by contamination of the matrix or porcelain is magnified by vacuum firing. The crown is preheated and placed in the furnace.

The surface texture of the patient's natural teeth should have been observed, and the glaze on the crown must be in harmony. This can be developed through variation in the terminal temperature of the glaze firing, or by varying the holding time (Fig. 23-40).

It must be repeated that before removal of the matrix, the crown should be taken to the mouth to check contacts and occlusion; these will almost always be acceptable if it was tried in the mouth before glazing. If there is a prematurity or if a contact is lacking in pressure, the stoned or undercontoured proximal area can be built up with a special "add-on" porcelain. This is dried and placed in the furnace (Table 23-1). To remedy a minute discrepancy on a contact surface, a thick coating of Steele's Super Glaze may be applied and fired at 1945° F.; this will make the surface quite smooth and give the contact the anticipated strength. The matrix is removed.

When a crown is fabricated in a laboratory, the technician must be instructed to return it with the matrix in place. Otherwise no alterations are possible.

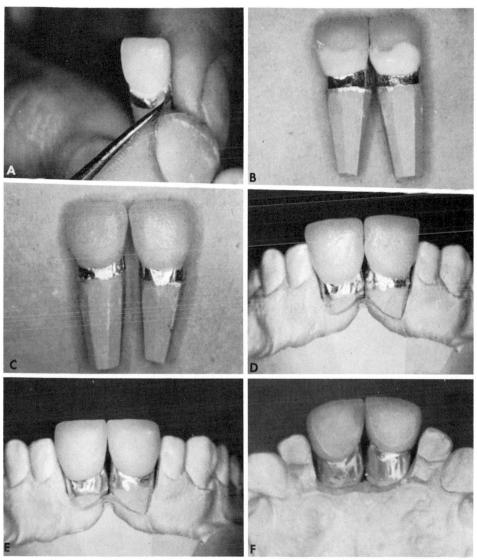

FIGURE 23–39. *A*, Readapting matrix to shoulder of die.
B, Ditches filled after crowns were contoured.
C, After second firing.
D, Contacts adjusted; dies seated.
E and *F*, Crowns contoured ready for third firing.

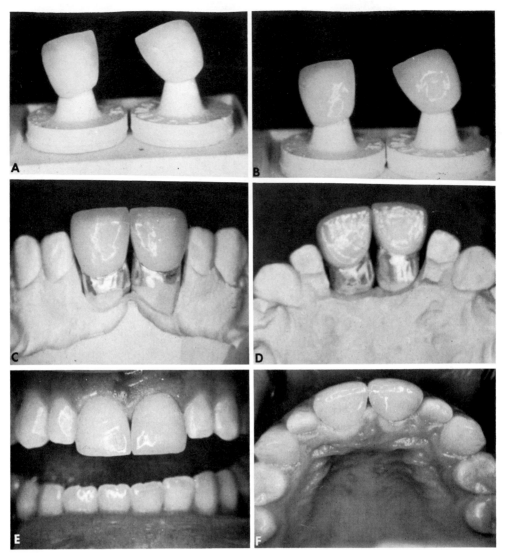

FIGURE 23–40.   *A*, Crowns have been checked for contacts and occlusion, contoured, and cleaned. Ready for glaze firing. Matrices were trimmed to facilitate seating crowns on teeth.

B, Crowns glazed.

C and *D*, Crowns on working cast.

E and *F*, Crowns cemented.

CEMENTATION

It is helpful to have at hand an assortment of zinc phosphate and silicophosphate cements so that there will be many shades from which to select the one, or the combination, that will enhance the coloring or harmony of the finished restoration.[9]

For a porcelain crown, the choice of a zinc phosphate cement can be made from trial mixes of powder and glycerin and water after the matrix has been removed. Silicate or resin cement may be chosen from a prepared shade guide.

The crown must be cleaned and dried and the tooth isolated and dried. The cements should be mixed not only for strength but also for less retarded extrusion. An excess of cement should be placed inside the crown and over the shoulder of the prepared tooth. When it has been seated, the crown should be held in position by the operator. After the hardened excess of cement has been removed, the gingival crevice should be examined for fragments (Fig. 23-40).

PATIENT RESPONSIBILITY

The patient must be instructed with regard to the normal care of the restoration and *his* part of the responsibility for the success of the case. The value of hygiene, gingival massage, and periodic examination to ascertain changes in occlusion must be emphasized. The patient should be admonished to avoid biting on thread or pipe stems or other hard objects that might act as a point contact.

BREAKAGE

When a porcelain jacket crown breaks in the mouth, it breaks from the inside out as a result of reciprocal pressures.[11, 18] Sharp line angles or corners cause more breakage than any other factor, owing to increased stress concentration in those areas. Moon-shaped breaks on the labial surface occur because of insufficient length in the prepared tooth. To afford support for the jacket, the abutment preparation at its longest portion should be close to two-thirds of the length of the finished restoration from shoulder to incisal. It must be remembered that an uninterrupted surface has a strength peculiar unto itself; interrupted, it becomes weakened. Therefore, before the platinum matrix is removed for cementation of the crown, all adjustments should be made and the crown reglazed to re-establish surface continuity. Even so, equilibration in the future may induce frail areas.

REFERENCES

1. Brecker, S. C.: The Porcelain Jacket Crown. St. Louis, The C. V. Mosby Company, 1951.
2. Johnston, J. F., Mumford, G., and Dykema, R. W.: Modern Practice in Dental Ceramics. Philadelphia, W. B. Saunders Company, 1967.
3. Theofilis, B. G.: The Porcelain Jacket Crown. Senior thesis, Indiana University School of Dentistry, June 1955.
4. Bartels, J. C.: Full porcelain veneer crowns. J. Pros. Den., 7:533, July 1957.
5. Bastian, C. C.: Porcelain jacket crown. Dent. Clin. N. Amer., March 1959, p. 133.
6. Rieser, J., and Aaronson, W.: Different technic of anterior porcelain jacket crown preparation. J.A.D.A., 56:559, April 1958.

7. Fairley, J. M., and Deubert, L. W.: Preparation of maxillary central incisor for a porcelain jacket restoration. British D. J., *104*:208, March 18, 1958.
8. Bartels, J. C.: Preparation of the anterior teeth for porcelain jacket crowns. J. South. California D. A., *30*:199, June 1962.
9. Nuttall, E. B.: Personal communication.
10. Malson, T. S.: Protection for jacket crown preparations. Ohio D. J., *33*:139, June 1959.
11. Pettrow, J. N.: Practical factors in building and firing characteristics of dental porcelain. J. Pros. Den., *11*:334, March-April 1961.
12. Pettrow, J. N.: Personal communication.
13. Baker, C. R.: Condensation of dental porcelain. J. Pros. Den., *10*:1094, Nov.-Dec. 1960.
14. Vines, R. F., and Semmelman, J. O.: Densification of dental porcelain. J. D. Res., *36*:950, Dec. 1957.
15. Dunton, H.: Personal communication.
16. Jones, R. J.: Personal communication.
17. Moskey, M. S.: Personal communication.
18. Nuttall, E. B.: Factors influencing success of porcelain jacket restorations. J. Pros. Den., *11*:743, July-Aug. 1961.

Bartels, J. C.: Porcelain as an esthetic restorative material. Dent. Clin. N. Amer., Nov. 1963, p. 831.

Bastian, C. C.: Restoration of lower anterior teeth. J. Pros. Den., 6:684, Sept. 1956.

Blancheri, R. L.: Optical illusions and cosmetic grinding. Rev. Association Den. Mexicana, 8:103, 1950.

Blazoudakis, C.: Personal communication.

Charlton, G.: A prefabricated post and core for porcelain jacket crowns. British D. J., 10:317-319, Aug. 1965.

Clarke, E. B.: The color problem in dentistry. D. Digest, 37:499; 571; 646; 732; 815; 1931.

Cowger, G. T., et al.: A non metal die for porcelain jacket crown fabrication. J. Pros. Den., 17:578-582, June 1967.

Felcher, F. R.: The Art of Porcelain in Dentistry. St. Louis. The C. V. Mosby Company, 1932.

Hobo, S.: A Study of the Fit of Porcelain Inlays Using Different Technics. Master's thesis, Indiana University School of Dentistry, 1964.

Lyon, D. M., et al.: Water swage for adaptation of platinum matrices. J.A.D.A., 73:1348-1350, Dec. 1966.

Manners, P.: Removal of jacket crowns. J. Pros. Den., 7:814, Nov. 1957.

Miller, C. J.: Inlays, Crowns and Bridges. Philadelphia, W. B. Saunders Company, 1962.

Sacchi, H., and Paffenbarger, G. C.: A simple technic for making dental porcelain jacket crowns. J.A.D.A., 54:366, March 1957.

Yock, D. H.: Porcelain jacket veneer crown preparation. Iowa D. J., 43:267, Oct. 1957.

chapter 24

THE PORCELAIN JACKET CROWN, PART II

CONSTRUCTING CROWNS USING ALUMINOUS PORCELAIN

During the past two decades there has been a marked renaissance in the use of fused porcelain in the construction of crown restorations and pontics. This could have occurred because of a growing awareness among dentists and patients of the deficiencies in the physical and hygienic properties of resins, and a desire for the ultimate in the esthetic effects to be achieved.

Owing to its relatively poor tensile strength, porcelain sometimes fails as a dental restorative material; its successful use may hinge on reinforcement by a metal substructure, as in the case of the porcelain-fused-to-metal restoration. When used for the jacket crown it is dependent on a balanced tooth preparation (see Chapter 23) that is planned and executed so that most of the forces directed against the restoration are compressive instead of tensile in nature.[1] Because of the great variations in tooth form and in the nature and location of occlusal contacts, preparations cannot always be made that will adequately support porcelain jacket crowns. It follows that there is a significant and disconcerting incidence of fracture. Such failures can be forestalled or corrected by using the porcelain veneered crown, but even the most skilled ceramists have been unable on occasion to endow these restorations with the fine harmonious qualities expected with porcelain jacket crowns.

For many years dental porcelains have been constituted from feldspar reinforced with quartz. Recently McLean[2] has experimented with the reinforcement of pigmented glasses with aluminum oxide (Al_2O_3) for use in the fabrication of jacket crowns. Alumina, as this material is called, is just below diamond on a standard hardness scale. When used as a reinforcing agent, alumina bonds chemically with the porcelain or glass. When a crack forms it must pass through the alumina crystal, and since the alumina particle is extremely hard it tends to inhibit the propagation of the crack and to make the porcelain measurably sturdier.

THE ALUMINA CORE

Alumina has one major disadvantage. It has an opacifying effect when mixed with a translucent material, which negates its use in quantity in the body porcelain. Instead, a core[3] of high alumina content porcelain (40 to 50 per cent) is formed (Fig. 24-1) over which the gingival and incisal porcelains are fused. The core is designed so that it is thick on the lingual surface, taking up about three-fourths of the bulk of the crown in this area, and extending to within about 0.5 mm. of the proximal contacts. The labial aspect is about 0.3 mm. thick. The incisal boundary of the core is kept short enough to allow 1.0 mm. or more of regular porcelain to extend beyond it. The form of the core makes it possible to place a mass of porcelain in the areas where shade and translucency must be developed, and at the same time strengthen the restoration in those parts where occluding forces are usually applied. The core is similar in shape to that of the metal substructure for a porcelain veneered crown, except for a slight undercontouring that calls for some porcelain to be fused over all surfaces.

The core material seems to be approximately twice as strong as conventional porcelain when subjected to flexural forces and is thought to increase the strength of a jacket crown about 50 per cent.

THE REINFORCED ALUMINA CORE

Pure alumina can be manufactured into sheets and other shapes for insertion into porcelain restorations. Its most useful application at present appears to be the inclusion of a sheet of the material in the lingual segment of a jacket crown (Fig. 24-2). The pure alumina sheet is fired into the aluminous core that has been described.

In some testing projects pure alumina coated with porcelain has been

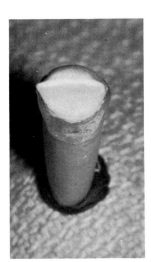

FIGURE 24-1. Incisal view of core built with high alumina content porcelain. Form of core much like metal substructure of porcelain veneered crown.

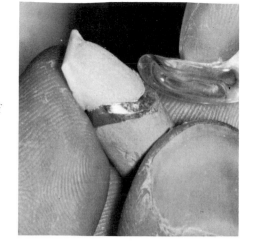

FIGURE 24–2. Core made using a sheet of pure alumina on lingual surface.

shown to have five times the durability of dental porcelain.[3] Whether it improves the resistance of a jacket crown to breakage by the same ratio is not known, but it is logical to assume that a pronounced lessening in fragility does occur, with a concomitant decrease in the number of fractures.

Prognosis. There is little indication that this new approach to jacket crown construction will make the porcelain veneered crown obsolete. Much more strength than has been realized so far would be required to eliminate all the fracture problems created by short teeth, adverse occlusion, and improper preparations. Although short bridges have been made using pure alumina reinforcement forms to join and reinforce the parts, such efforts need to be recognized as pure exercises in research and are not to be recommended for general use. When aluminous porcelain is used where the jacket crown is normally indicated and when care and skill have been engaged in the preparation of the tooth and fabrication of the restoration, there should be a notably elevated rate of success.[4]

The esthetic results with crowns made with the aluminous porcelains are quite good and should be equal to those fabricated with any popular vacuum-fired porcelain (Fig. 24-3). However, the opacifying effect of the alumina, together with the necessity at times to use a thin layer of the body

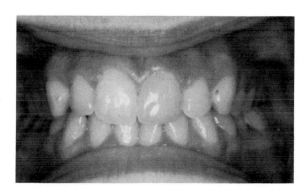

FIGURE 24–3. Jacket crown built of aluminous porcelain on maxillary left central incisor.

porcelain, may produce a bothersome lack of transulcence, but often this can be overcome by the artistic ability of the ceramist.

TECHNIQUE

The Materials

The available aluminous porcelains (several are being marketed) are similar to each other. The important differences are in the number of colored components needed to match the shade systems used, and in the firing temperatures.

Shades.   To match the Vita shade guide, Vitadur porcelain uses five shades of porcelain, plus a high alumina core material.

Steele's Aluminous Porcelains, both air-fired and vacuum-fired, are made with just the core material and two body porcelains, dentin and enamel.

Alumolain, Vita's aluminous porcelain preblended in Bioform shades, consists bascially of a core material and gingival and incisal shades.

All these porcelain systems provide modifiers to assist with characterization and modification of shades.

Firing Temperatures.   Vitadur core material is fired at 1975° F., while the body porcelains all fuse at 1725° F.

Both of Steele's Aluminous Porcelains have firing temperatures of 1650° F. for the body and enamel porcelains, but the air-fired has both a high-fusing core material (2010° F.) and a low-fusing core material (1920° F.). Steele's vacuum-fired Aluminous Porcelain is used only with a 1900° F. core material.

Alumolain porcelain core material fuses at 1990° F. and the body porcelain at 1740° F.

As with all porcelains, the firing temperatures given are approximate and not infrequently must be modified for a given furnace.

Since the technique for using Steele's vacuum-fired Aluminous Porcelain is the least complicated, the authors have concentrated on this material, technique for which is illustrated in Figures 24-4 through 24-23.

Preparation of Cast, Matrix, and Porcelain

The teeth on the stone cast approximating the die should be coated with lacquer. After this has hardened the cast will not absorb water from the porcelain being built on the die (Fig. 24-4 A). The matrix must be degassed and heated to approximately 100° above the fusing temperature of the porcelain so that all impurities from its surface will be burned off and so that it will not be brittle (Fig. 24-4 B).

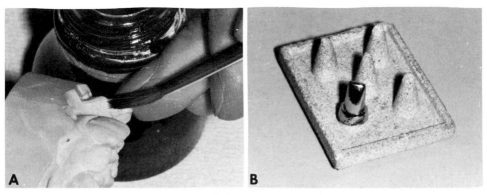

FIGURE 24–4. *A*, Painting cast with lacquer. *B*, Matrix on firing tray for annealing and purifying.

The core porcelain is placed on the glass slab and mixed with distilled water to a thick creamy consistency, using a glass stirring rod or spatula. Metal should not be used inasmuch as the porcelain will abrade metal. Should any abrasion occur with glass, the glass will be incorporated with the porcelain and should fuse and become an integral part of the finished restoration.

Building the Core

First Bake. The core material is mixed and built onto the crown 0.5 mm. thick on the labial and labioproximals and thicker on the lingual surface (Fig. 24-5 *A* and *B*). The material is blotted until dry and then the die is vibrated and moisture is removed with a gauze pad just as soon as it appears (Fig. 24–5 *C* and *D*). When the initial application has been dried and condensed to its fullest, the die is placed in the cast and the core is built laterally until it is in contact with the approximating teeth (Fig. 24-6 *A*). The lingual and incisal are now built in the same way (Fig. 24-6 *B* and *C*). The die is removed from the cast and the proximal indentations are filled (Fig. 24-6 *D*). When it has been condensed, it is ditched at the cervical so that there will be no porcelain adhering to the shoulder, then dried to one side and in front of the open furnace door for 4 to 8 minutes and gradually introduced into a hot 1550° F. (or below) muffle, which is closed and sealed. The temperature should be raised not more than 50° per minute while being elevated to 1900° F. under vacuum, where it is held in atmosphere for 1 minute. It should have an eggshell sheen. It is cooled slowly, preferably under glass.

Second Bake. The matrix is reburnished over the shoulder (Fig. 24-7 *A*). The cervical ditch and any cracks are filled. The drying and firing cycles are repeated, with the temperature being raised not more than 50° per minute.

Shaping the Core. The core is trimmed proximally (Fig. 24-7 *B*) and is checked for occlusion (Fig. 24–7 *C*). Clearance when closed should be 0.3 or

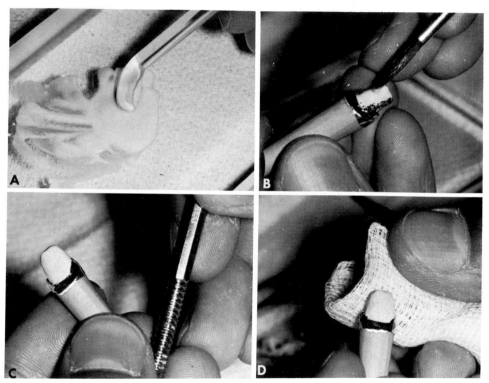

FIGURE 24–5.   *A*, Mixing powder and distilled water with glass rod.
B, Painting core porcelain on labial of matrix.
C, Vibrating die to bring moisture to surface.
D, Blotting moisture with gauze pad. This dries and pulls liquid from opposite surface, packing particles.

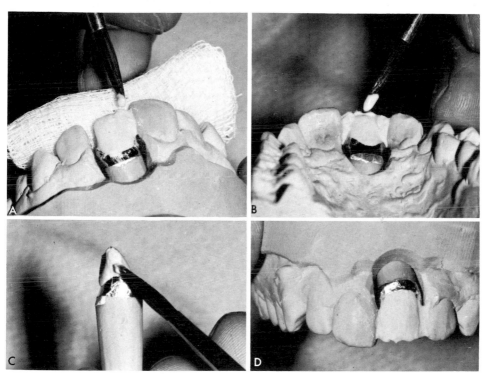

FIGURE 24–6. *A, B,* and *C,* Building core porcelain on proximals, lingual, and incisal. *D,* Filling proximal grooves to make wider and to counteract shrinkage.

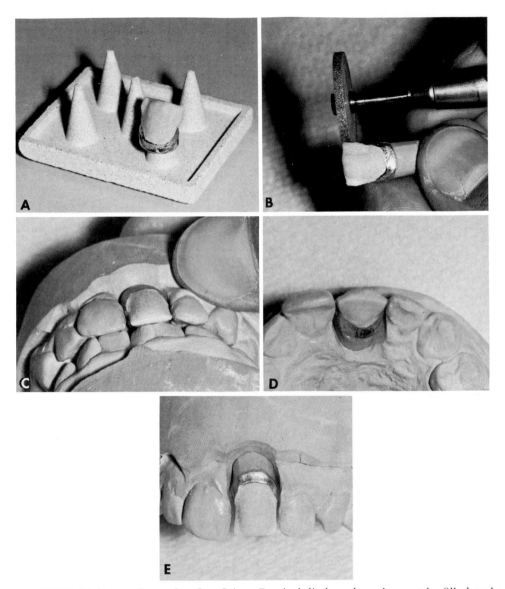

FIGURE 24–7.   *A*, Core after first firing. Cervical ditch and cracks must be filled and re-fired.

   B, Trimming proximals of core after second firing.

   C, Checking occlusion.

   D and *E*, Core, incisal and labial views.

0.4 mm. There is space on the proximals for body and enamel porcelain to be added (Fig. 24-7 *D* and *E*) and on the lingual for a layer of enamel porcelain that will take a glaze. The incisal edge must be trimmed 1.0 mm. or more short of the length of the approximating teeth. The core is now ready for the application of the body and enamel porcelains and for finishing the crown.

The Core Reinforced with Sheet Alumina

The core may be fabricated by using a curved sheet of pure alumina over the lingual surface, covering everything from the incisal edge to the cervical margin. This probably is the better of the two methods for making the core, since it gives a stronger, more fracture-resistant lingual surface.

Preparing and Attaching the Sheet Alumina. A piece of sheet alumina is measured for mesiodistal width, the outline of the lingual surface is made with a pencil, and it is trimmed (Fig. 24-8). Core porcelain is mixed and applied to the lingual surface (Fig. 24–9 *A*), and is dried, vibrated, dried,

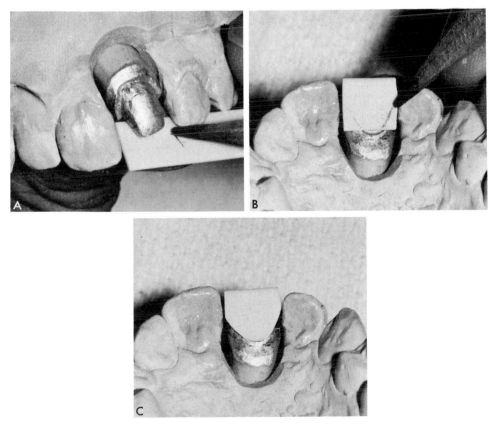

FIGURE 24–8. *A* and *B*, Outlining dimensions for lingual sheet of alumina. *C*, Lingual sheet of alumina trimmed to form.

and condensed (Fig. 24-9 *B*). The piece of sheet alumina is placed against the lingual surface (Fig. 24-9 *C*) and porcelain is added, filling the cracks between it and the matrix, and carried around past the line angles on the mesial and distal (Fig. 24-9 *D*). A strip of platinum foil is wrapped around the sheet alumina and the matrix and is fastened in front with a tinner's joint (Fig. 24-9 *E* and *F*). This is fired, using the formula for 1900° F. core porcelain, and the platinum strip is removed.

Shaping the Core.   Porcelain core powder, 1900° F., is added to the

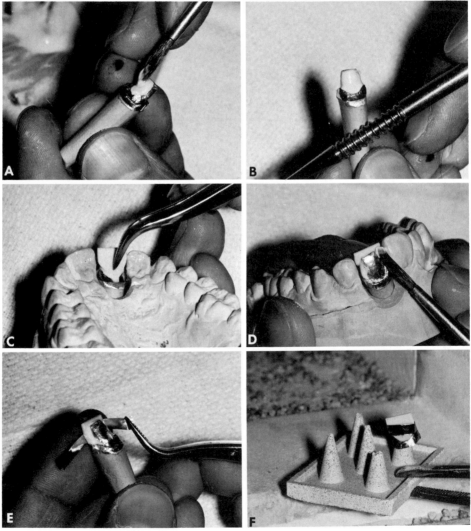

FIGURE 24–9.   *A*, Covering lingual of matrix with core porcelain.
B, Condensing porcelain; vibration followed by blotting.
C, Placing sheet alumina on lingual.
D, Filling gap with core porcelain.
E, Encircling sheet alumina and matrix with strip of platinum.
F, Alumina sheet secured to matrix and placed on tray for firing.

labial surface (Fig. 24-10 *A*), and the core is contoured, dried, and fired (Fig. 24–10 *B, C, D,* and *E*). After cooling the matrix is reburnished over the shoulder (Fig. 24-11 *A*), the final contour is given to the core (Fig. 24-11 *B*), and it is fired. Angles are rounded, it is trimmed to dimension, occlusion is checked, and the desired clearance in closure and in all excursions is made on the lingual surface (Fig. 24–11 *C, D,* and *E*). The finished core is shown in Figure 24-12.

Porcelain may be built and fired over the core (Fig. 24-13), using either

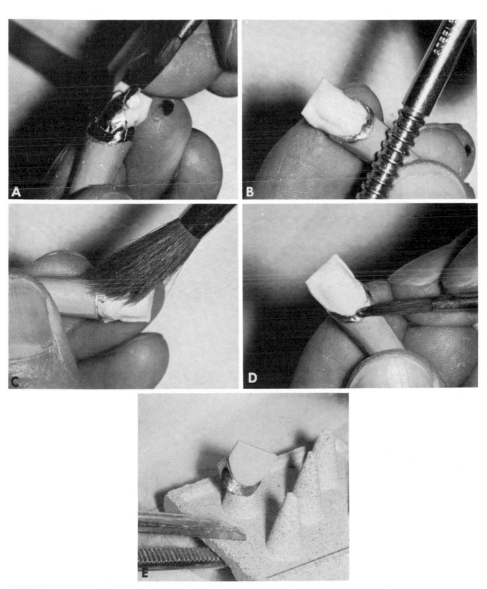

FIGURE 24–10. *A, B, C,* and *D,* Adding and condensing core powder. *E,* Core after firing.

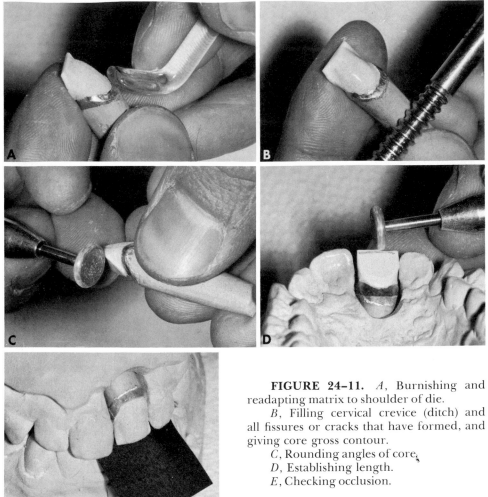

FIGURE 24–11. *A*, Burnishing and readapting matrix to shoulder of die.

B, Filling cervical crevice (ditch) and all fissures or cracks that have formed, and giving core gross contour.

C, Rounding angles of core.

D, Establishing length.

E, Checking occlusion.

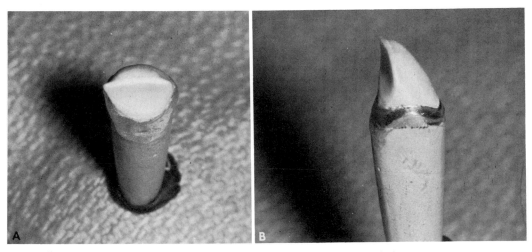

FIGURE 24–12.   *A* and *B*, Finished core, incisal and proximal views.

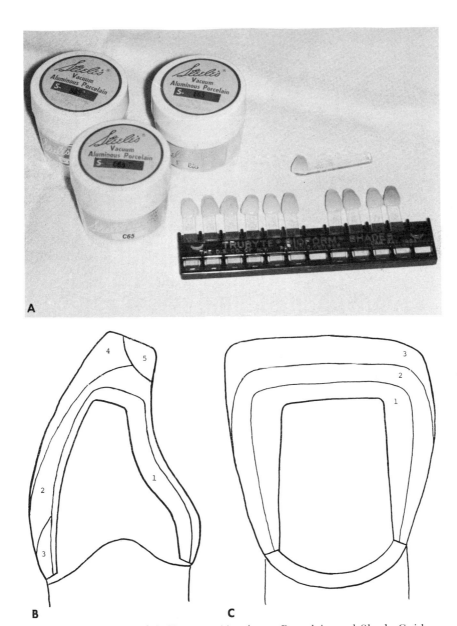

FIGURE 24–13. *A,* Steele's Vacuum Aluminous Porcelain and Shade Guide.

B, Diagram of cross section of crown, illustrating how porcelain is added for firing: (1) core; (2) body; (3) neck dentin, which may not be covered with enamel porcelain; (4) enamel porcelain, which usually covers all of labial except neck dentin; (5) translucent porcelain; this may not be required, depending on shade pattern.

C, Diagrammatic cross section from mesial to distal: (1) core; (2) body porcelain; (3) enamel porcelain.

the cervical ditching technique or the cervical contact technique, the latter being used most often by the authors.*

Building the Crown

First Bake. Body porcelain is added in quantities around the cervical (Fig. 24–14 *A* and *B*) and is condensed and fired (Fig. 24–14 *C*, *D*, and *E*).

---

*The detailed techniques for furnaces with either horizontal (discussed here) or vertical muffles are described in the booklet "Steele's Aluminous Porcelain Technique," which can be obtained from The Columbus Dental Mfg. Co., Columbus, Ohio.

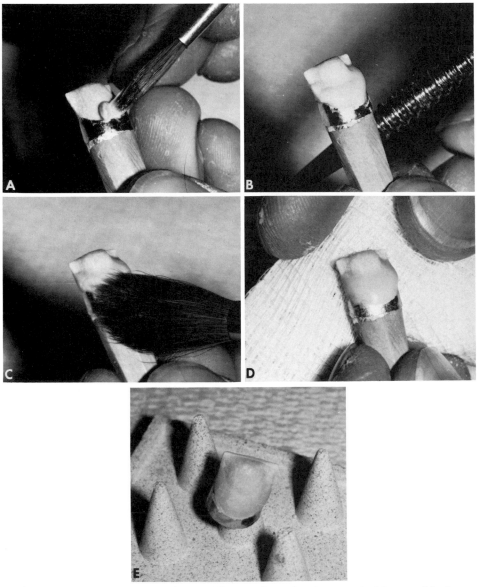

FIGURE 24–14.   *A, B, C,* and *D,* Adding and condensing cervical layer of body porcelain. *E,* Cervical layer fired; shrinkage was toward shoulder of matrix.

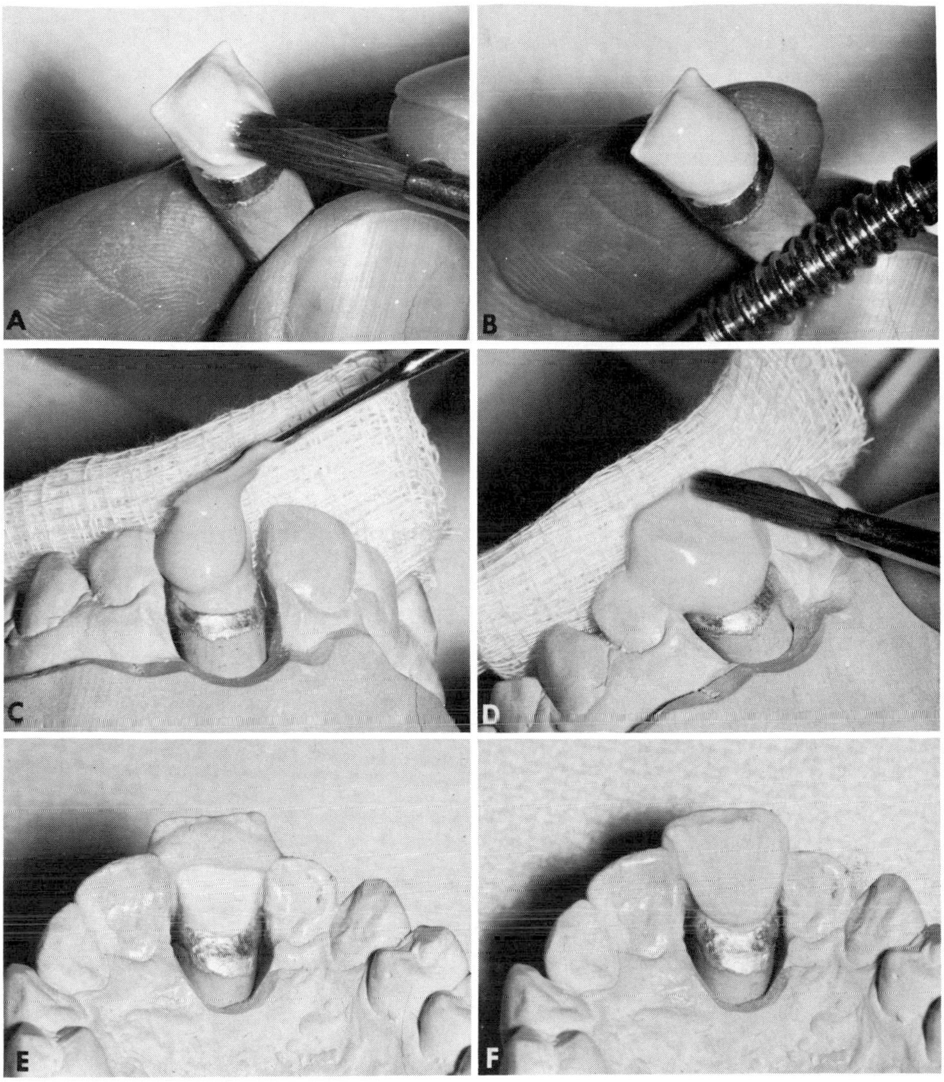

FIGURE 24–15. *A, B, C,* and *D,* Building body porcelain over buccal surface. *E* and *F,* Building body porcelain over lingual surface.

Body and enamel porcelains are dried and preheated in the same way as the core porcelain, but for a little longer time. The piece is placed in the muffle at 1290° F. and sealed, and the vacuum switch is turned on. The temperature is advanced no more than 50° per minute to 1650° F., where it is held for 1½ minutes. The crown is cooled under glass. Only a very small portion of this dentin porcelain will be visible after the crown is fully contoured.

Second and Third Bakes. Body porcelain is added to the labial and lingual and is dried, vibrated, dried, and condensed (Fig. 24-15). A portion of the incisal two-thirds of the body porcelain is carved away at an angle so that the junction between it and the enamel porcelains, at about the height of contour on the labial surface, will feather into each other without a line of demarcation (Fig. 24-16 *A* and *B*). The surface of the porcelain is wetted, angles are trimmed, and enamel porcelain is added labially and a little to the lingual (Fig. 24–16 *C, D,* and *E*). The lingual of the incisal edge is made concave (Fig. 24-17 *A* and *B*) and is filled with translucent porcelain all along the incisal edge (Fig. 24-17 *C*). The extent to which this is done is based on judgment and observation of the approximating natural teeth. The concavities on both the mesial and distal are filled with both enamel and body porcelain and the crown is built out to excessive contour (Fig. 24-17 *D*). The crown is brushed, vibrated, and dried; the apron is cleaned flush with the

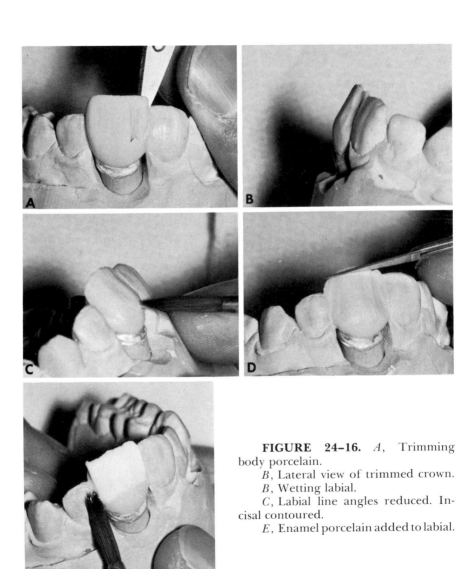

FIGURE 24–16. *A*, Trimming body porcelain.
B, Lateral view of trimmed crown.
B, Wetting labial.
C, Labial line angles reduced. Incisal contoured.
E, Enamel porcelain added to labial.

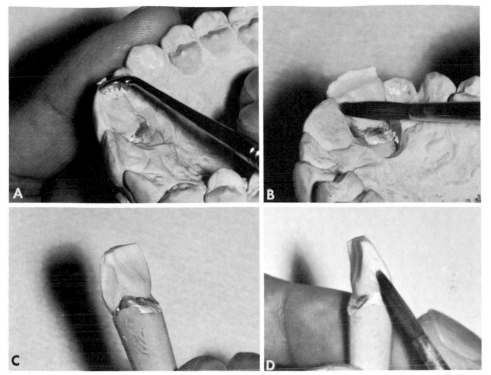

FIGURE 24-17. *A* and *B,* Hollowing linguoincisal to receive translucent porcelain.

C, Incisal filled with translucent porcelain. Note proximal concavity caused by porcelain overlapping approximating tooth.

D, Filling proximal concavities to overextend dimensions of crown and compensate for shrinkage.

margin; the surface of the crown is burnished and placed on the firing tray (Fig. 24-18); and the body cycle is repeated.

Shaping for the Glaze Firing. The cervical is contoured and finished, contacts are tested, and the width of the crown is established (Fig. 24-19). The incisal length is marked with a pencil and trimmed (Fig. 24-20 *A*). Proximal convexities are marked (Fig. 24-20 *B*), and the labial incisal contour is outlined with pencil (Fig. 24-20 *C* and *D*). Anatomical markings on the labial surface are outlined with pencil (Fig. 24-20 *E*), and the occlusion is checked (Fig. 24-20 *F*) and equilibrated.

After the surface of the crown has been smoothed (Fig. 24-21 *A*), it is placed in a solution of chloroform to dissolve any wax (Fig. 24-21 *B*) and then in a beaker of detergent water in an ultrasonic cleanser so that all debris may be removed.

Glazing. The crown may be glazed either by refiring or by using Steele's Super Glaze. The surface is rubbed with either 1650° F. porcelain powder or Super Glaze (Fig. 24-21 *C*), and the crown is fired. If Super Glaze is used, a coating is painted on also.

To glaze, the crown is slowly moved into a hot furnace and, in atmos-

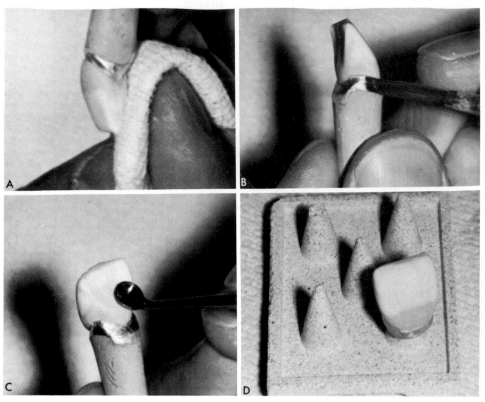

FIGURE 24–18. *A*, Drying and condensing porcelain.
B, Cleaning overlying porcelain from collar of matrix.
C, Burnishing and smoothing concave lingual surface.
D, Crown on stilt ready for drying and firing.

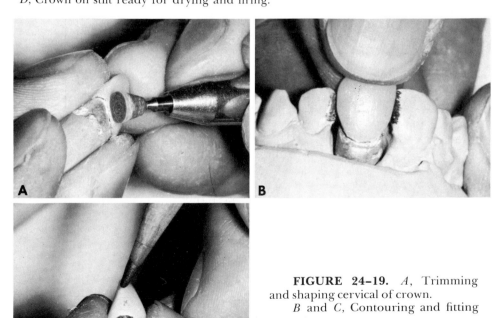

FIGURE 24–19. *A*, Trimming and shaping cervical of crown.

B and *C*, Contouring and fitting contact areas.

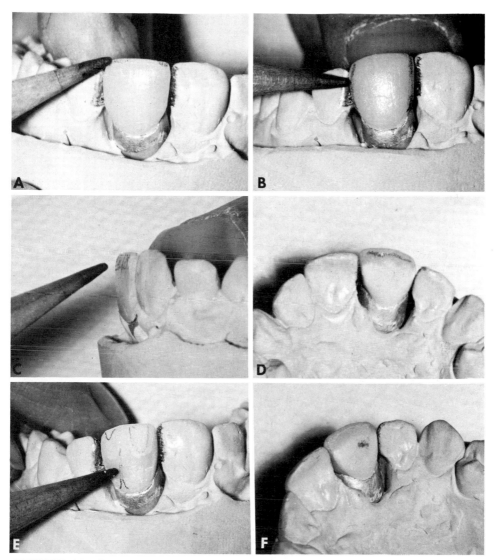

FIGURE 24–20.   *A*, Marking incisal outline.
B, Sketching labial line angles.
C and *D*, Indicating extent of labioincisal convexity.
E, Outlining labial markings.
F, Checking occlusion.

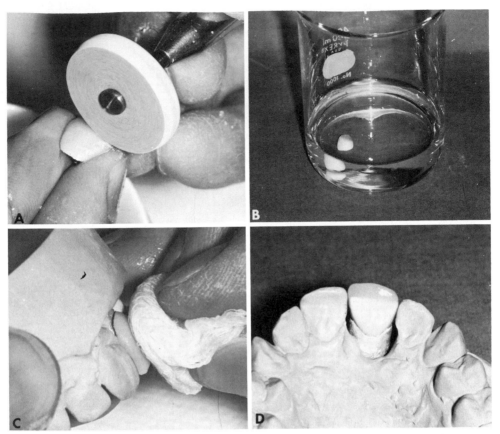

FIGURE 24–21. *A*, Smoothing surface after grinding in all anatomic markings.
B, Cleaning debris from surface.
C, Rubbing powder onto surface.
D, Lingual of fired crown.

phere, the temperature is gradually elevated to a level of 1650 to 1750° F. and held for 4½ to 5 minutes. If Super Glaze has been used, the surface texture and sheen should be checked after 1 and 2 minutes. Figure 24-21 *D* shows the lingual surface with the amount of translucent porcelain that was added in the incisal. The crown should be tried in the mouth, before the matrix is removed, to check and correct contacts and occlusion before the glaze firing.

The matrix is removed by prying the platinum away from the shoulder of the crown with a pointed instrument (Fig. 24–22 *A*) and by grasping at the joint area of the matrix with pliers. With a twisting rotary motion toward the center of the crown the platinum loosens easily if it has been smoothly burnished (Fig. 24–22 *B* and *C*).

Figure 24-23 shows three clinical cases, each with maxillary central incisor crowns built of Steele's Aluminous Porcelain.

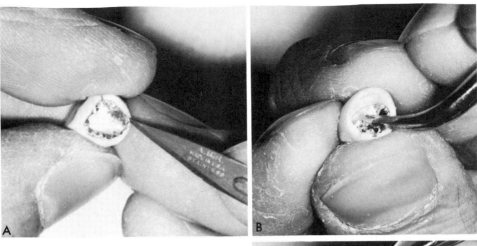

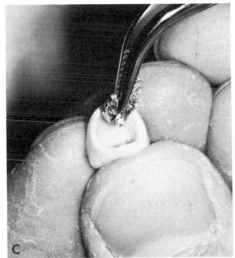

FIGURE 24-22. *A, B,* and *C,* Removing platinum matrix. Platinum loosens more readily if piece is wet.

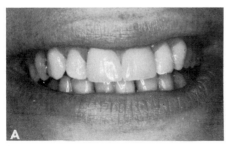

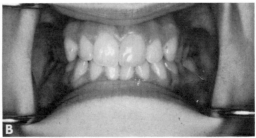

FIGURE 24-23. *A, B,* and *C,* Crowns built of aluminous porcelain.

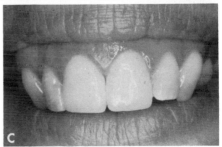

REFERENCES

1. Johnston, J. F., Mumford, G., and Dykema, R. W.: Modern Practice in Dental Ceramics. Philadelphia, W. B. Saunders Company, 1967, pp. 35–58.
2. McLean, J. W., and Hughes, T. H.: The reinforcement of dental porcelain with ceramic oxides. Brit. D. J., *119*:251, Sept. 21, 1965.
3. McLean, J. W.: The alumina reinforced porcelain jacket crown. J.A.D.A., *75*:621, Sept. 1967.
4. Brecker, S. C.: Aluminous porcelain, a new strong ceramic material for esthetic restorations. D. Digest, *73*:449, Oct. 1967.

Dykema, R. W.: Aluminous Porcelain Crowns. Indiana University School of Dentistry Alumni Bulletin, Spring 1970.

McLean, J. W.: A higher strength porcelain for crown and bridge work. Brit. D. J., *119*:268, Sept. 21, 1965.

McLean, J. W.: The alumina tube post crown. Brit. D. J., *123*:87, July 18, 1967.

Tylman, S. D.: Theory and Practice of Crown and Fixed Partial Prosthodontics (Bridge). St. Louis, The C. V. Mosby Company, 1970.

chapter 25

THE CONSTRUCTION OF VENEERED CROWNS, JACKET CROWNS, AND BRIDGES, USING RESINS

For more than three decades, resins have been used to restore individual teeth and to veneer crowns and bridges. As with many materials and processes achieving wide popularity almost instantaneously, there have been widespread abuses in application and expectations, extravagant claims for suitability and for improved physical properties, and on occasion unwarranted and unjust criticisms. Because of its adaptability and seeming successes, and in spite of its conspicuous failures, acrylic resin remains a part of the armamentarium of the dental profession.

In addition to acrylic resin, other materials are also available for veneering purposes. These include acrylic copolymers, vinyl, and epoxy resins. Each type has merits and demerits in terms of the inherent physical properties. However, none has been shown to be markedly superior, and all have the general characteristics that will be described here.[1, 2]

The authors do not use resins in the construction of crowns and bridges except for temporary coverings and space maintainers, where they are serviceable materials.

PHYSICAL PROPERTIES OF ACRYLIC RESIN

Acrylic resin is translucent in varying degrees, sometimes a desirable trait in a tooth-colored restoration. This translucent quality gives it a natural look in the mouth because it is capable of assuming shade values from the approximating teeth. The esthetic appearance of a veneered restoration may be affected considerably by the underlying metal, but this can be controlled in some measure by using opaquing or masking materials. The veneer helps

513

to serve as its own mask if it is at least 1.0 mm. thick. Properly manipulated, most of the resin materials procurable today are reasonably color-stable. Resin will flow and alter its shape when subjected to even light loads over long periods of time, and it undergoes elastic deformation under intermittent stresses that may be too light to cause permanent change.[3] Therefore, a resin veneer must be shielded from occlusal forces by a plate of gold that, with few exceptions, is visible.

Acrylic resin does not bond to the metallic portion of the restoration.[4] It must depend on some kind of mechanical lock. This constitutional weakness, coupled with a higher coefficient of thermal expansion than in gold, may form a space at the interface between the gold and the veneer, even though the veneer is protected by metal from the forces of occlusion. Debris from the oral cavity can filter under the veneer and discolor it, or induce tarnish and corrosion of the underlying metal, either of which could cause discoloration of the veneer.[5] Adequate retention and protection, and technique in packing and curing, will minimize such a space, although it can never be eliminated completely. The veneer is readily applied or removed for remaking if the shade is unsatisfactory.

Since pure gold is a relatively inert material, gold-plating the area to be veneered will lessen the chance of tarnish of the underlying metal. Gold-plating may be done by the usual electrical process or by flash-plating.*

The greatest single virtue of resin over porcelain as a veneering material on a gold restoration is the facility with which it can be worked. The fabrication of the veneer is less of an "art." The principal disadvantage, besides lack of an adhesive bond between the two materials, is low resistance to abrasion. The patient should be advised to use a soft toothbrush and a nonabrasive dentifrice, but even so wear does occur in time.[6] Discoloration and abrasion are all too commonly observed in the resin veneer.

Most resin veneering materials are composed of heat-cured acrylic and vinyl-acrylic copolymers. Recently thermosetting dimethacrylate resins have been introduced to the profession, e.g., Pyroplast.† Its physical properties are comparable to those of the conventional acrylic material. This resin is not flasked and molded as is a typical acrylic resin. Admittedly the technique is a convenient one, since the veneer can be fabricated within 8 minutes.

The clinical performance of a veneering material most often is based upon the proficiency exercised in fabricating the veneer. No one resin excels.

There is little or no difference in the preparation[7] of a tooth for a crown to be veneered with resin and one to be veneered with porcelain, *except* in length. For a resin veneer crown the prepared tooth, under ideal conditions, can be left 0.5 to 0.8 mm. longer than when a bonded porcelain veneer crown will be used (Fig. 25–1).

The Die. Any acceptable method of obtaining the dies and working casts may be used for constructing resin veneer crowns and bridges, but

*Gold Plating Solution, The L. D. Caulk Company, Milford, Del.
†Williams Gold Refining Co., Inc., Buffalo, N.Y.

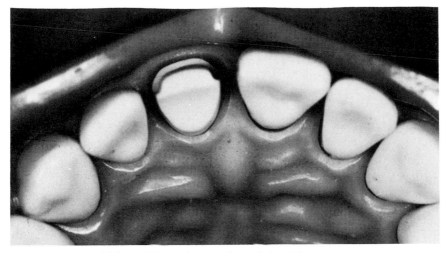

FIGURE 25–1. Width and lingual extension of shoulder.

there are obvious benefits in using an indirect technique. Metalized dies are excellent; stone dies and intact working casts, poured in one impression, give splendid results.

The Shade.   The shade should be determined by use of the shade guide that the manufacturer of each acrylic resin provides. The choice may be influenced by the shade of the tooth, and possibly by the resin favored by the technician.

A shade distribution chart, made with care, should be sent to the laboratory.

THE RESIN VENEER CROWN

The Wax Pattern

It is advisable that the pattern for the casting be carved to full anatomic form (Fig. 25-2) before an attempt is made to shape the area to be veneered, because correct contour cannot be visualized when dealing with only a

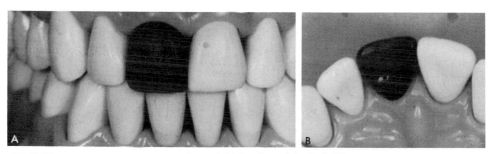

FIGURE 25–2. Wax pattern from labial (*A*) and incisal (*B*).

portion of a tooth. After form, contact, and occlusion have been attained, the veneer outline should be drawn on the wax pattern with a sharp instrument. Then the wax in the area of the veneer may be either completely removed to the labial surface of the die, and a single layer of 28-gauge sheet wax adapted to the die surface and sealed to the pattern, or a uniform layer of the original wax, about 0.5 mm. thick, may be left (Fig. 25-3). The latter method is preferable, since carving wax resists deformation during handling more effectively than the softer sheet wax.

The occlusal and cervical peripheral wax around the area to be veneered is not cut down as far as the gold casting will be reduced. This excess wax will cause molten metal to be fed into the thin labial portion of the casting from a surrounding area of heavier bulk, and will make certain a complete casting in the thin section that will back the veneer. An accessory wax sprue rod, or vent, joining the labial surface of the pattern and the sprue former, may be helpful in getting a complete casting. The proximal outlines should be established in the wax, since the proximal retentive loops will make it impossible to alter the outline here after the casting has been made.

Retention.   Retentive wire loops, 27-gauge or 28-gauge, incorporated in the proximal of the pattern, offer maximal retention for the veneer.[5] They can be purchased or they may be formed from wire of the appropriate size and physical properties. The wire must be nonoxidizing in order to form a union with the casting, soft enough so that adjustments can be made after the casting has been completed, and must have a fusing range high enough for gold to be cast to it without changing its physical properties.* The loops should be stapleline in shape, about 1.0 mm. in diameter and 1.5 mm. in length, and should be placed approximately 0.7 to 1.0 mm. inside the peripheral margin of the veneer area, perpendicular to the surface of the wax at that point (Fig. 25-4).

If the loops are warmed in a flame while being held by tweezers, the wire can be forced into the wax sufficiently far to be held securely. Then a

---

*Zephyr wire, The J. M. Ney Company, Bloomfield, Conn.
Pliant wire, J. F. Jelenko & Co., Inc., New Rochelle, N.Y.

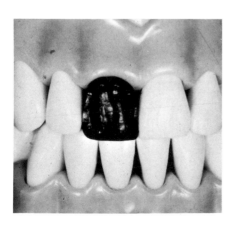

FIGURE 25-3.   Labial of pattern reduced.

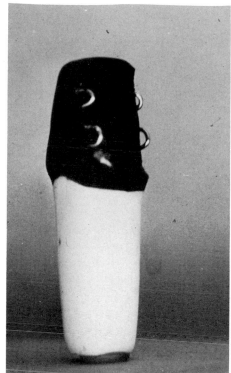

FIGURE 25-4. Retentive loops.

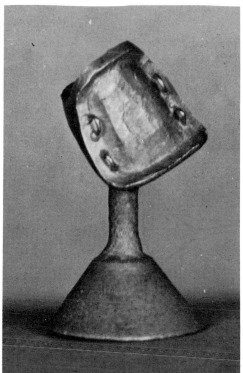

FIGURE 25-5. The casting.

small instrument should be heated and placed in contact with the wire loop. Heat will be conducted from the instrument and will melt the wax around the points of the wire, making it a simple matter to guide the loop to place. At no time should the hot instrument contact the wax.

The wire should extend into the pattern about 0.5 mm., leaving an exposed loop 1.0 mm. high and 1.0 mm. wide. The number of loops will depend on the length of the tooth involved; in most instances two loops can be inserted on each side. The wire must not be placed so far incisally on an anterior crown that it will show through the thin resin in that area.

Plastic beads may be added to the surface to be veneered, forming irregular nodules to supplement the loops and undercut retention and reduce the amount of percolation. Retention for the veneer should not depend on beads alone.

The Casting

A veneered gold crown has almost parallel walls and a small inside diameter, making it imperative that an investment and casting technique be

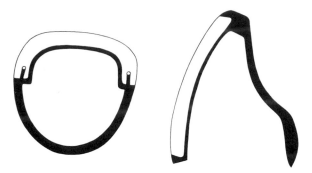

FIGURE 25-6. Diagram of retention form for acrylic resin veneer.

employed that will cause maximal expansion. A hard crown and bridge or partial denture gold should be used (Fig. 25-5).

The final peripheral outline of the casting is made by reducing the incisal plate and the cervical collar of gold, using a No. 557 or 558 steel bur. To augment the retention derived from the wire loops and assure that the bulk of resin in these areas will provide the required color in the veneer, undercuts must be placed incisally and cervically (Fig. 25-6) by a No. 33½ or 34 inverted cone, No. ½ round, and No. 14 wheel burs. After the undercuts have been made, the thickness of metal remaining between the opposing teeth and the resin veneer, which should be a minimum of 1.0 mm., must be checked. If the unit is a part of a bridge or splint, it should be soldered, and then the surface to be veneered should be cleaned and smoothed with a metal bur.

If it is suspected that the tips of the loops will be visible through the resin, they may be bent toward the midline of the restoration (Fig. 25-7),

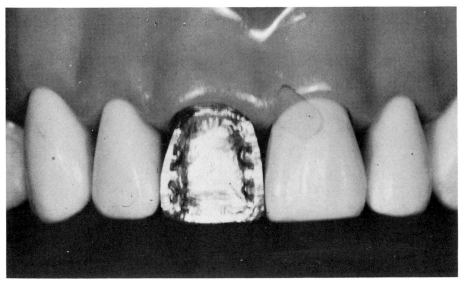

FIGURE 25-7. Peripheral outline established in casting. Loops bent toward center of crown.

thereby increasing the thickness of the veneering material over the wires. Bending must be done in the majority of cases and will not appreciably affect the retentive qualities of the loops. If the veneered area is to be plated, it must be done at this time, after which the restoration can be polished and scrubbed clean.[8]

The Mold

The wax for the preliminary veneer must be tooth-colored so that the mold, and subsequently the resin veneer, will not be impregnated with unwanted pigment. It must be carved with the exact contour and specific surface markings desired. The restoration should be invested in a small amount of stone, labial or buccal surface up, with the stone approaching but not in contact with the wax veneer. No undercuts on the metallic portion may be left unfilled by stone, because they would induce fracture of the second half of the mold when the flask was opened, or even worse they might effect deformation of the casting. If the restoration is complicated, of five, six, or more units, those not to be veneered may be wrapped in a thin layer of wet asbestos or heavy tin foil to make removal from the stone easier. All areas to be veneered must be supported by hard stone to ensure commensurate resistance to the high pressures that these sections must withstand during packing.

After the first layer of stone has set, it must be trimmed circumferentially to within approximately 2.0 mm. of the restoration and then invested in plaster or stone in the bottom half of the flask. This double-investing technique makes it possible to remove the crown or bridge from the bulk of the investing stone without danger of damage to the restoration. The surface of the investing stone in the first half of the flask should be lubricated with petroleum jelly and the excess wiped away without lessening any undulation or margin of the wax veneer.

The second half of the mold must be poured with well-spatulated bubble-free stone, without trapping air bubbles over the wax pattern. When it has set, the mold should be warmed in a water bath to prevent the wax from sticking to the mold, the flask opened, and the surface examined for imperfections (Fig. 25–8). If there are no bubbles or voids in the counterdie, the wax can be flushed from the mold by a stream of boiling water and all traces of the wax residue removed with a solvent such as chloroform. The case may be veneered with resin when the mold has cooled to room temperature.

Veneering Resins

There are a number of acrylic resins manufactured for use by the dental profession. The majority are satisfactory; selection will be governed solely by

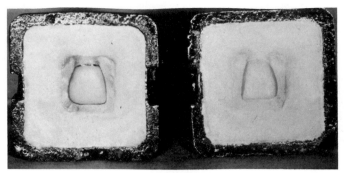

FIGURE 25–8.   Wax pattern flasked and flask opened.

inclination. There are opaque or masking materials also, but the resin ones appear to be the most successful. The paint and lacquer opaques seem to act as contaminating agents or to produce discoloration of the veneer. A resin masking material has the salutary property of becoming an integral, inseparable part of the veneer during the process of polymerization, permitting masking in the retentive areas of the casting without loss of retention. The autopolymerizing or self-curing resin restorative materials are not suitable for veneers, being very difficult to handle and not so color-stable as heat-cured resins.

Masking.   It is not always necessary to use a masking material. The darker shades especially should not be altered by the underlying metal. Nevertheless, masking probably will improve the shade of a veneer if it is no thicker than 1.0 mm.

The medium chosen should be approximately the same color or should be blended to complement the shade selected for the finished veneer. If a close match is out of the question, a darker opaque will be of more assistance than a lighter one, separate colors being used for masking the cervical and incisal sections. A thin, uniform coating, just ample to obliterate the color of the metal, should be applied, with no build-up of masking material around the peripheral margin of the veneer. As soon as the masking layer has set, the main body of the veneer may be applied.

The Veneer—Gingival.   The gingival portion of the veneer should be prepared first, placing the resin powder or blended powders of the preselected shade in a small, covered mixing jar. Only enough monomer should be added to wet all particles of the powder. The powder and liquid must be mixed slightly to assure uniform color, the jar covered tightly to avert evaporation of the liquid, and then set aside until the resin has reached a doughy consistency. Several sheets of cellophane should be placed in a bowl of water so that a fresh piece will be at hand each time the flask is to be closed.

Gingival resin, roughly equal to the bulk of the veneer, should be placed over the metal and shaped to approximate form with a stainless steel spatula. After a damp sheet of cellophane has been placed between the two halves of the flask, the mold must be closed with a bench press, then opened, and the veneer scrutinized for contour and surface markings. A lack of material, flow, or details would indicate the need for more resin, in which case a small amount is added, a fresh damp sheet of cellophane is placed for separation, and the flask is again closed in a press. Trial packing must be repeated until all contours and surface characteristics are registered and the resin has a firm consistency.

The Veneer—Incisal.   As soon as the flask is opened, the incisal area must be trimmed with a sharp instrument to remove the bulk to be replaced by the incisal shade; that which remains may be reshaped with a flat instrument. The incisal powder, mixed in a Dappen dish, will have a sandlike consistency when all particles have been wet by monomer. After it has been carried to place and patted to form, a moist sheet of cellophane is placed over the first half of the flask and the top portion is positioned without pressure and kept there for approximately 5 minutes. This will cause the two shades to blend without displacing the gingival portion. The flask should be opened to check the shade distribution. If the incisal has reached a doughy consistency, it is ready for the application of packing pressure. If more incisal must be added or an excess removed, corrections are made before the flask is closed under pressure. The flask must be opened for a final check, all excess trimmed from the periphery of the veneer, and a new sheet of cellophane inserted between the halves before the flask can be closed for processing.

Processing and Finishing

Processing should be completed by immersing the flask and press in a room-temperature water bath and raising the temperature of the water to 212° F. over a period of 30 minutes. Then the case must be boiled for an additional 30 minutes, after which press and flask should be removed from the boiling water and allowed to bench-cool to room temperature (Fig. 25-9). Only then should the flask be opened and the restoration cautiously removed from the investing stone so that the margins will not be harmed or the restoration distorted. If the packing was done meticulously and all excess removed before the final closure of the flask, there will be only a little additional flash of resin at the margins of the veneer, which can be removed with a sharp knife or a fissure bur. These areas are now polished. The cellophane used between the two halves of the flask will give the veneer a surface texture that should be undisturbed while polishing the margins.

The finished restoration should be stored in water until it can be cemented so that the veneer may attain equilibrium with water and thus be dimensionally stable when it is placed in the mouth and is subject to sorption of fluids.

Other special processing techniques that have been advocated include curing the resin in a vacuum oven, and an additional cure at an elevated temperature of approximately 600° F. Resin processed in such ways is not

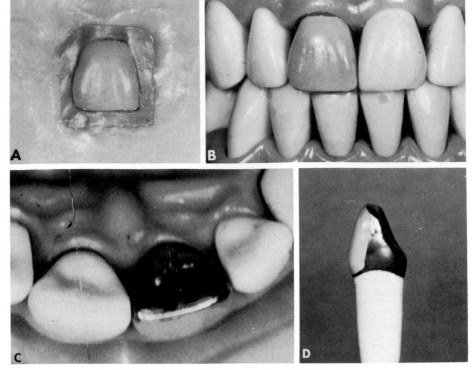

FIGURE 25–9. *The processed and finished crown.*

A, Crown in flask.
B, *C*, and *D*, Finished crown.

perceptibly harder or more resistant to abrasion, nor is it less irritating to tissue.

Resin veneer crowns may be cemented by the technique elected by the operator.

THE RESIN JACKET CROWN

It must be noted that the novice or student can learn readily to construct a jacket crown of resin that fits and is, at the time of seating, esthetically and biologically acceptable. With use of products now available, an acrylic resin crown seems to have serviceable color stability, and the wear on the contact areas of an anterior jacket does not constitute a hazard to arch length or embrasure form.[9, 10] It is true that a resin crown will abrade on the labial and linguoincisal, but it is not a restoration to be looked on with scorn or to be seated apologetically if its fundamental shortcomings are openly recognized. In almost all instances it will give extended service and will be in harmony with the approximating teeth for a protracted period.

A more adverse reaction from occlusal pressure and abrasion will be found on posterior resin crowns. Pressure will be generated in many directions during mastication, tending to break adhesion of cement, or after a period of wear to split the crown. Therefore, resin jacket crowns should be limited to maxillary incisors where there is at least a normal overjet in the maxillomandibular relationship.

Preparation

With one exception the preparation to receive a resin jacket crown is identical to that for a porcelain jacket. Areas of contact in centric occlusion and eccentric excursions should be cut 0.35 mm. deeper than for porcelain, to minimize the effects of wear and to inhibit flexing of the crown.

Selecting the color for a resin jacket crown is done in the same way as for a resin veneer. Dies and working casts are obtained in the same manner as those for porcelain jackets and porcelain veneered crowns. Platinum foil serves better than tin foil for the matrix. The wax pattern may be carved on the die and working cast or in the mouth.

Flasking. The acrylic resin jacket crown may be invested, packed, and processed in a two-section flask. A small amount of die stone is mixed with a mechanical spatulator and vacuumed to remove the air bubbles. The inside of the crown is filled and the pattern is positioned, lingual side down, in a small mass of stone placed on a glass slab or other smooth surface. The stone is carried to a point lingual to the labial line angles on the proximal and incisal surfaces so that the polished flash line will not be visible. No matter how well polished, this line can be detected if it is to the labial of the interproximal shadow. At the cervical, the investment is carried flush with the apron of the platinum matrix. After the stone has set completely, the mass is trimmed so that it is no more than 3.0 mm. thick at any point. This procedure makes for greater control of flasking materials and prevents the pattern from settling too far into the flask (Fig. 25-10).

With use of a fresh mix of stone, the pattern is set in the bottom section

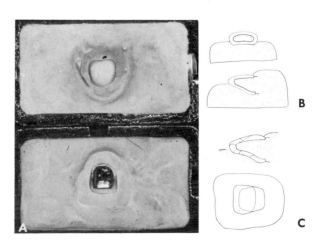

FIGURE 25–10. *Packing in two-piece flask.*

A, Pattern invested in flask; wax washed away.

B, Cross section of flasked pattern.

C, Increments of resin are added to blend gingival and incisal shades.

of the flask, just above the level of the edge of the flask. After the hardened stone has been smoothed, the surface is lubricated with petroleum jelly and the second half is poured. Any excess separating medium or air bubbles trapped on or near the pattern will cause defects on the surface of the crown.

Packing.   When the stone in the top half of the flask has set, it is warmed in hot water, opened before the wax has melted, and all wax is flushed away with a stream of clean, boiling water. When the case may be comfortably held in the bare hands, the portion of the mold in the bottom section of the flask is coated with a single layer of a foil substitute, such as Al-Cote.* If this were done while the case is hot, the foil substitute would peel from the surface of the stone after it dries.

When the acrylic resin has reached a relatively thick doughlike state, the mold is packed completely with the gingival shade, trial packing being employed and more material being added if wanted. Except that attention must be given to forcing resin into the lingual portion of the mold, the technique of packing and processing is the same as for the resin veneer crown, discussed early in this chapter.

Deflasking and Polishing.   After the flask has air-cooled to room temperature, it is taken from the press and opened. With a sharp knife the stone is removed from around the restoration until it may be freed from the flask with little effort. Resin is not a strong material and may be damaged by prying. Any stone remaining on the surface of the resin can be flaked off with a sharp instrument.

The stone inside the crown may be partially eliminated with a small round bur inserted into the mid-portion of the material, and the remainder may be chipped away with a small pointed instrument.

The platinum is loosened by grasping the apron of the matrix at the lap joint with tweezers and pulling toward the center of the crown. Then with a twisting motion the matrix can be wound onto the beaks of the instrument and freed. If the matrix was adapted to the die without wrinkles, the foil will separate intact by this one operation. Any bits of remaining platinum may be effaced with a round bur.

The flash is cut from the crown with either small fissure burs or carborundum stones. To protect the margin, flash at the cervical should be removed with the crown in place on the die. The crown can be polished with fine pumice in a rubber cup or on a small felt wheel. Wet whiting on a felt wheel, or a prepared resin polishing agent on a small dry rag wheel, will produce a luster on the surface. To avoid abrading the resin, a handpiece, rather than the speedier lathe, should be used for polishing (Figs. 25-11 and 25-12). If the labial half of the flask is covered with tin foil, burnished to be without wrinkles, the surface texture of the crown will be pleasing and need not be polished except at the cervical where the flash was trimmed.

---

*The L. D. Caulk Company, Milford, Del.

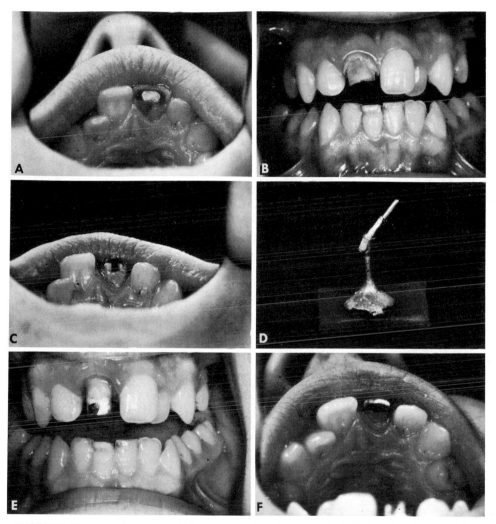

FIGURE 25–11. *Sequence of steps in constructing a resin jacket crown for a pulpless maxillary central incisor, using amulgam die, wax transfer, and plaster impression.*

A, Fractured central following endodontic therapy.

B, Shoulder partly formed in preparation of tooth.

C, Post of high-fusing clasp wire fitted into root canal and extending out to what will be the incisal edge of prepared tooth.

D, Cast core.

E and *F*, Finished preparation with cast core cemented.

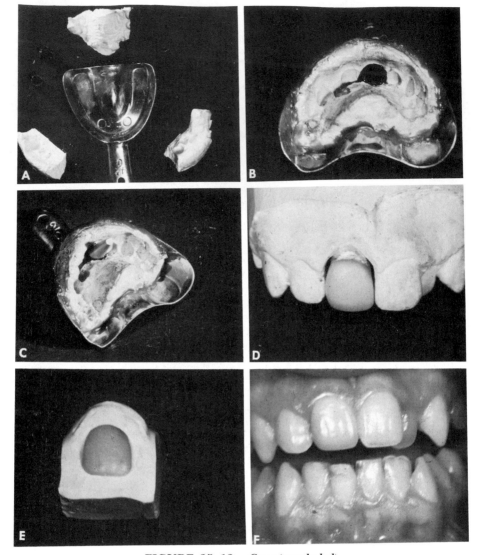

FIGURE 25–12.   *Case (concluded).*

A, B, and *C,* Plaster impression with amalgam die seated, ready to pour working cast.
D, Working cast and wax pattern.
E, First step in flasking pattern.
F, Finished crown on tooth.

CEMENTATION

Before a resin crown is seated permanently, it should be tried on the tooth and examined for color, shape, position, occlusion, contact areas, soft-tissue relationship, and fit. Zinc phosphate cement is preferred and the shade may be chosen after making test mixtures of the powders with water and glycerin. The cement should be mixed at a ratio that will give maximal physical properties, but should not be so thick that undue pressure must be applied when the crown is seated (Figs. 25–13 and 25–14).

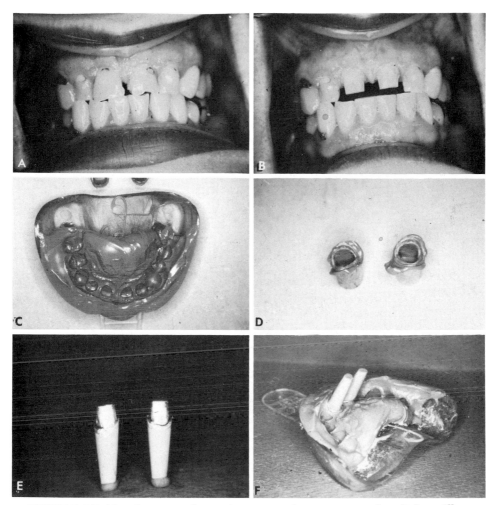

FIGURE 25–13.   *Sequence of steps in constructing two crowns for vital maxillary central incisors, using silver-plated dies and a polysulfide rubber impression.*

A, Central incisors before preparation.

B, After preparation; this is an end-to-end occlusion, making it necessary to have greater incisal clearance.

C, Polysulfide rubber impression for working cast was stored in a humidifier until dies were completed.

D, Polysulfide rubber impressions for metalized dies.

E, Dies.

F, Dies in impression ready for boxing.

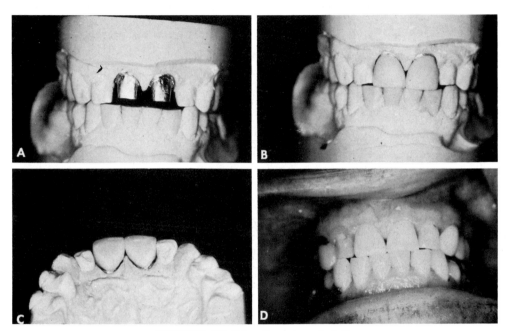

FIGURE 25–14. *Case (concluded).*

A, Working and opposing casts before mounting.
B and *C*, Wax patterns.
D, Completed crowns.

BRIDGES VENEERED WITH RESIN

Resin veneers are attached to bridge retainers and pontics by the same mechanical devices as with crowns, although pontics may be hollow, with the resin built around crossed wires or rods and into very irregular spaces (Fig. 25-15).

It is the considered observation of the authors that the ridge-contacting areas of pontics, since the relationship is static, should not be veneered with resin because of tissue irritation. However, Eich[11] and others have contended that this does not occur to a greater degree with resin than with porcelain or metal (Figs. 25-16, 25-17, 25-18, and 25-19). In the event that this procedure becomes necessary, ridge contact must be reduced to the minimum.

When both retainers and pontics are to be veneered with resin, shading will be more uniform if all veneers are approximately the same thickness. This is especially true in an anterior fixed prosthesis. It becomes progressively less important when pontics are posterior to the cuspid.

When veneering long prostheses or splints, a sectional flask should be used in order that the counterdie may be divided and opened and closed laterally on hinges (Fig. 25-20).

Packing, trial packing, and curing follow the routine for the single-unit crown.

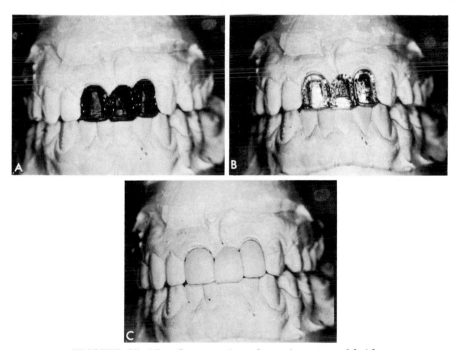

FIGURE 25-15. *Construction of a resin veneered bridge.*

A, Three wax patterns with retentive loops. They were cast individually.
B, Soldered bridge.
C, Waxed labial veneers.

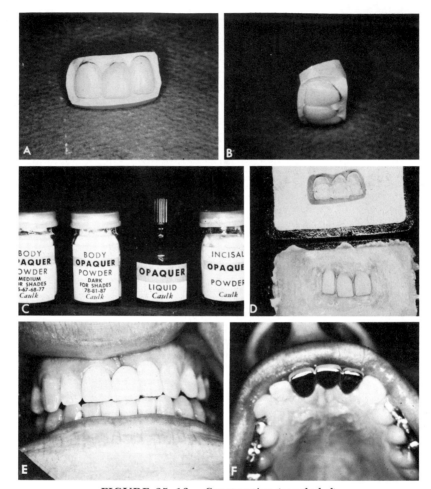

FIGURE 25–16.   *Construction (concluded).*

A, Bridge invested, ready for flasking.
B, Side view, showing investment extended just to height of contour.
C, Opaque.
D, Flask separated, wax eliminated, opaque applied.
E and *F*, Bridge seated.

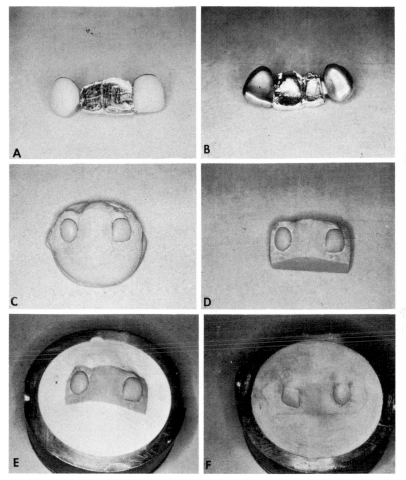

FIGURE 25–17.   *Maxillary bridge with resin veneers on cuspid and central incisor retainer.*

A and *B*, Pontics wrapped in heavy tin foil to aid in removing bridge from flask.

C and *D*, First step in flasking.

E, Bridge flasked.

F, Top half of flask. Note absence of bubbles near veneering areas.

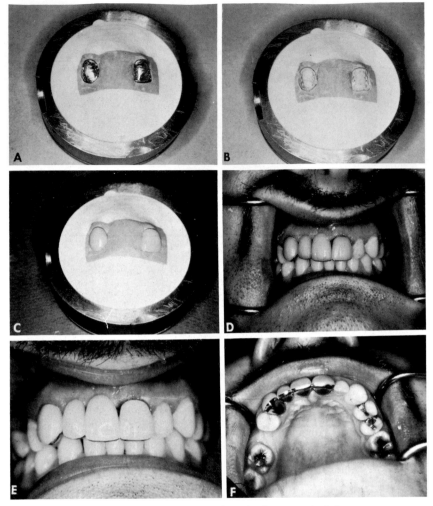

FIGURE 25–18. *Maxillary bridge (concluded).*

A, Wax has been flushed away with boiling water.
B, Opaque applied to retainers.
C, Veneers have been cured.
D, Bridge seated to cheek for possible distortion.
E and *F*, Bridge cemented.

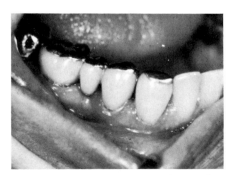

FIGURE 25–19.   Mandibular three-unit bridge and cuspid crown with resin veneers.

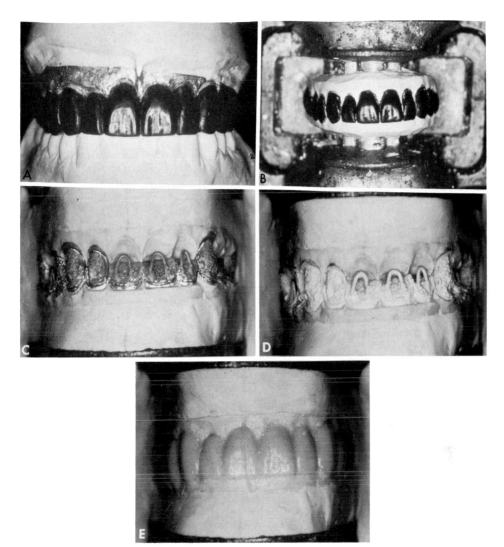

FIGURE 25-20.   *A*, Complete arch maxillary splint. Wax veneers carved.
B, Splint invested in sectioned flask.
C, Wax removed.
D, Opaque applied to metal.
E, Veneers cured.
(Courtesy of Dr. Frank A. Eich, Tufts University School of Dental Medicine.)

REFERENCES

1. Kafalias, M. C., Swartz, M. L., and Phillips, R. W.: Physical properties of selected dental resins, Part I. J. Pros. Den., *13*:1087, Nov.-Dec. 1963.
2. FitzRoy, D. C., Swartz, M. L., and Phillips, R. W.: Physical properties of selected dental resins, Part II. J. Pros. Den., *13*:1108, Nov.-Dec. 1963.
3. Peyton, F. A., and Craig, R. G.: Current evaluation of plastics in crown and bridge prosthesis. J. Pros. Den., *13*:743, July-Aug. 1963.
4. Swartz, M. L., and Phillips, R. W.: A study of adaptation of veneers to cast gold crowns. J. Pros. Den., 7:817, Nov. 1957.

5. Skinner, E. W., and Phillips, R. W.: The Science of Dental Materials. 6th ed. Philadelphia, W. B. Saunders Company, 1967.
6. Coy, H. D.: An evaluation of acrylic resin as a restorative material. J.A.D.A., *48*:266, March 1954.
7. Davis, M. C., and Klein, G.: Combination gold and acrylic restorations. J. Pros. Den., *4*:510, July 1954.
8. Cohn, L. A.: The acrylic-faced cast gold crown. J. Pros. Den., *1*:112, Jan.-March 1951.
9. Chevalier, P. L.: Personal communication.
10. Pincus, C. L.: Esthetic variations in jacket crowns and bridge restoration involving periodontal and other deformities. Its application to oral rehabilitation. New York J. Den., *24*:132, March 1954 (Abstract).
11. Eich, F. A.: Personal communication.

Fairhurst, C. W., and Ryge, G.: Effect of tin-foil substitutes on the strength of denture base resins. J. Pros. Den., *5*:508, July 1955.
Hedegard, B.: Evaluation of materials for anterior bridges with special reference to acrylic resins. Internat. D. J., *12*:33, March 1962.
Long, A. C.: Acrylic resin veneered crowns: The effect of tooth preparation on crown fabrication and future periodontal health. J. Pros. Den., *19*:370, April 1968.
McCune, R. J., et al.: An evaluation of a new resin veneering material. J. South. California D. A., *36*:496, Dec. 1968.
Pincus, C. L.: New concepts in mold techniques and high temperature processing of acrylic resins for maximum esthetics. Technical procedure. J. South. California D. A., *24*:26, Feb. 1956.
Ryge, G., and Foley, D. E.: Effect of dry heat processing on the physical properties of acrylic crowns. J.A.D.A., *66*:672, May 1963.
Vieira, D. F., and Phillips, R. W.: Influence of certain variables on the abrasion of acrylic resin veneering materials. J. Pros. Den., *12*:720, July-Aug. 1962.
Yock, D. H.: Indications for the use of plastic resins in crown and bridge prosthesis, J.A.D.A., *46*:505, May 1953.

chapter 26

BRIDGE PATTERNS

There is a divergence of opinion among dentists concerning the use of complete coverage of the abutment tooth. It is the contention of some men that the dentist is not fully aware of his responsibility, or, if he is aware of it, that he does not meet his responsibility if any surface of the abutment is permitted to remain uncovered so that it may be susceptible later to a carious lesion.

The authors do not subscribe to this philosophy. A noteworthy number of bridges, held in place by inlays, pinlays, or partial veneer crowns, have served for such long periods that the occluding surfaces have been worn to a point necessitating replacement of the original bridges. Many teeth that have been prepared for partial veneer crowns and other types of retainers not covering all the enamel surfaces have resisted caries so effectively that they are now supporting the third bridge.

It is true that there are numerous situations in which caries, movement of teeth, a short clinical crown, or the need for maximal retention makes a full veneer gold crown the retainer of choice. Periodic clinic surveys* have disclosed that full veneer or veneered gold crowns constitute between 55 and 60 per cent of all retainers used. These, it must be remembered, were placed in mouths that cannot be considered exactly typical of those to be found in practices in which fixed partial denture construction may be one of the major efforts. Oral hygiene concepts and routine clinical care render mouths of patients in private practice far more receptive to the construction of bridges.

In the following review of bridge patterns, it will be observed that a variety of retainers have been suggested. Selection was governed by *tooth form, tooth position, space length, occlusion,* and *caries* (either existing or previously treated).

MAXILLARY PATTERNS

Absence of a **single central incisor** is one of the patterns seen most frequently, doubtless because of the embarrassment that it causes the patient

---

*Indiana University School of Dentistry

(Fig. 26-1). In private practice, barring accident, this plight generally can be alleviated by inserting a temporary partial denture at the time of extraction, which is preferable to the immediate construction of a fixed prosthesis. This will help to mold the gingival tissue and will maintain the approximating and opposing teeth in their natural positions, provided it is not worn indefinitely.

Unless the teeth are exceedingly thin and unless the proximal surfaces or incisal angles are restored or carious, a pinledge retainer may be used on each abutment. If the distal surfaces are carious or have small restorations, such areas can be filled with gold foil, or possibly with resin or silicate cement, and the pinledge may still be used. Caries on the mesial surfaces presents somewhat greater difficulties, but again gold foil may be used to rebuild the teeth to normal form, after which they can be treated as sound.

There is no valid argument against using partial veneer crowns with this central incisor pontic except that in many cases it is useless to destroy so much tooth surface. The pinledge retainer is less conspicuous than the partial veneer crown, although the special types of partial veneer preparations advocated by Vedder,[1] Grubb,[2] and Willey[3] work beautifully.

The pinledge can be used on either a long or a short tooth, but some bulk labiolingually in the incisal half is a requisite. Now and then a modification that does not bring the preparation onto the incisal fourth of the lingual

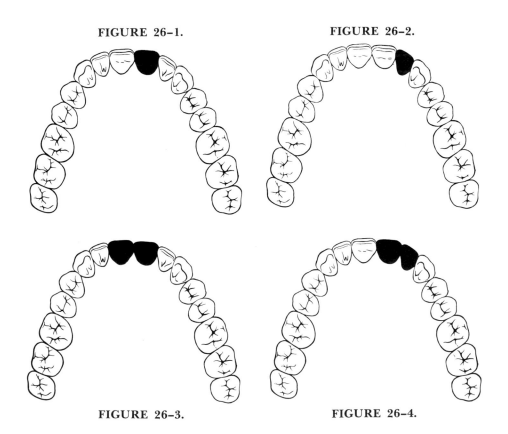

FIGURE 26–1.   FIGURE 26–2.

FIGURE 26–3.   FIGURE 26–4.

surface can be used. While the pins will be more centralized in their locations, if they are given maximal length and are cast, stability will not be jeopardized.

The veneered gold crown must be used, of course, when the caries index is high. Inlays seldom, if ever, provide satisfactory retention in this space. A broken-stress bridge or a cantilever pontic is contraindicated.

A missing **single lateral incisor** (Fig. 26-2) can produce a sizable problem for the student of crown and bridge prosthodontics.[4, 5] Very often a lateral incisor is replaced by cantilevering the pontic from a partial veneer crown retainer on the cuspid, with no rest at the mesial of the pontic. Some students, and some practitioners as well, believe that the teacher is being merely theoretical when he insists that this practice is detrimental to the tissue surrounding the single abutment, or when he asserts that alignment cannot be sustained throughout the lifetime of the bridge. Rotation to the labial is bound to occur and the mesiolingual margin of the lateral pontic will overlap the distolabial line angle of the central incisor. This is unsightly. Even more serious is the change that the anterior movement of the cuspid will bring about in the contact relationships of all posterior teeth in the quadrant.

When the space is narrow, when the forces from the opposing teeth are weak, or when the cuspid root is long and the alveolar recession is slight, there may be some justification for the two-unit bridge. However, a distolingual inlay in the central incisor, with a rest extending from the mesial of the lateral pontic into a recess previously prepared in this inlay, is favored in the event that two soldered retainers cannot be used.

The pinledge is indicated on each abutment unless caries, tooth position, or pulp size prohibits its use. A partial veneer crown is acceptable unless, as in the central incisor pattern, the caries index, shortness of the teeth, or leverages demand that the veneered gold crown be used.

A bridge replacing **both central incisors** (Fig. 26-3) will require more support than can be secured ordinarily from the lateral incisors, which usually have short and frail roots. Splinting the lateral incisors and cuspids as multiple abutments, and using partial veneer or veneered gold crowns as retainers, will insure gratifying results for the longest period.

When the lever arm is short and the clinical crowns are relatively short and stubby, four pinledge retainers can be used. Cast pins will furnish ample resistance to displacement. The partial veneer preparation cannot be adapted readily to such tooth form. Proximal caries that weakens an incisal angle, or a high caries index, would point to the veneered crown.[1]

The replacement of the **approximating central and lateral incisors** (Fig. 26-4) ordinarily will involve only two abutment teeth, namely, the remaining central incisor and the cuspid approximating the space. Much success has been experienced with this type of bridge, using a partial veneer crown on the cuspid and a pinledge or partial veneer retainer on the central.

If the alveolus around the central incisor has receded markedly, the lateral incisor should be included. While a lone lateral incisor is not a strong tooth and does not afford maximal retention, when it is splinted to the central incisor, the ensuing two-rooted multiple abutment will resist rotation and displacement greater than the sum of the two. When the lateral incisor is badly aligned and three abutments are needed, the prosthesis may be attached to the central incisor, cuspid, and first bicuspid, with a partial veneer or veneered crown on the central.

Building a bridge to replace the **central incisor on one side of the median line and the lateral incisor in the adjacent quadrant** (Fig. 26-5) is an entirely different matter from the one just discussed. The cuspid and central incisor will have an equal amount of periodontal membrane area, but, because of distribution, the support will not be comparable to that derived from the two abutments in the preceding pattern. The proximity of the central incisor to the cuspid would allow a cantilever central pontic to exert too much leverage on the central incisor; consequently, the remaining lateral incisor must be used as a terminal abutment. The option between pinledge, partial veneer, or veneered gold crown retainers will be decided by proximal caries, incisal angles, tooth form, long-axis relationship, and incidence of caries.

In a case where **both lateral incisors** are missing (Fig. 26-6), two three-unit bridges should be constructed, rather than one of six units, but the continuous replacement might be in order if recession has added as much as 25 per cent to the crown length of the central incisors. Pinledges, partial veneer, or veneered gold crowns could be used for the longer bridge. Condition and form of the abutments will dictate the choice.

When the **two centrals and one lateral incisor** have been lost (Fig. 26-7), removal of the remaining lateral and construction of a six-unit bridge are sometimes proposed. Unless this action is warranted by resorption of the alevolus, the lateral incisor should be retained. Its extraction will elongate the lever arm, and often the first bicuspids must be included as abutments. The teeth should be prepared for partial veneer or veneered crowns, depending on the restorations, caries index, or the length of the clinical crowns.

Replacing **one central and two lateral incisors** (Fig. 26-8) is not an exacting task unless the remaining central has drifted out of position. If there is harmony in the long-axis relationship, this bridge can be constructed by using partial veneer or veneered crowns on the cuspids and remaining central incisor. If the teeth are short, with contact areas very close to the gingival line, the retention of the partial veneer preparations must be increased with two extra pinholes in each lingual surface.

When replacing **four incisors** (Fig. 26-9), it has been the custom to use only the cuspids as abutments. Many bridges so constructed have failed, and faulty preparations or fit of castings cannot be held accountable for all these failures. The lever arm extends too far beyond the line of rotation. Retention and balance must be obtained through posterior extension. The cuspids and the first bicuspids, with partial veneer or veneered crowns as the retainers, will have compensating resistance to incising and rotating thrusts, and the life of the prosthesis will be prolonged. In a few cases, when the lever

FIGURE 26–5.   FIGURE 26–6.

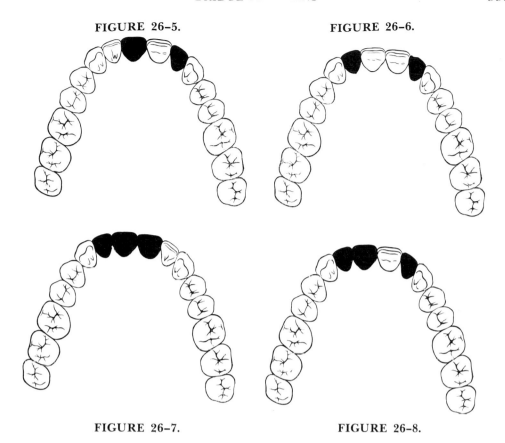

FIGURE 26–7.   FIGURE 26–8.

arm was very long, the second bicuspids have been included also. When the cuspids are of average length and the bicuspids are short, a combination of retainers may be indicated, partial veneer crowns being used on the cuspids and veneered gold crowns on the bicuspids.

Replacement of a **single cuspid** (Fig. 26–10) may become necessary for one of several reasons. With the increase in orthodontic treatment, cuspids are being extracted because of impaction or malposition. They are also lost through mishap or extensive caries, or they may be congenitally missing.

In a young patient the alveolar process will be pliable and the cusps of all teeth will retain much of the angulation present at the time of eruption. A bridge constructed here must have more abutments than would be used in the mouth of the adult, where the alveolus will be rigid and clinical crowns will be shortened by abrasion.

If a bridge is built for an adolescent, using only the first bicuspid and lateral incisor as abutments, the unit usually will move labially and forward into such a position that the mesiolingual portion of the lateral will overlap the distolabial line angle of the central incisor. This, in turn, causes loss or alteration of contact between the first and second bicuspids and the first molar. Even in a young adult, three abutments must be used to prevent such movement. Some authorities approve the use of the two bicuspids and the lateral incisor. Others feel that the central and lateral incisors and the first bicuspid will maintain the pontic in correct position more competently. Notwithstanding some difference of opinion, there is general agreement on the number of abutments.

To reach a decision, tooth form and occlusion must be studied. If the bicuspids are short occlusocervically, they will serve poorly; if the central and lateral incisors are thin labiolingually, with an excessive vertical overlap, their use may be contraindicated. If anterior retainers can be made that will be pleasing in appearance, the central and lateral incisors and the first bicuspid are preferred.

When the caries index is low, pinledge retainers on the central and lateral and a partial veneer crown on the first bicuspid will hold the bridge. However, if diagnostic casts and mouth examination reveal that considerable torque will be manifested in lateral excursions, partial veneer or veneered crowns should be used on the central and lateral incisors. Veneered crowns are obligatory if the caries index is high or if the teeth to be used as abutments are badly mutilated. If the first and second bicuspids and the lateral incisor are used, partial veneer or veneered crowns would be advisable.

In older patients, when abrasion has reduced the oblique forces from lateral excursions, the first bicuspid and lateral incisor may be ample for support. A few bridges replacing the cuspid have been retained for long periods by using an MO inlay in the first bicuspid and a pinledge on the lateral incisor, but the majority have been built with two partial veneer or veneered crowns.

When **both cuspids** are missing (Fig. 26-11), two fixed prostheses should be made, rather than an unbroken bridge from first bicuspid to first bicuspid.

The stringent measures proposed in the replacement of the cuspid are imperative because of the tremendous forces that bear on this tooth. Being situated at the corner of the arch, it receives anterior thrusts from the posterior teeth during mastication, and lateral force from the incising and protrusive movements of the opposing teeth. These are transferred to the cemented retainers and to the abutments.

Fortunately the absence of the **cuspid and approximating lateral incisor** (Fig. 26-12) occurs infrequently. While Ante's law can be satisfied in the replacement of these two teeth, resistance to the lever arm is not readily obtained. No less than three abutments should be used. If three will suffice, the two bicuspids and the central incisor are recommended. When the crown-root ratio, the contour of the arch, or the occlusion is abnormal, the second central incisor should be used, also. Partial veneer or veneered crowns must be used as the retainers.

A bridge to replace a **first bicuspid** (Fig. 26-13) must be constructed for many people. Sometimes, when the occlusion is receptive, an MO inlay in the second bicuspid and a pinledge on the cuspid will retain this prosthesis. The primary objectives, along with esthetic considerations, should be protection

FIGURE 26-9. FIGURE 26-10.

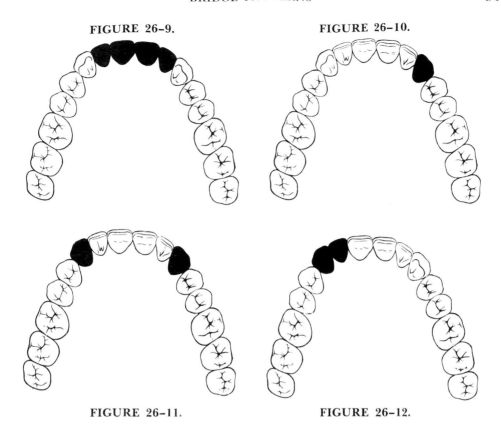

FIGURE 26-11. FIGURE 26-12.

of the abutment teeth and retention. These can be assured by using a partial veneer or veneered crown on each abutment tooth.

In replacing the **cuspid and first bicuspid** (Fig. 26-14), the opposing forces are more powerful than those against the cuspid and the lateral. As a rule, the first molar, second bicuspid, and lateral and central incisors must be used as abutments. Even if the teeth are short, partial veneer crowns can be used unless the caries index makes veneered or full veneer gold crowns mandatory.

Inlays may be used to replace the **second bicuspid** (Fig. 26-15) unless one (or more) of the specific contraindications for inlays exists; then retainers must be partial veneer or veneered or full veneer gold crowns.

When the **cuspid and second bicuspid** are missing (Fig. 26-16), the bony structure around the first bicuspid and lateral incisor must be examined critically. If the occlusion is normal and the crown-root ratio of the first bicuspid is no worse than one-to-one, three abutments will be sufficient. The lateral incisor, first bicuspid, and first molar retainers may be partial veneer or veneered or full veneer gold crowns, subject to tooth form, long-axis relationship, and caries index. If the alveolus encircling the lateral incisor and first bicuspid is reduced, but still may be considered safe, the central incisor should be added. Partial veneer or veneered crowns may be used on the central and lateral incisors and first bicuspid, with a full veneer gold crown as the retainer on the molar.

FIGURE 26–13.   FIGURE 26–14.

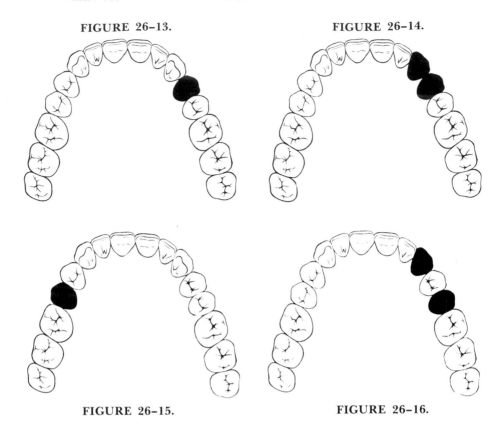

FIGURE 26–15.   FIGURE 26–16.

When **both central incisors and one first bicuspid** are missing (Fig. 26–17), it is to be hoped that a survey of the diagnostic cast will show that the long-axis relationship of the two cuspids, two laterals, and second bicuspid is harmonious. The most desirable method of restoration will be an extension of the pattern advised for the two central incisors, using partial veneer or veneered gold crowns as retainers on the five abutments. Occasionally the terminal cuspid can be excluded.

When the **lateral incisor and first bicuspid** have been lost (Fig. 26–18), it can be expected that the second bicuspid and cuspid will withstand migration or destructive stimulation; but if the alveolar process around the cuspid has receded more than one-third, the central incisor should be used as the terminal abutment. Partial veneer or veneered crowns will be required for retainers.

When the **first bicuspid and central incisor in the same quadrant** are to be replaced (Fig. 26–19), two three-unit bridges should be built, because there is no purpose in complicating construction by having to parallel four abutments. Nevertheless, if the alveolar process has receded and the abutments must be splinted, the same abutments, namely, the second bicuspid, cuspid, and lateral and central incisors, can be prepared for either partial veneer or veneered crowns.

A bridge replacing the **approximating bicuspids** (Fig. 26–20) is quite successful if a full veneer gold crown is used on the first molar and a partial veneer on the cuspid. In case the anterior abutment cannot be prepared for this retainer, a veneered crown must be used.

When the **approximating bicuspids and a lateral incisor** have been lost (Fig. 26-21), the normal periodontal membrane area of the first molar and cuspid will exceed that of the missing teeth. The occlusion of the lateral pontic will demonstrate whether the central incisor must enter into the plan of treatment. If the relationship is benign and the crown-root ratio of the cuspid is favorable, the lateral pontic can be cantilevered without adversely affecting the cuspid.

However, if these three teeth are missing, there will of necessity be some resorption of the alveolus around the cuspid. Construction must be guided by the amount remaining and its capacity to resist the forces against the abutment teeth. The first molar and the cuspid should be capable of holding this bridge, using a full veneer gold crown on the molar and a partial veneer on the cuspid. The acceptability of the partial veneer crown will depend on tooth form and caries index.

Two bridges should be constructed for replacing **two bicuspids and the central incisor in the same quadrant** (Fig. 26-22) for the same reasons discussed under the first bicuspid and the central incisor patterns.

Is it possible that the **four incisors and a first bicuspid** can be lost (Fig.

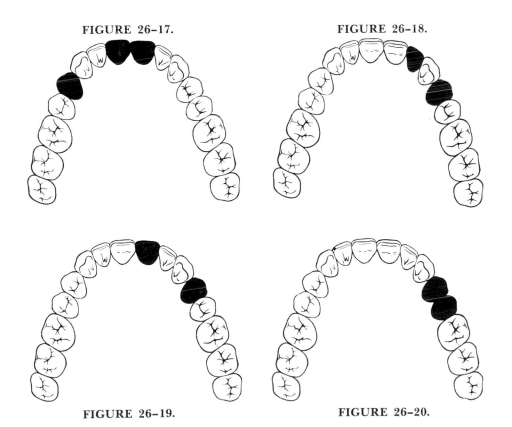

FIGURE 26-17.　　　　　　　　FIGURE 26-18.

FIGURE 26-19.　　　　　　　　FIGURE 26-20.

26-23), leaving an isolated cuspid with a suitable crown-root ratio? Ordinarily the answer would be No. Still, extraction of the cuspid would be no solution. If the crown-root ratio is close to one-to-one and not further complicated by an active atrophy, and if clinically the cuspid is not mobile, it should be used as a "pier," with the first molar and second bicuspid on the same side of the median line, and the cuspid and first bicuspid on the other, being used as the terminal multiple abutments.

The degree of the lower cuspid "lift" and the possibility of balancing the occlusion on each side of the isolated cuspid should be calculated. Every effort should be made to promote a wide distribution of the load, to protect the cuspid and to ensure its long life. Some enlargement or thickening of the periodontal membrane may be expected and need not be viewed with alarm, provided there is no discomfort.

In a mouth in which recession is minimal, the cuspid and first bicuspid on one side are prepared for abutments; on the opposite side, the cuspid and second bicuspid. Partial veneer or veneered crowns are constructed for the retainers, contingent on the condition of the individual tooth.

When the **four incisors and the four bicuspids** must be replaced (Fig. 26-24), a removable bridge merits consideration. Support and retention may be found on the cuspids and the first molars. Usually the cuspids must be reshaped with partial veneer or veneered crowns and the molars must be

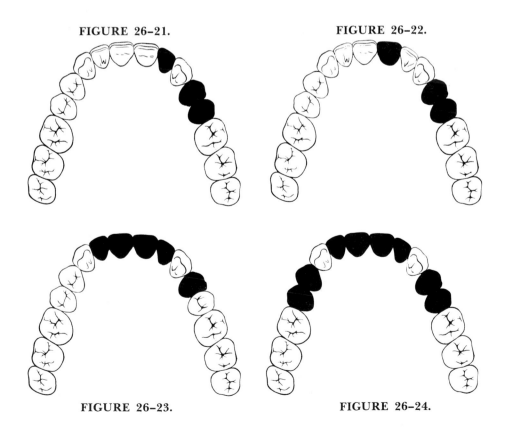

FIGURE 26-21.   FIGURE 26-22.

FIGURE 26-23.   FIGURE 26-24.

recontoured or realigned with full veneer gold crowns to supply rest seats and undercuts.

Except when the alveolus has receded around one of the cuspids, a fixed partial denture is more utilitarian and comfortable. This prosthesis should be retained by partial veneer or veneered and full veneer gold crowns.

If there are missing the **two bicuspids and the lateral and central incisors in one quadrant** (Fig. 26-25), a fixed prosthesis should be constructed if half of the alveolar process remains around the cuspid. Even if a bicuspid or molar is missing on the opposite side, a removable partial denture would not take precedence over two bridges. In the latter situation, retainers for the longer bridge would be a full veneer gold crown on the first molar and veneered or partial veneer crowns on the cuspid and on the central and lateral incisors across the median line.

When a bridge is being constructed to replace a **first molar** (Fig. 26-26), the second molar abutment should be crowned and the second bicuspid prepared to receive a partial veneer or veneered crown, because the occluding surface of the first molar pontic would be so much larger than the occlusal seat of a second molar inlay retainer. An inlay-supported bridge would be feasible only under ideal circumstances and if precisely constructed.

When the **approximating first molar and second bicuspid** have been lost (Fig. 26-27), the second molar retainer should be a full veneer gold crown. Coronal length and the caries index will control the first bicuspid retainer, either a partial veneer or veneered crown. If this space appears bilaterally (Fig. 26-28), bridges should be constructed unless the alveolar process has receded so far that bracing would be helpful, in which case a removable prosthesis must be considered.

When the **first molar and first bicuspid on the same side** are missing (Fig. 26-29), three teeth should be used as abutments, because there would be excessive leverage on the second bicuspid from a cantilever first bicuspid pontic. A full veneer gold crown retainer is indicated for the second molar. If the cuspid and second bicuspid are short, a veneered crown may be necessary on the bicuspid, with pin retention on the cuspid. If the caries index is high, veneered crowns will be mandatory. If this pattern is bilateral (Fig. 26-30), and if it is possible to insert bridges, a removable partial denture is contraindicated.

Occasionally there will be missing the **two bicuspids and central incisor on one side and the lateral incisor, second bicuspid, and first molar on the opposite side of the median line** (Fig. 26-31). A removable prosthesis is contraindicated unless the supporting structure of the remaining teeth has receded grossly. Even then the central and lateral incisors should be replaced by an immovable bridge, and a removable bridge should be constructed to replace the molar and bicuspids.

If 50 per cent or more of the alveolus remains, three separate fixed units should be built. This treatment plan enlists the first molar and cuspid as abutments for the missing first and second bicuspids; the lateral, central,

FIGURE 26–25.   FIGURE 26–26.

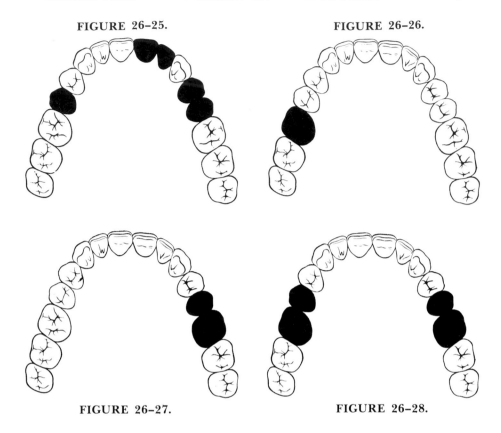

FIGURE 26–27.   FIGURE 26–28.

and cuspid for the anterior prosthesis; and the first bicuspid and second molar for the third bridge. Because of the great number of teeth missing, partial veneer, veneered, and full veneer gold crowns should be used for retainers.

If a mouth is presented with the **four incisors lost and the second bicuspid missing on one side and the second bicuspid and first molar missing on the other** (Fig. 26–32), a removable partial denture might be contemplated if the anterior ridge has resorbed abnormally. It is practicable to construct a continuous bridge using the first molar, first bicuspid, cuspid, cuspid, first bicuspid, and second molar as abutments, and veneered and full veneer gold crowns as retainers. There will be no more mouth preparation in making a bridge than would be needed for the stabilization of a removable prosthesis, and esthetically the bridge probably will be superior.

To replace a **second molar** (Fig. 26–33), full veneer gold crown retainers should be placed on the third and first molars. When the third molar is useless as an abutment, it should be extracted. A fixed prosthesis can be constructed, using the first molar and second bicuspid as abutments, with a cantilever second molar pontic.[4] Such a pontic must be smaller and have harmonious occlusion in all excursions. Its primary function is to keep the opposing tooth in position, not to furnish additional surface for mastication.

FIGURE 26-29.   FIGURE 26-30.

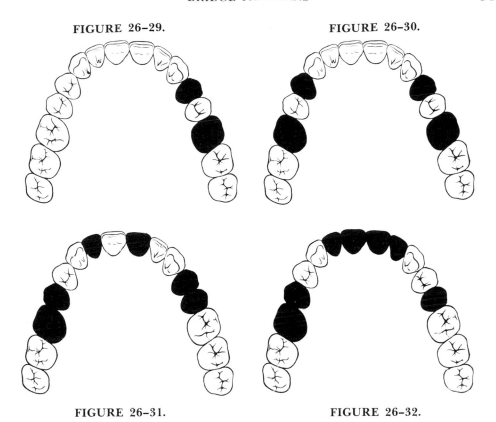

FIGURE 26-31.   FIGURE 26-32.

On a few occasions when the **approximating first and second molars** (Fig. 26-34) have been lost and the third molar has remained in position, it has been used as an abutment for a fixed prosthesis. Such treatment rarely can be sanctioned unless in position, crown, and root form the third molar closely resembles the second molar. Otherwise it should be removed and the area restored with a Class II partial denture.

When a **second bicuspid and second molar** are missing (Fig. 26-35), probably the third molar has been or should be extracted. In the rare event that it qualifies as an abutment, the third molar, first molar, and first bicuspid must be used for stability, with full veneer and veneered gold crowns as retainers. If the first bicuspid is long and substantial, it can be prepared for a partial veneer crown. In a majority of cases, the third molar should be extracted and a bridge constructed having a cantilever second molar pontic. Usually the cuspid will not be included as a third abutment.

If this condition occurs bilaterally, the third molars should not be retained. Bridges should be constructed supplying the second bicuspids, with full veneer gold crown retainers on the first molars and partial veneer or veneered crowns on the first bicuspids. The second molars can then be attached to a Class I removable prosthesis.

When the **approximating first molar, second bicuspid, and first bicus-**

pid have been lost (Fig. 26-36), a bridge from second molar to cuspid may not fulfill all requirements. However, if the occlusion is favorable, if the musculature of the face is not extremely powerful, and if the second molar and cuspid to be used as abutments are rugged, in good alignment, and well supported, a bridge can be made that will be comfortable and efficient for a worth-while period.

Although the span is long, the lever arm will be negative. The pontics must be modified drastically through increased embrasure size, exaggerated spillways, and a decreased buccolingual measurement. Alveolar response will be good if equilibration is maintained. Some bridges of this type have been retained by a full veneer gold crown on the second molar and a partial veneer on the cuspid, but often a veneered crown can be used to advantage on the cuspid.

When there are missing the **third molar, second molar, second bicuspid, and first bicuspid on the right side, and the central incisor, second bicuspid, and first molar on the left side** (Fig. 26-37), two bridges and a Class II, Modification I, partial denture should be built. One bridge will supply the right bicuspids, using the first molar and cuspid as abutments; the other, the left central incisor, with the approximating central and lateral as the abutment teeth. The molar retainer should be a full veneer gold crown. The others will be dictated by mouth conditions. After the left first bicuspid

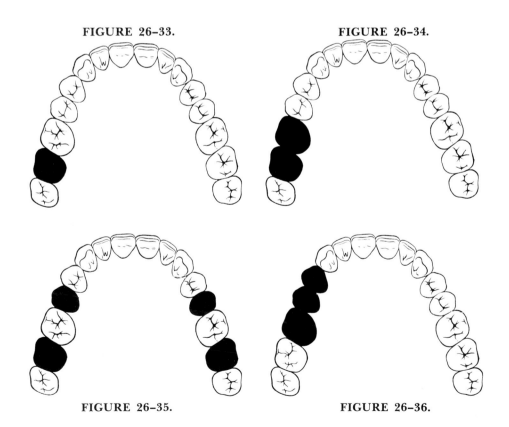

FIGURE 26-33.

FIGURE 26-34.

FIGURE 26-35.

FIGURE 26-36.

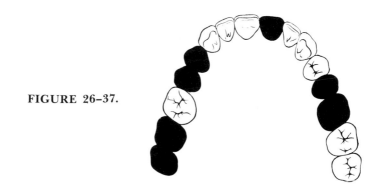

FIGURE 26-37.

and second molar have been prepared or recontoured for retention and support, the left second bicuspid and first molar and right second molar spaces should be filled by the removable partial denture.

MANDIBULAR PATTERNS

Lower incisors are not easily prepared for partial veneer or veneered gold crowns. These teeth are small, and the preparations must be delicately done; but when veneered crowns for these teeth are well made, the effect is pleasing.

Replacement of a **single central incisor** by a bridge (Fig. 26-38) can be complicated by proximal caries, rotation, or angulation of designated abutments, an end-to-end occlusion, or frail crown form. If the alveolus on the adjacent central has resorbed more than one-fourth in linear measurement, three abutments should be used. The MacBoyle or veneered crown retainer will overcome either proximal caries or rotation; caries-free teeth in regular alignment will accept the pinledge.

A mandibular cantilever **single lateral incisor** pontic (Fig. 26-39) has even less merit than the maxillary cantilever lateral. The adjacent cuspid and central incisor must be used, and if one central incisor will not be adequate, the two centrals must be splinted. There are times when the life of the remaining incisors can be prolonged by a continuous splint running from cuspid to cuspid, adding one tooth and rigidly joining the five remaining. Caries, alignment, and patient acceptance of metal display will guide the dentist in choosing between pinledge, MacBoyle, or veneered crown retainers.

Replacing a **single cuspid** can pose many problems, especially when it has been extracted because of an eccentric position. This space will be reduced through the contact area but be normal or near-normal in width at the cervical, and any pontic built for it will have to be narrow. The approximating bicuspid and lateral incisor seldom will have compatible long axes, and often it will be necessary to extract one of these teeth before a suitable bridge can be built.

If the lateral incisor is removed (Fig. 26-40), the first bicuspid and two central incisors should be able to carry the prosthesis; if the first bicuspid is lost (Fig. 26-41), the central and lateral incisors and the second bicuspid probably will suffice. A survey of the alignment of the abutment teeth will show which tooth should be sacrificed. According to tooth condition, the retainers would be pinledges and a partial veneer or veneered crown, or veneered crowns throughout.

When **both lateral incisors** have been lost (Fig. 26-42), the alveolar process must be measured. If they have been removed because of lingual or labial malpositions, enough bony tissue should remain to give support to the centrals; but if they were extracted for any other reason, it might be better to remove the centrals also and to construct four pontics between the cuspid abutments. If the centrals can be retained, a continuous unit still is desirable, using partial veneer crowns on the cuspids and MacBoyles or pinledge retainers on the centrals. When the pulps have receded and the caries index is high, all abutments can be prepared for veneered crowns.

A bridge replacing **both central incisors** (Fig. 26-43) ordinarily can be capably supported by the mandibular laterals. They are larger than the centrals, with root surface and form a little more adapted to resisting an added load. Pinledges, partial veneers, MacBoyles, or veneered crowns can be used for retainers, and preference is in the order named if there is no caries.

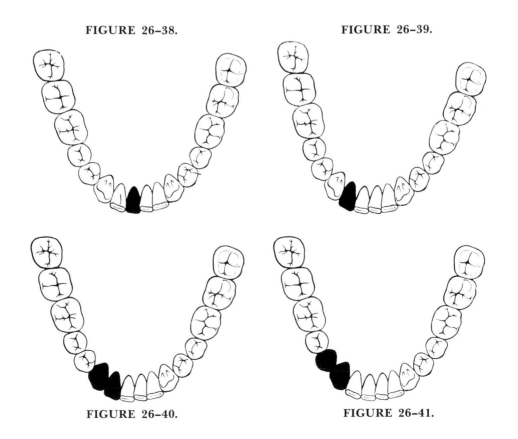

FIGURE 26–38.

FIGURE 26–39.

FIGURE 26–40.

FIGURE 26–41.

If the **central and lateral incisors in one quadrant** are missing (Fig. 26-44), three teeth must serve as abutments, namely, the remaining central and lateral, which should receive pinledge retainers (provided caries and alignment permit such preparations), and the cuspid, which may be prepared for either the partial veneer crown or the pinledge.

In the lower arch, replacing a **central incisor on one side of the median line and a lateral incisor on the other** (Fig. 26-45) calls for a solution similar to that for the same pattern above. The remaining central and lateral incisors and the cuspid will be needed for support. Pinledge retainers or MacBoyles on the central and lateral and a partial veneer crown or pinledge on the cuspid will stabilize the prosthesis, although veneered crowns may be used on all abutments. It may be expedient to include the remaining cuspid if it will blend the shading or if realignment will improve esthetic appearance. If the supporting tissue is minimal, it will be advisable to remove the central and lateral and to build a six-unit prosthesis anchored on the cuspids.

If **three incisors** have been lost, it is logical to extract the one that remains (Fig. 26-46), so that a cuspid-to-cuspid bridge may be built.

A **first bicuspid** (Fig. 26-47) can be replaced by using partial veneer or veneered crowns as retainers on the cuspid and second bicuspid. The type of construction in which a porcelain veneer is fused to the gold structure may be advocated here.

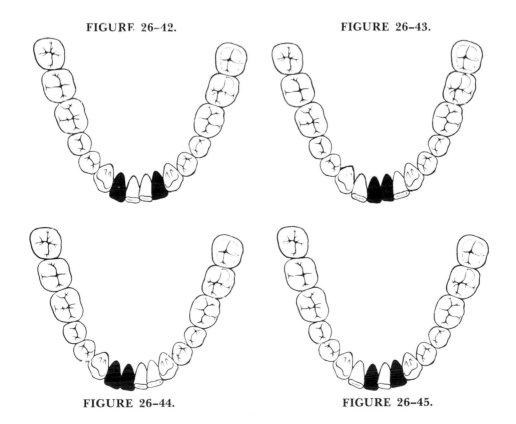

FIGURE 26-42. **FIGURE 26-43.**

FIGURE 26-44. **FIGURE 26-45.**

Inlays will retain a **second bicuspid** pontic (Fig. 26-48) unless the occlusion, the occlusocervical measurement of the crowns, or the caries index contraindicates their use. Such a bridge should have a broken-stress joint between the pontic and the first bicuspid inlay. If the first bicuspid has been weakened by caries and a partial veneer or a veneered crown must be employed, a full veneer gold crown should be placed on the first molar and two solder joints should be used.

Frequently the **first molar** (Fig. 26-49) can be replaced by using inlay retainers. However, if the abutment teeth have drifted so that the occlusion has been disarranged, a full veneer gold crown on the second molar and either a partial veneer or veneered crown on the second bicuspid will be essential.

When the third and first molars can be used in the replacement of the **second molar** (Fig. 26-50), the retainers should be full veneer gold crowns. If the clinical crown of the third molar has insufficient length, surgery may be warranted to remove some of the overlying soft tissue. If this is impracticable, the construction of a bridge is contraindicated.

When the **approximating bicuspids** (Fig. 26-51) have been missing for an extended period of time and the molars have moved forward, with a resultant mesial inclination, often all posterior teeth on that side of the mouth must be rebuilt or reshaped to regain maximal occlusion and func-

FIGURE 26-46.   **FIGURE 26-47.**

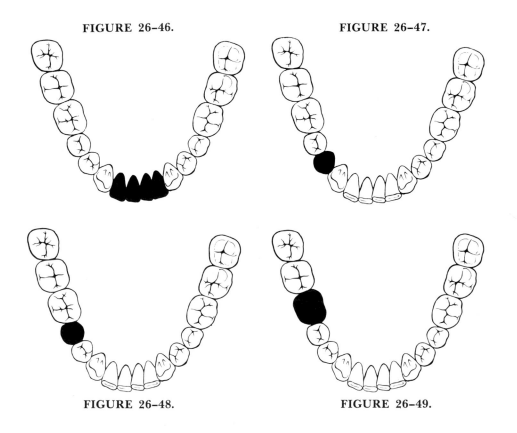

FIGURE 26-48.   **FIGURE 26-49.**

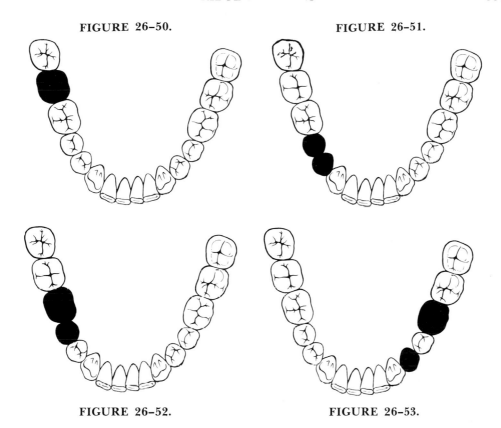

FIGURE 26-50.

FIGURE 26-51.

FIGURE 26-52.

FIGURE 26-53.

tion. Even under initial receptive conditions, a full veneer gold crown on the molar and a partial veneer or veneered crown on the cuspid will be the preferred retainers.

When the **second bicuspid and first molar** have been removed (Fig. 26-52), the first bicuspid is not a good single abutment. It should be splinted to the cuspid. Veneered and full veneer gold crowns will be required to retain this bridge except when the cuspid and first bicuspid are appropriate for partial veneer crowns.

When supplying the **first bicuspid and first molar** (Fig. 26-53), the second molar, second bicuspid, and cuspid should be used as abutments. A full veneer gold crown and two veneered or partial veneer crowns may be used for retainers.

When the **first and second molars** are missing (Fig. 26-54) and the third molar is suitable as an abutment, under most circumstances both bicuspids will be indispensable to stabilize the anterior end of the bridge. Full veneer and veneered gold crowns must be used as the retainers. If the opposing teeth have extruded, the occlusal plane must be restored or be recontoured to eliminate eccentric interference.

It is hazardous to construct a mandibular bridge that substitutes for **both bicuspids and the first molar** (Fig. 26-55). The span is too long, even if the opposing teeth have not extruded or can be restored to their former occlusal

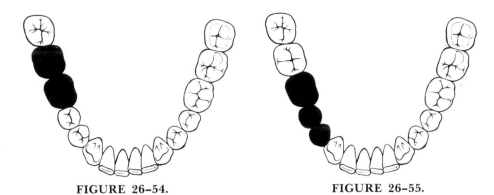

FIGURE 26–54.   FIGURE 26–55.

plane. A noticeable lever arm may be developed, owing to the position of the cuspid. Without losing embrasure space through an increase in size of the solder joints, there might not be strength to withstand breakage or flexing that would destroy cement adhesion.

A removable bridge will be safer. The cuspid should be recontoured with a partial veneer or veneered crown, to support as well as to retain the prosthesis, and the second molar should be rebuilt with a full veneer gold crown to afford retention and depth for an occlusal rest seat. Two approximating teeth on the opposite side should be prepared to receive an embrasure clasp. The masticating efficiency of such a prosthesis will be equal to that of a bridge.

*   *   *   *   *   *

Innumerable patterns may be encountered. It is felt that the principles of retention and stabilization and the combinations of abutment teeth set forth in this chapter can be applied to restore effectively any single space or combination of spaces.

REFERENCES

1. Vedder, F. B.: Personal communication.
2. Grubb, H. D.: Fixed bridgework. J. Pros. Den., 3:121, Jan. 1953.
3. Willey, R. E.: Preparation of abutments for veneer retainers. J.A.D.A., 53:141, Aug. 1956.
4. Ewing, J. E.: Re-evaluation of the cantilever principle. J. Pros. Den., 7:78, Jan. 1957.
5. Moulton, G. H.: Esthetics in anterior fixed bridge prosthodontics. J.A.D.A., 52:36, Jan. 1956.

Adams, J. D.: Planning posterior bridges. J.A.D.A., 53:647, Dec. 1956.
Klaffenbach, A. O.: Biomechanical restoration and maintenance of the permanent first molar space. J.A.D.A., 45:633, Dec. 1952.
Schweitzer, J. M., et al.: Free-end pontics used on fixed partial dentures. J. Pros. Den., 20:120, Aug. 1968.

chapter 27

SPLINTING TEETH

The term "splinting" denotes a rigid or semirigid attachment of one tooth to another, or the comparative immobilization or support of a series of teeth by either a removable or attached appliance. The extent, and perhaps the number, of individual tooth movements usually is restricted because of the union.

Teeth are splinted in the construction of fixed partial prostheses, in preparing mouths to support and retain removable partial prostheses (see Fig. 27–9 *D*), and for mutual or individual support in periodontally affected mouths. When two or more approximating or separated teeth are joined, forces from mastication, whether against the teeth themselves or transmitted from a prosthesis, will be shared to some degree. Splinting is also useful for long-range retention following orthodontic treatment.

Splinting is indicated in fixed partial construction when the space is long or when an individual abutment tooth at one or both ends of the space will yield to the torque from the lever arm of the prosthesis. Because of counterbalancing, two teeth splinted will provide support, and resistance to forces, in excess of the sum of the support or the resistance of the individual teeth (Fig. 27-1).

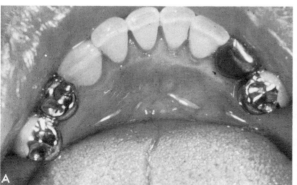 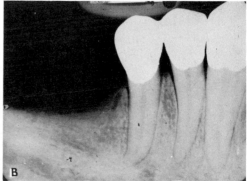

FIGURE 27–1. *Two examples of splinting.*

A, Note occlusal rest seats, small solder joints, and normal embrasures.

B, Second bicuspid radiograph shows evidence of the torque from a poorly designed clasp. The recontoured and splinted tooth became comfortable.

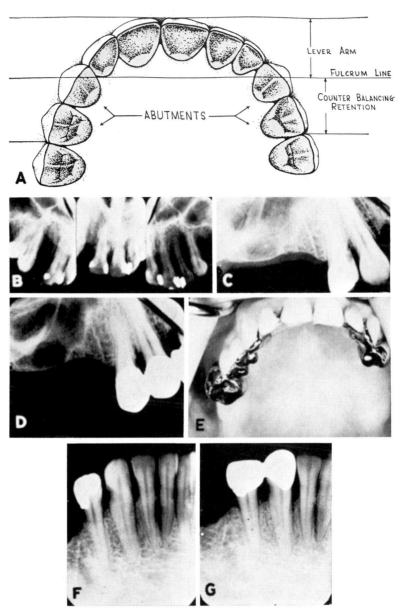

FIGURE 27–2.   *Splinting.*

A, Cuspid and bicuspid retainers splinted to form "multiple abutments."

B and *C*, Good alveolar process and crown-root ratio on cuspid and first bicuspid. Lateral incisor space.

D, Splinted cuspid and bicuspid abutments; cantilever lateral incisor pontic.

E, The three-unit bridge.

F, Reduced support around first bicuspid; too weak for partial denture abutment.

G, Splinted first bicuspid and cuspid; now a strong abutment.

If splinted teeth are to be used as abutments for either fixed or removable partial prostheses, the occlusion table should be reduced; the embrasures should be kept as large as feasible; the solder joints should be as small as is consistent with strength, and round rather than oblong; and the joints should be placed at the normal points of contact between the teeth. Any periodontal involvement should be eradicated. Teeth with short crowns or those irregularly aligned are very poor subjects for splinting.

Splinting may be effected by solder joints (Figs. 27-2 and 27-3), by precision attachments, or by simultaneous support from extensive clasps or adapted bars that are a part of a removable framework.

When teeth are joined rigidly by solder joints, any force directed against one tooth will be in part passed on to the one (or the others) to which the recipient is splinted. When two teeth are interlocked by a precision attachment, lateral pressures and any force in line with its path of insertion, except one directed solely to the tooth containing the female attachment, will be felt by the other. Splinting by clasping minimizes lateral movement or rotation by the involved teeth, but they can move into and out of their sockets, one by one, on the application or release of pressure.

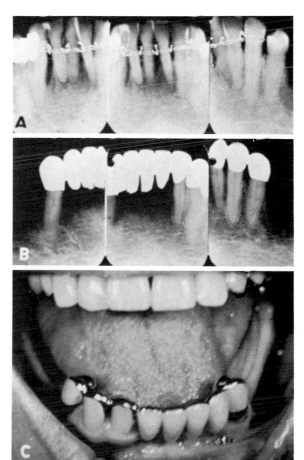

FIGURE 27-3. *Bridge constructed with four abutments.*

A, Situation not acceptable radiographically. Did not respond to periodontal treatment. Three incisors and one cuspid removed.

B, Radiographs showing embrasures.

C, Bridge shown in *B.* The three splinted abutments will stabilize the single bicuspid on the left side of the arch. It has good bony support and will receive bilateral bracing from removable partial denture.

When teeth are splinted, there are potential hygienic and periodontal risks. If teeth are short, the solder joint will occupy much of the cervical embrasure, thus reducing the amount of stimulation for the underlying gingival tissue. If in addition the solder joint is wide buccolingually, overprotection for the septal gingival tissue is increased. Therefore it is axiomatic in splinting with solder joints that the joint be kept to minimal size, that without obliterating the occlusal embrasure it be placed at the maximal height occlusally (proximally), that it be round for easy cleansing, and that its structure be such that maximal strength will accrue from minimal size.

Teeth may be splinted in sections when there is a variable long-axis relationship, and the sectional splints may be joined and mutually supported by a precision or semiprecision attachment. The precision attachment has some features that contraindicate its use in splinting. First is the amount of tooth structure that must be cut away to receive the female portion. Secondly, if it is to have the greatest effectiveness, the attachment must run the full length of the crown occlusocervically or linguocervically. This effaces the cervical embrasure and seriously encroaches on the lingual space. Hygiene is very difficult to achieve with the fixed precision attachment splint, and invariably periodontal disturbances will follow its use.

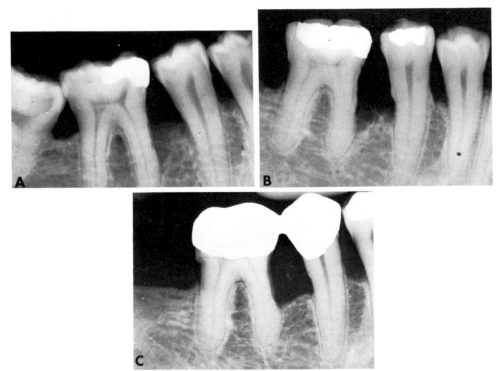

FIGURE 27–4.   A, Radiograph showing pocketing around mesial root of mandibular first molar.

B, Second molar lost due to carious exposure. First molar and second bicuspid separated. Pocket advanced.

C, Three years following periodontal surgery, reshaping of alveolar process, and splinting. Molar has served during this time as an abutment for a removable partial denture. Notice reduced masticating area on molar.

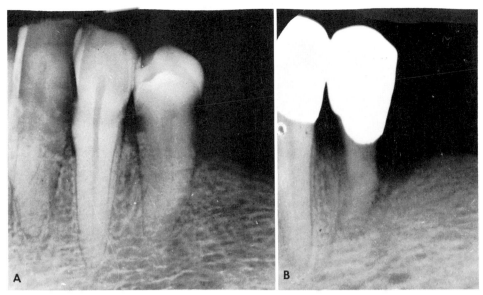

FIGURE 27–5. *A*, Radiograph of bicuspid and cuspid to be splinted in the preparation of mouth for removable partial denture.

B, Seventeen months later. Bicuspid must be extracted. Masticating area increased in size and crown-root ratio altered. Marginal ridges too high.

Splinting with clasps is occasionally indicated, but bulk, exaggerated contours, and temporary food retention all tend to make this approach unpopular with the patient if used for an extended period of time. This method is more often employed to contribute temporary support during periodontal treatment or as a means of retaining severely affected teeth until it is possible to remove and replace them. The prolonged retention of periodontally affected dentition by means of a removable splint would seem to indicate that the mouth might have been treated more advantageously otherwise.

Posterior teeth should be splinted by using full or partial veneer crowns (Fig. 27–4). Special attention must be given to the preparation of the teeth proximally. These areas must be reduced more than is normal so that the casting will have strength even though lingual and cervical embrasures are enlarged. The approximating occlusal margins of the preparations must also be deepened slightly so that spillways may feed into the lingual embrasure between the splinted teeth. Intercuspal distance sometimes may be constricted buccolingually to reduce leverage loads further (Fig. 27–5).

Anterior teeth are splinted, using veneered crowns, partial veneer crowns, and pinledges (Fig. 27–6). Each has its peculiar set of indications, although these may be interrelated. Veneered crowns are used when teeth must be rebuilt, appearance improved, or a tooth clasped or used to house a precision attachment (Fig. 27–7). Partial veneer crowns will suffice to support a partial denture or an abutment tooth. Much of the time pinledges are used to build lingual surfaces into occlusion or when teeth are periodontally affected.

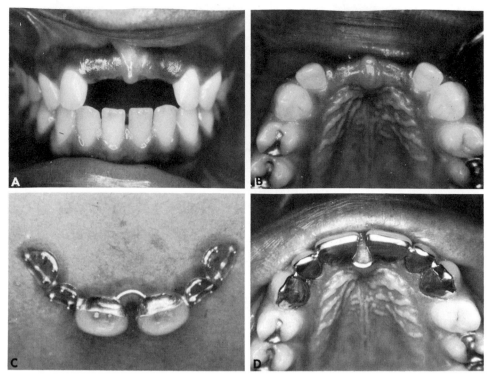

FIGURE 27–6.   *A* and *B*, Anterior space too wide for prosthesis to be supported by lateral incisors only.

C and *D*, Six-unit anterior bridge. Lateral incisors and cuspids splinted on each side, providing counterbalancing retention to offset lever arm and to bring strong cuspid abutments into support of bridge. There will be no labial drifting.

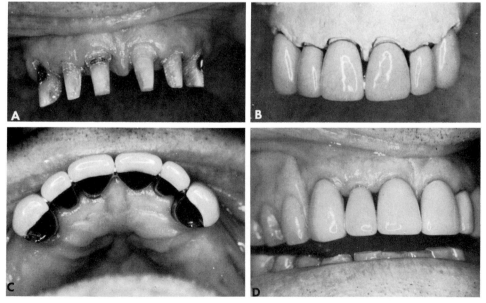

FIGURE 27–7.   *A*, Six maxillary anterior teeth following removal of splint made previously.

B and *C*, Six-unit splint. Cuspids house precision attachments.

D, Splint and partial denture in mouth.

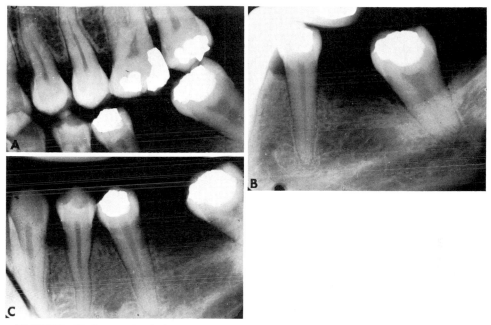

FIGURE 27–8. *A*, Occluding teeth; mandibular first molar missing, with second molar inclined mesially. Maxillary first molar extruded on distal.

B, Considerable loss of supporting alveolar bone around molar.

C, Bicuspids, if splinted, would provide excellent support for bridge and against lateral forces on molar. Periodontal surgery would give bicuspids sufficient crown length for splinting.

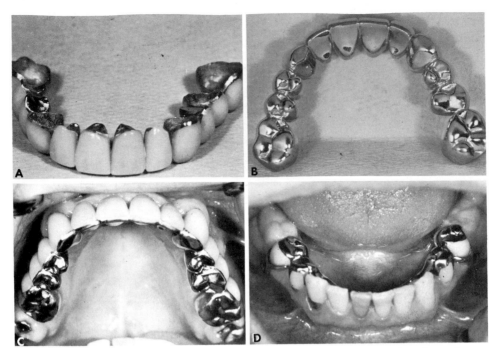

FIGURE 27–9.   *A* and *B*, Two views of twelve-unit maxillary prosthesis. Three abutments on patient's left, two on right. Embrasures are open. Ridge-contacting areas are small. Buccolingual dimensions of pontics reduced. Joints as small as possible, consistent with needed strength.

C, Twelve-unit splint cemented.

D, Occluding arch. Bicuspids on each side joined. Second bicuspids, the abutments, support and retain removable prosthesis. First bicuspids have rest seats to receive secondary retainers of Class I partial denture.

Many times, of necessity, teeth must be splinted (Figs. 27-8 and 27-9). When selecting patients for whom it is to be done, maintenance of adequate hygiene and assurance of arrested atrophy must be determined or success may be uncertain.

REFERENCES

Glickman, I., Stein, R. S., and Smulow, I. B.: Effect of increased functional forces upon the periodontium of splinted and non-splinted teeth. J. Periodont., *32*:290, Oct. 1961.

Hudson, W. C.: Provisional coverage and splinting procedures in crown and bridge ceramics and rehabilitation. D. Practitioner & D. Record, *8*:198, March 1958.

Karlstrom, S.: The Pontostructor Method. Stockholm, A. B. Nordiska Bokhandelns, 1955.

Morris, M. L.: The diagnosis, prognosis and treatment of the loose tooth. Oral Surg., Oral Med. & Oral Path., *6*:957, 1037, Aug.-Sept. 1953.

Sanell, C., and Feldman, A. J.: Horizontal pin splint for lower anterior teeth. J. Pros. Den., *12*:138, Jan.-Feb. 1962.

Shooshan, E. D.: Pin-ledge casting technique—its application in periodontal splinting. Dent. Clin. N. Amer., March 1960, p. 189.

Weinberg, L. A.: Force distribution in splinted anterior teeth. Oral Surg., Oral Med. & Oral Path., *10*:484, May 1957.

Weinberg, L. A.: Force distribution in splinted posterior teeth. Oral Surg., Oral Med. & Oral Path., *10*:1268, Dec. 1957.

Winslow, M. B.: Fixed splint and bridge assembly. J.A.D.A., *51*:47, July 1955.

chapter 28

THE CONSTRUCTION OF CROWNS AND BRIDGES IN THE PREPARATION OF PARTIALLY EDENTULOUS MOUTHS FOR CLASP-RETAINED REMOVABLE PROSTHESES

In the rebuilding of a partially edentulous mouth, the philosophy should be one of rendering a real oral health service, not one of merely "filling the space."[1] A fixed partial denture is the restoration of choice when existing conditions and space length will permit (Fig. 28-1). In many instances, however, a removable prosthesis must be employed for a portion or all of the replacement (Fig. 28-2).[2, 3]

Restoration, preservation, and prevention are all of vital concern. Appearance, mastication, speech clarity, and comfort should be restored, at the same time preserving teeth, alveolar process, gingival tissue, tooth position, occlusion, and oral and systemic health. Finally, any further loss of teeth and injury to supporting tissues must be prevented by bringing the forces acting on the removable partial denture within the limits of tissue tolerance.[4, 5]

The most important step in achieving these objectives is adequate preparation of the mouth before construction of a prosthesis. Mouth preparation can be defined as the series of operations that will enable a mouth to accept and to support a partial denture for the maximal period of time with minimal adverse reaction on the remaining natural teeth and supporting tissues.[6, 7, 8]

A clasp-retained prosthesis can contribute much to oral health, provided

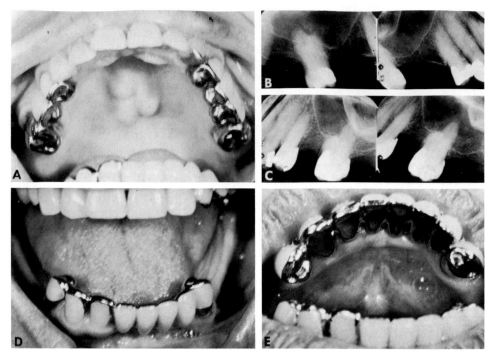

FIGURE 28–1.   *A*, Maxillary arch in which two bridges have been placed. Such spaces are restored frequently with one removable partial denture. While this could be done, it would require rebuilding each of the abutment teeth for support and retention, and would require bars (major connectors) crossing the palate anteriorly and posteriorly to the torus. The plane of occlusion was made acceptable to the construction of the mandibular prosthesis.

B and *C*, The radiographs substantiate the treatment plan. There are properly distributed healthy abutment teeth to support fixed replacements.

D and *E*, A bridge was placed in the anterior of the mandibular arch of this mouth. Four teeth are supporting four pontics. The bony process was good, and the first bicuspid, cuspid, and lateral incisor on the right will give the needed support to the left first bicuspid. Also through the splinting action of the bridge, the bicuspids will be much stronger in their role of abutments for the Class I partial denture. The elimination of the anterior modification space simplifies construction of the removable prosthesis.

the mouth is correctly prepared for its retention and support and for positioning its parts. Otherwise it can be an instrument of destruction.

Restorative dentistry, which plays a major part in mouth preparation, includes rebuilding individual teeth with crowns, inlays, or other restorations; splinting teeth by connecting adjacent restorations with a solder joint; and placement of fixed prostheses before the removable partial denture is constructed. Often it is advisable to restore an anterior space with a bridge before building the removable prosthesis, to avoid restrictions in selecting the most desirable path of insertion, and to make construction more simple, design more efficient, and maintenance and repair easier.[9, 10]

The extent of caries, caries index, quantity and quality of remaining supporting tissue, and tooth contours seen in each individual case will dictate the amount and kind of restorative dentistry.

Carious teeth must be restored and caries controlled by whatever procedures are feasible. A high caries index will make it necessary to cover the

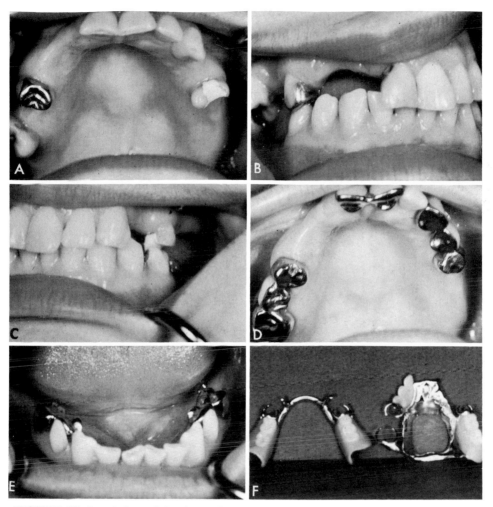

FIGURE 28–2. *A, B,* and *C,* Views of Class II, Mod. III, maxillary arch. The two isolated bicuspids were vital and well supported. The molar was inclined buccally so far that clasping was contraindicated without major recontouring.

D, The preparation of the arch for a removable prosthesis included two fixed restorations and one splint. This stabilized all abutment teeth, eliminated two modification spaces, and changed the classification to Class II, Mod. I. The forms of the molar and the bicuspids were made suitable for clasping and support, and the incisors were splinted and recontoured to give support and to receive force parallel to their long axes.

E, The opposing arch was prepared by splinting the bicuspids on each side with a crown and a partial veneer crown. Note the occlusal rest seats for the clasps on the distals of the second bicuspids and for the secondary retainers on the mesials of the first bicuspids. Guiding planes were made also on the distal surfaces of the second bicuspids and at the mesiolingual line angles of the first bicuspids.

F, The prostheses built for this mouth. The mandibular has two retainers and four rests; the maxillary, three retainers and four rests.

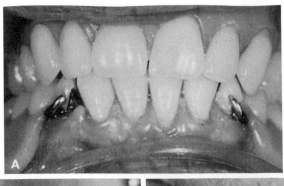

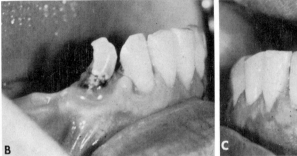
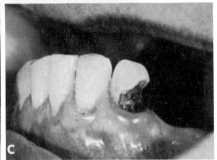

FIGURE 28-3.   Carious abutment teeth. Endodontic therapy was necessary. This was followed by building the teeth to prepared form with cast cores retained by posts in the root canals.

abutment teeth with crowns (Figs. 28-3 and 28-4). Splinting may be essential to distribute the forces that will be brought to bear on the remaining teeth. This service is indicated in numerous mouths, but is seldom delivered, yet it is one of the best methods available for distributing forces over a wider area (Fig. 28-5). (See Chapter 27, Splinting Teeth.)

Although many phases of dentistry may be pursued in properly preparing a partially edentulous mouth, it is the purpose of this chapter to discuss what is probably the most neglected phase of treatment in all dentistry, the construction of crowns and bridges that *fulfill* the specific requirements of support, retention, and ideal design for partial dentures and removable bridges.[11, 12, 13]

These requirements encompass (1) the establishment of abutment tooth contour that will remove any interference with the rigid portion of the partial denture framework and reciprocal clasp arms during insertion or removal (Fig. 28-6); (2) protection of the abutment tooth against caries; (3) restoration of a favorable occlusal plane and harmonious occlusion; and (4) elimination of modification areas that might complicate design, tolerance, and maintenance.

INDICATIONS

Crowns or bridges (or both) for the support and retention of removable partial prostheses are indicated

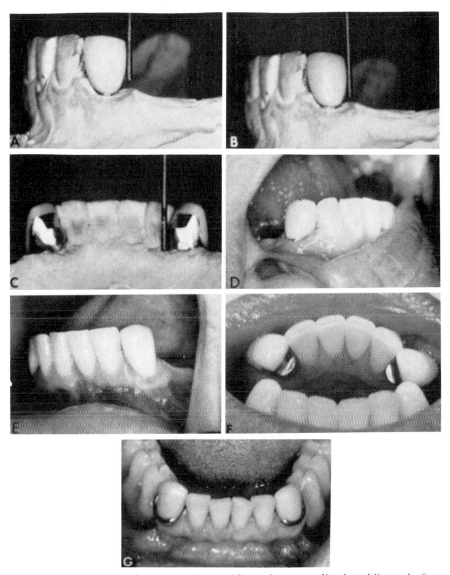

FIGURE 28–4. *A, B,* and *C,* Surveying guiding planes on distal and lingual of crown: *A,* before glazing; *B* and *C,* after glazing.

D and *E,* The crowns built to reconstruct and recontour abutments shown in preceding figure. The frameworks are cast gold; the veneers are porcelain bonded to the castings. Retentive undercuts of the desired depth, and specifically positioned at the mesiocervical, were located with a surveyor and ground into the porcelain. Guiding planes, partly on gold and partly on the veneer, were placed at the distal. An overglaze was used.

F, The type of lingual contour in the castings. The prosthesis will be supported, the gingival tissue protected, and the force directed along the long axes of the abutments.

G, Partial denture in position.

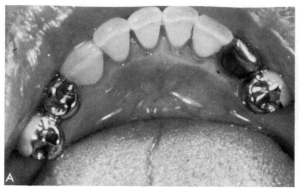
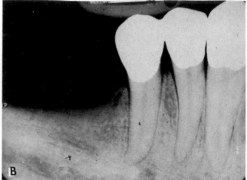

FIGURE 28–5. *Examples of splinting.*

A, Note occlusal rest seats, small solder joints, and normal embrasures.

B, Second bicuspid radiograph shows evidence of the torque from a poorly designed clasp. The recontoured and splinted tooth became comfortable.

(1) when abutment teeth are carious or the caries index is high;

(2) when crown form must be changed on either normal or tipped teeth to accommodate a benign clasp design (see Fig. 28-7);

(3) when splinting is imperative because of alveolar recession or root form;

(4) to restore occlusion or to level the occlusal plane when teeth have extruded, and to regain occlusal harmony in the finished partial denture;

(5) to allow more freedom in making a decision on the path of insertion when an anterior modification space exists;

FIGURE 28–6. *A,* Left, survey line produced on buccal of recontoured tooth brings clasp arm low on tooth and forms a retentive undercut that accepts only the flexible portion of the clasp arm. Center, survey line (or height of contour) on lingual is low. Reciprocal, non-retentive clasp arm can contact and support tooth at all times while retentive arm is flexing and going over height of contour into or out of retentive undercut. Right, clasp close to cervical line and closer to point of rotation in root.

B, Recontouring tooth for Roach-Akers clasp. Buccal shows survey line, or height of contour, developed to produce retentive undercut next to edentulous area. Under force of mastication, retentive tip moves away from tooth. Proximal and lingual views show stabilizing, or nonretentive, clasp arm above a height of contour placed down very near but not on gingival line.

C, Guiding planes on lingual and proximal of recontoured abutment. Occlusal and cervical margins of lingual plane are above and below point where buccal clasp arm begins to flex over height of contour and into undercut. Thus, stabilizing lingual arm supports tooth during seating of prosthesis.

D, Convexity above and below height of contour the same in length and depth.

E, Heavy lines show guiding planes opposite retentive undercuts.

F, Three incorrect and one correct occlusal rests and rest seats. Top left: Seat too angular and rest too thin crossing margin. Will fracture. Top right: Not enough bulk. Will fracture. Bottom left: Too sloping. Tendency to slide will cause clasp arms to exert adverse pressure. Bottom right: Correct as to bulk and contour.

G, Framework on cast. Guiding plane surfaces on distal of molar, lingual of molar, and mesiolingual of bicuspid. Strut for secondary retainer placed in mesiolingual embrasure. Lingual clasp arm low on tooth, but entirely above height of contour.

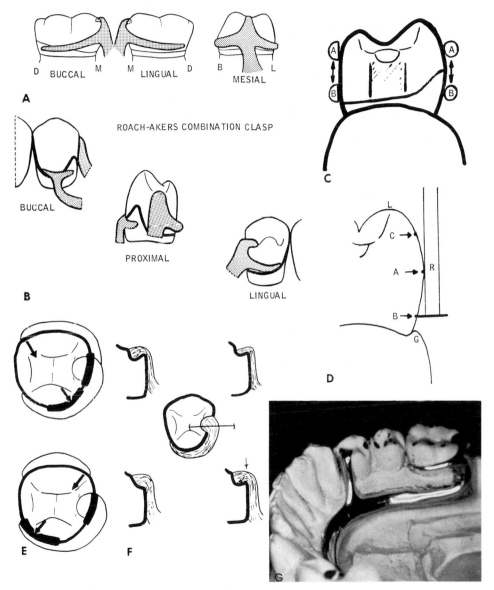

FIGURE 28–6. *See legend on facing page.*

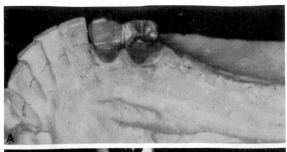

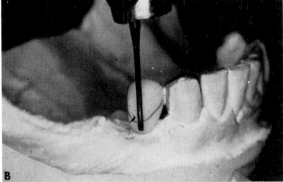

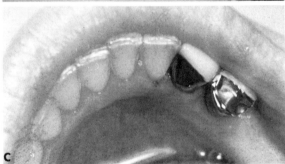

FIGURE 28–7. *A*, Splinted castings for removable partial denture. Rest seat in bicuspid and shelf on cuspid. Line on cast shows height of proposed lingual plate.

B, Marking survey line and developing height of contour and mesiobuccal retentive undercut on a bonded porcelain veneer.

C, Finished retainer shown in *A*.

(6) to splint a bicuspid that is standing alone so that it may resist torque or leverage; and

(7) for esthetic reasons. (See Figures 28–8 and 28–9.)

PRELIMINARY DESIGN AND TREATMENT PLANNING

Before the preparations are started, the diagnostic cast should be surveyed, a preliminary design made for the cast metal framework, and the path of insertion established. At the same time the amount of recontouring of teeth to be used for retention or support of the prosthesis should be diagrammed. If one (or more) of the abutment teeth does not require recontouring, the path of insertion should be selected with this in mind. Reduction of the abutments can be guided by the space measurements when the analyzing rod is in contact with the height-of-contour line.

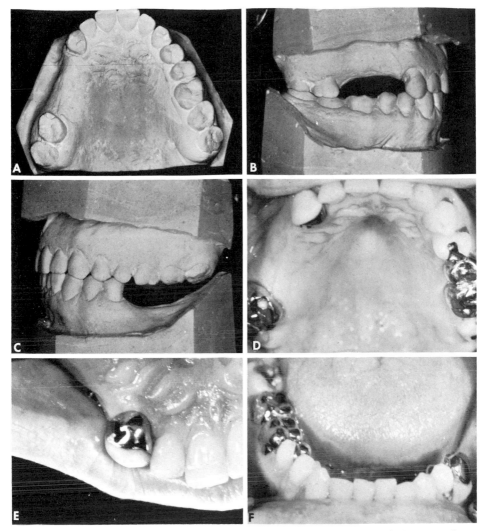

FIGURE 28–8. *A* and *B*, Cast of maxillary Class III arch. Cuspid abutment has poor crown-root ratio because of apicoectomy.

C, Class II occluded mandibular arch.

D, Maxillary mouth preparation. Bonded porcelain veneer on cuspid housing precision attachment. Recontoured molar with rest seat and distobuccal retentive undercut. Recontoured molar and bicuspid on opposite side. Back-to-back clasps will cross occluding surfaces above contacts.

E, Mirror view of cuspid crown.

F, Mandibular mouth preparation. First and second molars to be clasped. Occluding surfaces grooved for crossing clasp. Rest seat in mesiolingual occlusal of bicuspid. Bicuspid crowned for clasping.

The crown surfaces that are to be contacted by minor connectors and nonretentive sections of clasps must be parallel to each other and to the path of insertion to form planes that will guide the prosthesis along the predetermined path of insertion. They will provide, also, for balanced and equalized retention, strategically located and of the accepted, but not excessive, depth for the designated clasp design. This can be accomplished by using a sur-

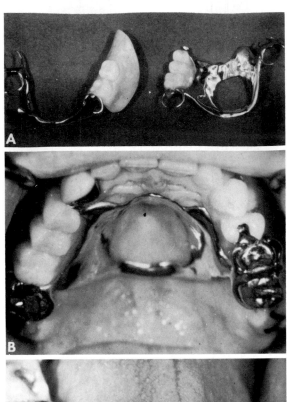

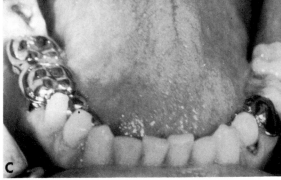

FIGURE 28–9.   *A*, Removable partial dentures.
B and *C*, Prostheses in position.

veyor while carving the wax pattern. Thus it will be possible to procure bracing and reciprocation. Since secondary retainers should never be placed on inclined planes, the cingulum areas of anterior teeth must be elevated to create ledges (see Fig. 28-4 *C*), which will direct the forces parallel to the long axes of the roots.

TOOTH PREPARATION

In the preparation of a tooth to be clasped or to support a secondary retainer, there must be more reduction of the marginal ridge so that an occlusal rest seat in the finished crown may have enough depth (Fig. 28-10). Rest seats are located in the marginal ridge areas of the occlusal surfaces and

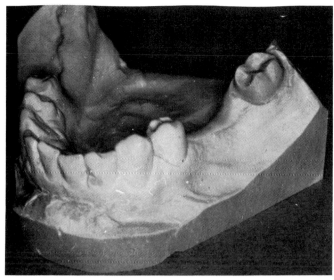

FIGURE 28-10. Preparation of molar to make room for adequate rest seat in casting.

over the crests of the alveolar ridges. Rest seats should be spoon-shaped (see Fig. 28-5 *A*), slanting slightly toward the center of the teeth, and must be a minimum of 1.5 mm. deep, 2.0 mm. wide, and 2.5 mm. long.[14]

The axial preparation of a tooth to be reshaped must be done so that the right contour for clasping can be built into the completed restoration.

The gingival margin of the crown, barring gingival recession, should be extended into the sulcus. When one (or more) of the surfaces of the tooth is not covered, inhibiting treatments of stannous fluoride should be used.

TAKING THE IMPRESSIONS

An accurate indirect technique will aid in producing such exact contour in the restoration. After the teeth have been prepared and adequate tissue displacement has been obtained, a full arch polysulfide rubber impression is made. Two casts are poured, one being sectioned for dies and the other left intact, to be used as a working cast (Fig. 28-11). The working and opposing casts are occluded, using a face-bow and a Kerr Bite Frame or an occlusion rim, so that occlusion and contact may be established on the wax patterns. The working cast must be removable so that the patterns can be surveyed. Alginate may be used for the opposing cast impression.

SURVEYING THE WAX PATTERNS

The wax pattern for either a crown or a pontic that will retain or support a removable partial denture must first be carved to have harmonious form and occlusion. Then the working cast is transferred to a sur-

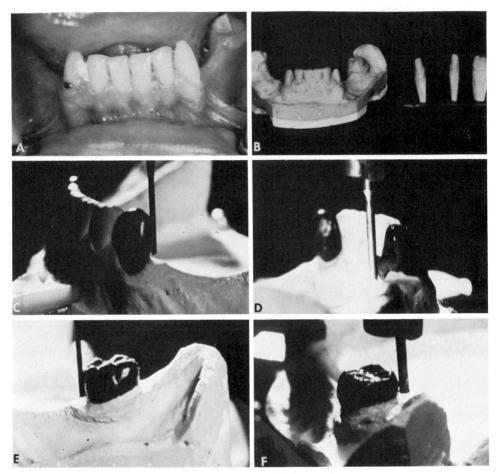

FIGURE 28–11.   *A*, A Class II, Mod. I, mandibular arch.

B, The working cast and dies for mouth preparation.

C, Placing distal guiding plane on pattern for left cuspid crown; surveyor table is set at correct tilt for predetermined path of insertion.

D, Carving guiding plane on lingual of raised cingulum, mandibular right cuspid.

E, Checking guiding plane, parallel to path of insertion, with warmed analyzing rod of surveying instrument.

F, Checking position and depth of retentive undercut of mandibular molar crown.

veying table (Fig. 28-12), where guiding plane areas, to be contacted by a minor connector and a reciprocal clasp arm, will be formed with a warmed analyzing rod. These must be parallel to the path of insertion. The predetermined amount of undercut should be measured and located ideally on the pattern, eliminating all interfering contours except the measured suprabulge above the undercut. Also, while the cast is on the surveying table, any modifications should be made in the height of contour and the buccal and lingual surfaces that are needed to form supporting areas that will balance and stabilize the tooth during insertion and removal of the partial denture.[15] (See Figure 28–11 *C, D. E,* and *F.*)

After occlusion, contact areas, and contour have been obtained, the wax pattern is returned to the die for correction or completion of the cervical margin and for polishing. The polished casting is placed on the working cast and checked with the surveyor analyzing rod for exactness of guiding planes, and with an undercut gauge for depth of undercut. It is then cemented on the abutment tooth, completing the restorative phase of mouth preparation (Fig. 28-13).

Removable partial dentures should not be built around isolated bicuspids or incisors. Such teeth may be splinted with bridges to cuspids anteriorly, molars posteriorly, or to cuspids or other incisors laterally.[6] A bridge built for this purpose gives superb support to the abutment tooth, closes an

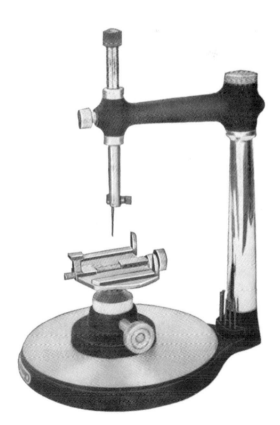

FIGURE 28–12.   Surveyor (Ney).

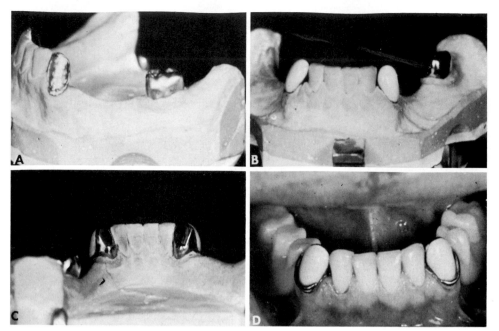

FIGURE 28–13.   *A*, Castings from wax patterns shown in Figure 28–11; note guiding planes.

B, Veneered cuspid crowns and polished molar crown.

C, Lingual form of cuspid crowns.

D, Class II, Mod. I, mandibular partial denture that occludes with maxillary complete denture.

awkward modification space, enhances incising if in the anterior, and provides rest seat, guiding plane, and embrasure areas for secondary retainers and minor connectors.

A crown on an abutment tooth may be undercontoured, with a shelf as a supporting area for clasp arms that restore normal contour to the tooth. Pontics or connectors may be contoured or grooved for clasps that cross the occlusal surface. Preparation of abutment teeth or pontic design must be planned to facilitate such a clasping situation. Cingulums of retainers or pontics may be contoured or recessed to support lingual plates or rests.[16]

A tooth with receded alveolar process may be doubly supported by another bridge abutment and the bilateral bracing from a removable partial denture.

*   *   *   *   *   *

From the foregoing discussion, it is evident that before a student or dentist is qualified to prepare mouths and to construct biologically acceptable partial dentures, he must have a good foundation in crown and bridge prosthodontics. These two fields of dentistry are inseparable, since the success of the partial denture will depend entirely on the quality of the preparatory crown and bridge work (Figs. 28–14, 28–15, and 28–16).

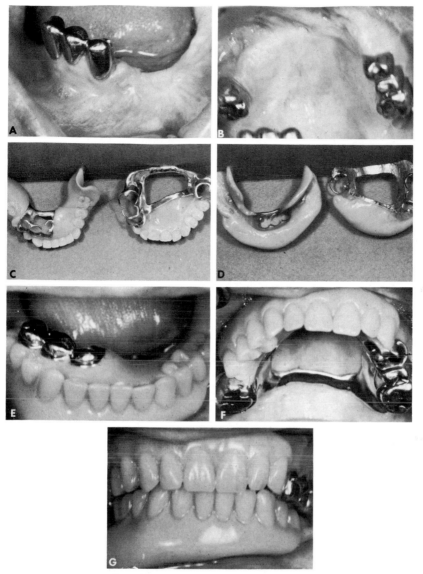

FIGURE 28–14. *Rebuilding a mutilated mouth. Preservation of the seven remaining teeth is essential if the patient masticates and has normal appearance. Portions of both mandibular and maxillary arches shot away. Repaired by bone grafts and plastic surgery.*

A, Mandibular cuspid treated endodontically. Crowns extended as far as possible cervically. Guiding planes on buccal surfaces, retention on lingual. Rest seats mesially and distally on splint.

B, Three teeth splinted and contoured for buccal and lingual retention. Clasp arms reciprocate. Mesial and distal occlusal rests. Grooves for crossing occlusion. Right molar contoured for ring clasp and two occlusal rests.

C and *D,* The mandibular and maxillary prostheses.

E, Mandibular prosthesis in mouth, built around three abutment teeth to restore contour to face.

F, Maxillary prosthesis in mouth. It is supported by four rests, one strut, and scar tissue.

G, Mastication, appearance, and enunciation satisfactory to patient. Without recontoured crowns and splinting, such a case is hopeless.

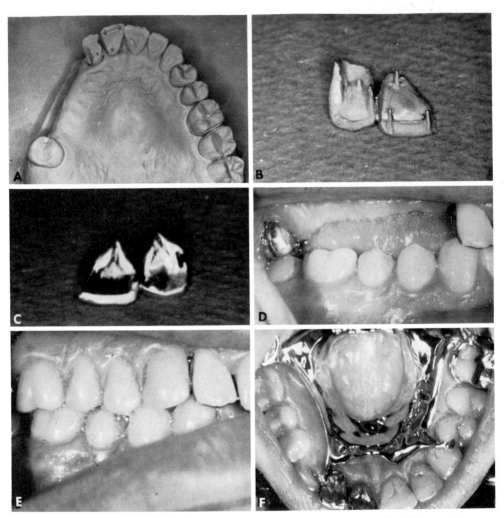

FIGURE 28–15.   *A*, Cast of maxillary arch. Right molar crowned, with mesial rest seat. Left molars prepared for clasping. Lateral and central incisors prepared for splinting. Lateral will house precision attachment. Same preparation, although less deep, would be required for Sherer rest seat.

    B, C, and *D*, Splinted retainer for lateral and central.

    E, Partial denture in place. Esthetic appearance acceptable.

    F, Mirror view of partial denture. Four points of support and stabilization. Four areas of retention.

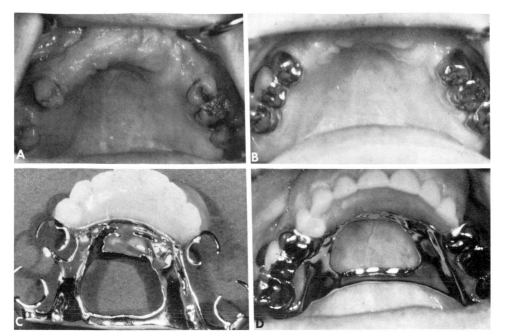

FIGURE 28–16.   *A*, Class IV maxillary arch resulting from accident.

B, Mouth preparation. Bridge on right splinting molar and bicuspid. Abutments will be clasped and provide support as well as retention. All teeth on left crowned. Retention and support pattern same as on right side.

C and *D*, Partial denture before seating, and seated. Class IV removable partial denture must have retention as far as possible behind the fulcrum line. Anterior support must be rugged.

REFERENCES

 1. Jordan, L. G.: Designing removable partial dentures with external attachments (clasps). J. Pros. Den., *2*:716, Nov. 1952.
 2. Frechette, A. R.: Partial denture planning with special reference to stress distribution. J. Ontario D. A., *30*:318, Oct. 1953.
 3. Smith, G. P.: Factors affecting the choice of partial prosthesis—fixed or removable. Dent. Clin. N. Amer., March 1959, p. 3.
 4. Dykema, R. W., Cunningham, D. M., and Johnston, J. F.: Modern Practice in Removable Partial Prosthodontics. Philadelphia, W. B. Saunders Company, 1969.
 5. Eich, F. A.: Role of removable partial dentures in the destruction of the natural dentition. Dent. Clin. N. Amer., Nov. 1962, p. 717.
 6. Johnston, J. F., and Bogan, R. L.: Partial denture design and related mouth preparation. Bull. Virginia D. A., *40*:25, March 1963 (Abstract).
 7. Johnston, J. F.: Preparation of mouths for fixed and removable partial dentures. J. Pros. Den., *11*:456, May-June 1961.
 8. Cunningham, D. M.: Mouth preparation for removable appliances. Arizona D. J., *2*:154, Dec. 1956.
 9. Steffel, V. L.: Planning removable partial dentures. J. Pros. Den., *12*:524, May-June 1962.
10. Johnston, J. F.: Preparation of mouths for fixed and removable partial dentures. Alumni Bulletin, Indiana University School of Dentistry, Sept. 1960, p. 4.
11. Towle, H. J., Jr.: Mouth preparation for removable partial dentures. New York J. Den., *31*:119, April, 1961.
12. Glann, G. W., and Appleby, R. C.: Mouth preparation for removable partial dentures. J. Pros. Den., *10*:698, July-Aug. 1960.

13. Mills, M. L.: Mouth preparation for the removable partial denture. J.A.D.A., *60*:154, Feb. 1960.
14. Perry, C.: Importance and preparation of the occlusal rest. J. Michigan D. A., *42*:97, March 1960.
15. DeRisi, M. C.: Surveying for removable partial denture prosthesis. J.A.D.A., *63*:603, Nov. 1961.
16. McCracken, W. L.: Partial Denture Construction; Principles and Techniques. 3rd ed. Ed. by Henderson, D., and Steffel, V. L. St. Louis, The C. V. Mosby Company, 1969.

Block, P.: Indirect-direct method for constructing crowns to fit existing partial dentures. D. Digest, *71*:500, Nov. 1965.

Martone, A. L.: A challenge of the partially edentulous mouth. J. Pros. Den., *8*:942, Nov.-Dec. 1958.

McCracken, W. L.: Mouth preparation for partial dentures. Bull. Alabama D. A., *39*:37, Oct. 1955.

McCracken, W. L.: Mouth preparation for partial dentures. J. Pros. Den., *6*:39, Jan. 1956.

Metty, A. C.: Obtaining efficient soft tissue support for the partial denture base. J.A.D.A., *56*:679, May 1958.

Perry, C.: Philosophy of partial denture design. Bull. St. Louis D. Soc., *25*:48, May 1954 (Digest).

Schuyler, C. H.: Analysis of the use and relative value of the precision attachment and the clasp in partial denture planning. J. Pros. Den., *3*:711, Sept. 1953.

Steffel, V. L.: Postgraduate course, Ohio State University School of Dentistry, 1953.

Steffel, V. L.: Clasp partial dentures. J.A.D.A., *66*:803, June 1963.

Terkla, L. G., and Laney, W. R.: Partial Dentures. 3rd ed. St. Louis, The C. V. Mosby Company, 1963.

chapter 29

ORTHODONTIC POSITIONING OF ABUTMENTS AND ASSOCIATED TEETH

Abutment alignment is one of the most important factors influencing the design, esthetic effect, and longevity of a fixed partial denture. Improved axial directions of the abutment teeth not only will provide a more suitable foundation for the prosthesis—that is, one better able to accept additional forces—but also will make it possible to utilize teeth that otherwise would be unusable as abutments (Figs. 29–1, 29–2, 29–3, and 29–4).

Reorientation of abutment teeth will enable the prosthodontist to cope with many uncertainties associated with pathologic axial inclinations of abutments. The purpose of this chapter, therefore, is to demonstrate a few of the more typical problems that may exist because of poor alignment of the abutment teeth and to suggest methods of treatment. It is not the intent here either to discuss all the abnormalities that may be present or to elaborate on the various techniques that may be used to correct them.

Considerations that may be used as the basis for a successful solution for some of these situations will be set forth. Only one technique will be outlined, namely, that of the so-called "working retainer." This appliance is sufficiently versatile to effect a majority of the tooth movements that the prosthodontist may wish to do himself. However, it does have limitations, which must be recognized. These will be mentioned in the section on technical procedures.

SOME TYPICAL PROBLEMS

It may be desirable to alter the positions of the abutment teeth for one or more of the following reasons:

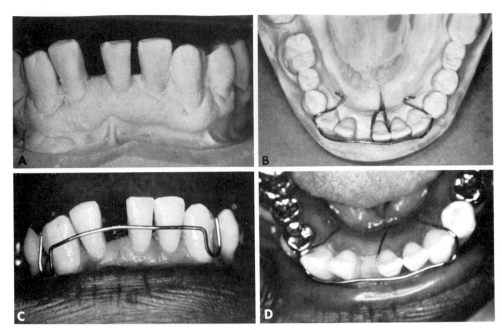

FIGURE 29–1.   *A*, Cast of mandibular arch.
B, C, and *D*, Incisor abutments were first moved lingually, then laterally (*D*).

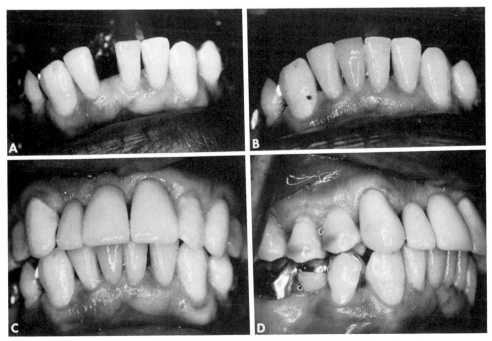

FIGURE 29–2.   *A*, Repositioned abutments.
B, C, and *D*, Views of mandibular anterior bridge and occluding maxillary bridge.

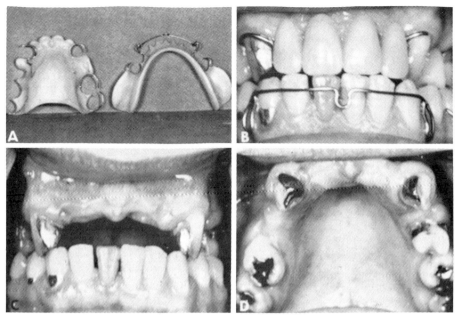

FIGURE 29–3. *A*, Working retainers that were used to improve tooth position. The maxillary left cuspid clasp is free of acrylic resin over most of its length so that it can be activated to cause labial movement of the tooth. The labial wire on the mandibular anteriors will be used to move the incisors lingually and together.

B, Appliances in the mouth. The mandibular posterior supplied teeth are set high to increase the vertical dimension so that the left cuspid will be free to move into proper position.

C, Left cuspid has moved to position. Teeth have temporary amalgam restorations.

D, Occlusal view of *C*.

1. A lack of contact with adjacent teeth, if uncorrected, can result in a food trap if the retainer is overcontoured in an attempt to make contact.

2. Axial tilting can lead to a crushing of the periodontal membrane under an additional load, with subsequent periodontal and alveolar atrophy.

3. Teeth can display occlusal interference in eccentric excursions. (An example of this is a mandibular second molar tipped forward into a first molar space, the mesial of the tooth rotating to the lingual, the distobuccal being elevated above the occlusion table, and cuspal interference with the mesiolingual cusp of the maxillary second molar occurring during lateral excursions.)

4. When there is a rotation effecting disturbances in inclined-plane relationships, it might be difficult to design the preparation of the abutment tooth so that it will meet the demands of both appearance and mechanics.

5. When teeth are tipped labially or lingually, or when anterior teeth are flared labially with an unsatisfactory esthetic effect, preparations could result in overreduction.

This list is incomplete, but these are the abnormalities most frequently encountered (Figs. 29-5 and 29-6).

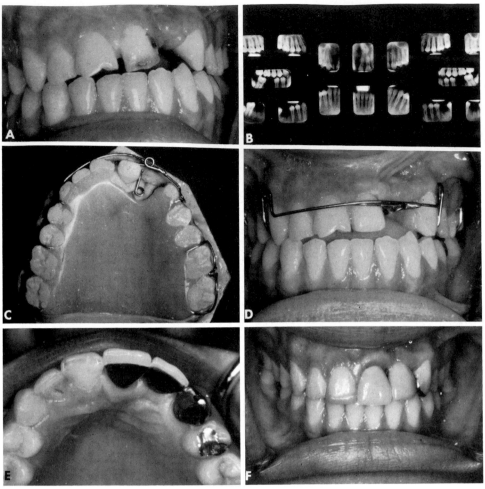

FIGURE 29–4.   *A* and *B*, Mouth of adolescent. Lateral incisor missing, owing to repaired cleft. Axial inclination and pulp size of central made preparation impossible.

C, Appliance to correct inclination of central. Tooth will be tipped instead of being moved bodily, but this will suffice.

D, Repositioning almost completed.

E and *F*, Bridge on realigned abutments.

PHYSIOLOGIC CONSIDERATIONS OF TOOTH MOVEMENT

The periodontal membrane is composed primarily of collagenous fibers, and the majority of the fibers are oriented obliquely and directed apically as the cementum of the tooth is approached. Orban[1] states that the blood supply for this structure is derived from the blood vessels (1) entering the apical foramen, (2) passing over the alveolar crest from the gingivae, and (3) penetrating the wall of the alveolus, with the major supply coming from the last mentioned.

The periodontal membrane is more vascular on the side next to the

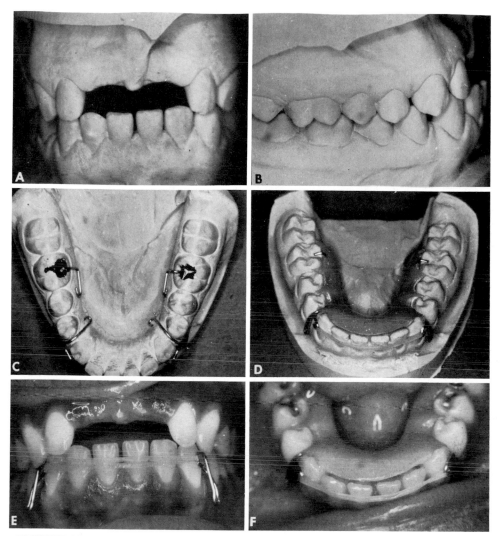

FIGURE 29–5. *A* and *B*, Casts of opposing arches. Observe relationship of incisal edges of mandibular teeth to maxillary ridge. This position and width of space made situation very difficult.

C and *D*, Appliance to move mandibular incisors lingually. Force exerted lingually by elastic band stretched over labial surfaces. Resin contoured to give freedom of movement and to maintain alignment.

E and *F*, Appliance at work. Movement short of that desired.

alveolus, and this characteristic is greater in the apical third than in the coronal portion. Bone is a highly vascular tissue, but cementum is an avascular structure. It is quite possible that the resorption differences of bone and cementum are due to these dissimilarities in vascularity and that the more common presence of resorption in the region of the apex may be traced to the higher vascularity of the periodontal membrane at this point.

Hemley[2] believes that the actual resorptive mechanism stems from pH changes in the periodontal membrane as force is applied to it. As a consequence of such compression, stasis of the blood at the compression site

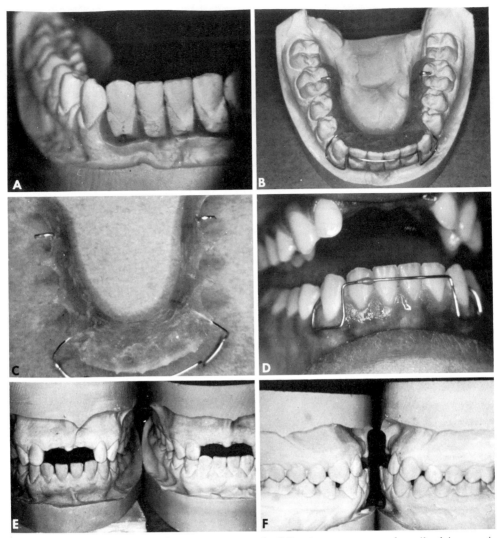

FIGURE 29–6.   *A*, *B*, and *C*, Cast was made following treatment described in previous figure. It was sectioned, teeth were aligned, and a Hawley retainer made.

D, Second appliance pushed mobile teeth into alignment. Patient was uncomfortable for about two hours.

E and *F*, Contrasting casts showing realigned mandibular incisors. Occlusion now suitable for maxillary bridge. (See Case History 1 in Chapter 36.)

lowers the pH, which in turn causes an increased solubility of the mineral salts of the bone, resulting in resorption. Relief of the stasis allows a resumption of the normal pH, and local calcium is deposited in the formation of new bone.

Oppenheim[3] has found that a force applied to the crown of a tooth causes a tipping movement, the fulcrum of which is located approximately at the beginning of the apical third of the root. The distance of this fulcrum point from the apex is a function of the degree of force applied to the tooth. This creates four areas of activity in the periodontal membrane, two of resorption and two of deposition (Fig. 29-7).

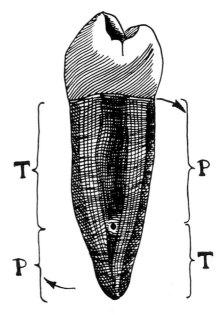

FIGURE 29–7. Diagram showing the areas of pressure (P) and tension (T) along the root of a tooth receiving a buccal tipping force.

Reitan[4] has noted a cellular increase in the periodontal membrane within the first to second day of tooth movement in humans, and also an increase, particularly marked around the ninth day, in the osteoid present on the alveolar wall. Under pressure there occurs either direct resorption of bone or hyalinization of the periodontal membrane with resorption in adjacent areas of the bone. Cellular proliferation is stated to be a response to tension of the fibers of the periodontal membrane.

Owing to the thickening of the periodontal membrane around the tooth during movement, mobility to the extent of approximately 1.0 mm. may ensue. To enable the tissues to reorganize around the root, active treatment is followed by a period of retention[5] in which the teeth are held during undisturbed reparative processes. This is accomplished by having the working appliance adjusted passively to maintain the new positions of the abutment teeth. One alternative would be to prepare the abutment teeth and then to stabilize them with a temporary acrylic resin bridge to be worn during fabrication of the prosthesis.

DIAGNOSIS, ANALYSIS, AND TREATMENT PLANNING

"Diagnosis," as used here, refers to the recognition of an existing incongruity concerning the position of the abutment teeth. The simple recognition of such disturbance is followed by a scrutiny of the abnormality, which is termed "analysis." Information from the analytical process is the basis for the formulation of the treatment plan, which may include repositioning of the abutment teeth.

Abutment position must not be considered separately from the design of the prosthesis. It is one of the factors that dictate this choice and should enter into the treatment planning much the same as does the caries index of the mouth. Malpositions of teeth to be used as abutments are only one phase that must be contemplated in the restoration of a mouth to an optimal level. For instance, a complete denture opposing the arch to be restored would decrease the forces on a bridge and might make it unnecessary to reposition the abutment teeth for better resistance to stresses.

In the analysis, information is gleaned from diagnostic casts, intraoral radiographs, and oral examination. The diagnostic casts, plus the radiographs, will show the axial inclinations of the teeth in a mesiodistal direction. The casts also will divulge faciolingual axial inclinations, abnormal rotations, and resistance to orthodontic movement of abutment teeth caused by interlocking cuspal relations, unerupted teeth, or ankylosis. Ankylosed teeth cannot be moved, but cuspal interferences may be minimized either by spot grinding of the offending cusps or by the construction of a bite plane against which the lower incisors occlude, thus prohibiting articulation in the posterior segments.

Examination of the mouth will disclose cuspal relations in lateral excursions. If an excessive curve of Spee exists, a view of the interocclusal space in rest position will show whether the excessive vertical overlap is due to infraclusion of the posterior teeth or to supraclusion of the anterior teeth.

Isolation of the reason for the exaggerated vertical overlap will help to formulate the ideal solution. If the interocclusal space is more than 3.0 to 5.0 mm., undereruption of the buccal segments, especially the mandibular bicuspids and maxillary molars, is the probable cause. Sometimes a bite plane, occluding against the lower incisors, will prevent the occlusion of the posterior teeth and facilitate their eruption, thereby reducing the vertical overlap. If the interocclusal space is within the 3.0 to 5.0 mm. range, usually there is an overeruption of the anterior teeth. Such a situation should be handled by an orthodontist, inasmuch as it requires depression of teeth, the most challenging type of movement, and involves procedures not within the scope of the restorative dentist.

After completion of the analysis, the form of the appliance is considered. To the maximal extent permitted by limiting factors, it must correct the problem as it has been visualized. The analytical process should show the directions and the distance sought in tooth movement. The limiting factors include those inherent in the appliance, the patient, and the operator.

A tooth may undergo movement in three planes of space simultaneously, as, for example, distally, lingually, and occlusally. The appliance to be described will not perform bodily movement of teeth and will not actively erupt teeth. Tissues may not respond as anticipated in some patients, and movement may be extremely difficult if not impossible. In other individuals, eruption is not easily obtained when using bite planes, and the new positions may be unstable. **Lack of skill and comprehension of the potentialities of the appliance definitely can preclude achievement of the result expected.**

APPLIANCE DESIGN

Factors presented by each individual case determine the pattern of the appliance. It is constructed of an acrylic resin base, the working arms being formed from stainless steel wire varying from 0.025 to 0.030 inch. Mostly the smaller wire is used instead of its heavier counterpart to produce a lighter force that will act for a longer time and through a greater distance.

The passive wire to be activated should be deformed 1.0 mm. in the direction toward which movement is desired (Fig. 29-8). Therefore, by opening slightly the primary coil (Fig. 29-8 at *1*), the free arm of this coil, which extends to the secondary coil, is displaced 0.5 mm. An additional 0.5 mm. is then gained by opening the secondary coil (Fig. 29-8 at *2*). The result is a displacement paralleling the direction sought in the movement (mesial in this instance).

If only the primary coil were opened in this case, the resultant movement would have a labial component that might be undesirable. The degree of displacement of the working arm will vary with the size of the wire being used, customarily with more displacement being placed in the thinner wires.

Types of tooth movement and some basic designs that can be realized with the working retainer are illustrated.

Labiolingual Movement of Incisors

Lingual tipping of an incisor can be effected by utilizing a labial arch wire that is deformed to place a force on the labial surface of the tooth to be moved. One application of this arch wire is shown in Figure 29-9.

The acrylic resin is cut away on the lingual surface of the central to be repositioned, and the pressure is kept on the central incisor by gradually building an inset into the arch passing over it, or closing the vertical loops, or both (Fig. 29-10). This is done by making minor adjustments in the arch wire at two-week intervals. This inset will keep the arch from being in contact on the labial surface of the other incisors and cuspids.

Force is then generated in the loops overlying the cuspids and is trans-

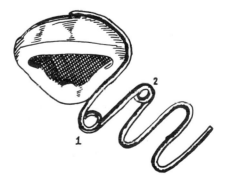

FIGURE 29–8. Double cantilever spring as used to apply a direct proximal thrust on an incisor. 1, The primary coil; 2, the secondary coil.

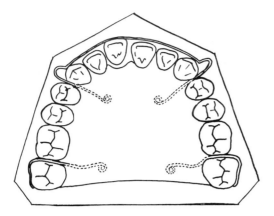

FIGURE 29–9. Design of appliance to tip an incisor lingually. The acrylic resin, as shown, is relieved on the lingual of the incisor to allow movement.

mitted to the central incisor. The wire should rest in contact across the labial surface of the central if there is no reason to rotate this tooth. This can be checked by drawing a length of dental floss between the wire and the tooth to test the accuracy of fit.

Labial tipping of an incisor is achieved by placing a double cantilever spring on the lingual surface, as suggested by Adams[6] and shown in Figure 29-11. With this type of movement, owing to the slope of the lingual surface, there is a tendency for a force on the lingual of most incisors to unseat the appliance because of a component directed downward; but usually this can be counteracted with wire clasps on the labial surfaces of the cuspids. As a rule, the posterior end must be retained with clasps around a molar on each side.

Mesial and Distal Tipping of Anterior Teeth

This is done with a lever, as shown in Figure 29-12. The labial arch wire is contoured to curb rotation of the tooth being tipped to the distal. Rotation is also controlled by the judicious relief of the acrylic resin on the mesiolingual as the tooth tips distally. As the tooth moves distally, the resin is relieved to make space.

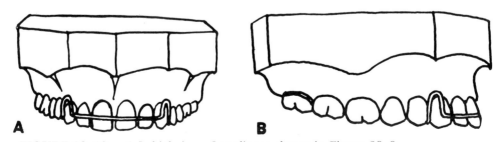

A   **B**

FIGURE 29–10.   *A*, Labial view of appliance shown in Figure 29–9.
B, Buccal view of appliance shown in Figure 29–9; closure of the vertical loops applies a distal thrust to any teeth contacting the labial arch.

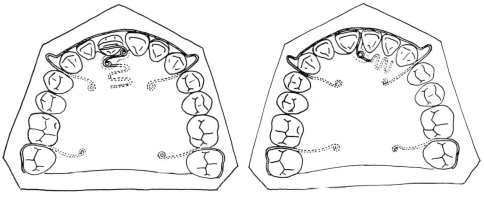

FIGURE 29–11.   **FIGURE 29–12.**

FIGURE 29–11.   Diagram showing the use of a double cantilever spring to effect labial tipping of an incisor.

FIGURE 29–12.   Distal tipping of a central incisor using a single cantilever spring.

Mesiodistal Movement of Posterior Teeth

The same appliance plan used for the anterior teeth fulfills the needs of this operation. In general, a heavier wire will be used on a molar than on an incisor, since the root area is larger. As an illustration, a 0.025 inch wire might be used for an incisor, whereas in most cases a molar would call for a 0.028 or 0.030 inch wire for the lever.

Frequently the occlusion must be freed when tipping a posterior tooth, since cuspal interdigitation can counteract the force exerted by the appliance. To avert full closure, the resin on the lingual of the incisors on a maxillary retainer is built up to act as a stop against the mandibular incisors. A posterior opening of 1.0 to 2.0 mm. should be ample.

Buccolingual Movement of Posterior Teeth

Molars and bicuspids may be tipped buccally or lingually with the working retainer. While this is being executed, it may be necessary to keep the posterior teeth out of occlusion. Buccal movement may be induced with a single-armed or double-armed cantilever spring (Fig. 29–13).

When using the double cantilever spring, both the primary and the secondary coils must be freed from the base to obtain a direct buccal thrust. The single lever spring can be used when rotating molars by having the free end of the lever resting on the surface that is to be moved the farthest. As in Figure 29–13 *A*, the mesial of the second molar will be pushed farther buccally than the distal.

Lingual movement of the posterior abutment tooth may be brought about by a single lever or an inset in a buccal arch. This inset is placed in the wire in the same manner as in the labial arch wire used to tip incisors lingually. The force is generated in the vertical loops (Fig. 29–14).

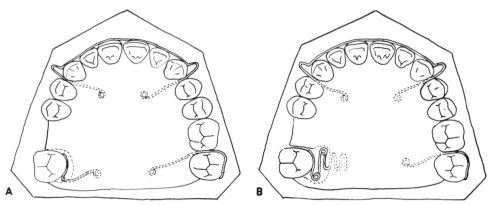

FIGURE 29–13.   *A,* Single cantilever spring to tip a molar buccally.
B, Double cantilever spring as used to tip a molar buccally.

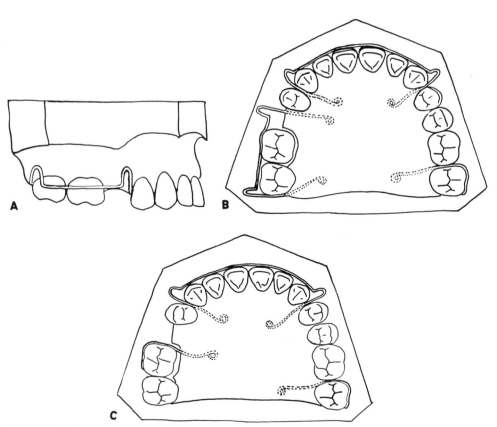

FIGURE 29–14.   *A,* Buccal view of appliance used to effect lingual tipping of a molar.
B, Occlusal view of appliance in *A.*
C, Diagram showing the use of a single cantilever spring to effect lingual movement of a
molar.

FIGURE 29–15. Diagram showing necessary force application to effect rotation of an incisor.

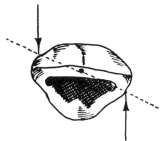

Rotation of Incisor Teeth

Rotation of incisor teeth with the working retainer presents some difficulties. It is essential to apply two forces to the tooth, one from the labial and one from the lingual, with the distance between the two points of application as great as possible (Fig. 29-15).

There are two methods. The first consists of a labial arch wire acting on the labial surface, and selective relief of the acrylic resin on the lingual, to force the tooth to rotate instead of tipping lingually (Fig. 29-16). The second is to have a spring acting from the lingual instead of having a fulcrum point on the base (Fig. 29-17).

The tooth is braced on the mesial by an acrylic resin tooth, which fills the edentulous space. This double action will cause the tooth to rotate in situ rather than being tipped lingually to some degree, as in Figure 29-16. Therefore, the choice of design will depend on the type of correction desired.

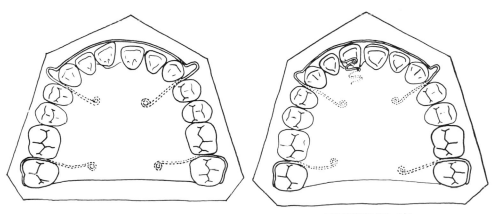

FIGURE 29–16.   **FIGURE 29–17.**

FIGURE 29–16. Design of appliance used to reposition the mesial of the incisor lingually.

FIGURE 29–17. Use of labial arch and double cantilever spring to rotate an incisor in situ.

Eruption of Posterior Teeth

The final type of tooth movement to be considered is that of eruption of posterior teeth. This can be brought about by using a bite plane to the lingual of the maxillary incisors, which serves as a stop to prevent the posterior teeth from occluding. There should be an opening in the posterior segments of approximately 1.0 mm. As these teeth erupt into occlusion, acrylic resin is added to the bite plane to keep the interocclusal space 1.0 mm. in height.

Detailed instructions for fabrication are purposely omitted from this chapter. Reference to the standard texts on this subject will supply such information.

REFERENCES

1. Orban, B. J.: Textbook of Histology. 4th ed. St. Louis, The C. V. Mosby Company, 1957.
2. Hemley, S.: Orthodontic Theory and Practice. New York, Grune & Stratton, 1953.
3. Oppenheim, A.: Human tissue response to orthodontic intervention of short and long duration. Amer. J. Orthodont. & Oral Surg., 28:263, May 1942.
4. Reitan, K.: The initial tissue reactions incident to orthodontic tooth movement. Acta Odont. Scand., Suppl. 6, 1951.
5. Salzmann, J. A.: Principles of Orthodontics. 2nd ed. Philadelphia, J. B. Lippincott Company, 1943.
6. Adams, C. P.: The design and construction of removable orthodontic appliances. Bristol, John Wright & Sons, Ltd., 1955.

Jarabak, J. R.: Orthodontic treatment preparatory to fixed partial denture prosthesis. Dent. Clin. N. Amer., March 1959, p. 31.

chapter 30

CROWN AND BRIDGE PROCEDURES FOR THE YOUNG-AGE GROUP

Until very recently construction of fixed partial prostheses for the preadolescent or adolescent patient was thought to be ill advised. Such restorative procedures were considered wholly acceptable only for a period starting with the early twenties and ending in the middle fifties. Reflecting on the difficulties formerly attending the preparations of abutment teeth, these limitations may have been warranted. However, with the advent of speedier operations, indirect techniques, and the clinical research directed by Castaldi, Mink, Davis, Starkey, and other advanced pedodontists, the scope of the fixed prosthesis has been widened. To construct at least short-span bridges for young patients as soon as permanent teeth have erupted into occlusion, and even for very young patients when deciduous teeth are congenitally missing, is now recognized as safe and advantageous (Fig. 30-1).

The authors have been privileged to observe rather extensive fixed partial prostheses and crowns placed in the mouths of patients as young as four years, and have watched or have participated in the construction of many bridges for patients 16 years of age and younger. For the very young, because the deficiencies responsible for the spaces probably will have affected the contours of the teeth, it is usually necessary to use full gold or veneered gold crowns. Often, except at the cervical margin, little preparation will be needed (Fig. 30-2).

When newly erupted permanent teeth are used as abutments, clinical experience has dictated that inlays are better retainers biologically than either partial veneer or full veneer gold crowns. Almost always the preparations for inlays will be two-surface and will be much like those described in Chapter 7, The Inlay Retainer. Proximal and occlusal depth of the cavities must be governed by information obtained from carefully made radiographs. Pinholes must be judiciously positioned (Fig. 30–3 E and F).

Because of the potential mobility of teeth in the adolescent patient, bridges should be constructed with rigid joints. It is of the utmost impor-

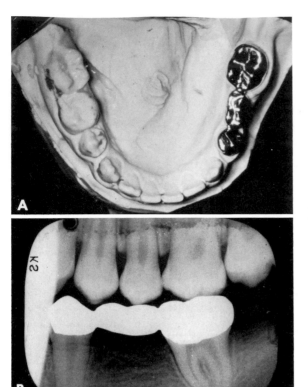

FIGURE 30–1. Bridge restoring continuity of mandibular arch for patient 14 years of age. Built in late 1960.

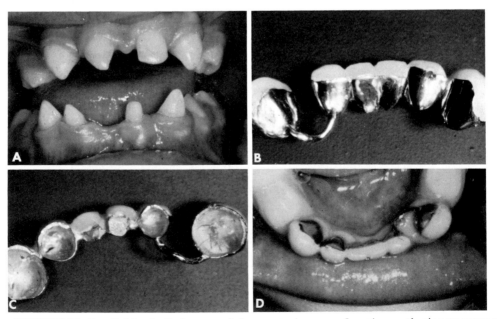

FIGURE 30–2. Bridge built for preadolescent to improve function, esthetic appearance, and attitude. Approximate age, 4 years.

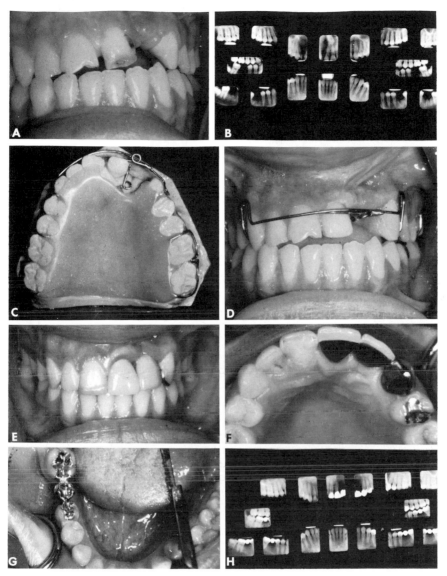

FIGURE 30-3. *A* and *B*, Patient, female, 17 years old, with operated cleft. Central incisor abutment realigned orthodontically. Pulp was large.

C, Appliance used to reposition abutments.

D, Appliance in mouth. Left central incisor and cuspid moved laterally from space.

E and *F*, Anterior maxillary bridge. Right central incisor restored with a porcelain incisal edge bonded to a pinlay casting.

G, One mandibular bridge with inlay retainers.

H, Radiograph of completed mouth. Constructed in early 1962.

tance that bridges built for young patients have adequate embrasure form and *minimal* ridge contact under the pontic. Before and after cementation, owing to the rapidly changing jaw relationships in the growing patient, these bridges must be critically equilibrated and should be examined at approximately three-month intervals so that the occlusion may be checked and corrected.

Anterior bridges are less easy to construct because of shorter clinical crowns and large pulps (Fig. 30-3), but if the abutment teeth are analyzed and meticulously prepared for pin-supported retainers, many extraordinary replacements may be accomplished.

When a first molar is lost at a very early age, a decision must be made about maintaining the space and holding the opposing teeth in position (Fig. 30-4). If the second molar has already erupted, a space maintainer should be built and cemented; this will stabilize the prospective abutment teeth and also should prevent extrusion of the opposing tooth or teeth. If the first permanent molar has erupted and the first and second deciduous molars are lost, unilaterally or bilaterally, a removable space maintainer should be built to provide occlusion for the opposing teeth. It should be constructed of a material that will permit an opening to be made later to accommodate the eruption of the underlying tooth or teeth (Fig. 30-5).

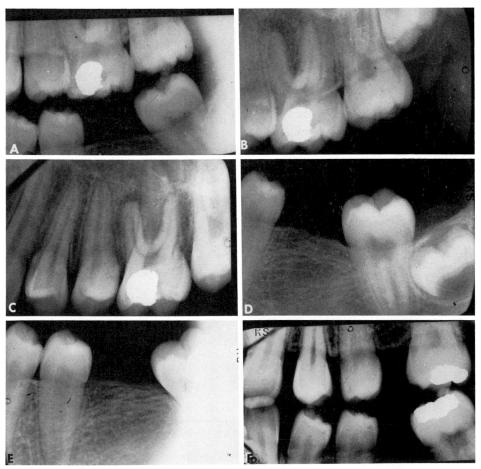

FIGURE 30–4. Radiographs of preadolescent patient with mandibular first molar already lost and condemned maxillary first molar, which was extracted. *F*, Situation 13 months later. This patient is a dental cripple, needlessly.

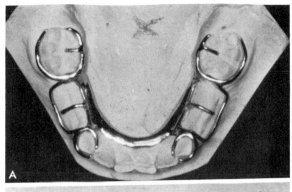

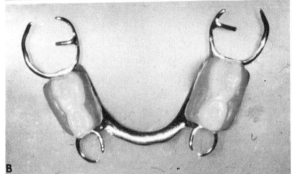

FIGURE 30–5. *A*, Frame for combination space maintainer and masticating prosthesis. Retentive arms for resin base are spaced so that areas may be cut out to permit eruption of bicuspids.

B, Completed temporary partial denture.

(Figures 30–1, 30–2, and 30–5, courtesy of Dr. Bailey Davis.)

The span of life of such bridges is difficult to predict. Many have been in the mouth five or more years. Some of the early ones were built using full veneer gold crowns as retainers. Gingival acceptance of these retainers was often unsatisfactory, particularly at the linguocervical margins; as yet it has not been possible to determine the etiology. There also has been some, and similarly located, tissue disturbance from partial veneer crowns. Such reactions seemingly do not occur with much severity following puberty, and do not appear at all when inlays are used as the retainers.

This is the type of fixed partial prosthodontic service that should be practiced zealously.

REFERENCES

Mink, J. R.: Restorative dentistry for children. J.A.D.A., *66*:227, Feb. 1963.

Mink, J. R.: Crown and bridge for the young adolescent. Dent. Clin. N. Amer., March 1966, p. 149.

Scures, C. C.: Porcelain baked to gold in pedodontics. J. Den. Child., *30*:9, 1st quar., 1963.

chapter 31

THE RESTORATION OF MUTILATED ANTERIOR TEETH

Mutilations of anterior teeth can be caused by fracture, by caries, or by excessive cutting away of tooth structure (sometimes unavoidable) for access in endodontic treatment.

The vitality of a fractured tooth often can be maintained if the pulp is not actually traumatized and if the patient can be treated very soon after the injury. The exposed fractured surface immediately over the pulp should be coated with a palliative or neutral dressing and all the surface covered with cement. This, in turn, is shielded by some device that has been made compatible with the occlusion. Steel crowns or plastic crown forms may be used, but cemented orthodontic bands, extending 0.3 to 0.5 mm. to the incisal of the fracture, are beginning to be substituted for crowns of all types and will keep the dressing on the fractured surface. Protection should be continued until it can be determined whether vitality has been preserved or whether, through no response to the accepted stimuli, it seems that the tooth is no longer vital.

When a tooth has gross carious lesions that undermine one or both incisal angles, it must be explored by removing the caries and be insulated against shock throughout a waiting period long enough to ascertain whether endodontic therapy will be needful.

There are three highly recommended means by which vital fractured teeth may be rebuilt:

1. If a portion of a proximal surface and an angle are involved, a wire-retained-and-supported resin restoration may suffice, making it unnecessary to resort to a less conservative repair, such as the jacket or veneered gold crown.

2. When all the incisal edge is missing, but without extensive involvement of the labial and proximal surfaces, the remaining tooth structure can be prepared for a partial veneer crown and the incisal portion of the casting filled with either silicate cement or resin. This is a well-established and meritorious method.

600

3. If a major portion of the incisal edge has been broken away, particularly if the fracture is a diagonal one across the labial surface, a casting to which porcelain has been bonded will restore contour, function, and usually appearance, in a most gratifying manner.

The objective of each of these three techniques is definitive and not solely an intermediate treatment preliminary to the construction of a jacket or veneered crown. Future developments in individual mouths may eventually make the latter approach mandatory.

CLASS IV RESIN RESTORATIONS

Resin restorations, retained and supported by wire, have been widely accepted for rebuilding proximal surfaces and incisal angles, and portions of incisal edges of incisors. Such restorations must be replaced periodically, but if this is anticipated and is done when indicated, radical restorative measures can be postponed indefinitely.

Cavity Preparation. When a tooth is to be restored by this technique, a box-type preparation is made on the proximal surface. A typical Class IV step may be extended approximately three-fourths of the way across the incisal edge, or a retentive angle can be cut on the axial wall just inside the dentinoenamel junction. A pinhole capable of accepting an 0.020 inch stainless steel wire is placed in the cervical seat, somewhat to the lingual of the center of the tooth. The second pinhole is placed in the tooth structure supporting the remaining incisal angle, or on the proximal surface, parallel to the incisal edge, to the lingual of the center of the tooth but inside the dentinoenamel junction. These holes should be 1.0 mm. deep (Fig. 31-1).

Threaded wire is cut and shaped so that it will extend into the holes for their full depth. With the holes filled with cement, the wire is placed first in the cervical hole and then flexed so that it may be pushed into the hole at the incisal. As a precaution against the possibility that a shadow will show through the labial surface of the restoration, the wire should be bent slightly toward the lingual half of the tooth. The excess of hardened cement is chipped away and the restoration is built to form.

Building Restoration. Either the brush or the crown form technique may be used to build up the resin to contour. It is important that the occluding surface be equilibrated to accommodate mandibular movements. The restoration should be checked regularly and replaced if there is any evidence of marginal seepage. Opposing incisal edges and angles should be rounded to minimize shearing.

VENEERED PARTIAL VENEER CROWN

When a partial veneer crown with a window is to be used, the proximal and lingual surfaces are reduced without extending the proximal margins

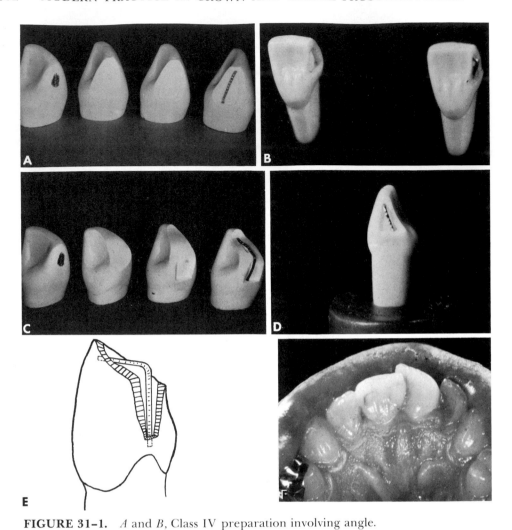

FIGURE 31-1.   *A* and *B*, Class IV preparation involving angle.
C and *D*, Class IV preparation involving angle and incisal edge.
E, Diagram of preparation in *C* and *D*.
F, Both centrals restored with wire-supported acrylic resin restorations.
(Courtesy of Department of Operative Dentistry, Indiana University School of Dentistry.)

labially beyond the line angles. The grooves may run parallel to the long axis of the tooth, they should be shallow, and their retentive properties should be supplemented by two or three shallow pinholes 0.7 mm. deep in the lingual surface. Lingual clearance should be approximately 0.5 mm., and reduction of the proximal surfaces should be minimal. Labial extension for prevention can be disregarded. If caries should ever develop around the proximal margins, the tooth can then be restored with a jacket or veneered crown (Fig. 31-2).

An indirect technique is indicated. In order that the metal casting can be contoured to function without premature contact in any position, full arch casts must be occluded. The area of the prepared tooth should be poured first. When this stone has set for 1 hour it is removed; from it the die will be

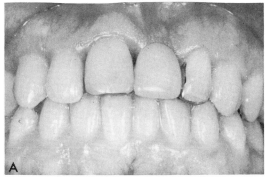

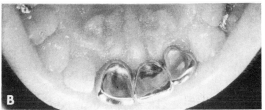

FIGURE 31-2. Bridge replacing maxillary left central incisor. Mesial angle of central abutment and incisolingual of lateral were fractured. Patient was immature; pulps were large. Shallow partial veneer preparations were made and exposed areas of castings were veneered with acrylic resin. Silicate cement could have been used and would have been equally effective.

made. The full arch working cast is then poured. The casts may be mounted with a face-bow on an adjustable articulator, although the occluding unprepared anterior and posterior teeth should adequately guide the casts for carving the pattern even if freehand mounting has been used.

The wax pattern should be carved to cover the incisal edge. Lingual and incisal contours must be exact; otherwise, when equilibrating the casting, holes may appear in the metal through which the resin or silicate can be distorted or abraded. There must be a greater thickness of wax to ensure casting and bulk of metal for equilibration. The casting can be thinned at the labial margins for esthetic purposes. If the casting is to have minimal bulk, a hard crown and bridge or partial denture alloy is indispensable.

When the casting has been equilibrated and polished, it is cemented on the tooth, undercuts are made in both the tooth structure and the metal, and the resin or silicate veneer is built.

PORCELAIN INCISAL BONDED TO A METAL SUBSTRUCTURE

When the operator understands the fabrication of ceramic restorations, a casting with a bonded porcelain incisal edge probably is the most satisfactory restoration for the vital fractured anterior tooth. Assuming that he has the skill to make castings that fit, the first requisite is a sound ceramic technique. Second, and even more consequential, is a discerning sense of shade and shade matching. Third, the clinician must have a concept of tooth form and the ability to mold the restoration into harmony with the surface contours remaining.

A workable and productive ceramic technique is not beyond the grasp of the average diligent and determined dentist or technician. Matching shades is a skill that even those who lack true color sense can acquire. In such cases as these, there is a great deal of remaining tooth surface that should guide the operator in contouring his restoration with comparative ease.

A bite-wing radiograph, or one that shows minimal coronal distortion, is essential (Fig. 31-3 B).

Preparation of Tooth. When a fractured tooth is prepared for a bonded porcelain restoration (Fig. 31-3 C, D, and E), the incisal edge should be smoothed and any abrupt angles or curves eliminated. If the fracture line is close to or bisects one of the incisal angles, this portion of the tooth should be shortened to provide not less than 1.5 mm. of space.

The lingual surface of the tooth is prepared in the same way as for a pinledge retainer (0.5 mm. clearance is sufficient) except that the incisal pinholes are placed on the fractured incisal edge, mesially and distally to the pulp horns. However, when bulk of tooth structure permits, a ledge is cut cervically to the linguoincisal edge of the tooth to increase the area of bonding. Although the pinholes, 2.0 mm. in depth, can be made with a tapered fissure bur, a spiral drill is preferable. When a long 0.023 inch drill is being used, a paralleling instrument may be helpful.

The Working and Firing Casts. Nylon bristles 0.022 inch in diameter are placed in the pinholes and a silicone rubber impression is taken in a custom-built tray (Fig. 31-3 F). The path of removal should be parallel to the direction of insertion for the pins. A stone master cast is poured and allowed to set for 1 hour. The impression is very carefully removed and a second cast is made of porcelain investment.* This should not be separated sooner than 60 minutes or later than 2 hours after pouring (Fig. 31-4).

Waxing and Investing the Pattern. The wax pattern is made on the original stone die after 0.020 inch nylon bristles have been cut, roughened, and placed in the pinholes. It should cover all the lingual preparation except the extension over the incisal edge, where it should be approximately 0.35 mm. short of the proximal and labial peripheral margin.

A large sprue pin is attached to the center of the wax pattern, parallel to the path of withdrawal, and the pattern is removed from the die. The investing and casting technique is the same as for crowns to be veneered with porcelain, with the exception of the vents. The casting is made from a gold in balance with the porcelain to be used. The authors have always used Ceramco alloy and porcelain.

Building Technique with Ceramco Alloy and Porcelain. The casting is seated on the stone master cast, and the surface that will be exposed is polished; that which is to receive the porcelain is ground with a coarse wheel stone. It is immersed in hydrofluoric acid for 8 hours, or this time may be reduced to 30 minutes if the acid container is placed in an ultrasonic cleaner.

The casting is placed on the porcelain investment cast and both are degassed in the porcelain furnace. (For degassing cycle, see Chapter 21,

---

*Loma Linda Porcelain Inlay Investment, Surgident, Ltd., Los Angeles, Calif.
Whip-Mix Porcelain Inlay Investment, Whip-Mix Corporation, Louisville, Ky.

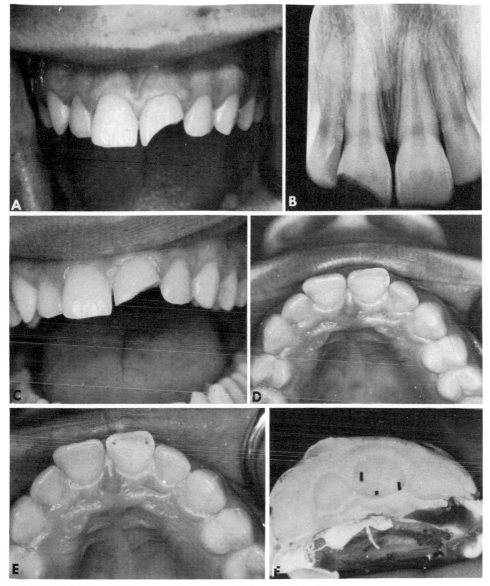

FIGURE 31–3.   *A*, Fractured maxillary left central incisor.
   B, Fracture is in close proximity to pulp. Faint color was visible but there was only nominal sensitivity. Tooth did and does test normally.
   C and *D*, Preliminary preparation.
   E and *F*, Prepared tooth and elastic impression.

The Construction of Bonded Porcelain Veneer Crowns.) They are cooled, and opaque is applied to the metal only. It has not been found necessary to extend the opaque application beyond the edge of the metal casting.

With use of the firing cycle described in Chapter 21, the opaque is fired in vacuum. The vacuum is released and the temperature is increased in air. The assembly is cooled and the body and incisal-colored porcelains are applied. The cast is wetted and the porcelain is condensed by capillary

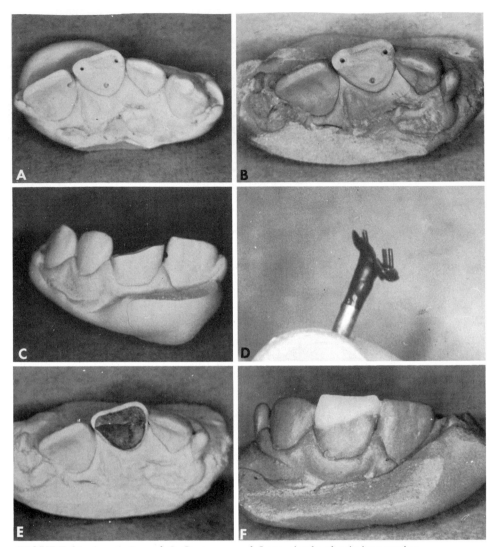

FIGURE 31–4. *A*, *B*, and *C*, Casts poured from single elastic impression.
D, Wax pattern.
E, Casting on stone cast.
F, Porcelain fired and bonded to casting.

action. It is built about 1.0 mm. high but *not* to full contour *at this time,* as shrinkage will pull the porcelain from the labial margin.

The porcelain is dried and fired in vacuum, then in air. The second application of porcelain is built to an overcontour and the firing cycle is repeated.

After it has cooled, the restoration is deinvested and cleaned with hydrochloric acid in an ultrasonic cleaner, after which it is roughly ground to form on the stone master cast. Contour and occlusion are refined in the patient's mouth, using fine disks for contouring and small stones for adjusting occlusion (Fig. 31-5).

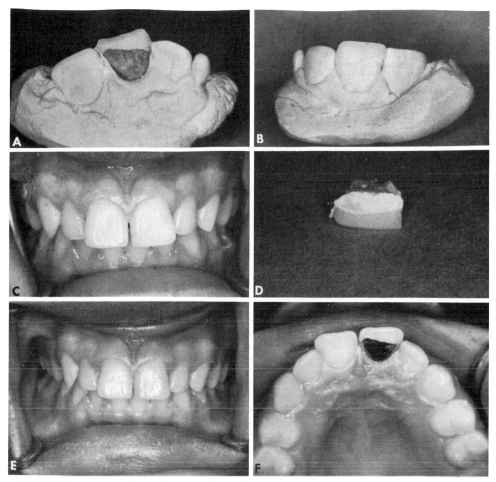

FIGURE 31–5.   *A*, Lingual view of bonded porcelain and casting.
B, Porcelain contoured on stone cast.
C, Porcelain contoured and equilibrated in mouth.
D, Restoration reinvested for glaze firing.
E and *F*, Cemented restoration.

The restoration is reinvested in ceramic investment up to the porcelain margin and is left to set for 30 minutes. After drying, it is fired in air to bring the desired glaze to the surface. After deinvesting, the cavity surface is again cleaned in hydrochloric acid in the ultrasonic cleaner. It may be cemented with either zinc phosphate or silicophosphate cement.

Pulpless Teeth

Teeth in which much dentin has been lost, through caries and endodontic therapy, require other means of restoration than those that may be applied to the vital fractured incisor. Following preparation of the tooth structure that still remains, the tooth stump must be built to prepared form so that the subsequent restoration will be amply supported, and also as insurance against the fracture of the remaining coronal tooth substance.

A pulpless tooth will best resist fracture if the restoration and tooth structure are supported by a post extending into the root canal for a distance equal to the coronal length of the restoration, and with a core rebuilding the tooth to prepared form. Even though a pulpless tooth has an intact labial surface and incisal angles, some endodontists and restorative dentists feel that a post should be inserted in the root canal to extend approximately one-half the distance from the opening of the pulp chamber to the apex. Despite the fact that there is considerable insistence that pulpless teeth are *not* more brittle than vital teeth, it has been the clinical observation of the authors that they are more prone to fracture unless supported internally by a post (Fig. 31-6). This is especially true when a tooth is serving as an abutment.

Direct Technique for Cast Post and Core.   The root canal is enlarged with a round bur (or with a reamer) to a depth the same as or greater than the incisocervical coronal measurement of the restoration. A post of high-fusing, nonoxidizing wire* is fitted and cut to extend from the extreme depth of the hole to approximately 3.0 mm. beyond the incisal edge of the prepared tooth.

Casting wax is softened and forced into the posthole. The wire post, serrated in the coronal two-thirds, is heated and forced as far as possible through the wax into the root canal. The wax is built and carved to the form of the prepared tooth. The casting may be made with a regular crown and bridge gold if the pattern has bulk, or with a partial denture gold if the incisal half is thin (Figs. 31-7 and 31-8).

Indirect Technique for Cast Post and Core.   When using an indirect technique, the wire post may be serrated throughout its entire length. The apical portion is coated with wax and is repeatedly seated in the root canal until it can be removed with minimal resistance. The serrated coronal portion will be so firmly gripped by the rubber base impression material that an accurate relationship will be maintained when the cast is poured. Since the

---

*Ney PGP wire; Jelenko No. 6 wire.

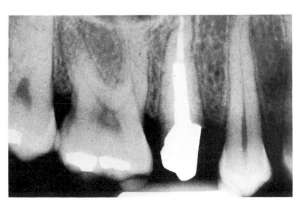

FIGURE 31-6. Relationship of post to crown-root ratio.

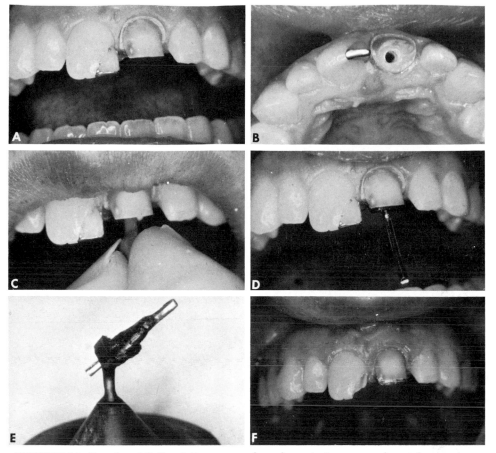

FIGURE 31–7.   *A* and *B*, Partially prepared tooth ready for wax and post for carving core.
C, Placing wax in enlarged canal.
D, Serrated wire post forced through wax into canal.
E, Wax pattern.
F, Post and core cemented.

wire has been coated with wax, it can be warmed and readily removed from
the cast.

   The core is waxed, cast, polished, and cemented. Then the preparation
is refined.

   Rebuilding Vital Tooth to Prepared Form.   When there has been
much loss of coronal dentin and enamel and the tooth is still vital, the
favored restoration will be a jacket or veneered crown. The remaining tooth
structure should be prepared for the type of crown selected. The core, which
will rebuild the tooth to prepared form, can be retained by pins, or a ferrule,
or both. Pinholes, running in a long-axis direction, must extend into the
dentin from 1.0 to 2.0 mm. Although tapered fissure burs can be used, drills
are more effective, because the diameter of the holes will be smaller and there
can be more and longer pins extending into the dentin.

   The pattern can be made by direct waxing. If an indirect technique is

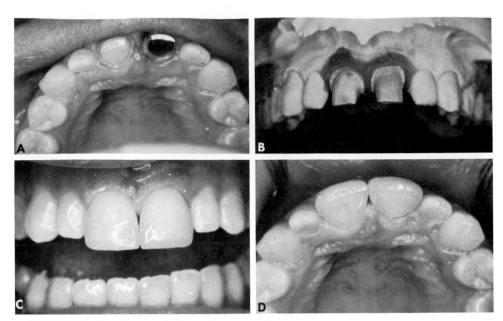

FIGURE 31–8.   *A*, Incisal view of prepared incisors.
B, Cast and dies of prepared incisors.
C and *D*, Teeth restored with porcelain jacket crowns.

elected, nylon pins must be placed in the nontapered pinholes before a silicone rubber impression is taken. Dies, working casts, patterns, and castings are made as described previously.

Some operators complete the crown before cementation of the casting, but it is considered wiser to cement the casting and to check and make any needed refinements in the preparation before proceeding with the construction of the restoration.

REFERENCES

Baum, L., Hayden, J., Jr., and Bonlie, D.: Cast restorations with baked porcelain incisal edges for fractured young permanent incisors. J. Den. Child., *28*:177, 3rd quar., 1961.
Starkey, P.: The use of self-curing resin in the restoration of young fractured permanent anterior teeth. J. Den. Child., *34*:15, Jan. 1967.

chapter 32

OCCLUSION FACTORS IN BRIDGE CONSTRUCTION

Occlusal disharmony, either before or after the construction of a bridge, or the added load on the abutments subsequent to the building of a prosthesis, can definitely alter the attachment apparatus. The manifestation of expanded function upon the periodontium may be divided into clinical symptoms and radiographic and histologic changes in supporting structures.

Clinically there may be a more pronounced mobility of the teeth, tenderness to masticating pressure, hyperemia of the soft tissues, and eventually, according to some authorities, a cleftlike formation of the gingiva. More acute sensitivity to heat, cold, and sweets can be experienced, also.

Radiographic differences may include a widening of the periodontal membrane space, a more discernible and compact lamina dura, an increased trabeculation of the alveolar bone, and a wedge-shaped radiolucent area, or funneling, of the alveolar crest at the coronal third.

Histologically the cementum may be thickened, even to the point at which "spurs" will be formed; the periodontal membrane may become wider and heavier (Table 32–1), with more dense bundle fibers; and the alveolar bone may be recontoured.

Following the placement of a dental restoration, a patient may report discomfort ranging from a feeling of "lameness" to severe and constant pain. Sensitivity is due, in most cases, to pulp irritation from traumatic contact or greater leverages. When the occlusion has been adjusted, each type of discomfort may be relieved almost instantly and should disappear shortly.

The thought has been advanced that a tooth with hypercementosis and irregular projections, or spurs, will have an enlarged root surface and a strengthened root attachment and thus will be a better abutment. Within limits this may be true.

In the process of making the adjustment to supplemented or varied activity, the alveolar bone often recontours. Resorption occurs first, then the periodontal membrane and cementum widen, the lamina dura of the

Table 32-1   THICKNESS OF PERIODONTAL TISSUES IN VARYING CONDITIONS OF FUNCTION*

	ALVEOLAR CREST MM.	MIDROOT MM.	APEX MM.	AVERAGE MM.
Teeth in heavy function, 44 teeth from 8 jaws	0.20	0.14	0.19	0.18
Teeth not in function, 20 teeth from 12 jaws	0.14	0.11	0.15	0.13
Embedded teeth, 5 teeth from 4 jaws	0.09	0.07	0.08	0.08
Malposed and drifting teeth	0.22	0.16	0.18	0.19

*From Coolidge, E. D., and Hine, M. K.: Periodontology, 3rd ed. Philadelphia, Lea & Febiger, 1958, p. 359.

alveolar bone becomes more compact, and trabeculae multiply. All these are physiologic responses to additional stresses placed on the teeth.

With a fixed partial prosthesis, it is possible to stabilize a tooth, minimize or eliminate shock from occlusion, and improve the health of the supporting structure in every way, especially if the tooth in question can be made an intermediate abutment. However, unless everything has been done that will further a tranquil functional relationship between the abutments and occluding teeth, the opposite may ensue, with the clinical symptoms of tenderness becoming magnified.

The histologic picture of periodontal traumatism may include hyperemia, hemorrhage and thrombosis, tearing and hyalinization of fibers, both osteoclastic and osteoblastic activity, and necrosis of bone or periodontal fibers, or both. In short, injury of tissues and physiologic tissue response is seen. There is little inflammatory cell infiltration and, therefore, no inflammation in the true sense of the word.

The adaptability of the periodontium may result in satisfactory adjustment that takes care of the additional burden, but later in life, because of changes in local or systemic conditions, a breakdown may take place.

In the construction of crowns and bridges and in the preparation of mouths for removable partial dentures, occlusal equilibration, reduction of occlusal areas, and accentuation of spillways are frequently mandatory to lessen occlusal forces.

Teeth subjected to intemperate stress may be more mobile than is normal. The simplest test for detecting mobility is to grasp the tooth with the index finger of each hand and apply force laterally. Sometimes such movement can be noted by retracting the lips and watching the chewing cycle. Also, the gingiva may blanch as pressure displaces the tooth. A check must be made not only for excessive lateral but also for increased vertical movement.

The patient's history can reveal symptoms indicative of temporomandibular joint disturbance, habit neuroses, wandering teeth, and pain. These factors usually can be related to some form of intercuspal malrelationship.

To aid in the detection of occlusal disharmonies and in the study of wear patterns and facets, and to enable the operator to design restorations that will not create interferences, diagnostic casts of the patient's dental arches should be mounted on an instrument capable of simulating, if not actually duplicating, the motions of the mandible.

The accuracy with which records must be obtained for this procedure probably is related to the patient's individual needs. Almost all persons have some occlusal discrepancies, and few people possess dentitions in which centric occlusion and centric relation coincide. Unless the patient has conditions such as periodontal disease, temporomandibular joint disturbance, extreme wear, mobile or tender teeth, or a large majority of the teeth carious or missing, it seems sensible to let the mandible continue to function in its acquired relationship and to make no gross change in the dentition other than to correct the clinically evident occlusal disharmonies, to restore mutilated teeth, and to replace any missing teeth.

In symptom-free cases, diagnostic casts often may be related on an articulator by an arbitrary face-bow mounting and a centric occlusion registration (such as the Kerr Bite Frame and impression paste registration). The condylar guidance mechanism may then be set by the use of wax eccentric interocclusal registrations or even by merely observing the patient's mandibular movements and adjusting the articulator to conform while at the dental chair. Minor wear facets seen on the casts may also be used in setting the instrument. Although restorations planned or executed on an instrument adjusted by such patently empirical means cannot relate to the opposing dentition in the mouth exactly as on the articulator, the discrepancies in the mouth should be within remediable limits.

For a patient who has one or more of the previously mentioned conditions, a more precise method of relating diagnostic casts and adjusting the articulator must be sought. The opening and closing center of rotation for each condyle should be found with a hinge axis locator and an arbitrary third reference point chosen, such as the infra-orbital notch (Fig. 32–1). Casts then may be mounted in the right relationship to the hinge axis formed by the two centers of rotation and to the plane formed by this axis and the third reference point. If there must be more than one mounting of diagnostic apparatus or casts, the three reference points may be marked permanently on the patient's skin. This is done so that later mountings will not require the relocation of these points, taking new registrations, and readjustment of the instrument. As a matter of convenience, the infra-orbital point is placed on the side of the nose rather than at the rim of the orbit.

A face-bow is adjusted to the three marked reference points and to the maxillary arch and used to mount the maxillary cast on the articulator (Fig. 32–1D). In this way the maxillary cast is related to the opening and closing axis of the instrument in the same way as the maxillary teeth are related to the hinge axis of the patient. (See Figure 31–3A.)

The mandibular cast is related to the maxillary cast by a wax centric relation registration (Figs. 32–2 and 32–3). This registration is procured by

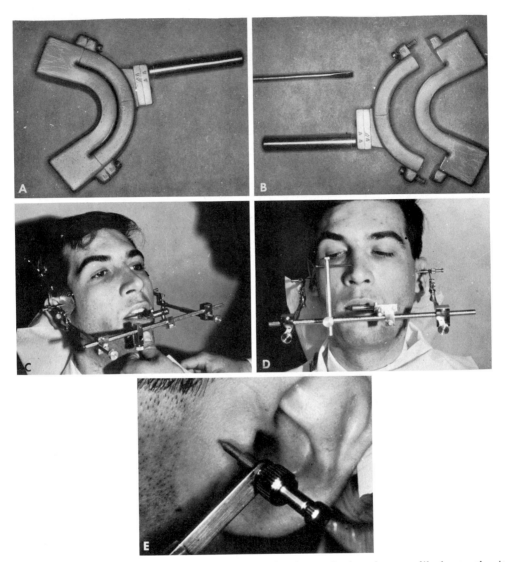

FIGURE 32–1. *A* and *B*, Two-piece clutch that is attached to the mandibular teeth with impression plaster in order to join the hinge axis locator to the mandible rigidly. The clutch is separable to allow easy removal from the mouth.

C, Locating the hinge axis by gently guiding the patient in pure rotary opening and closing movements of the mandible. When the points of the axis rods have been adjusted so that they rotate without arcing against the grids just anterior to the patient's ears, the axis of rotation has been located. The points then may be marked on the skin.

D, The face-bow related to the maxillary teeth by means of a bite fork covered with wax. The axis rods are adjusted to the hinge axis marks on the skin over the condyles and infra-orbital marker to the mark on the patient's nose.

E, Axis rod adjusted to axis mark on left side.

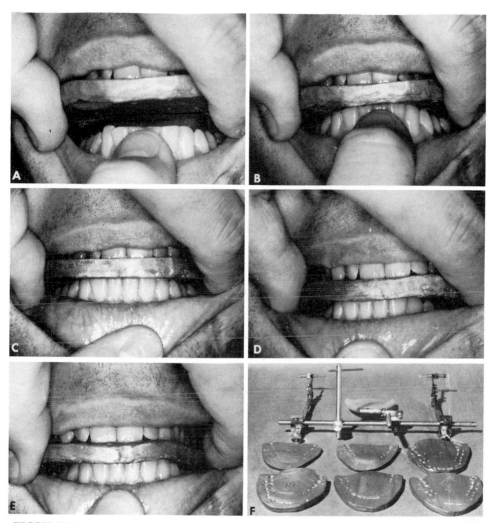

FIGURE 32–2. *A* and *B*, Guiding the patient in a hinge closure into a wax wafer to obtain a centric relation registration. Opposing teeth should not make contact. Three of these records are made. Note that upper and lower midlines do not coincide.

C, Obtaining a protrusive registration in wax. The anterior teeth are in an end-to-end relationship but do not touch through the wax.

D, Right lateral registration being made. The right posterior teeth are in a cusp-to-cusp relationship. They do not touch.

E, Left lateral registration.

F, The face-bow transfer, three centric relation registrations, and right lateral, left lateral, and protrusive registrations in wax.

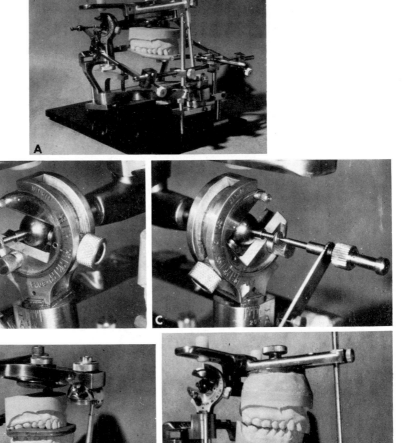

FIGURE 32–3.   *A,* The articulator related to face-bow transfer by means of a mounting board. The articulator is adjusted so that the axis-orbital plane indicator aligns with the axis-orbital pointer on the face-bow and the extendible axis rods of the articulator with the axis rods on the face-bow. When this is accomplished, the upper cast is attached to the instrument with low expansion dental stone or plaster. (Hanau face-bow, Hanau 130–13 articulator, Hanau mounting jig.)

B and *C,* The axis rods on the articulator equally extended to meet the axis rods of the face-bow.

D, The upper cast has been mounted. The lower cast is related to the inverted assembly by means of one of the centric relation registrations and fastened with stone or plaster.

E, Both casts mounted on the instrument.

guiding the patient in a hinge movement and, while so doing, having him close part way into softened strips of double-thickness hard baseplate wax or into a wafer of Aluwax* (Fig. 32–2 *A* and *B*). The wax should not be perforated during the procedure, since contact between opposing teeth invariably results in a false centric relation registration. The best wax registrations are those indented only by the cusp tips. Three separate centric relation records are made, one of which is used in mounting the lower cast on the articulator, the other two being used to verify the first. If the mounted casts seat properly in all three registrations, the records are accurate (Fig. 32–4 *A*). Since the wax records cannot be identical in thickness, it is only with a suitable relationship of both casts to the hinge that the instrument can accept all three centric relation registrations. Inaccuracy demonstrated at this point necessitates new centric registrations and remounting of the lower cast. Existing premature contacts in centric closure may now be demonstrated on the instrument (Fig. 32–4 *B* and *C*).

When an articulator is used to study prematurities in eccentric movements, the instrument must be adjusted to the patient's individual condylar guidance. The recording device used will depend on the precision with which the dentist wishes to do this operation. The most uninvolved technique uses wax eccentric interocclusal records, which are acceptable with articulators having straight or simple paths of motion.† Such instruments will not reproduce jaw movements without some latitude, and the errors introduced by wax records are likely no greater than those inherent to the articulators themselves.

The wax records generally consist of protrusive, right lateral, and left lateral registrations, with some clinicians recommending the use of three of each. (See Figure 32–2 *C, D, E,* and *F*.) It must be recognized that since the operator cannot control the patient to a degree that will ensure that the mandible is in the same position for each registration, these registrations may not be interchangeable.

The registrations are made in a hard baseplate wax or Aluwax, with the patient's teeth in an end-to-end or cusp-to-cusp relationship. To avoid rocking or shifting of the mandible, no teeth should make actual contact.

The condylar guidance is made to conform first to the protrusive record. The Bennett movement adjustment is opened about 15 degrees to allow for a possible deviation by the patient from a pure protrusive movement and the wax protrusive record is placed between the casts (Fig. 32–5*A*). The condylar guidance is set and locked on each side so that the teeth on the casts make maximal interdigitation with the wax record (Fig. 32–5*B*). Next, the left lateral record is placed between the casts, and the lateral adjustment is made for the Bennett movement on the right side of the instrument, or the side representing the gliding condyle (Fig. 32–5*C, D,* and *E*). The condylar

---

*Aluwax Dental Products Co., Grand Rapids, Mich.

†Instruments such as the Hanau #130–13 (Hanau Engineering Co., Inc., Buffalo, N.Y.), the Dentatus (distributed by the Kerr Mfg. Company, Romulus, Mich.), and the Whip-Mix articulator (Whip-Mix Corporation, Louisville, Ky.).

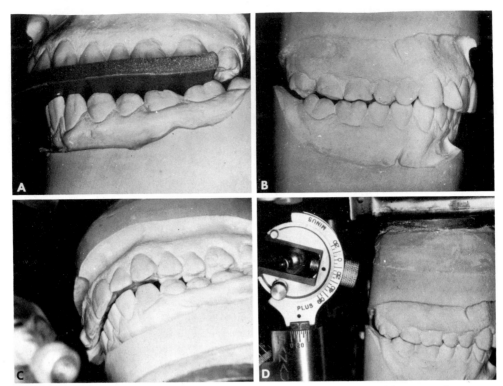

FIGURE 32–4. *A*, A second centric relation registration inserted between the mounted casts with the condylar guides locked in centric relation. The perfect interdigitation of the teeth into the wax record indicates an accurate centric relation mounting.

B, The articulator closed to find the first contact during hinge closure. The only contact is made by the right mandibular second molar with the right maxillary third molar.

C, Amount of opening in anterior region caused by the centric prematurity.

D, Release of the right condylar ball allows the mandibular cast to move forward with the teeth interdigitating similarly to the patient's acquired centric occlusion.

guidance adjustment is checked against that made with the protrusive record. The right lateral record is then used to adjust the left side of the instrument, and again it may be used as a check against the protrusive record (Fig. 32–5*F*). There are some who obtain only a single protrusive record, which is used to adjust the condylar guides, with the Bennett setting being arbitrarily selected. The articulator settings should be recorded in order that the instrument may be realigned in case of inadvertent movements of parts, or because more than one patient's casts must be mounted on the same articulator.

The patient's occlusion in both centric and eccentric relationships of the mandible may now be studied and occlusal prematurities located (Fig. 32–6).

The purpose of equilibration should be relief of traumatic occlusion and establishment of improved function. These objectives can be attained by removing premature contacts, both centric and eccentric, and the working of facets against facets.

Some operators prefer to remedy all discrepancies on the articulated casts before going to the mouth. If this is done, a written record is made of all changes on the casts. Centric prematurities should be removed first. Since

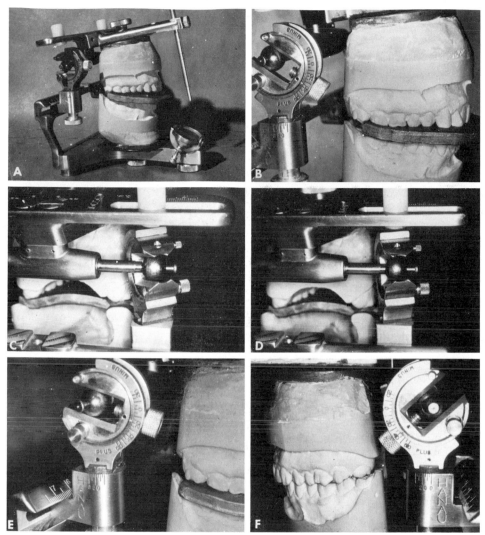

FIGURE 32–5. *A*, Protrusive registration placed between the casts on the articulator before adjustment. The anterior teeth cannot be placed into the indentations made in the mouth.

B, After increasing the condylar guidance, all teeth go to place in the registration. This adjustment must be made on both sides of the articulator.

C, Left lateral wax registration in the instrument with excessive rotation of the condylar posts to allow easy insertion of the record. Note that the condylar ball does not make contact with the shoulder on the instrument's axle.

D, Condylar ball brought into contact with the shoulder on the axle. This limits the sideward or Bennett shift to that which occurred during taking the wax registration.

E, Adjustments completed on right side: 18 degrees of condylar inclination, 21 degrees of rotation of condylar post to accommodate the lateral shift.

F, Left adjustments made in manner described for the right side of instrument: 42 degrees of inclination of condylar guide, 7 degrees for the lateral shift.

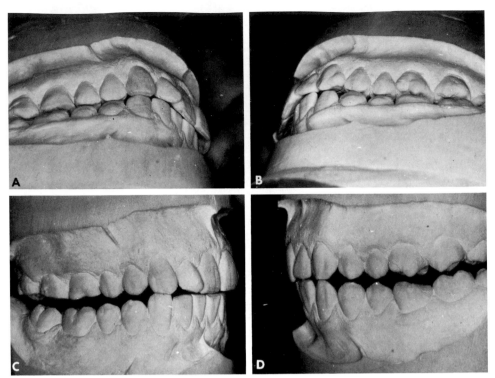

FIGURE 32–6. *A*, In right lateral movement the two first bicuspids are the only teeth that make contact. Note wear on tip of buccal cusp of the maxillary first bicuspid.

B, Casts on adjusted articulator moved into left lateral excursion. There is excessive contact between the maxillary and mandibular laterals and the two first bicuspids as well. There is no contacting of the two cuspids.

C and *D*, Right and left lateral protrusive movements. The articulated casts closely follow the facets of wear on the cuspids.

all prematurities involve at least two opposing teeth, a decision must be made as to which offender is to be recontoured. If one of the surfaces is also in a traumatic relationship in an excursive movement, it is the one to be changed. For instance, if the prematurity exists between a cusp of one tooth and a fossa of another, and the cusp is also making excessive contact in an eccentric position, the cusp should be shortened (Fig. 32–7). Conversely, if no eccentric prematurity exists, either the cusp may be reshaped or the sulcus deepened. In this circumstance, re-forming the sulcus may be indicated to maintain existing excursive relationships and chewing efficiency, which might be reduced if the cusp were shortened or blunted (Fig. 32–8).

A more obvious illustration is traumatic centric occlusion involving anterior teeth. If the teeth have a good incising relationship, the premature contact is removed by grinding the lingual aspect of the maxillary tooth, since shortening the mandibular tooth would take the teeth out of occlusion in protrusive movement (Fig. 32–9). If both centric and protrusive relationships are traumatic, the lower incisal edge is altered (Fig. 32–10). Should

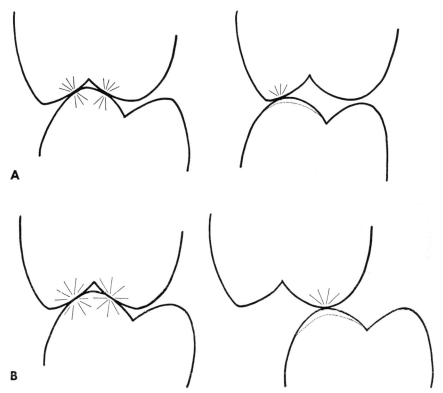

FIGURE 32–7. *A*, Traumatic relationship in centric occlusion relieved by reducing the lower buccal cusp, which is also striking excessively in the working or functional relationship.

B, Another traumatic relationship in centric occlusion relieved by reducing the lower buccal cusp, which is also in a traumatic relationship in the nonfunction movement.

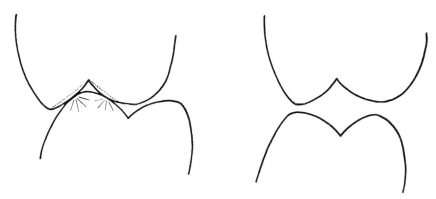

FIGURE 32–8. Sulcus is reduced as indicated to eliminate a centric prematurity, rather than reducing the lower buccal cusp, causing it to pass still farther away from its opponent in working excursion.

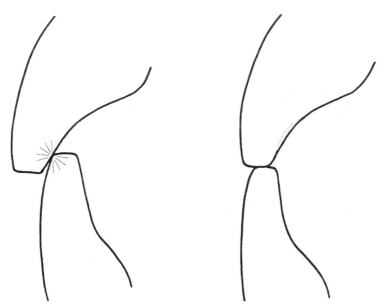

FIGURE 32–9.   An anterior centric prematurity between teeth with a satisfactory protrusive relationship is corrected by altering the upper lingual surface.

removal of the faulty centric contact fail to eradicate the protrusive interference, the incisal edge of the maxillary tooth is ground also.

Once centric occlusion has been corrected, along with removal of any directly related excursive prematurities, a check is made for other eccentric traumatic relationships. Since centric occlusion has been established, all subsequent improvements must be made on surfaces *not* making centric con-

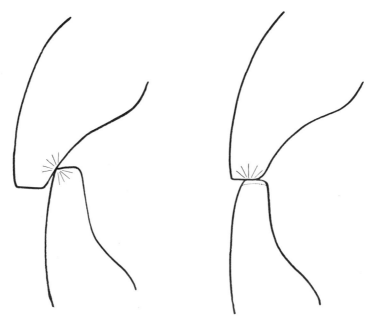

FIGURE 32–10.   An anterior traumatic relationship that occurs in both centric and protrusive relationships is corrected by reducing the lower incisal edge.

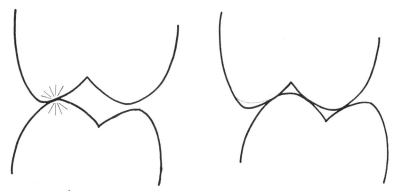

FIGURE 32–11. Excessive contact between buccal cusps in lateral excursion is eliminated by shortening the upper buccal cusp while maintaining the original centric occlusion.

tact. To destroy centric contact while adjusting lateral and protrusive relationships would create an unstable occlusion, making eruption of teeth and recurrence of eccentric prematurities possible.

If, for example, during the masticating stroke, the buccal cusp of a mandibular bicuspid strikes the buccal cusp of its opposing tooth, the buccal cusp of the maxillary tooth is shortened (Fig. 32–11). To recontour the buccal cusp of the lower tooth would take it out of centric occlusion, perhaps inviting the teeth to extrude and causing the lateral prematurity to recur.

It has been claimed that premature contact on the nonworking side (often called balancing side) is the most destructive of all occlusal defects. This contention is reasonable, since the posterior tooth relationships that occur during this phase of chewing do not direct forces along the long axes of the participating teeth. Whether such contacts should be eliminated completely, or just reduced enough to make them no more forceful than those on the working side, is open to argument. However, it seems logical to err on the side of no contact rather than to gamble on forces that may exceed the physiologic limits of the supporting structures.

Nonworking contacts involve the lingual cusps of maxillary posterior

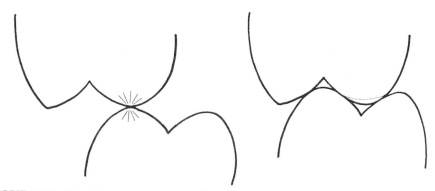

FIGURE 32–12. Traumatic nonworking or "balancing side" contacts at times may be eliminated by reducing the cusp tips without interfering with centric stops.

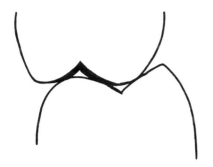

FIGURE 32–13. If a cusp loses its centric stop following removal of cuspal interference, the opposing sulcus or marginal ridge will have to be built up by means of a restoration.

teeth and the buccal cusps of mandibular teeth. Both areas form centric contacts. Fortunately, centric contact generally occurs on cusp planes instead of on the tips of the cusps. Consequently, shortening the cusp to rid it of a nonworking contact will not necessarily cause loss of centric occlusion (Fig. 32–12). If this should occur, there is no recourse other than to place a restoration that builds up the sulcus or the marginal ridge area of the opposing surface, or both (Fig. 32–13).

The type of occlusion that is best for most patients is a subject of much controversy. In the past, completely balanced occlusion has been widely advocated. Recently there is growing support for a tooth arrangement having an anterior guidance that permits little contact of posterior teeth away from centric occlusion. Most natural dentitions appear to be some modification of the latter type.

The principles briefly outlined here can be applied to both the equilibration and the restoration of natural dentitions. There is only scant evidence to support the use of either procedure as a prophylactic measure in the absence of a pathologic condition.

REFERENCES

D'Amico, A.: The canine teeth. J. South. California D. A., *26*:64, 1958.

Granger, E. R.: Practical Procedures in Oral Rehabilitation. Philadelphia, J. B. Lippincott Company, 1962.

Kemper, W. W., et al.: Periodontal tissue changes in response to high artificial crowns. J. Pros. Den., *20*:160, Aug. 1968.

Lucia, V. O.: Modern Gnathological Concepts. St. Louis, The C. V. Mosby Company, 1961.

Moulton, G. H.: Importance of centric occlusion in diagnosis and treatment planning. J. Pros. Den., *10*:921, Sept.–Oct. 1960.

Pruden, W. H., II: Development of occlusion where total reconstruction is contraindicated. J. Pros. Den., *16*:549, May–June 1966.

Schuyler, C. H.: Considerations of occlusion in fixed partial dentures. Dent. Clin. N. Amer., March 1959, p. 175.

Schweitzer, J. M.: Masticatory function in man. J. Pros. Den., *12*:262, March–April 1962.

Stallard, H.: Functions of the occlusal surfaces of the teeth. J.A.D.A., *13*:401, 1930.

Stallard, H., and Stuart, C. E.: Eliminating tooth guidance in natural dentitions. J. Pros. Den., *11*:474, May–June 1961.

Wilson, W. H., and Lang, R. L.: Practical Crown and Bridge Prosthodontics. New York, McGraw-Hill Book Company, Inc., 1962.

chapter 33

BRIDGE FAILURES: INDICATIONS AND CORRECTIVE MEASURES

The prosthodontist who constructs bridges must be well aware of both gross and subtle indications of failure and have some knowledge of remedial procedures. The failure of a bridge can be manifested in various ways. There may be discomfort, the bridge may become loose, caries may recur, the supporting structure may atrophy or a pulp degenerate, the framework or a facing may fracture, a veneer may be lost, the prosthesis may have ceased to function, or there may be a complete loss of tissue tone or tissue form.

Changes in environment may necessitate the removal and remaking of a bridge. Also, a bridge simply may wear out. After all, no bridge, nor the teeth approximating or opposing it, can carry a lifetime guarantee. Replacement for these two reasons cannot be classified under failures.

DISCOMFORT

It is only natural that discomfort will claim the attention of the patient more readily than any other type of failure, with the possible exception of fracture. Discomfort may be caused by

(1) malocclusion or premature contact;

(2) an oversize or poorly positioned masticating area, with retention of food by pontics or retainers;

(3) torque produced from the seating of the bridge or from occlusion;

(4) an excess of pressure on the tissue;

(5) plus or minus contact areas;

(6) overprotected or underprotected gingival and ridge tissue;

(7) sensitive cervical areas;

(8) thermal shock; and

(9) certain intangible sources, usually relatively unimportant and easily rectified if diagnosed.

Discomfort from *malocclusion* can be traced to a high marginal ridge, central fossa, cusp tip, or an inclined surface on one of the cusps in lateral excursion, and also to mobility and extrusion from loss of supporting bone. *Areas of premature contact* will be indicated by burnished metal. All or any of these can be corrected by equilibration, using either a small knife-edge stone or a round bur. Mobility from lack of support may have occurred because of faulty diagnosis and planning; that is, from too much having been expected of too few abutment teeth. There is no cure except to rebuild the bridge, including a greater number of abutment teeth, or to construct a removable prosthesis with bilateral bracing.

An *oversize or poorly positioned masticating area* is difficult to correct if the operation requires grinding porcelain, which cannot be reglazed. When the food table is too wide, an attempt may be made to narrow the distance between the cusp tips by reducing the buccolingual measurement, often at the expense of the lingual cusp; by opening the embrasures, again at the expense of the lingual cusp or cusps; and by cutting auxiliary escape grooves through the marginal ridges to both the lingual and the buccal of the connectors.

Tenderness during chewing and a reluctance to utilize the bridge will be evidence that food is being retained on the occlusal surface of a crown or a pontic. The height and form of the marginal ridges and the contour of the inclined surfaces of the cusps must be examined. It is often necessary to widen the embrasures, diminish the lingual cusp, and increase the number and size of the grooves crossing the marginal ridges and emptying into the embrasures. Occasionally auxiliary grooves to the buccal of the solder joint will aid the escape of food from the occlusal surface of a pontic or retainer.

Torque, generated when the bridge was seated, may be eliminated in time by resorption and rebuilding of the alveolar process. It must be remembered that no bridge should be cemented if seating changes the natural long-axis relationship of the abutments. Torque from occlusion stems from a cusp extended too far buccally or lingually, or a premature contact at the extremity of a lateral excursion. This can be helped by reduction of the buccolingual dimension or by equilibration.

Pressure on tissue may have been present at the time the bridge was seated, or it may be caused by a foreign body, such as food or cement particles lodging under the pontic ridgelap.[1] For the first of these two conditions there is no cure other than removal and reconstruction of the bridge. If the pressure results from a removable irritant, the area should be cleansed by passing dental floss mesiodistally between the pontic and mucous membrane, and treated by flushing with a mild antiseptic and painting the surrounding tissue with a mild counterirritant.

The *strength of contact areas* may be increased or diminished by malocclusion, which would tend to force the bridge either toward or away from an approximating tooth. Equilibration, either on the occluding surfaces of the bridge or the opposing teeth, is the remedy. No bridge should be seated if contact with an approximating tooth is faulty. However, to correct such a situation, it may not be necessary to remove the bridge. Sometimes it is possible to prepare a small proximo-occlusal cavity in the retainer and to make and cement an inlay that will bring the strength and location of the contact to the desired point.

Overprotected gingival tissue probably will show some swelling and hemorrhage. The overcontoured areas of a crown or pontic may be reduced, reshaped, and repolished. For *underprotection of gingival tissue* there is no treatment except reconstruction of the prosthesis.

Exposed sensitive cervical areas are caused by overdisplacement of gingival tissue before taking impressions, by overextended temporary crowns worn for too long a period during construction of the prosthesis, and by recession due to exposed margins of preparations or ill-fitting, underextended, overpolished, or overextended castings. Zinc chloride and stannous fluoride seem to be effective medicaments. Frequently a cavity preparation can be made at the margin of the restoration and a restoration placed that will protect the patient from further inconvenience. Although this is a makeshift operation, it is better than removing an otherwise satisfactory bridge.[2, 3]

Thermal shock, if it persists for many days following the seating of the crown or fixed partial denture, may point to a serious pulpal involvement, premature contact, or an exposed margin or cementoenamel junction. Malocclusion is indicated not only by tenderness of the supporting structure but also by sensitivity to sweets and cold. A reaction to heat is more significant, since it seldom occurs without pulpal abnormality. Correction of malocclusion and exposed margins has been discussed. Sensitivity to heat now and then is corrected by natural reparative action; therefore, the sensible procedure could be to wait for more definite developments before deciding on a course of treatment that might necessitate endodontics or extraction.

LOOSENESS OF BRIDGES

When a bridge becomes loose at one end, it may be feasible to remove and recement it, provided the cause of failure is correctable. More often it will be necessary to reprepare the abutments and rebuild the prosthesis.

A bridge becomes loose because of
(1) deformation of the metal casting on the abutment;
(2) torque;
(3) technique of cementation;
(4) solubility of cement;
(5) caries;
(6) mobility of one or more abutments;
(7) lack of full occlusal coverage;
(8) insufficient retention in the abutment preparation; or
(9) poor initial fit of the casting.

Deformation of a retainer may result when the yield point of the alloy is low, or when the casting is too thin because of insufficient reduction of the abutment in the areas that will receive forces from opposing teeth. Deformation may also be caused by wear or equilibration brought about or necessitated by reduction of vertical dimension in other quadrants; by a sharp cusp on an opposing tooth, which should have been rounded or reshaped prior to the construction of the bridge; or by an opposing restoration, made of a harder metal or of unglazed porcelain, which will bring about undue wear. Deformed cast retainers must be corrected by reconstruction of the restoration.[4]

Torque, which will break the cement bond and let a retainer become loose, generally is caused by a premature contact in lateral excursion, or by different types of occlusion; that is, a natural tooth opposing one end of the bridge with a tissue-supported removable partial denture opposing the other, or an absence of any occlusion on a terminal abutment. Torque may be eliminated by equilibration, by recontouring or reducing occluding areas, or by the construction and insertion of an occluding prosthesis.

If a bridge becomes loose because of the *technique of cementation*, it can be assumed that either the abutment tooth (or teeth) or the inside surface of the retainer was not dry or clean, or that the cement was improperly mixed. If the bridge can be removed and recemented, with the field, the abutment teeth, and the retainers dry, and if it is *held in position without movement* until cement has hardened, success may be expected.

Cement dissolves for one of three reasons: the margins were open originally; the retainer has been deformed, creating an open margin; or a hole has been worn through an occluding surface of the retainer. There are no means of improving this condition except by remaking the bridge.

When a bridge becomes unseated, partially or totally, because of *recurrent caries*, it must be removed, the abutment teeth must be reprepared, if possible, and the bridge must be reconstructed. Caries will develop because of a leaking margin, gingival recession, or an exposed cervical margin. Also, there are many cases on record in which illness seemingly has predisposed the patient to caries, and exposed enamel areas, healthy at the time the bridge was seated, have become susceptible to caries.

Mobility of an abutment may cause a bridge to loosen. Lack of judgment by the prosthodontist, an increased load on the abutment teeth due to malfunction in another segment of the arch, or periodontal disease from an undetermined origin might be responsible. The bridge and the area should be evaluated carefully to ascertain whether more abutment teeth and splinting will correct the fault, or whether the offending abutment must be lost.

Sometimes *when the buccal cusp of a bicuspid has not been covered* in the construction of a retainer, because of esthetic demands, a force applied directly to the occluding enamel surface will tend to drive the tooth out of the retainer. Unless the bridge is very short, with inlay retainers and one broken-stress joint to allow greater individual tooth movement, all occluding surfaces of all abutment teeth should be covered by metal that will absorb and dissipate forces from the occluding teeth.

If a bridge comes off because of *too little retention* in the prepared abutments, a new bridge is mandatory. Even though teeth are short or conical, auxiliary grooves and pins may be used to increase parallelism and frictional retention.[1]

A bridge that becomes loose because a *retainer casting did not fit* should not have been seated in the first place.[5] Often only one retainer will move on its abutment, and the patient will not be cognizant of the condition or the potential sequelae. It is the duty of the dentist to recall the patient periodically for prophylaxis and examination, at which time any fixed prosthesis should be thoroughly inspected for signs or evidence of loosening, or of developments that might terminate in such a situation. Precautionary equilibration, polishing, or a small restoration may forestall failure of this type.

RECURRENCE OF CARIES

Caries may recur because of
(1) overextension of margins;
(2) short castings;
(3) open margins;
(4) wear;
(5) a retainer coming loose;
(6) pontic form that fills the embrasures;
(7) poor oral hygiene;
(8) use of the wrong type of retainer, which will promote caries susceptibility; or
(9) because temporary protection of the abutment uncovered the neck of the tooth by a prolonged or permanent displacement of the gingiva.

Overextended margins cannot be adapted to the converging convexity of the enamel at the cervix of the tooth. While the space between the margin of the casting and the tooth may be filled with cement at the time the bridge is seated, cement is soluble, and later a crevice may appear that will be filled with saliva or food debris. This can stimulate recession of the gingival tissue and induce disintegration of enamel and cementum, and caries. Occasionally it is possible to polish off the excess casting, prepare a cavity, and place a restoration. Usually, however, the affected area will go so far occlusally beyond the margin of the retainer that it becomes necessary to remove the bridge, explore the tooth, and be guided in reconstruction by what remains.

A *short casting* leaves the cervical margin of the prepared tooth surface exposed. This rough enamel or dentin collects debris, and caries results. Sometimes it may be removed and the area can be restored with a casting or a resin restoration.

Open margins, regardless of the cause, encourage the entry of saliva and cariogenic organisms, and require the remaking of the prosthesis.

Wear, producing an opening through the occluding surface, will expose cement or tooth structure, and caries may occur. If detected in time, a plastic restoration or an inlay may be sufficient to return the tooth to normalcy.

Saliva and food particles that infiltrate into the space between a *loose retainer* and the tooth have no means of escape. Through the pumping action or movement of the casting, especially if there are pinholes in the preparation, the destruction is accelerated, and within only a very short time the entire coronal dentin may be affected.

When cleaning embrasures is impossible, owing to overcrowding from *poor pontic form,* and this results in caries, the only remedy is to remove the bridge and build one of correct design.

Oral hygiene should be stressed and preventive therapy should be employed when retainers are used that do not cover all surfaces of the crown.

Many times *small carious areas* on the labial or buccal surface of a tooth carrying a partial veneer crown, or on a proximal surface supporting an inlay retainer, may be restored without disturbing or unseating the casting. Judgment must be exercised in this respect. If there is any doubt at all about the stability of the retainer or the depth of the caries, the bridge should be removed and the tooth reprepared. In mouths showing a relatively high caries index, partial veneer crowns, pinledges, MacBoyle-type restorations, and inlays should not be used unless the dentist is reasonably sure that the tendency toward caries has been arrested, or is being controlled by frequent prophylaxis, stannous fluoride treatments, and correct diet. Otherwise, retainers with long marginal lines are susceptible to recurrent caries in a period of time shorter than the normal life of the restoration or prosthesis.

When the *temporary protection* for the prepared abutment has uncovered the neck of the tooth because of overextension, or because it was used for too long a period of time, this area may be attacked by caries. In such a case, repreparing the abutment tooth and extending the cervical margin of the preparation to a less susceptible point should be seriously considered.

RECESSION OF SUPPORTING STRUCTURE

Loss of the supporting alveolar process[6] may result from overloading due to

(1) length of the span;

(2) size of the occlusion table;

(3) embrasure form;

(4) contour of the retainers; or

(5) too few abutment teeth;

or it may develop because of

(6) an overextension of the cervical margins of the preparation, which interferes with or traumatizes the peripheral attachment of the periodontal membrane.

(7) Indiscreet band impression technique can also stimulate recession of the alveolar process. Too much pressure might have been exerted in taking the impression, forcing the band up beyond the attachment of the periodontal membrane and either cutting or tearing it loose. These same things will

happen if the band is not contoured to the proximal curvatures of the gingival line.

Overloading can be avoided by correct diagnosis and planning of the restoration. If the *span is too long,* or if there are not enough teeth suitable for abutments, a fixed partial denture should not be constructed. Often the *size of the occlusion table* can be reduced, *embrasure form* can be changed, or *contour of the retainers* can be altered to decrease the load during mastication. If *too few abutment teeth* have been used, the bridge must be removed and remade with multiple terminal abutments. If these are not available, the prepared abutment teeth should be recontoured for the support and retention of a removable prosthesis. An *overextended margin* must be ground and polished to contour. If this cannot be done, the restoration should be removed and rebuilt. *Loss of the alveolar process* often can be retarded or removed by periodontal treatment, re-establishing the right occlusal plane, or equilibrating the existing occlusion.

DEGENERATION OF PULP

Supporting structure, or root length, may be lost owing to periapical involvement brought about by the method of preparation, lack of protection of the prepared abutment teeth during construction, hidden caries, and malocclusion. It seems that a latent, low-grade pulp infection can be activated by the preparation of the abutment tooth and the building of the bridge, irritation from temporary coverage, lack of temporary coverage, or malocclusion. There is no method by which such a pulp condition may be discovered, and discomfort or pulp degeneration, occurring several months after the insertion of a fixed prosthesis, may be the result of such infection.[7]

A *pulp might degenerate* because of too-rapid preparation of the tooth or because of improper lubrication during preparation. Teeth unprotected during the construction of a bridge are exposed to saliva and the resulting irritation. Caries under a retainer sometimes cannot be discovered by radiographs. Marginal examination with a mirror and explorer should supplement radiographic examination.

Endodontic therapy may be possible without removing the bridge. However, if apical resection, rather than apical curettage, is deemed better, the change in crown-root ratio can create the need for splinting. If such treatment is not in order, the prosthesis must be cut, the pontics and the affected retainer removed, and the abutment extracted. The casting should be left on the remaining abutment until a new plan of treatment has been established.

FRACTURES OF BRIDGE COMPONENTS

A *bridge framework will fracture*[8, 9, 10] because of (1) a faulty solder joint, (2) incorrect casting technique, and (3) overwork of the metal due to the length of the span or to struts or parts that are too small. *Imperfections in solder joints* or from *casting technique* have been discussed in the appropriate chapters. *Overwork* or *strain hardening* caused by *a span being too long*, with springing in the center of the bar, may result in brittleness, loss of strength and ductility, and subsequent fracture. When *parts are too small*, there is a similar situation and result. Redesigning and remaking the prosthesis will be necessary.

A *facing may fracture* because, in its final form, a shelf of porcelain was left exposed to opposing surfaces or cusps and was subjected to either *leverage* or *spot contact*. Checks in a facing, or susceptibility to fracture, may be caused by *over-rapid heating* or *cooling* during glazing. A satisfactory replacement can be made in most instances without disturbing the bridge, provided it is given correct form.

When a pontic has been constructed so that the metal protecting the porcelain facing is insufficient to resist deformation from occluding teeth, fracture or loosening will ensue. Under such conditions equilibration is indicated before another facing, or perhaps a different type of facing or veneer, can be substituted. The force that caused the deformation must be directed to another area, or the tooth supplying the force must be reshaped to eliminate the force, malocclusion, or premature contact.

LOSS OF VENEERS

Veneers are lost from the labial and buccal surfaces of crowns or pontics because of
(1) too little retention;
(2) badly designed metal protection;
(3) deformation of the protecting metal;
(4) malocclusion; and
(5) improper curing or fusing technique.

If a resin veneer is lost because of *insufficient retention*, a resin substitute must be constructed. Usually it will be retained by incorporated metal pins and projections from the veneer fitting into holes in the metal structure. If a porcelain veneer fractures or comes off, a resin substitute frequently will be necessary.

Lack of metal protection or *deformation of metal protection* calls for equilibration, reduction of the force from occlusion, some change in the form of the occluding areas, and an increase in the number of pinholes supplying the retention.

If *malocclusion* has been responsible for the loss of a veneer, a change in occlusal form is in order.

A veneer that becomes unsatisfactory because of *curing or fusing technique* may be replaced with some expectation of success (Fig. 33–1).

Broken facings and lost veneers do not always suggest the removal of the prosthesis, but if the plight recurs consistently, rebuilding the bridge is the only solution.

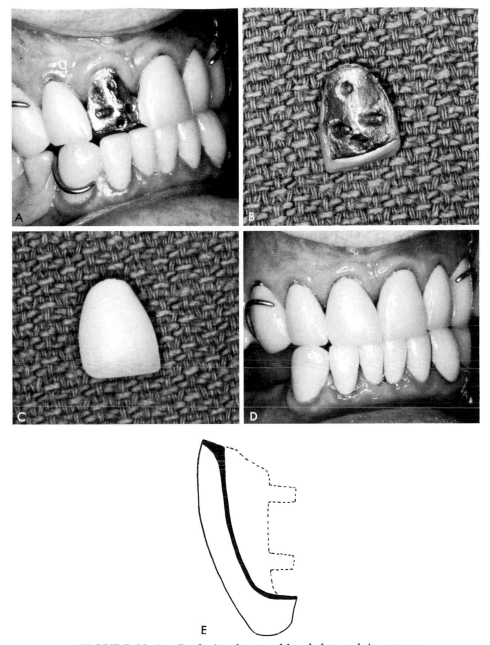

FIGURE 33–1. *Replacing fractured bonded porcelain veneer.*

A, All porcelain has been removed from labial surface of central incisor crown. Some of metal casting has been ground away. Four postholes were placed in metal and into supporting coronal structure. Wax pattern for plate (*B*) was carved direct.

B, Inner surface of casting after porcelain veneer was added. Technique for veneering was standard.

C, Labial view of replacement veneer.

D, Repaired prosthesis.

E, Cross-section drawing showing casting (black) with veneer. Dotted lines show outline of repair before sectioning.

LOSS OF FUNCTION

Bridges are failures at times because
(1) they do not function in occlusion;
(2) they have no contact with opposing teeth; or
(3) they have premature contact.
(4) Overcarved or undercarved occlusal surfaces may impair efficiency, as may
(5) loss of opposing or approximating teeth.

The esthetic effect that the patient expected may have required that the bridge be built in such a way that *function is at a minimum or lacking completely.*

"No contact with the opposing teeth" need not indicate failure of the bridge. Loss of a tooth in the opposing arch without subsequent replacement may permit drifting, rotation, and tilting of teeth occluding with the bridge. Such movement reduces the efficiency of the occlusion, and the opposing arch must be reconstructed.

When function is reduced because of *premature contact* with an opposing tooth, either the occlusal plane of the bridge or the offending cusp of the opposing tooth should be recontoured.

When a bridge performs with subpar efficiency because of an *overcarved occlusal surface*, it must be rebuilt. If the *occlusal surface is undercarved*, usefulness will be increased by cutting grooves and spillways and by sharpening cusps, so long as this recontouring does not destroy contact with the opposing teeth in centric occlusion and in lateral movements.

If function is lost because of the *extraction of the opposing teeth*, replacement of those teeth is mandatory.

LOSS OF TISSUE TONE OR FORM

Loss of tissue tone or form may be due to
(1) pontic design;
(2) position and size of the joints;
(3) embrasure form;
(4) overcontouring or undercontouring of retainers; or
(5) the oral hygiene practiced by the patient.

The health of the tissue can be affected by too much pressure from the *pontic*, by improper clearance between the pontic and the ridge tissue, or because the cervical half of the pontic is oversize. In such cases the bridge must be removed, the tissue given time to reorganize, and the bridge reconstructed.

If tissue is overprotected by the *position and size of the solder joints*, these joints probably can be reduced in contour, which in turn will increase the size of the embrasures and allow more adequate massage of the tissue by the food bolus during mastication.

If *embrasure form* is too small, lingual portions of the pontic[11] and bulky retainers may be recontoured. Nevertheless, when a bridge was so *badly designed* that considerable change is required in the form of the pontic or of the retainer to make it biologically acceptable, everyone concerned would be better off if the bridge were removed and rebuilt.

Oral hygiene is largely up to the patient, provided the bridge is built in such a way that oral hygiene can be effectuated. He should be instructed in methods of using dental floss, Stim-U-Dents,* and toothbrushes. If, at a later visit, there is evidence that the patient is not following advice concerning mouth cleanliness, instructions should be repeated and their importance emphasized in no uncertain terms.

FAILURE TO SEAT

Why is it that occasionally a bridge will fail to seat, even though constructed with some care over abutment preparations that contained no undercuts and had been checked to verify the seating and fit of the retainer castings? (1) The abutment preparations may not be parallel, or (2) the soldering assembly may have been incorrect, or the relationship of the retainers may have been altered during soldering.

If the abutment preparations are *not parallel*, one or more teeth must be reprepared and the associated retainers reconstructed. It is relatively easy to check parallelism of the abutment teeth by taking an alginate impression and pouring a cast in impression plaster, which sets quite rapidly. After transferring the cast to a surveyor, the acceptability of all prepared surface planes on the abutments may be substantiated with the analyzing rod of the surveying instrument.

When castings do not fit, *undercuts* may be detected on one or more surfaces of the preparations by using the surveyor. The tooth or teeth must be reprepared and new retainers constructed.

If the individual parts of a bridge have been incorrectly related in the *soldering assembly*, or if alignment has been changed during soldering, one or more joints must be broken and the bridge must be reassembled and re-soldered.

Such discernible factors as poor preparations, bad waxing and casting techniques, incorrect assembly and application of heat during the soldering operation, and a general lack of attention to pertinent details may be to blame when a bridge does not fit. It is true that intangible or unknown factors do crop up; for instance, it is not always possible to control the shelf life of materials being used, or to prevent contamination. Likewise, there are inherent variables in the casting procedure and other manipulative steps in the bridge fabrication that cannot be controlled perfectly. For the most part, however, failures in bridge construction are due to attempted short cuts or positive indifference and inexcusable ignorance on the part of those concerned with building the prosthesis.

---

*Stim-U-Dents, Inc., Detroit, Mich.

REFERENCES

1. Willey, R. E.: Why do bridges fail? J. Florida D. Soc., *31*:110, Fall 1960.
2. Agnew, R. G.: Impregnation of tooth surfaces with zinc chloride and potassium ferro-cyanide. California D. J., *26*:228, Sept. 1950.
3. Pelton, W. J.: The effect of zinc chloride and potassium ferrocyanide as a caries prophy-laxis. J. D. Res., *29*:756, Dec. 1950.
4. Rieser, J.: Periodontal aspects of fixed bridge failure. J. Pros. Den., *5*:677, Sept.–Oct. 1955.
5. Teteruck, W. R.: A study of the fit of certain dental casting alloys using different investing materials and technics. Master's thesis, Indiana University School of Dentistry, 1963.
6. Dykema, R. W.: Fixed partial prosthodontics. J. Tennessee D. A., *42*:309, Oct. 1962.
7. Brecker, S. C.: How to prevent failures in crowns and bridges. D. Practitioner & D. Record, *14*:261, March 1964.
8. Dykema, R. W.: A study of the effects of certain variables on the comparative strengths of soldered and cast bridge joints. Master's thesis, Indiana University School of Den-tistry, 1961.
9. Simpson, R. L.: Failures in crown and bridge prosthodontics. J.A.D.A., *47*:154, Aug. 1953.
10. Pokorny, D. K.: Fixed bridge failures. J. Michigan D. A., *43*:203, July–Aug. 1961.
11. Henry, P. J.: An investigation into the changes occurring in the oral mucosa beneath fixed bridge pontics. Master's thesis, Indiana University School of Dentistry, 1963.

Bull, A. W.: Diagnosis: A factor in the success of fixed partial dentures. J. Pros. Den., *24*:498, Nov. 1970.

Mahalick, J. A., Florian, F. J., and Weiter, E. J.: Occlusal wear in prosthodontics. J.A.D.A., *82*:154, Jan. 1971.

Schwartz, N. L., Whitsett, L. D., Berry, T. G., and Stewart, J. L.: Unserviceable crowns and fixed partial dentures: Life-span and causes for loss of serviceability. J.A.D.A., *81*:1395, Dec. 1970.

Thin, Vu thi: A study of the Brinell hardness of metals used in conjunction with the por-celain fused to metal technic. Master's thesis, Indiana University School of Dentistry, 1962.

chapter 34

FORMING FUNCTIONAL OCCLUSAL RELATIONSHIPS IN WAX

The reproduction of acceptable occlusal form in gold restorations and the renewal of masticatory function are difficult to achieve even under the best circumstances. This task becomes more troublesome in ratio to the amount of tooth mass that is missing or is in unnatural relationships with adjacent or opposing surfaces.

Development of properly organized occlusal components is especially laborious when both opposing surfaces are to be rebuilt. Not only do the cusps, ridges, fossae, and grooves need to relate correctly in centric occlusion, but they also must have desirable interrelations during all movements of the mandible. These working relationships cannot be consummated in a haphazard trial-and-error manner. They can be created only by using a highly systematic series of steps.

Dr. Everett Payne introduced a method of waxing that truly integrates occlusal components, in both centric occlusion and eccentric relationships. Called the "add on," "wax added," or "wax-to-wax" technique, it is being used successfully by many dental schools in the teaching of functional occlusal morphology. It is in widespread use, usually in modified form, for the evolution of functional occlusion in oral rehabilitative operations when all posterior occlusal surfaces are rebuilt simultaneously. Originally Payne's technique brought about what is basically a cusp-to-embrasure relationship (Fig. 34–1). The gnathological approach to oral rehabilitation customarily employs a modification of Dr. Payne's waxing procedures, which produces a cusp-to-fossa arrangement for all working cusps (Fig. 34–2). Very often existing tooth orientation does not permit an ideal cusp arrangement for either philosophy, and alterations must be practiced to obtain a workable occlusion if the teeth are not to be rearranged orthodontically.

The knowledge and skill gained by mastering this method of waxing

637

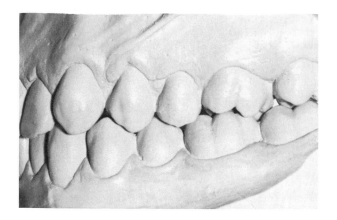

FIGURE 34–1. Cusp to embrasure occlusion. The buccal cusps of the mandibular premolars and the mesial buccal cusps of the mandibular molars fit into the occlusal embrasures of the maxillary teeth.

may be beneficial in numerous ways even if it is never used in advanced oral rehabilitation. As a diagnostic procedure this system may be utilized for pre-waxing a case before final determination of treatment. The method may be used in its entirety at any time that opposing posterior surfaces are to be restored with castings. Also, many of the steps in the procedure may be employed to refine the occlusal anatomy of wax patterns even though the location, height, and basic form of components may be decided in advance by an existing opposing surface that is not to be altered. Learning this operation increases appreciation for the functional aspects of occlusal morphology and thereby helps to improve the ability to attain a benign occlusion regardless of the restorative material being placed or the extent of the restoration being made.

Developing a functional occlusion in wax is begun by establishing the peripheral form and dimensions of the restorations or pontics except for the occlusal surfaces. (In teaching exercises, this condition frequently is simulated by grinding or carving away the occlusal one-third of the posterior teeth on appropriate stone casts.) Cusps are located and their lengths fixed by the placement of wax cones. The various ridges leading away from the cusps are added in small increments of molten wax. Each cone representing a cusp, and

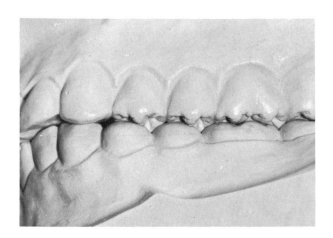

FIGURE 34–2. Cusp to fossa occlusion. The buccal cusps of the mandibular premolars fit into the mesial fossae of the opposing premolars. The buccal cusps of the molars fit into the three fossae in each of the maxillary molar teeth.

each addition to a ridge, is scrutinously evaluated as it is formed to insure a satisfactory working relationship with its antagonists. This systematization reduces greatly the possibility of errors and allows corrections and alterations at a point in the technique when the changes require minimal time and effort. An occlusion developed in this way should never call for major changes near the end of the procedure.

ORDER OF PROCEDURE

The order in which the basic components are added in waxing a functional occlusion can be outlined as follows:
(1) mandibular buccal cones (cusp tips);
(2) maxillary buccal cones (cusp tips);
(3) buccal ridges of mandibular buccal cusps;
(4) buccal ridges of maxillary buccal cusps;
(5) triangular ridges of maxillary buccal cusps;
(6) mesial and distal ridges of all buccal cusps;
(7) maxillary lingual cones (cusp tips);
(8) all ridges of maxillary lingual cusps;
(9) maxillary mesial and distal marginal ridges;
(10) triangular ridges of mandibular buccal cusps;
(11) mandibular lingual cones (cusp tips);
(12) all ridges of mandibular lingual cusps; and
(13) mandibular mesial and distal marginal ridges.

Establishing Mandibular Buccal Cones

The mandibular buccal cusps, which are centric holding (or working) cusps, contact the maxillary posteriors midway buccolingually (Fig. 34–3A). Also, the mandibular buccal cusp tips are located approximately at the line of junction between the buccal one-third and the middle one-third of the occlusal surface (Fig. 34–3B). Mesiodistally the buccal cone for a mandibular first premolar is located to fall on the mesial marginal ridge of the maxillary first premolar. The mandibular second premolar contacts the distal marginal ridge of the maxillary first premolar and the mesial marginal ridge of the second premolar. The mesiobuccal cusp of the mandibular first molar touches the marginal ridges of the maxillary second premolar and first molar, while its distobuccal cusp goes into the central fossa of the maxillary first molar. A similar arrangement exists between the mandibular second molar and the maxillary first and second molars. Figure 34–4 shows completed mandibular cones held against an intact maxillary arch to illustrate their relationships to opposing tooth contours. With these relationships in mind, cones representing the mandibular buccal cusps are located and adjusted for length. Usually the distal cusp of the mandibular first molar is placed at a later time.

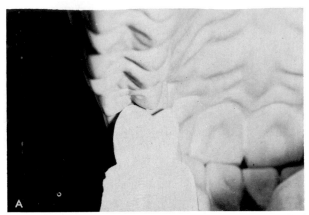

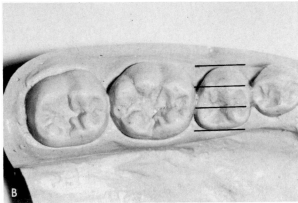

FIGURE 34-3. *Locating mandibular buccal cusps.*

A, Cross section of mandibular premolar making contact with an opposing proximal marginal ridge at about the center of the bucco-lingual dimension of the opposing premolars.

B, Mandibular buccal cusps located at junction of buccal one-third and middle one-third of tooth dimension.

Each cone pre-establishes the height as well as the location of its cusp. Permissible cusp height is decided by the following factors:

(1) condylar guidance (condylar inclination);
(2) anterior guidance (combination of vertical and horizontal overlap);
(3) the relationship of condylar guidance to the occlusal plane;
(4) occlusal curves (curves of Spee and Wilson);

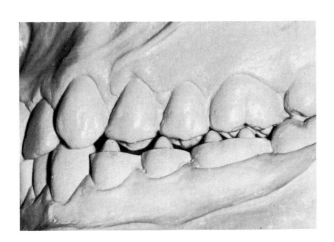

FIGURE 34-4. Cones representing mandibular buccal cusps in their relationships to an intact opposing occlusion. This is done for illustrative purposes only and is not normally part of the procedure in developing occlusion in wax.

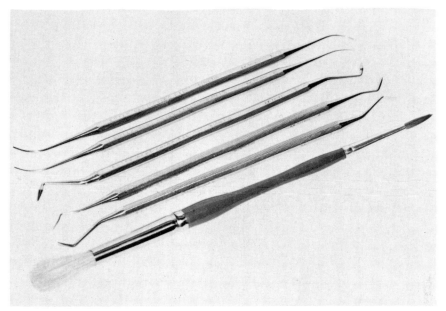

FIGURE 34–5.   Instruments as seen from top to bottom:
No. 1 PKT waxing instrument;
No. 2 PKT waxing instrument;
No. 3 PKT carving instrument;
No. 4 PKT carving instrument;
No. 5 PKT carving instrument.
The brush, which is a Whip-Mix plate type, double-ended brush, is used in cleaning wax shavings from the patterns and also in applying zinc stearate for checking occlusal contacts.

(5) the amount, direction, and character of the sideshift (Bennett shift); and

(6) the philosophy of occlusion being followed.

Obviously, in order to be aware of some of the above factors and to be able to control others, the casts must be properly related to an adequately adjusted articulating instrument.

Dr. Peter K. Thomas has designed a set of five waxing instruments* that are very helpful in waxing functional occlusion (Fig. 34–5).

The mandibular buccal cones are formed with the No. 2 PKT waxing instrument and altered, if needful, with the No. 4 PKT carving instrument (Fig. 34–6).

Establishing Maxillary Buccal Cones

The maxillary buccal cusp tips are located just inside the buccal outline (Fig. 34–7*A*), and when the casts are in centric relation about midway between a pair of mandibular buccal cusps (Fig. 34–7*B*). They are built up with the No. 2 PKT waxing instrument and may be contoured with the No. 4 PKT carving

*O. Suter Dental Mfg. Company, Chico, Calif.

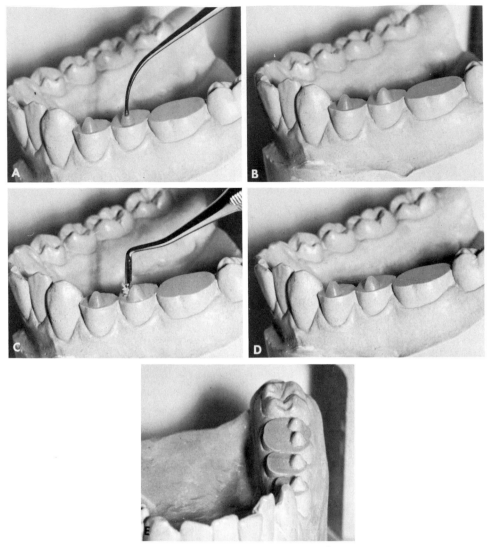

FIGURE 34–6.   *Mandibular buccal cones.*

A, Applying wax in the shape of a cone with the No. 1 PKT waxing instrument.

B, Wax cone applied.

C, Carving cone to proper form and size.

D, Cones completed for mandibular premolar buccal cusps.

E, All mandibular buccal cones completed as viewed from the anterior aspect. Notice the placement of the cones at the junction of the buccal one third with the middle third of the buccolingual dimension.

instrument. The heights of these cusps are fixed by moving the articulated casts into a lateral-protrusive relationship so that a pair of opposing cones will be end-to-end as each maxillary cone is established. If either a balanced occlusion or a group function is to be established, the cones are adjusted to just touch in this position. If posterior disclusion is an objective, cones are adjusted in height to pass each other by the amount felt to be optimal for the particular patient being treated (Fig. 34–7C). Since completely balanced occlusion, or even posterior group function, is almost never seen in the

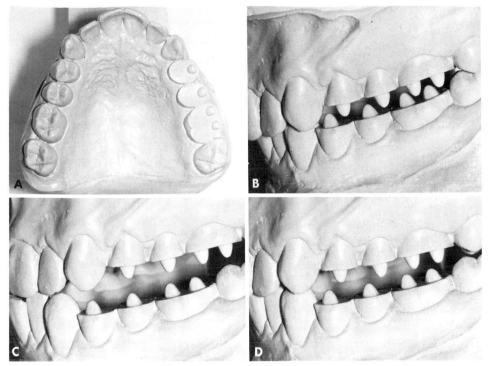

FIGURE 34–7. *Maxillary buccal cones.*

A, Occlusal view showing relationship of buccal cones to the buccal outline of the maxillary teeth.

B, Relationships of maxillary and mandibular cones in centric relation.

C, Lateral-protrusive movement showing clearance of the cones representing cusp tips during eccentric movement.

D, Straight lateral movement showing the way the cusps pass between each other during this movement.

natural dentition, it seems logical to avoid, whenever possible, all eccentric posterior tooth contacts when rebuilding the posterior occlusion. Sometimes it is convenient and somewhat simpler to create tip-to-tip buccal cusp contacts when using this waxing technique as an initial learning exercise, even though the same approach to occlusion may never be used clinically. The illustrations in this chapter depict an occlusal relationship having buccal cusps that clear when brought into the lateral-protrusive position.

The maxillary buccal cones are located by the method just described. They will be smaller and a little shorter than the mandibular buccal cones and, therefore, are formed best with the smaller end of the No. 1 PKT waxing instrument.

Because the mesiodistal distances between the buccal cusps many times diminish progressively posteriorly, in a given lateral-protrusive position all the opposing cones seldom will be exactly aligned (Fig. 34–7C).

In pure lateral excursion the mandibular cones should pass between the maxillary cones (Fig. 34–7D).

As the maxillary cones are added it may be necessary to readjust the heights of the mandibular cones. Cones may be carved down or added to as required to eradicate interferences and to establish the occlusal plane.

Buccal Ridges of the Mandibular Buccal Cusps

The buccal ridges are arbitrarily added to the mandibular buccal cones without melting the cones. The mandibular buccal cusps are somewhat rounded in form (Fig. 34–8A). The addition of this ridge involves the central one-third of the mesiodistal dimension of the buccal surface (Fig. 34–8B). Each cusp is checked in the lateral-protrusive position to make certain that cusp height has not been molested (Fig. 34–8C).

Buccal Ridges of the Maxillary Buccal Cusps

This addition also is limited to the center one-third of the buccal surface (Fig. 34–9A). Maxillary buccal cusps are quite pointed (Fig. 34–9B). Again, any change in the present cusp height, as fixed by the cones, is avoided.

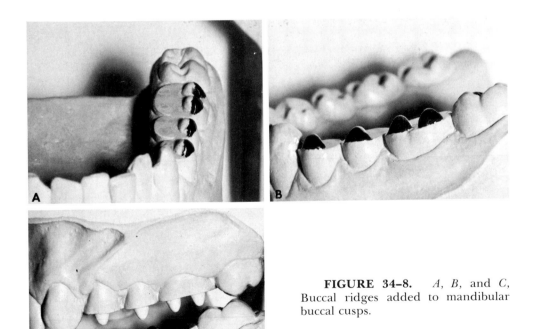

FIGURE 34–8. *A, B,* and *C,* Buccal ridges added to mandibular buccal cusps.

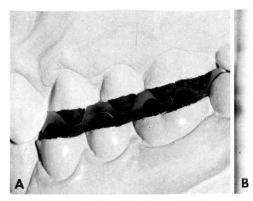
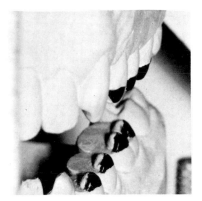

FIGURE 34–9.   *A* and *B*, Buccal ridges added to maxillary buccal cusps.

Triangular Ridges of Maxillary Buccal Cusps

A triangular ridge is extended from the tip of a maxillary buccal cusp to the central groove, which is located about midway buccolingually (Fig. 34–10*A*). This ridge is triangular, being narrow near the cusp tip and broad at its base in the groove (Fig. 34–10*B*). Its form is convex both mesiodistally and buccolingually. The triangular ridges of the buccal cusps of the maxillary premolars run straight buccolingually. However, the triangular ridge of the first buccal cusp of a maxillary molar is angled distally, and that of the distal cusp toward the mesial, both pointing toward the central fossa.

The triangular ridges are formed by adding wax to the lingual aspects of the maxillary buccal cones with the No. 1 or 2 PKT waxing instrument. After the addition of each increment of wax the articulator is closed to judge the relationships being formed with the opposing surfaces (Fig. 34–10*C*). The triangular ridges of the premolars do not create centric stop areas in a cusp-ridge occlusion, but the triangular ridges of the maxillary molar buccal cusps do provide centric stops for the distal buccal cusps of the mandibular molars. Inasmuch as the mesial and distal ridges of the mandibular cusps have not yet been added, no contact should occur at this time, but after the addition of wax the approximate relationships that will exist at completion can be estimated by observing closed casts. Superfluous wax is removed and the triangular ridges are shaped with the No. 5 PKT carving instrument (Fig. 34–10*D*).

Form and bulk of the triangular ridge that may be permitted are arrived at by the paths of the mandibular buccal cusps in protrusive and lateral-protrusive movements. As wax is added to the triangular ridges the area is dusted with zinc stearate powder and, with the anterior teeth contacting, the articulated casts are manipulated to go through protrusive and lateral-protrusive motions (Fig. 34–10*E*). Interferences will cause marking where the powder is rubbed away. These areas can then be adjusted by carving the ridges until the desired harmony is obtained. Balanced occlusion and group function require light contacting of these areas as the anterior teeth rub

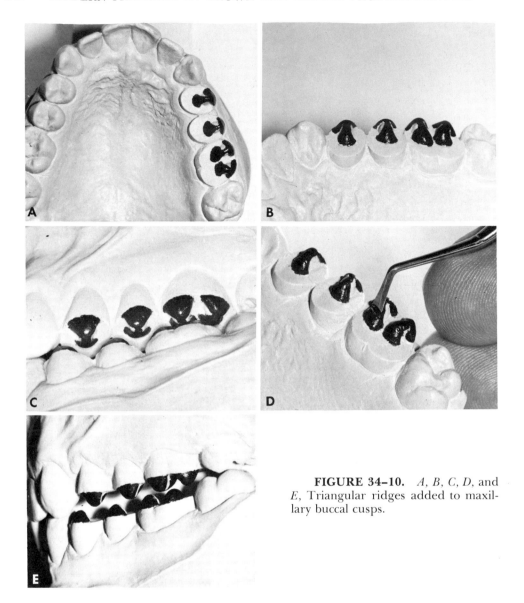

FIGURE 34–10. *A, B, C, D,* and *E,* Triangular ridges added to maxillary buccal cusps.

together. Normal functional occlusion would have these areas clearing at least by an amount that would not cause marking on the powdered surface.

Mesial and Distal Buccal Cusp Ridges

In the next step the mesial and distal ridges are added to the buccal cusps of both arches. This is done with the large end of the No. 2 PKT waxing instrument, beginning with the mesial buccal ridge of the mandibular first premolar. The maximal height this ridge may have is decided by its working compatibility with the distal incisal arm of the maxillary cuspid in the course of lateral movement. In a balanced occlusion it would touch the cuspid during movement, but in most clinical applications there will be a discernible clearance (Fig. 34–11A). The ridge is formed and carved to full contour, completing that portion of the buccal surface and the shape of the buccal and occlusal embrasures (Fig. 34–11B). Hopefully the junction between the cusp ridge and the triangular ridge will automatically produce the supplemental groove separating these two parts (Fig. 34–11C).

The distobuccal ridge is added in a similar manner, arbitrarily forming a contour that is symmetrical with the mesial ridge.

Next, the mesiobuccal ridge is added to the buccal cusp of the maxillary first premolar. Depending on the type of occlusal relationship being sought, it will either clear or just touch in lateral excursion.

Subsequently the order of procedure is to form the mesial ridge of the lower, the distal ridge of the upper, the distal ridge of the lower, and the mesial ridge of the upper, until the two opposing quadrants are completed.

There will be no centric contacts formed by the mandibular premolars at this time, since the maxillary proximal marginal ridges are not yet made; yet there will be centric contacts made between the cusp ridges of the disto-

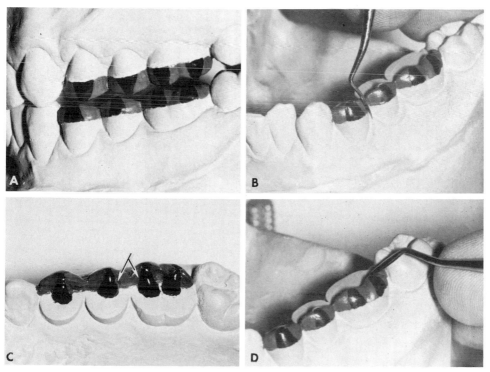

FIGURE 34–11. *Mesial and distal buccal cusp ridges.*

A, Clearance established in lateral movement.

B, No. 4 carving instrument used for contouring.

C, Supplemental grooves formed by the junction of cusp arms and triangular ridges.

D, Forming developmental groove between mandibular molar distobuccal cusp and distal cusp.

buccal and distal cusps of the mandibular first and second molars and the triangular ridges of the maxillary buccal cusps. The triangular ridge of the maxillary mesiobuccal cusp falls in the developmental groove between the mesiobuccal and distobuccal cusps of the opposing mandibular molar. The triangular ridge of the maxillary distobuccal cusp falls in the developmental groove between the distobuccal cusp and the distal cusp of the mandibular molar. As a rule, the distal cusp is not completely formed at this time, but the distobuccal developmental groove may be marked by flowing wax into this area when building the distal ridge of the distobuccal cusp and closing the articulator and making a lateral movement before the wax hardens completely. The indentation formed is then shaped by carving with the curved blade of the No. 4 PKT carving instrument (Fig. 34–11D).

Establishing Maxillary Lingual Cones

In centric occlusion the maxillary lingual cusps, which are the centric holding cusps of the maxillary arch, are placed midway buccolingually as related to the mandibular cusps (Fig. 34–12A). Mesiodistally, in the cusp-embrasure arrangement, these cusps fall in (or over) the fossae except for the distolingual cusps of the molars (Fig. 34–12B). These occlude with the proximal marginal ridges of their respective antagonists. The lingual cusp of the maxillary first premolar is located in the distolingual fossa of the mandibular first premolar. If the lingual cusp of the lower first premolar is normally underdeveloped, actual contact may not be made. The lingual cusp of the maxillary second premolar contacts the distal fossa of the mandibular second premolar. The mesiolingual cusp of the maxillary first molar is located in the central fossa of the mandibular first molar. The distolingual cusp of the maxillary first molar touches the distal marginal ridge of the mandibular first molar and the mesial marginal ridge of the mandibular second molar. The mesiolingual cusp of the maxillary second molar contacts the central fossa of the mandibular second molar and the distolingual cusp occludes with the distal marginal ridge of the mandibular second molar.

Wax cones for the maxillary lingual cusps are placed in the relationships just described (Fig. 34–12C, D, and E). The lengths of these cusp tips are established more or less arbitrarily. With the arch related to a horizontal plane, the lingual cusp of the maxillary first premolar is a little shorter (about 1.0 mm.) than the buccal cusp, but the lingual cusp of the second premolar is the same length as the buccal cusp. The mesiolingual cusp of the first molar is about 1.0 mm. longer than the mesiobuccal cusp, while the distolingual cusp is the same length as the distobuccal cusp (Fig. 34–12F). The same criteria are used to fix the length of the second molar lingual cusps.

Ridges of the Maxillary Lingual Cusps

All ridges of the maxillary lingual cusps are now formed. As their occluding surfaces have not yet been developed, these ridges are fashioned by flow-

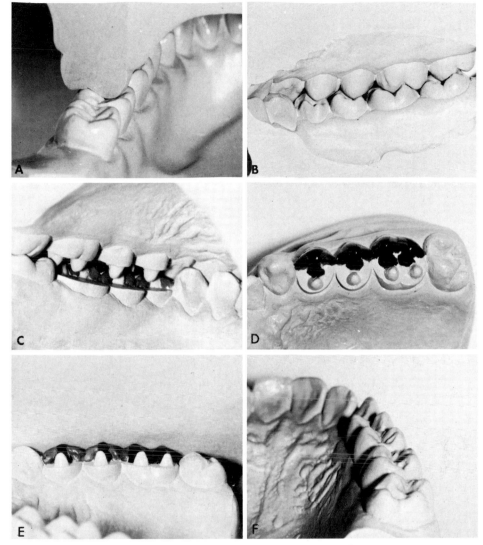

FIGURE 34–12. *Locating maxillary lingual cusps.*

A, Maxillary lingual cusp located midway buccolingually between mandibular cusps.
B, Mesiodistal relationships of maxillary lingual cusps to the mandibular teeth.
C, D, and *E,* Maxillary lingual cones established.
F, Natural teeth showing the progressive lengthening of maxillary lingual cusps as compared to the buccal cusps.

ing one ridge at a time to standard anatomical form. This must be done with great accuracy, since the location and contour of the opposing ridges will be subject to the correctness with which this is accomplished.

The mesial and distal ridges of the first premolar are formed first, avoiding any change in the cusp height as set by the cone. The lingual ridge is placed next, followed by the triangular ridge (Fig. 34–13*A*). If each addition of wax is made artfully, the supplemental grooves dividing the mesial and distal ridges from the triangular ridge will be formed automatically. Should this not happen, these grooves can be carved with the No. 3 PKT instrument

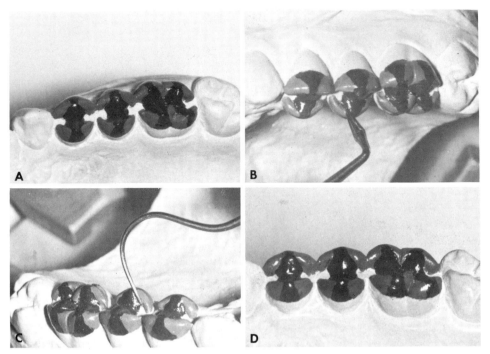

FIGURE 34–13.   *A, B, C,* and *D,* Formation of maxillary lingual cusp ridges.

(Fig. 34–13*B*) or a No. 23 explorer (Fig. 34–13*C*). The first and second premolars are made approximately alike. Because they fit into the distal fossae of the mandibular premolars, they must incline slightly to the mesial.

In completing the mesiolingual cusps of the maxillary molars the mesial ridge is made first. This ridge is much larger and longer than the same ridge on a premolar because of the distal position of this cusp. Next, the oblique ridge is added. It runs diagonally from the tip of the mesiolingual cusp to the base of the triangular ridge of the distobuccal cusp (Fig. 34–13*D*). The buccal and lingual sections complete the cusp, which is much broader buccolingually and more rounded than the lingual cusp of a premolar.

A like sequence of steps is used to complete the distolingual cusp, which is separated from the mesiolingual cusp by the lingual developmental groove. The occlusal portion of the groove angles distally and extends into the distal fossa.

Maxillary Mesial and Distal Marginal Ridges

In the cusp-embrasure concept of dental occlusion the mandibular buccal cusps, except the distobuccal and distal cusps of the molars, touch the proximal marginal ridges of the opposing teeth (Fig. 34–14*A*). This is a common occurrence in natural dentitions. The next step in the waxing is to produce these cusp-to-ridge centric stops by completing the maxillary marginal ridges to make contact with the mesial and distal cusp ridges of the mandibular buccal cusps.

The ridges are applied with the No. 1 or 2 PKT waxing instrument. Before the wax hardens completely it is dusted with zinc stearate powder and the articulator is closed. If there is an excess of wax, a dark imprint outlined by the white powder will be seen where contact has been made. The essential carving of the ridge is done with the No. 4 or 5 PKT carving instrument to create normal marginal ridge form and to reduce to a minimum the area of contact. The contact area should be barely to the outside aspect of the marginal ridge. As each contact area is formed it is mandatory to check the occlusal contacts on the opposite side of the arch to make certain that the additions of wax are not increasing the vertical dimension. If an incisal guide pin is being used, this can be checked also to insure that it continues to be in contact with its stop when the articulator is in centric relation. Zinc stearate powder should be applied to the lower waxup also, in order to reveal the contact areas on the mesial and distal ridges of the buccal cusps. The mandibular first premolar has only one stop on the buccal cusp; it occurs just distal to the cusp tip. The buccal cusp of the second premolar and the mesiobuccal cusps of the molars each have two, one on each side of the cusp tip. Buccolingually these contacts will be found on the crests of the mesial and distal cusp ridges.

The marginal ridges are formed one at a time. As pairs are completed, both may not be exactly the same height. This happens because the occluding mandibular cusp was incorrectly made. The offending lower cusp should be corrected and the maxillary marginal ridges re-formed (Fig. 34–14A and B).

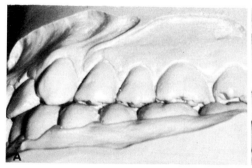
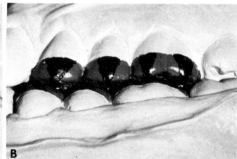
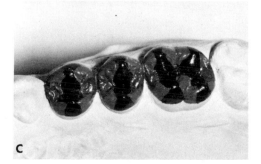

FIGURE 34–14. *Forming the maxillary mesial and distal marginal ridges.*

A, Stone casts of mandibular buccal cusp relationships in cusp-embrasure occlusion.

B and *C,* Maxillary marginal ridges completed.

Triangular Ridges of Mandibular Buccal Cusps

The next step is the creation of the triangular ridges of the mandibular buccal cusps. These ridges make up some of the centric stops for those maxillary lingual cusps that occlude into mandibular fossae (premolar lingual cusps and the mesiolingual cusps of the molars) (Fig. 34–15A).

The premolar triangular ridge runs lingually, straight to the center of the tooth (Fig. 34–15B and C). In order that it may make contact with the lingual cusp of the maxillary first premolar, the triangular ridge of the mandibular first premolar may have to be overcontoured. In some clinical cases this may not be feasible. Actually, in most cases, if contact is to be made in the distal fossa of a mandibular first premolar, the distal half of this tooth must be formed to resemble a second premolar. Contact with the triangular ridge is made on its distolingual slope.

The triangular ridges of the mesiobuccal and distobuccal cusps of the mandibular molars converge toward the centers of the occlusal surfaces (Fig. 34–15B and C). While the triangular ridge of the mesiobuccal cusp of the mandibular molar has no centric contact and is formed arbitrarily, the corresponding ridge of the distobuccal cusp makes contact with the maxillary molar to the buccal of the crest of the mesiolingual cusp.

As each triangular ridge is added, it is dusted with zinc stearate powder and test movements are made in the nonworking direction. If rubbing occurs

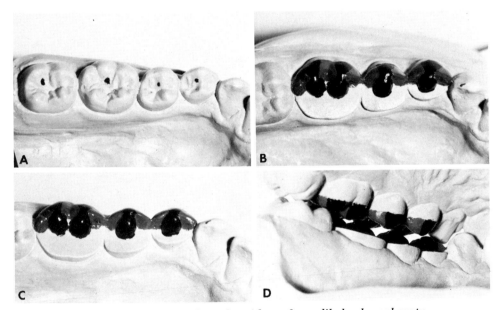

FIGURE 34–15. *Triangular ridges of mandibular buccal cusps.*

A, Centric stops for maxillary lingual cusps located on the triangular ridges of mandibular lingual cusps.

B and *C,* Triangular ridges of mandibular buccal cusps formed.

D, Clearance between maxillary lingual cusps and mandibular triangular ridges during nonworking lateral movement.

or the centric contacts are overly large, the form is corrected by carving. In these test movements the mesiolingual cusps of the maxillary molars should pass through the occlusal embrasures formed by the groove separating the mandibular distobuccal cusps from the distal cusps (Fig. 34–15D). The mandibular triangular ridges should be contoured so that, while no rubbing occurs in lateral movement, the centric contacts are retained.

Establishing Mandibular Lingual Cones

Like the maxillary buccal cusps, the mandibular lingual cusps are not centric holding cusps. Because of this they are sharp in form, and buccolingually the tips are positioned very near the lingual periphery (Fig. 34–16A).

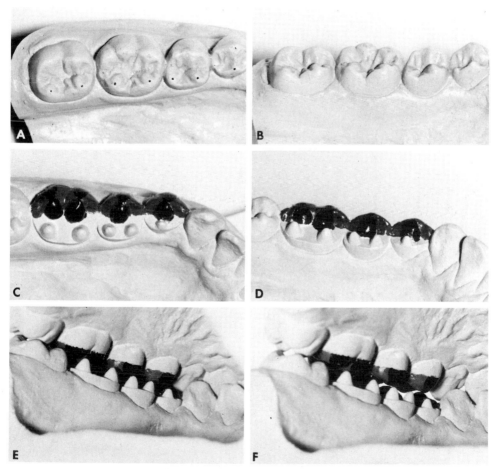

FIGURE 34–16. *Placement of mandibular lingual cones.*

A, Occlusal view of mandibular posterior teeth showing proximity of lingual cusp tips to the lingual outline.

B, Lingual view of mandibular posterior teeth showing mesiodistal separation of lingual cusps.

C, D, E, and *F,* Cones representing mandibular lingual cusps.

The tips of the molar lingual cusps must be widely separated to allow the passage without interference of the large mesiolingual cusp of the maxillary molar when a working movement is made (Fig. 34–16B). The mandibular lingual cusps are all shorter than their buccal counterparts.

Wax cones are made and positioned according to the outlined criteria (Fig. 34–16C and D). They should be smaller and shorter than the buccal cones. As each is formed, the articulator is checked in centric relation (Fig. 34–16E) and moved into the working relationships (Fig. 34–16F). There should be no contact in either position, and in a test movement in a working direction a maxillary lingual cusp should travel approximately midway between two wax cones.

Ridges of Mandibular Lingual Cusps

In completing the mandibular lingual cusps the triangular ridge or the buccal aspect of each cusp is formed first, starting with the first premolar. If the ridge is built high enough, a centric stop will occur on the distal slope in a location resembling the one on the triangular ridge of the buccal cusp. Contact here occurs very seldom in the natural dentition. In treatment of patients, clinical judgment will determine what is to be done. The second premolar can be given centric contact routinely (Fig. 34–17A). After each

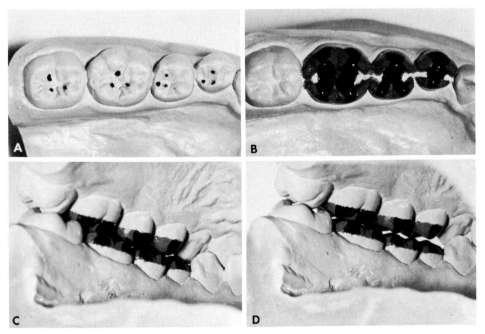

FIGURE 34–17.   *Mandibular lingual cusp ridges.*

A, Centric contacts formed by mandibular triangular ridges.
B and C, Lingual cusp ridges added.
D, Checking for eccentric contacts.

triangular ridge is made, the lingual ridge, and then the mesial and distal ridges, are added in the same manner as for the maxillary lingual cusps.

The triangular ridges of the lingual cusps of the mandibular molars converge toward the center of these teeth, and each ridge provides a centric stop for the mesiolingual cusp of the maxillary molar with which it occludes (Fig. 34–17B and C).

As each ridge is added it is checked for the right centric contact and for interferences in test working movements (Fig. 34–17D). Zinc stearate powder is used to help to delineate any contacting or rubbing.

Mandibular Mesial and Distal Marginal Ridges

The last major occlusal components to be added are the mandibular proximal marginal ridges. Since the mesial marginal ridges of the premolars and the first molar make no occlusal contacts, they are formed arbitrarily, following good tooth morphology. However, the distal marginal ridges of both premolars in some cases do form occlusal stops, as do the distal ridge of the first molar and the mesial and distal ridges of the second molar (Fig. 34–18A).

The distal marginal ridges of the mandibular first and second premolars furnish the third occlusal contacts for the lingual cusps of the maxillary premolars. As they are formed, zinc stearate powder is used to demonstrate the contacts formed in both arches and to detect any rubbing in eccentric movements.

In the cusp-embrasure occlusal scheme, the distal marginal ridge of the mandibular first molar and the mesial marginal ridge of the second molar

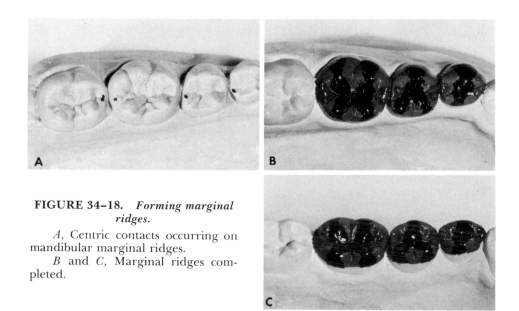

FIGURE 34–18. *Forming marginal ridges.*

A, Centric contacts occurring on mandibular marginal ridges.

B and *C,* Marginal ridges completed.

create a pair of centric stops for the distolingual cusp of the maxillary first molar. The mandibular second molar has a similar relationship with its antagonist.

As the distal marginal ridge of the mandibular first molar is formed, the distal cusp may also be completed; normally it does not make an occlusal contact. The ridge running from its tip toward the center of the tooth separates the distal fossa from the distobuccal developmental groove. Except for final corrections for all occlusal contacts, this completes the formation of the mandibular teeth (Fig. 34–18B and C).

Final Corrections

Any groove areas between ridges that have not been fully completed by this time are added and carved. The No. 3 PKT wax instrument is useful in delineating and smoothing these grooves.

Zinc stearate powder is used to check critically all centric contacts and to detect any eccentric interferences. Alterations that are needed are made systematically from anterior to posterior (Fig. 34–19).

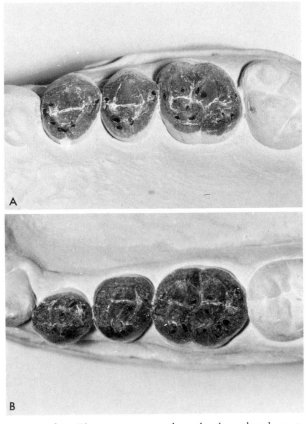

FIGURE 34–19.   *A* and *B,* Zinc stearate used to check occlusal contacts.

REFERENCES

Huffman, R. W., Regenos, J. W., and Taylor, R. R.: Principles of Occlusion (Manual). Colum-
    bus, H and R Press, 1969.
Lundeen, H. C.: Introduction to Occlusal Anatomy (Manual). Lexington, Kentucky, H. C.
    Lundeen, 1969.
Thomas, P. K.: Syllabus on Full Mouth Waxing. Technique for Rehabilitation Tooth-to-Tooth
    Cusp-Fossa Concept of Organic Occlusion. 3rd ed. San Francisco, School of Dentistry,
    Postgraduate Education, University of California, 1967.
Wilson, W. H., and Lang, R. L.: Practical Crown and Bridge Prosthodontics. New York,
    McGraw-Hill Book Company, Inc., 1962.

chapter 35

COMPLETE ORAL REHABILITATION

To rehabilitate means "to restore to a former capacity." Oral rehabilitation is the restoration of the form, function, and esthetic qualities of the masticatory mechanism. The rehabilitation of a mouth, therefore, can be the *satisfactory* placement of a single restoration, or it can encompass the rebuilding of the remaining teeth and replacing of any number of missing teeth. It follows then that not all oral rehabilitation procedures entail complete restoration and not all full mouth reconstructions can be correctly called oral rehabilitation.

Unfortunately the terms "oral rehabilitation," "oral reconstruction," "full mouth rehabilitation," "full mouth reconstruction," "occlusal reconstruction," and "occlusal rehabilitation" are used interchangeably by members of the dental profession. Even the word *gnathology* is used by some in place of these terms. However, the definition of gnathology is "the *science* of the masticatory system, including physiology, functional disturbances, and treatment." While gnathological principles may form a basis for complete oral rehabilitation, all full mouth reconstruction operations cannot be considered to be the practice of gnathology.

Perhaps the best term to designate extensive restorative treatment that involves most or all of the teeth and that is accomplished according to sound anatomic and physiologic concepts might be "complete oral rehabilitation."

The indications for complete oral rehabilitation are:

1. Loss of large amounts of tooth structure necessitating the replacement or restoration of most or all of the dentition.

2. Temporomandibular joint disturbances that can be attributed to the patient's faulty occlusion.

3. The treatment of periodontally diseased mouths in which defective occlusion seems to play a major role as a contributing factor.

Many techniques have been advocated and used in endeavors to achieve complete oral rehabilitation. In the early 1920's McCollum and his group of investigators attempted to demonstrate the existence of rotational centers about which the mandible moved. They designed apparatus for the purpose of locating and recording these centers of rotation with extraoral tracing

658

devices, transferring this information to a dental articulator, which was then adjusted to follow the recorded motions of the mandible. In an effort to minimize the amount of force on any one tooth during mastication, McCollum taught the usage of balanced occlusion; that is, synchronous contact of all teeth in centric occlusion and during all movements of the mandible.[1]

Granger,[2] Stuart,[3, 4] and Guichet each have produced tracing equipment and articulators intended to be improvements over those of McCollum.* Granger[5] has been an advocate of balanced occlusion; Stuart[6] teaches the use of tooth arrangement in which the posterior teeth have simultaneous contact in centric occlusion, but no contact in any eccentric position of the mandible.

These techniques and devices are complicated and time-consuming and not particularly well understood by the members of the dental profession as a whole. This has led many to continue the use of the simpler, albeit less accurate, procedures that came before, also has led to the development of other, sometimes simplified, methods that are expected to afford more exactness and control than altogether arbitrary approaches.

Mann and Pankey[7] and Schuyler make use of the Bonwill triangle and the Monson sphere to rebuild the lower arch, the upper arch being co-ordinated with the rebuilt lower by means of a functionally generated path obtained in the mouth. After the occlusion has been effected, it is altered to have some degree of "long centric" and barely to eliminate contact between cusps on the "balancing side." The proponents of this technique believe functional centric occlusion to be an area, *not* a point.

Several simplified articulators are on the market. Included among these are the Hanau and Dentatus instruments. These are characterized by having straight paths of motion, with the guiding elements on the lower member and the condylar ball on the upper, which is just the opposite of the human mechanism.

One of these, the Hanau #130, may be converted so that the condylar ball is on the lower member and most of the guiding mechanism on the upper, but with the paths of motion remaining straight lines. An instrument introduced by the Whip-Mix Corporation has the condylar elements on the lower and the guiding elements on the upper member.

Intraoral checkbites are used to set all three of these instruments, and casts may be mounted on them by either an arbitrary face-bow or a hinge axis transfer-bow.

A patient who suffers from any of the conditions requiring the rebuilding of his dental arches deserves the best his dentist has to offer. Since the successful handling of such patients may depend on the degree of accuracy with which the operator can capture and utilize the highly individual functional characteristics of the patient's masticatory mechanism, the dentist should use the most nearly faultless techniques and machines within his capabilities.

In most complete oral rehabilitation cases it is necessary to prepare and to restore *at the same time* many, if not all, of the teeth in order to have total

---

*Granger Gnatholator, Gnatholator Co., Inc., Pelham Manor, N.Y. Stuart Articulator, Charles E. Stuart, Ventura, Calif. Denar D4 Articulator, Denar Corporation, Anaheim, Calif.

control over the occlusal relationships that are to be established. Once this is done, the patient's original occlusal relationship, be it good or bad, is destroyed forever. Under these circumstances, it seems wise, if not imperative, that the patient's diagnostic and working casts be related exactly to the hinge axis through hinge axis transfer and centric relation registrations.

The care with which eccentric records are made and transferred to the instrument is probably related equally to the patient's needs and the dentist's skills. One such method is discussed in Chapter 32, Occlusion Factors in Bridge Construction. It is logical to assume that since the precision required for individual patients cannot be wholly comprehensible, it would be better to err on the side of too much, rather than too little, effort in this direction; conversely, that the operator is well advised not to employ techniques over which he does not have unqualified control, owing to lack of proficiency or understanding.

As in the case of occlusal equilibration or adjustment, there appears to be no excuse for the use of complete oral rehabilitation as a prophylactic measure.

REFERENCES

1. McCollum, B. B.: Fundamentals involved in prescribing restorative dental remedies. D. Items Interest, *61*:522; 641; 724; 852; 942; 1939.
2. Granger, E. R.: Practical Procedures in Oral Rehabilitation. Philadelphia, J. B. Lippincott Company, 1962.
3. McCollum, B. B., and Stuart, C. E.: Gnathology, A Research Report. South Pasadena, Scientific Press, 1955.
4. Stallard, H., and Stuart, C. E.: Eliminating tooth guidance in natural dentitions. J. Pros. Den., *11*:474, May-June 1961.
5. Granger, E. R.: The establishment of occlusion. The articulator and the patient. Dent. Clin. N. Amer., Nov. 1960, p. 536.
6. Stuart, C. E., and Stallard, H.: Diagnosis and treatment of occlusal relations of the teeth. Texas D. J., *75*:435, Aug. 1957.
7. Mann, A. W., and Pankey, L. D.: Oral rehabilitation. Part I. The use of the P-M instrument in treatment planning and in restoring the lower posterior teeth. Part II. Reconstruction of the upper teeth using a functionally generated path technique. J. Pros. Den., *10*:135; 151, Jan.-Feb. 1960.

Courtade, G. L. (ed.): Symposium on occlusal rehabilitation. Dent. Clin. N. Amer., Nov. 1963.

D'Amico, A.: The canine teeth. J. South. California. D. A., *26*:6, 1958.

De Pietro, A. J.: Concepts of occlusion. Dent. Clin. N. Amer., Nov. 1963, p. 607.

Huffman, R. W., Regenos, J. W., and Taylor, R. R.: Principles of Occlusion (Manual). Columbus, H and R Press, 1969.

Kazis, H., and Kazis, A. J.: Complete Mouth Rehabilitation through Crown and Bridge Prosthodontics. Philadelphia, Lea & Febiger, 1956.

Lucia, V. O.: Modern Gnathological Concepts. St. Louis, The C. V. Mosby Company, 1961.

Schweitzer, J. M.: Masticatory function in man. J. Pros. Den., *12*:262, 1962.

Schweitzer, J. M.: Oral Rehabilitation Problem Cases. St. Louis, The C. V. Mosby Company, 1964.

Thomas, P. K.: Syllabus on Full Mouth Waxing. Technique for Rehabilitation Tooth-to-Tooth Cusp-Fossa Concept of Organic Occlusion. 3rd ed. San Francisco, School of Dentistry, Postgraduate Education, University of California, 1967.

chapter 36

CASE HISTORIES

This chapter includes three case histories depicted through illustrations and brief captions.

The first patient, an adolescent, required orthodontic treatment of the opposing arch and some recontouring of the repositioned teeth. The abutments were surveyed for the best path of insertion, construction was indirect on a cast, and dies were made from an elastic impression. One post-seating adjustment was made.

The second case was complicated by the skepticism of the patient and the intricacies of the abutment preparations. Extent of the cutting was determined after the facings were shaped, aligned, and approved. After this was accomplished, construction proceeded by the indirect technique. Three post-seating checks were made, only the first showing a minimal prematurity.

Each of these bridges was seated without interference.

The third patient, a young adult, needed a replacement for a congenitally missing mandibular incisor. A removable prosthesis had been worn for ten years following the removal of the ankylosed deciduous tooth. Four teeth were clasped. All were etched buccally and lingually and across the covered marginal ridges. Disintegration of the enamel occurred despite constant periodic prophylaxis and stannous fluoride treatments.

Final treatment included surgical intervention to increase the vertical dimension of the space and to expose small areas of the abutments. Orthodontic treatment widened the edentulous area and closed the contacts on the distals of the abutments. The abutments were very thin labiolingually.

There was some minor difficulty in holding the abutments in exact relationship during the construction period, and reassembly of the bridge was necessary. There has been no discomfort following cementation.

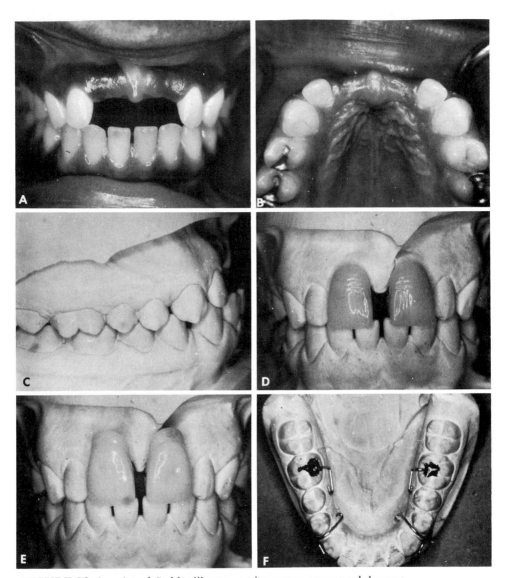

FIGURE 36–1.   *A* and *B*, Maxillary anterior space, young adolescent.
   C, Lateral view. Poor relationship between mandibular incisors and maxillary ridge.
   D, Largest facings. Diastema much too large.
   E, Large denture teeth. Diastema still overwide. Decision made to move mandibular
incisors lingually and to shorten them to improve situation for building bridge.
   F, Wires bent for a working retainer; those on molars to support appliance. The anterior
loops were to hold an elastic that would force incisors lingually.

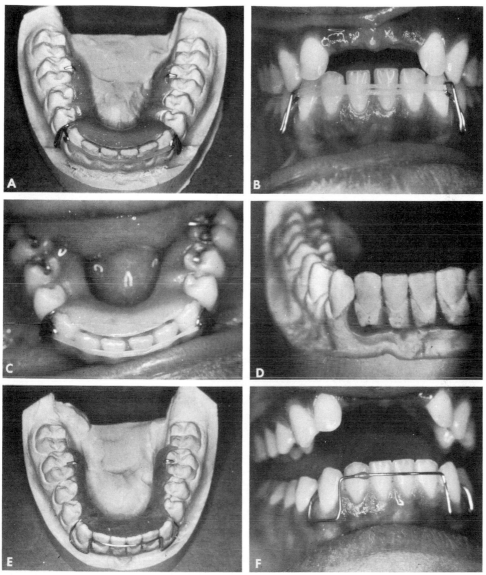

FIGURE 36–2.   *A*, *B*, and *C*, Appliance showing wire support on molars and elastic against incisors. Lingual movement by this method was 50 per cent of that desired.

D, Teeth sectioned and aligned for Hawley retainer.

E and *F*, Hawley retainer on cast and in mouth. Patient was uncomfortable for a few hours. This was worn for several weeks.

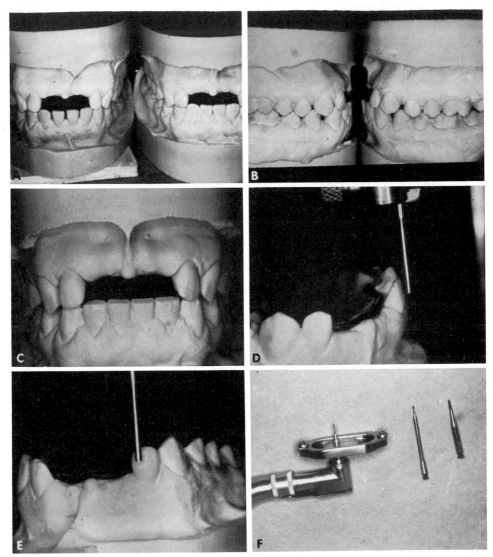

FIGURE 36–3.   *A* and *B*, Casts before and after orthodontic treatment. While mandibular incisors were tipped, instead of being moved bodily, realignment produced a situation readily treatable. Vertical overlap of bridge should maintain new positions.

C, Mandibular incisors shortened on cast. Radiographs showed this to be feasible.

D and *E*, Determining best path of insertion.

F, Loma Linda Parallelometer and drills for pinholes.

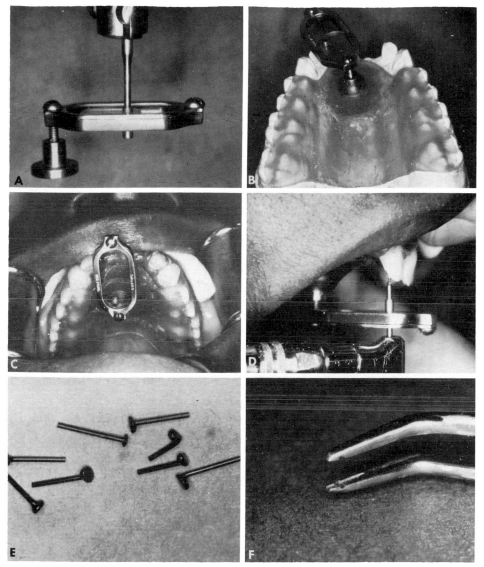

FIGURE 36–4. *A*, Parallelometer on analyzing rod of surveyor, ready to be attached to baseplate. Holes will be drilled in line with pre established path of insertion.

B and *C*, Device attached; on cast and in mouth. Plate covers parts of occlusals of posterior teeth and is well adapted to lingual surfaces and embrasures. It is quite stable when seated in mouth.

D, Disk with bur sleeve moves forward and back and rotates so that drill can reach any of the four anterior teeth.

E, Nylon bristles cut and headed.

F, Cross-grooved pliers for handling either headed or straight bristles.

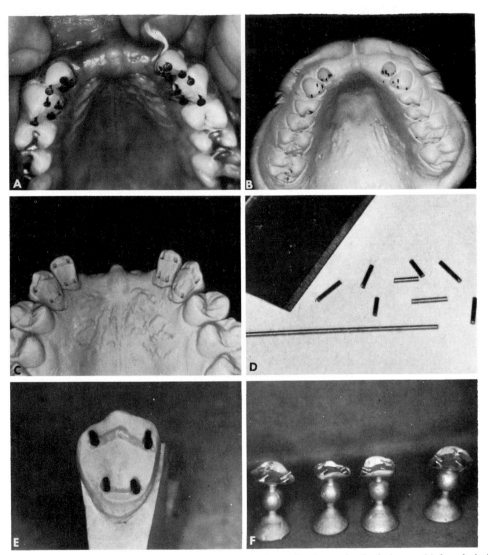

FIGURE 36–5.   *A* and *B*, Abutments packed to displace gingival tissue. Nylon bristles placed in pinholes. When cotton fibers were removed (*B*), impression was taken with silicone.

C, Cast of prepared arch. Another was poured prior to this one, to be sectioned for dies.

D, Cut nylon bristles. Drills were 0.023 inch in diameter. Bristles for impression were 0.022 inch. These are 0.020 inch.

E, Die, lubricated and with bristles in place, ready for waxing retainer patterns.

F, The retainer castings. Pinholes in teeth must be very slightly countersunk with round bur so that castings will seat. Investment breaks down minutely where pin and lingual plate join. This cannot be machined safely.

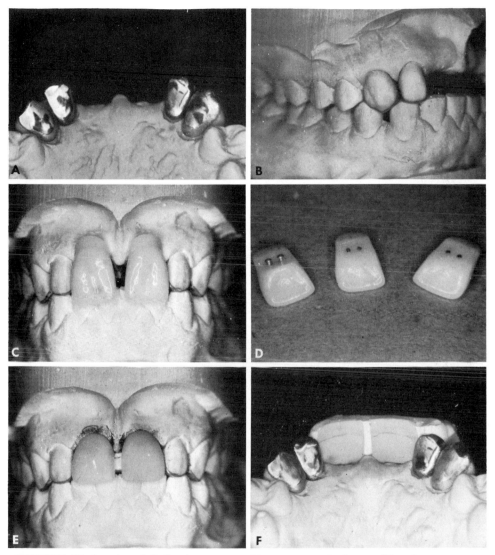

FIGURE 36–6. *A* and *B*, Castings on working cast, ready for equilibration.

C and *D*, Denture teeth from which facings will be made. Pins are cut off, are partly drilled out, and then are finally removed with aqua regia.

E and *F*, Facings ground to form and alignment. Pencil line shows extent of hollow-ground incisal bevel.

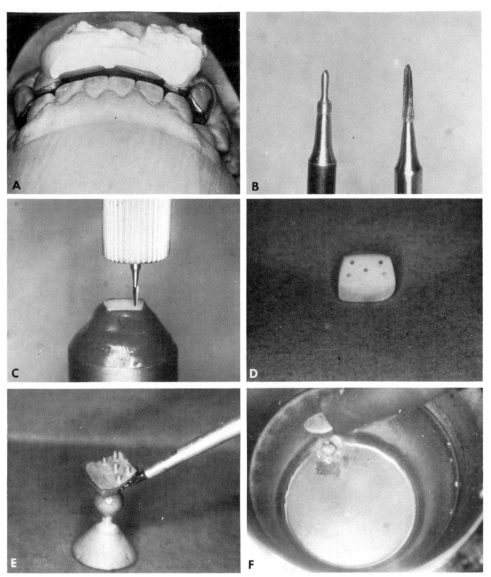

FIGURE 36–7.   *A*, Aligned facings, incisal view. Hollow-ground bevel gives room for bulk of metal to protect facing at incisal edge.

B, Drills made from carbide burs.

C, Facing mounted on table with modeling compound for drilling holes.

D, Completed facing.

E, Cast pontic being coated with lacquer before "stripping." This is necessary to reduce size of cast pins so that facing will seat without causing stress in porcelain. Also, holes must be countersunk very slightly with round-end diamond stone.

F, Casting in stripping machine. Stripper is Model 300 Stripper/Plater (Westwood Dental Mfg. Co., Inc., Van Nuys, Calif.).

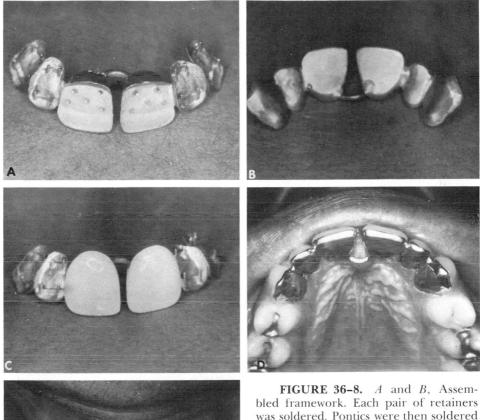

FIGURE 36–8. *A* and *B*, Assembled framework. Each pair of retainers was soldered. Pontics were then soldered to retainers. Loop was soldered to one pontic in third assembly. One pontic was cast to loop, but this joint was reinforced with solder to give better contour to joint.

C, Facings glazed and cemented.

D, Bridge from incisal. Loop is contoured from 17-gauge, high-fusing clasp wire and is set in a rugae depression. It contacts tissue without pressure.

E, Bridge in occlusion. Overlap is sufficient to maintain mandibular incisors in new alignment.

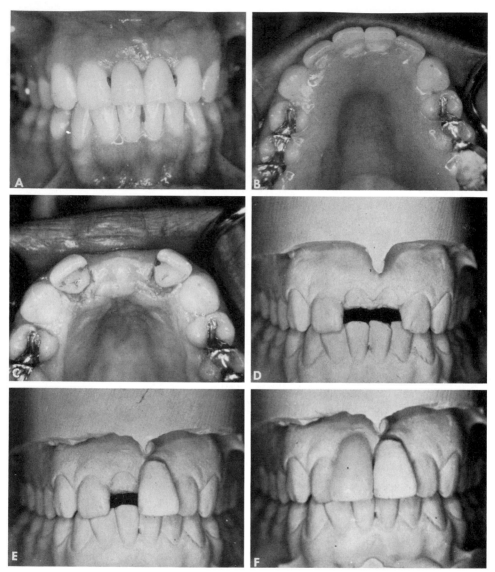

FIGURE 36–9. *A* and *B*, Maxillary arch showing patient wearing temporary partial denture replacing central incisors. Space is narrow. Centrals are in alignment but are narrower than laterals.

C and *D*, Upper arch and cast with denture removed.

E, Occluded casts with a stone replica of patient's extracted central incisor. Instead of recommending orthodontic treatment, patient had been advised to have overlapping centrals extracted.

F, A wax incisor has been added, closely duplicating alignment of maxillary teeth before extraction.

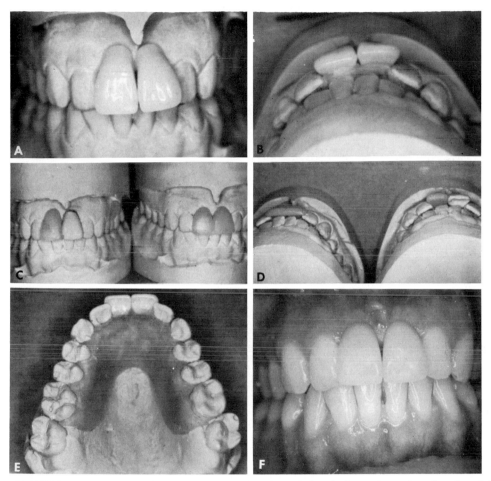

FIGURE 36-10. *A* and *B*, Denture teeth selected for facings. In a situation in which there must be irregular alignment or overlapping, the reverse-pin facing is very adaptable.

C and *D*, Two wax teeth have been carved and aligned to simulate expected esthetic result.

E and *F*, Denture teeth ground to contour and alignment and attached to resin base and seated in mouth (*F*). This was done to help persuade patient that end result would be desirable and to help plan preparations on lateral incisors.

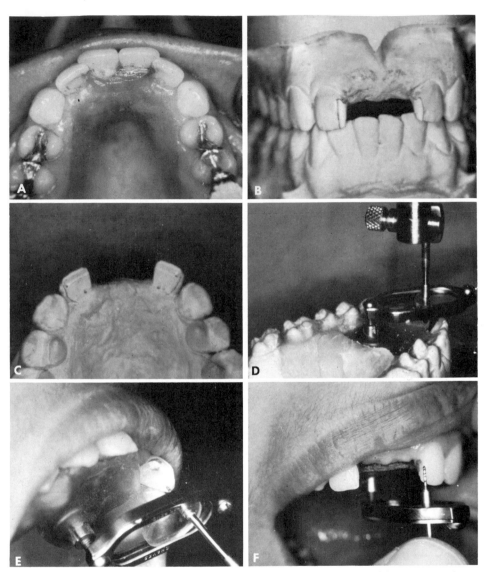

FIGURE 36–11. *A,* Incisal view. Central facings are same width as natural central incisors and have been adapted and aligned in a manner pleasing to patient.

B and *C,* Simulated preparations on diagnostic cast. Extensions on labial determined by contacting surfaces of the facings.

D, Loma Linda Parallelometer attached to baseplate parallel to calculated path of insertion so that preparations may be duplicated in mouth.

E and *F,* Drill used to cut labioproximal grooves.

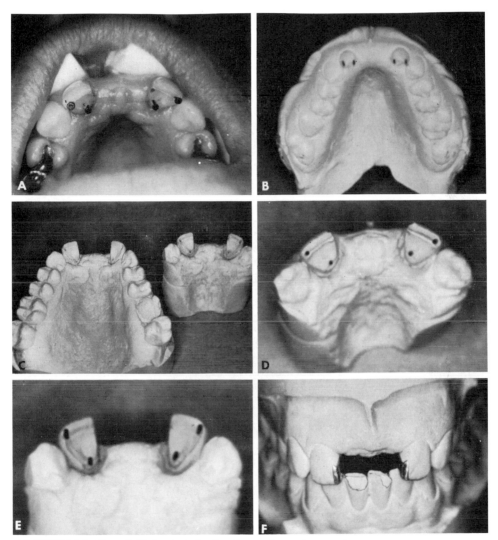

FIGURE 36–12. *A*, Nylon bristles in place prior to impression.
B, Silicone impression.
C and *D*, Working cast and cast to be used for carving patterns.
E, Nylon bristles on lubricated die cast.
F, Castings on working cast with reduced areas on occluding teeth outlined in pencil. This grinding was done when finished bridge was fitted.

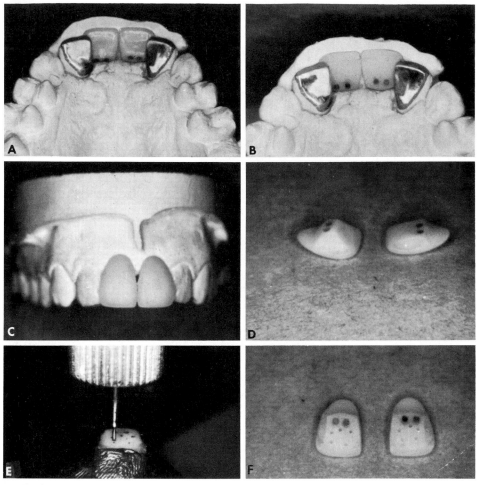

FIGURE 36–13.   *A* and *B*, Facings before and after preparing lingual surfaces and beveling and hollow-grinding incisal edges.
   C, Final alignment of facings.
   D, Showing concave grinding to effect overlapping.
   E and *F*, Holes for reverse-pins.

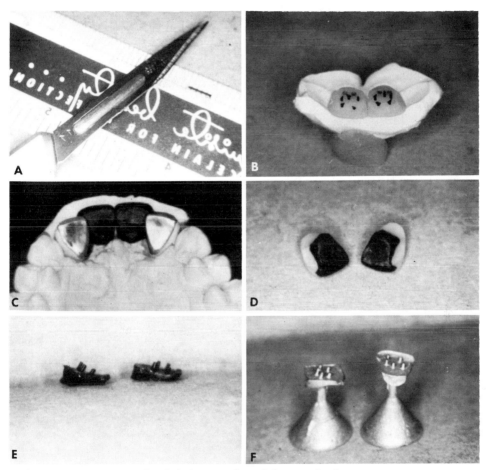

FIGURE 36–14. *A*, Nylon bristle cut to length for pontic pin.
B, Facings seated in labial index ready for waxing of pontic patterns.
C, D, and *E,* Pontic patterns carved.
F, Pontic castings.

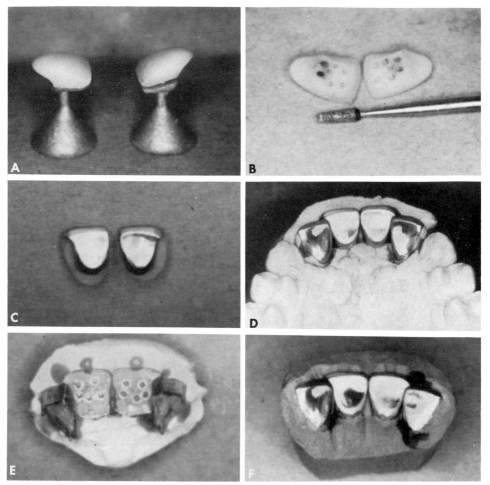

FIGURE 36–15. *A* and *B,* Facings will not seat on castings until castings have been "stripped" and (*B*) pinholes have been countersunk slightly with a round-tip stone.

C, Polished pontics.

D, Bridge aligned using labial plaster index.

E, Bridge assembled in lingual splint ready to pour soldering assembly after painting index with separating medium and soaking for 5 minutes.

F, Soldering assembly trimmed and washed.

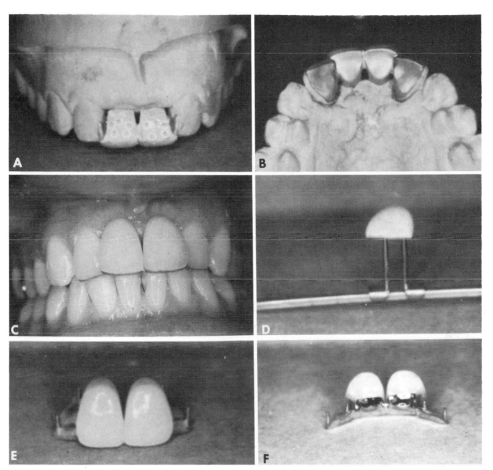

FIGURE 36–16. *A* and *B*, Soldered bridge on working cast. Size and location of solder joints and size and contour of embrasures correct.

C, Bridge, with unglazed facings, checked for occlusion.

D, Facing, on holder, ready for glazing.

E, Bridge with glazed and cervically stained facings.

F, Tissue-contacting surfaces highly polished and glazed.

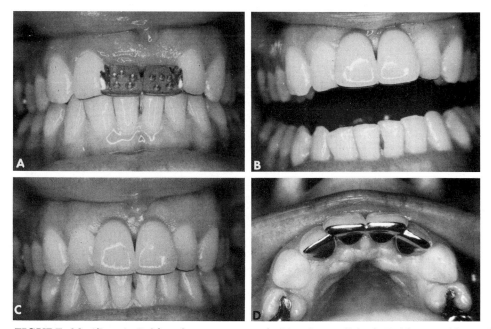

FIGURE 36–17. *A,* Bridge frame cemented. Margins polished. Bridge could not be seated with facings in place.

B, Facings cemented. Extra care needed to remove all particles of cement from labial embrasures and under pontics.

C and *D,* Bridge, labial and incisal views.

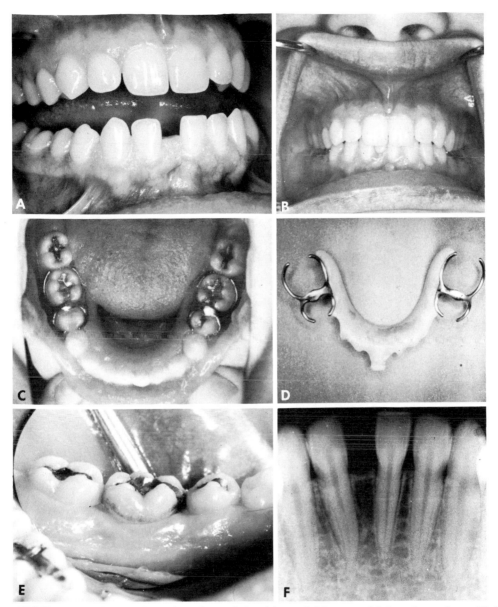

FIGURE 36–18. *A,* Anterior view of dentition of 23 year old female patient. Right mandibular central incisor congenitally missing. Ridge tissue very high. This was due, in some degree, to the stimulation from a removable replacement that had no other anterior support.

B and *C,* Labial and incisal views of mandibular arch with prosthesis in place.

D, The prosthesis replacing missing incisor. There had been no mouth preparation of any kind.

E, Lingual view of two abutments showing etched line on molar. Bicuspid was affected to a lesser degree. Buccal surfaces and marginal ridges of four abutments and linguals of other two had similar disintegration.

F, Radiograph of proposed abutments for three-unit fixed prosthesis. Teeth quite thin in incisal thirds.

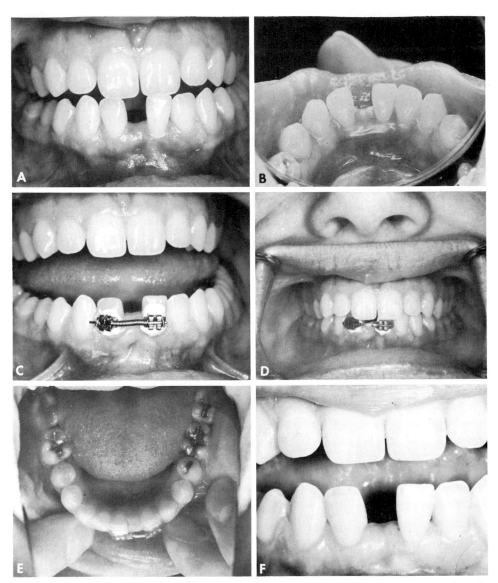

FIGURE 36–19.   *A* and *B*, Labial and lingual views of space after ridge was reduced and contoured to receive bridge.

C, D, and *E,* Orthodontic appliance cemented to labial surface of abutments with Durelon cement. Regular brackets, with a wire mesh on tooth-contacting area, were used. These were substituted for bands so that all possible space could be shifted to edentulous space.

F, Abutment teeth moved laterally into contact with approximating teeth. Long axes were tipped, but this did not interfere with building a pleasing replacement.

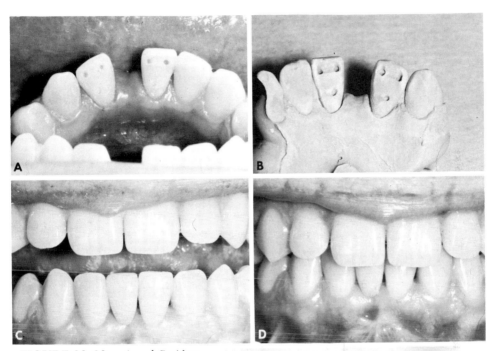

FIGURE 36–20. *A* and *B*, Abutment preparations—teeth and cast. Preparations are short of incisal edge because of very thin incisal thirds.

C and *D*, Labial views of cemented prosthesis. A yellow shade of silico-zinc phosphate was used to cement both the facing and the bridge, thus partially masking the gray shadow from the casting through the thin teeth. Prior to cementation the teeth were coated with Copalite cavity varnish.

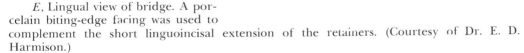

E, Lingual view of bridge. A porcelain biting-edge facing was used to complement the short linguoincisal extension of the retainers. (Courtesy of Dr. E. D. Harmison.)

September 28, 1661.

"Up betimes, and busied myself with my books."

Samuel Pepys, The Diary.

APPENDIX

Manufacturers of the materials mentioned in the text are listed below. Special thanks are due to those who helped in the assembly of illustrations and reference material.

Julius Aderer, Inc.
Long Island City, N.Y.

Aluwax Dental Products Co.
Grand Rapids, Mich.

American Dental Mfg. Co.
Missoula, Mont.

Claudius Ash, Sons & Co., Inc.
Niagara Falls, N.Y.

Barkmeyer Electrical Mfg. Co.
Yucaipa, Calif.
(The J. M. Ney Company)

Blue Island Specialty Co., Inc.
Blue Island, Ill.

Harry J. Bosworth Co.
Chicago, Ill.

Buehler, Ltd.
Evanston, Ill.

Buffalo Dental Mfg. Co., Inc.
Brooklyn, N.Y.

The Carborundum Company
Niagara Falls, N.Y.

The L. D. Caulk Company
Milford, Del.

Ceramco, Inc.
Woodside, N.Y.

Chayes Dental Instrument Corp.
Danbury, Conn.

The Cleveland Dental Mfg. Co.
Cleveland, Ohio

The Columbus Dental Mfg. Co.
Columbus, Ohio

Denar Corporation
Anaheim, Calif.

Dental Development & Mfg. Corp.
Brooklyn, N.Y.

The Dentists' Supply Company
York, Pa.

William Dixon, Inc.
Carlstadt, N.J.

Gnatholator Co., Inc.
Pelham Manor, N.Y.

Hanau Engineering Co., Inc.
Buffalo, N.Y.

Harmony Dental Products Corp.
Pasadena, Calif.

Howmedica, Inc.
Chicago, Ill.

K. H. Huppert Co.
Chicago, Ill.
(Julius Aderer, Inc.)

The Hygienic Dental Mfg. Co.
Akron, Ohio

J. W. Ivory, Inc.
Philadelphia, Pa.

J. F. Jelenko & Co., Inc.
New Rochelle, N.Y.

Johnson & Johnson
New Brunswick, N.J.

K and R Dental Products Co.
Blue Island, Ill.

Kerr Mfg. Company
Romulus, Mich.

683

L & R Mfg. Co.
Des Plaines, Ill.

Lever Bros.
New York, N.Y.

Midwest American
Melrose Park, Ill.

Mizzy, Inc.
Clifton Forge, Va.

E. C. Moore Company
Dearborn, Mich.

Motloid Co., Inc.
Chicago, Ill.

National Keystone Products Co.
Philadelphia, Pa.

The J. M. Ney Company
Bloomfield, Conn.

Pascal Company
Seattle, Wash.

Pfingst and Company, Inc.
New York, N.Y.

Precision Dental Mfg. Co.
Chicago, Ill.

Premier Dental Products Company
Philadelphia, Pa.

The Ransom & Randolph Co.
Toledo, Ohio

Star Dental Mfg. Co., Inc.
Philadelphia, Pa.

Stern Dental Co., Inc.
Mount Vernon, N.Y.

Stim-U-Dents, Inc.
Detroit, Mich.

Charles E. Stuart
Ventura, Calif.

Surgident, Ltd.
Los Angeles, Calif.

O. Suter Dental Mfg. Company
Chico, Calif.

Teledyne-Densco
Denver, Colo.

Tempil Corp.
New York, N.Y.

Torit Mfg. Co.
St. Paul, Minn.

Union Carbide Corp.
Speedway, Ind.

Unitek Corporation
Monrovia, Calif.

Dr. Wagner's Dental Specialties
Ellison Bay, Wis.

Western Gold and Platinum Co.
Belmont, Calif.

Westwood Dental Mfg. Co., Inc.
Van Nuys, Calif.

Whip-Mix Corporation
Louisville, Ky.

The S. S. White Dental Mfg. Co.
Philadelphia, Pa.

Williams Gold Refining Co., Inc.
Buffalo, N.Y.

INDEX

Page numbers set in *italics* indicate illustrations.

685